Current Researches in Drug Testing and Analysis

Current Researches in Drug Testing and Analysis

Edited by **Judith Baker**

SYRAWOOD
PUBLISHING HOUSE
New York

Published by Syrawood Publishing House,
750 Third Avenue, 9th Floor,
New York, NY 10017, USA
www.syrawoodpublishinghouse.com

Current Researches in Drug Testing and Analysis
Edited by Judith Baker

International Standard Book Number: 978-1-68286-227-8 (Hardback)

Printed in China.

Contents

Preface

The world is advancing at a fast pace like never before. Therefore, the need is to keep up with the latest developments. This book was an idea that came to fruition when the specialists in the area realized the need to coordinate together and document essential themes in the subject. That's when I was requested to be the editor. Editing this book has been an honour as it brings together diverse authors researching on different streams of the field. The book collates essential materials contributed by veterans in the area which can be utilized by students and researchers alike.

Pharmaceutical drug testing and analysis are conducted to explore whether the drugs are safe and effective in treatment of different medical disorders and problems. The chapters in this book brings forth researches and studies on drug testing and analysis in varied scenarios. The topics covered in this extensive book deal with the significant aspects such as adverse drug effects, classification and assessment of drugs, drug conception and design, etc. It presents contributions by internationally acclaimed scholars. Scientists and students actively engaged in this field will find this book full of crucial and unexplored concepts.

Each chapter is a sole-standing publication that reflects each author´s interpretation. Thus, the book displays a multi-facetted picture of our current understanding of applications and diverse aspects of the field. I would like to thank the contributors of this book and my family for their endless support.

Editor

Effectiveness of green tea mouthwash in postoperative pain control following surgical removal of impacted third molars: double blind randomized clinical trial

Majid Eshghpour[1], Hamed Mortazavi[2], Naser Mohammadzadeh Rezaei[3] and AmirHossein Nejat[4*]

Abstract

Background: Pain following surgical removal of impacted molars has remained an important concern among practitioners. Various protocols have been proposed to reduce postoperative pain. However, each one has special side effects and limitations. As green tea possesses anti-inflammatory and antibacterial properties, the aim of the current study was to evaluate the effectiveness of green tea mouthwash in controlling postoperative pain.

Materials and methods: In a study with split-mouth and double blind design, 44 patients in need of bilateral removal of impacted third molars underwent randomized surgical extraction; following one surgery patients rinsed with a green tea mouthwash from the first to seventh postoperative day and after other extraction rinsed with placebo mouthwash in the same duration. Both patients and surgeon were blinded to the type of mouthwash. The predictor variable was type of mouthwash and primary outcome variable was postoperative pain measured by visual analogue scale (VAS) during first week after surgery. In addition, number of analgesics patients used after surgery recorded. To measure the effect of green tea mouthwash, repeated measures test with confidence interval of 95% was performed.

Results: Total of 43 patients with mean age of 24 years underwent total of 86 surgeries. VAS value had no statistically difference prior rinsing among groups (P-value > 0.05). However, the mean value of VAS following rinsing with green tea was statistically lower than placebo in postoperative days of 3–7 (P-value < 0.05). In addition, while rinsing with green tea, patients took significantly lower number of analgesics after surgery (P-value < 0.05). No side effects reported.

Conclusion: Green tea mouthwash could be an appropriate and safe choice to control postoperative pain after third molar surgery.

Keywords: Camellia sinensis, Impacted third molar, Mouthwash, Oral surgery, Postoperative pain

Introduction

The main aim of dental practices is not only to provide appropriate treatment and restore function, but also is to remove pain and bring relief the to their patients [1]. On the other hand, changes in lifestyle have resulted in smaller human jaw and lack of enough space for third molar eruption [2]. Hence, incidence of third molar impaction has increased and postoperative pain following surgical removal of third molar teeth has remained an important concern in need of control for many practitioners [3,4]. In addition to the inconvenience, the perception of patient toward dental practice would change after pain experience [5,6].

Various medications have been used to control postoperative pain following surgical removal of impacted molar teeth [1,7-13]. Analgesics including paracetamole and diclofenac sodium in addition to non-steroidal anti-inflammatory drugs (NSAIDs) have been widely used to

* Correspondence: a_68_n@yahoo.com
[4]Member of Student Research Committee, School of Dentistry, Mashhad University of Medical Sciences, Mashhad, Iran
Full list of author information is available at the end of the article

control postoperative pain. However, gastrointestinal and renal complications are of possible side effects reported for NSAIDs [14].

Green tea (Camellia Sinensis) has been a popular drink in eastern countries for many years. Green tea is very rich in polyphenols including catechins which possess antioxidant, antidiabetic, antimutagenic, antiviral, antibacterial, and anti-inflammatory properties [15]. It has reported that green tea is effective on periodontal diseases and is also beneficial against cariogenic activities [16-19]. However, there exists no study to investigate benefits of green tea extract in controlling postoperative complications in oral surgeries.

The purpose of this study was to address the following question: is green tea mouthwash effective in relieving the pain following surgical removal of impacted mandibular third molars? The investigators hypothesized that the pain following rinsing with green tea after surgical removal of mandibular impacted third molar would equal to the pain following rinsing with placebo mouthwash.

Materials and method

This study was performed at Mashhad Oral and Maxillofacial Surgery Clinic. The Ethical Committee of Mashhad University of Medical Sciences approved the study protocol and all the patients provided a signed detailed informed consent.

Study design

To investigate the research hypothesis, the investigators performed a split-mouth, randomized, double-blind study based on the consent statement and Declaration of Helsinki.

Study sample

The study population consisted of 44 patients in need of bilateral impacted third molar surgery between April 2012 and September 2012.

The inclusion criteria were: be 18–30 years old; have bilateral mandibular impacted third molars; have moderate difficulty level of impacted teeth on both sides of mandible based on the sum score of values regarding the spatial direction of the teeth, depth of impaction, and relationship with the ramus on preoperative panoramic radiography (Table 1) [20].

Patients were excluded from the study if: were smoking, were lactating or pregnant, were using analgesic drugs, had received antibiotic during past 2 weeks, had systemic disorders, or had any lesions on panoramic radiography.

Study variables

The predictor variable was type of mouthrinse used in the study and control groups (green tea or placebo mouthwash). The outcome variable was self-reported pain (based on VAS). Other study variables were demographic variables (including age and sex), surgical variables (including operation time and extraction difficulty score), and post surgical variables (including number of analgesics used during first postoperative week). Operation time defined as time between the first incision till flap closure.

Table 1 Measurement of difficulty level of impacted teeth according to panoramic radiograph

Spatial direction (value)	Depth (value)	Ramus relationship (value)	Difficulty score (sum of values)
Mesioangular (1)	Level A (1)	Class I (1)	Minimally difficult (3–4)
Horizontal (2)	Level B (2)	Class II (2)	Moderate (5–7)
Vertical (3)	Level C (3)	Class III (3)	Very difficult (8–10)
Distoangular (4)			

Mouthwash preparation

Green tea extract prepared in the pharmacology laboratory of Mashhad University of Medical Sciences with the following protocol: Camellia Sinesis leaves were dried in 40°C for 45 minutes and powdered with electrical mortar; 100 grams of powder mixed with 500 ml of water; After 48 hours this mixture was filtered and the sediment was removed; The remnant solution was stored in room temperature; After 4 days the powder of green tea extract was obtained.

To obtain the green tea mouthwash, 5 g of extracted solved in 100 ml distilled water to produce 5% mouthwash. The rinse poured into 250 ml dark bottles. The placebo mouthwash consisted 250 ml distilled water. In addition, the mint flavor added to both study and placebo rinses to make the rinse type unidentifiable for patients.

Surgical procedure

All the surgeries performed by an experienced surgeon using the same protocol: povidone iodine solution was applied around the mouth; 2% lidocaine + 1:80,000 epinephrine carpules were used to block the inferior alveolar/long

Table 2 Demographic variables and surgical variables in two groups

Study variable	Green tea	Placebo	P - value
Sample size	43	43	-
Gender (M/F)	17/26	17/26	1.000
Surgical Difficulty Score			
5	21	19	0.896
6	17	18	
7	5	6	
Operation Time (min)	14.53 ± 5.12	15.07 ± 4.78	0.854
Age	23.67 ± 4.78	23.67 ± 4.78	1.000

Table 3 The mean score of VAS during 7 postoperative days in study and control groups

Day	Green tea		Placebo		P-value
	Mean	SD	Mean	SD	
1	57.26	10.13	56.65	10.27	0.784
2	45.16	8.91	48.79	9.48	0.071
3	35.26	8.01	40.98	9.00	0.012
4	24.72	7.01	31.11	8.11	0.009
5	18.05	6.42	23.37	7.90	0.007
6	10.25	5.15	16.42	7.34	< 0.001
7	4.03	3.99	9.69	6.66	< 0.001

buccal nerves; a mucoperiosteal envelop flap was created using a standard incision; if needed, bone removal, tooth sectioning, and bone recontouring were performed with a low-speed handpiece under sufficient sterile solution irrigation; following tooth removal the socket was irrigated with 60 ml of saline; the flap was sutured using 3–0 silk sutures. Patients were instructed to take two pills of Acetaminophen (325 mg) one prior the surgery and another 4 h after surgery. From the next day, patients instructed to take analgesics (Acetaminophen) after VAS assessment and also to record time and number of analgesics they had taken.

Patient allocation

Following each surgery, patients received a bottle containing 250 ml mouthwash. Each patient received both green tea extract and placebo mouthwash during study period; however, the type of rinse received for the first surgery was selected by flip of a coin. Randomization of surgical side in each patient was kept unknown to surgeon and patients till the end of the study period.

Data collection

Patients were instructed to rinse with 15 ml of mouthwash two times per day from one day after surgery till seven consecutive days. To record the pain, patients were instructed to quantify the level of their pain by using a 100 mm ruler as the visual analogue scale (VAS); 0 was no pain and 100 was severe and unbearable pain. Each VAS was recorded at the morning of 7 consecutive postoperative days before taking any analgesic medication and prior to rinsing.

Two follow-up appointments, two days and 7 days after surgery, were held after each surgery to evaluate the healing process. In addition, the patients were told to come back if they faced persistent or increasing pain.

Statistical analysis

Appropriate descriptive statistics (including mean, frequency, range, or standard deviation) computed for each variable. To analyze data, Chi-square, independent sample t-test, and repeated measures of ANOVA were performed using SPSS software version 11.5 with the confidence interval of 95%.

Results

Total of 44 patients met the inclusion criteria; however, one patient excluded as he did not participate second surgery during study period. The mean age of participants was 23.67 ± 4.78. There were no significant differences in

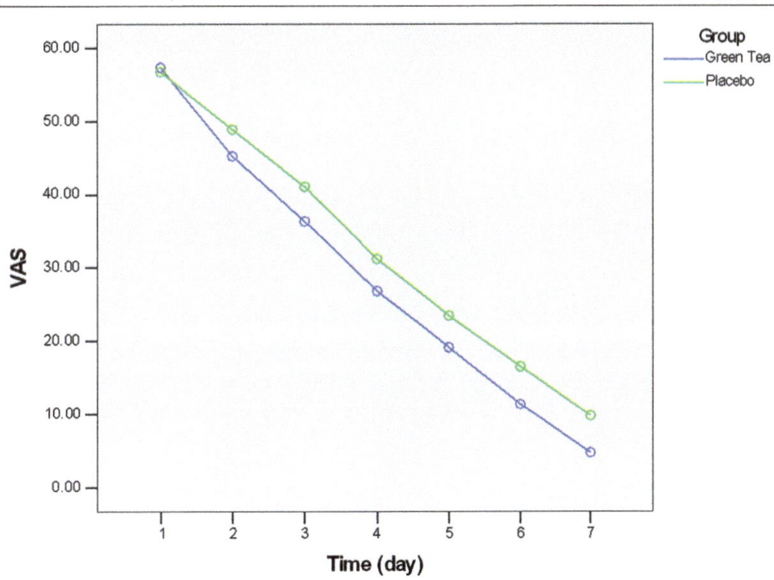

Figure 1 Changes in VAS during postoperative week. Pain was significantly lower in study group in comparison to control group during days 3–7 (P-value < 0.05).

Table 4 The mean number of analgesics used during 7 postoperative days in study and control groups

Day	Green tea		Placebo		P-value
	Mean	SD	Mean	SD	
1	2.14	0.41	2.77	0.78	< 0.001
2	0.65	0.69	1.81	0.66	< 0.001
3	0.37	0.49	0.93	0.59	0.001
4	0.05	0.21	0.32	0.47	0.002
5	0.00	0.00	0.09	0.29	0.041
6	0.00	0.00	0.02	0.15	0.323
7	0.00	0.00	0.02	0.15	0.323

age, gender, surgical difficulty, and operation time in both groups (Table 2).

According to the repeated measure analysis, significant difference observed in VAS values during first week after surgery (effect size = 0.971, P-value < 0.001). There were also significant changes in VAS values during the first week in both groups (effect size = 0.339, P-value < 0.001). Between groups analysis revealed that in study group the mean value of VAS was significantly lower in days 3 to 7 in comparison to control group (Table 3, Figure 1).

In addition, a significant decrease observed in number of analgesic tablets used in both groups over time (effect size = 0.910, P-value = 0.001). Also significant changes observed in number of analgesics during 7 postoperative days when considering grouping (effect size = 0.478, P-value = 0.003). Moreover, the number of analgesics used in green tea group was significantly lower than the control group in days 1–5 after surgery (Table 4, Figure 2). Most of the analgesics (80.2%) were used during first two days after surgery in both groups.

No side effects following rinsing with green tea or placebo mouthwashes reported.

Discussion

The aim of this study was to evaluate the effectiveness of green tea mouthwash on postoperative pain of impacted third molar surgery. The study hypothesis was rejected as the pain experienced by patients was significantly lower in study group when compared to control group.

Pain following surgical removal of impacted molars is a common complication which starts few hours after surgery as the effect of local anesthesia has eliminated. To relief this pain, various protocols have been proposed; none of which was based on herbal medicine [1,7-13,21-29].

The mechanism of postoperative pain has dedicated to trauma during surgery as it increases biochemical mediators of pain and inflammation including prostaglandins, histamine, bradykinine, and serotonin [1]. These mediators initiate the inflammatory process. As a result, anti-inflammatory drugs, including NSAIDs, are commonly prescribed to control postoperative pain [30,31]. However, peptic ulcer, gastrointestinal bleeding or perforation, renal function impairment, and platelet function inhibition are of possible side effects mentioned for NSAIDs [14].

Aromatic components of green tea have shown anti-inflammatory properties at the site of inflammation [15,32]. Results of the current study indicated that green tea extract effectively reduced the postoperative pain after initiation of rinsing. This could be dedicated to anti-inflammatory action of green tea components at the site of surgery.

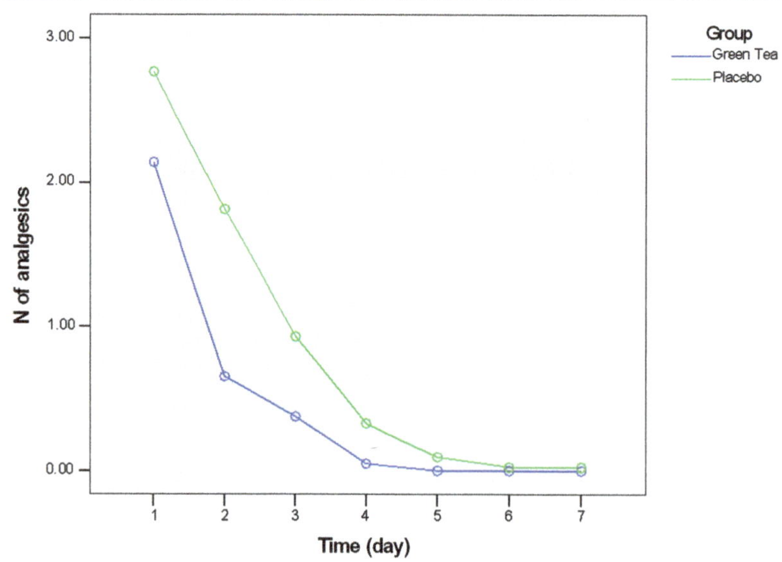

Figure 2 Number and time of analgesics used. Patients took significantly lower number of analgesics during days 1–5 when rinsing with green tea in comparison to placebo (P-value < 0.05).

In addition to inflammation, bacterial infection following impacted molar surgery increases postoperative pain [22,25]. Catechins of green tea (EGC, EGCg, and ECg) possess antibacterial activities and in vitro and in vivo studies have reported effectiveness of green tea against bacteria in periodontal diseases and caries [1,16]. Hence, the results of the current study could be also attributed to antibacterial properties of green tea mouthwash along with its anti-inflammatory activity.

The effectiveness of green tea mouthwash was in consistent with studies using antibiotics, chlorhexidine mouthwash, or low level laser therapy (LLLT) which have shown significant reduction in postoperative complications including pain [22,24-29]. However, rinsing with green tea does not possess the side effects of antibiotics (including bacterial resistancy) and chlorhexidine (including taste changes and oral discoloration). Moreover, green tea is commonly available in eastern countries and its accessibility and cost make it more appropriate in such countries in comparison to low level laser therapy.

This study was double blind as either the surgeon or the patient had no idea about rinsing solution. In addition, as the study was split-mouth, each patient served as his/her own control. This design led to elimination of age and gender as confounding variables. We also controlled for other confounding factors including difficulty of surgery, operation time, surgeon experience, and number of analgesics used after surgery.

Previous reports state that amount of trauma during surgery affect the magnitude of postoperative pain directly [25,33]. Two indices of trauma in molar extraction surgery are extraction difficulty score (based on radiograph) and operation time [33]. In the current study both factors had no significant differences in study and control group. Moreover, experience of surgeon could also affect the amount of trauma and hence postoperative complications [34]. This factor also eliminated as all the surgeries performed by one surgeon.

According to the results of this study, number of patients used analgesics and also number of analgesics taken, were lesser in study group in comparison to control group. This could be dedicated to effectiveness of green tea in controlling postoperative pain. In addition, as the greater proportion of analgesics was taken during first two days after surgery and control group used higher number of analgesics, the insignificant difference in VAS of second day in two study groups may be related to analgesic drugs.

Pain has a subjective nature and there exists difficulties to measure it. Seymour et al. reported that visual analogue scale (VAS) is a sensitive and reliable tool to evaluate the pain following surgical extraction of impacted molars [35]. This scale has been used widely in the studies that investigate the effectiveness of pain interventions after oral surgeries [36]. According to the essence of pain, in the most of the studies the personal differences in participants play as a confounding factor [36]. However, in the current study the pain scale of each participant compared to his/her own pain following rinsing with two types of mouthwash.

There were also some limitations in the current study. Rinsing with mouthwash during the day of surgery lead to blood clot resolution; hence, we had to prescribe analgesics at the day of surgery – as the postoperative pain reaches highest level 6–12 h after surgery – and instruct patients to start rinsing at the first postoperative day. This limitation is under research as investigators have designed a study to use green tea extract via slow releasing systems that is usable immediately after surgery.

Conclusion

The results of the current study indicated that daily rinsing with green tea may be beneficial to control postoperative complications of impacted molar surgery including pain. Moreover, the need for analgesics would become less and side effects following using antibiotics, NSAIDs, or chlorhexidine mouthwash could be escaped.

Competing interests

The authors declare that they have no competing interests.

Authors' contributions

ME and AN designed the study and wrote the study protocol. ME performed surgeries. NMR provided VAS and collected demographic and surgical data. AN performed randomization and kept it secret. HM analyzed the data and performed literature review. All authors participated in drafting, critical evaluation, and approval of final version of manuscript. All authors read and approved the final manuscript.

Acknowledgments

The authors would thank Oral and Maxillofacial Clinic staff and Pharmacology Faculty of Mashhad University of Medical Sciences.

Author details

[1]Dental Research Center, Department of Oral and Maxillofacial, Mashhad University of Medical Sciences, Mashhad, Iran. [2]Department of Oral Medicine, Dental School, Shahid Beheshti University of Medical Sciences, Tehran, Iran. [3]Mashhad University of Medical Sciences, Mashhad, Iran. [4]Member of Student Research Committee, School of Dentistry, Mashhad University of Medical Sciences, Mashhad, Iran.

References

1. Comfort MB, Tse AS, Tsang AC, McGrath C: **A study of the comparative efficacy of three common analgesics in the control of pain after third molar surgery under local anaesthesia.** *Aust Dent J* 2002, **47**:327–330.
2. Blum IR: **Contemporary views on dry socket (alveolar osteitis): a clinical appraisal of standardization, aetiopathogenesis and management: a critical review.** *Int J Oral Maxillofac Surg* 2002, **31**:309–317.
3. Osborn TP, Frederickson G Jr, Small IA, Torgerson TS: **A prospective study of complications related to mandibular third molar surgery.** *J Oral Maxillofac Surg* 1985, **43**:767–769.
4. Gobetti JP: **Controlling dental pain.** *J Am Dent Assoc* 1992, **123**:47–52.
5. Holt VP, McHugh K: **Factors influencing patient loyalty to dentist and dental practice.** *Br Dent J* 1997, **183**:365–370.

6. O'Shea RM, Corah NL, Ayer WA: **Why patients change dentists: practitioners' views.** *J Am Dent Assoc* 1986, **112**:851–854.
7. De Craen AJ, Di Giulio G, Lampe-Schoenmaeckers JE, Kessels AG, Kleijnen J: **Analgesic efficacy and safety of paracetamol-codeine combinations versus paracetamol alone: a systematic review.** *BMJ* 1996, **313**:321–325.
8. Irvine GH, Lutterloch MJ, Bowerman JE: **Comparison of diflunisal and paracetamol in the management of pain following wisdom teeth removal.** *Br Dent J* 1982, **152**:18–20.
9. Rodrigo MR, Rosenquist JB, Cheung LK: **Paracetamol and diflunisal for pain relief following third molar surgery in Hong Kong Chinese.** *Int J Oral Maxillofac Surg* 1987, **16**:566–571.
10. Scott R, Ellis E 3rd, Upton LG: **Double-blind evaluation of etodolac (200 mg, 400 mg) compared with zomepirac (100 mg) and placebo on third molar extraction pain.** *Oral Surg Oral Med Oral Pathol* 1986, **62**:638–642.
11. Giglio JA, Campbell RL: **Comparison of etodolac, zomepirac, and placebo for relief of pain after oral surgery.** *J Oral Maxillofac Surg* 1986, **44**:765–770.
12. Hutton CE: **The effectiveness of 100 and 200 mg etodolac (Ultradol), aspirin, and placebo in patients with pain following oral surgery.** *Oral Surg Oral Med Oral Pathol* 1983, **56**:575–580.
13. Seymour RA, Hawkesford JE, Sykes J, Stillings M, Hill CM: **An investigation into the comparative efficacy of soluble aspirin and solid paracetamol in postoperative pain after third molar surgery.** *Br Dent J* 2003, **194**:153–157.
14. Wallace JL: **Nonsteroidal anti-inflammatory drugs and the gastrointestinal tract. Mechanisms of protection and healing: current knowledge and future research.** *Am J Med* 2001, **110**:19S–23S.
15. Cabrera C, Artacho R, Gimenez R: **Beneficial effects of green tea–a review.** *J Am Coll Nutr* 2006, **25**:79–99.
16. Jenabian N, Moghadamnia AA, Karami E, Mir AP: **The effect of Camellia Sinensis (green tea) mouthwash on plaque-induced gingivitis: a single-blinded randomized controlled clinical trial.** *Daru* 2012, **20**:39.
17. Hirasawa M, Takada K, Makimura M, Otake S: **Improvement of periodontal status by green tea catechin using a local delivery system: a clinical pilot study.** *J Periodontal Res* 2002, **37**:433–438.
18. Otake S, Makimura M, Kuroki T, Nishihara Y, Hirasawa M: **Anticaries effects of polyphenolic compounds from Japanese green tea.** *Caries Res* 1991, **25**:438–443.
19. Chacko SM, Thambi PT, Kuttan R, Nishigaki I: **Beneficial effects of green tea: a literature review.** *Chin Med* 2010, **5**:13.
20. Pedersen GW: **Surgical Removal of Teeth.** In *Oral Surgery.* Edited by Pedersen GW. Philadelphia: WB Saunders; 1988:63.
21. Aznar-Arasa L, Harutunian K, Figueiredo R, Valmaseda-Castellon E, Gay-Escoda C: **Effect of preoperative ibuprofen on pain and swelling after lower third molar removal: a randomized controlled trial.** *Int J Oral Maxillofac Surg* 2012, **41**:1005–1009.
22. Happonen RP, Backstrom AC, Ylipaavalniemi P: **Prophylactic use of phenoxymethylpenicillin and tinidazole in mandibular third molar surgery, a comparative placebo controlled clinical trial.** *Br J Oral Maxillofac Surg* 1990, **28**:12–15.
23. Khorshidi Khiavi R, Pourallahverdi M, Pourallahverdi A, Ghorani Khiavi S, Ghertasi Oskouei S, Mokhtari H: **Pain control following impacted third molar surgery with bupivacaine irrigation of tooth socket: a prospective study.** *J Dent Res Dent Clin Dent Prospects* 2010, **4**:105–109.
24. Bamgbose BO, Akinwande JA, Adeyemo WL, Ladeinde AL, Arotiba GT, Ogunlewe MO: **Effects of co-administered dexamethasone and diclofenac potassium on pain, swelling and trismus following third molar surgery.** *Head Face Med* 2005, **1**:11.
25. Krekmanov L, Nordenram A: **Postoperative complications after surgical removal of mandibular third molars. Effects of penicillin V and chlorhexidine.** *Int J Oral Maxillofac Surg* 1986, **15**:25–29.
26. Sridhar V, Wali GG, Shyla HN: **Evaluation of the perioperative use of 0.2% chlorhexidine gluconate for the prevention of alveolar osteitis after the extraction of impacted mandibular third molars: a clinical study.** *J Maxillofac Oral Surg* 2011, **10**:101–111.
27. Minguez-Serra MP, Salort-Llorca C, Silvestre-Donat FJ: **Chlorhexidine in the prevention of dry socket: effectiveness of different dosage forms and regimens.** *Med Oral Patol Oral Cir Bucal* 2009, **14**:445–449.
28. Markovic A, Todorovic L: **Effectiveness of dexamethasone and low-power laser in minimizing oedema after third molar surgery: a clinical trial.** *Int J Oral Maxillofac Surg* 2007, **36**:226–229.
29. Fernando S, Hill CM, Walker R: **A randomised double blind comparative study of low level laser therapy following surgical extraction of lower third molar teeth.** *Br J Oral Maxillofac Surg* 1993, **31**:170–172.
30. Jung YS, Kim MK, Um YJ, Park HS, Lee EW, Kang JW: **The effects on postoperative oral surgery pain by varying NSAID administration times: comparison on effect of preemptive analgesia.** *Oral Surg Oral Med Oral Pathol Oral Radiol Endod* 2005, **100**:559–563.
31. Tiigimae-Saar J, Leibur E, Tamme T: **The effect of prednisolone on reduction of complaints after impacted third molar removal.** *Stomatologija* 2010, **12**:17–22.
32. Pan T, Jankovic J, Le W: **Potential therapeutic properties of green tea polyphenols in Parkinson's disease.** *Drugs Aging* 2003, **20**:711–721.
33. Van Gool AV, Ten Bosch JJ, Boering G: **Clinical consequences of complaints and complications after removal of the mandibular third molar.** *Int J Oral Surg* 1977, **6**:29–37.
34. Sisk AL, Hammer WB, Shelton DW, Joy ED Jr: **Complications following removal of impacted third molars: the role of the experience of the surgeon.** *J Oral Maxillofac Surg* 1986, **44**:855–859.
35. Seymour RA, Meechan JG, Blair GS: **An investigation into post-operative pain after third molar surgery under local analgesia.** *Br J Oral Maxillofac Surg* 1985, **23**:410–418.
36. Meechan JG, Seymour RA: **The use of third molar surgery in clinical pharmacology.** *Br J Oral Maxillofac Surg* 1993, **31**:360–365.

2

Effects of atorvastatin on plasma matrix metalloproteinase-9 concentration after glial tumor resection; a randomized, double blind, placebo controlled trial

Niayesh Mohebbi[1], Alireza Khoshnevisan[2], Soheil Naderi[2], Sina Abdollahzade[2], Jamshid Salamzadeh[3], Mohammadreza Javadi[1], Mojtaba Mojtahedzadeh[1] and Kheirollah Gholami[1*]

Abstract

Background: Neurosurgical procedures such as craniotomy and brain tumor resection could potentially lead to unavoidable cerebral injuries. Matrix metalloproteinase-9 (MMP-9) is up-regulated in neurological injuries. Statins have been suggested to reduce MMP- 9 level and lead to neuroprotection. Atorvastatin preoperatively administered to evaluate its neuroprotective effects and outcome assessment in neurosurgical-induced brain injuries after glial tumor resection. In this prospective, randomized, double-blind, placebo-controlled trial, 42 patients undergoing glial tumor surgery randomly received 40 mg atorvastatin or placebo twice daily from seven days prior to operation and continued for a 3 weeks period. Plasma MMP-9 concentration measured 4 times, immediately before starting atorvastatin or placebo, immediately before surgery, 24 hours and two weeks after the surgery. Karnofsky performance score was assessed before first dose of atorvastatin as a baseline and 2 months after the surgery.

Results: Karnofsky performance scale after surgery raised significantly more in Atorvastatin group (11.43 +/− 10.62 vs. 4.00 +/− 8.21) ($p = 0.03$). Atorvastatin did not significantly reduce MMP-9 plasma concentration 24 hours after surgery in comparison to placebo. No statistical significance detected regarding length of hospital stay among the groups. Significant reduction in MMP-9 plasma concentration was recorded in atorvastatin group two weeks after surgery ($p = 0.048$).

Conclusions: Significant statistical differences detected with atorvastatin group regarding MMP-9 plasma concentration, clinical outcome and Karnofsky performance score. Consequently, atorvastatin use may lead to better outcome after neurosurgical procedures.

Keywords: Atorvastatin, Matrix metalloproteinase-9, Neuroprotective effects, Brain injuries, Glial tumor resection

Introduction

Neurosurgical procedures could be complicated by a diverse spectrum of factors, such as direct trauma, hemorrhage, brain retraction, and electrocautery with subsequent morbidity and mortality. Blood–brain barrier (BBB) disruption and brain edema is one of the proposed causalities [1,2]. Discovering novel neuro-protective agents and suggesting pre-operative regimen can result in better outcome after brain surgeries. The matrix metalloproteinases (MMPs) are enzymes that play important roles in physiologic and pathophysiologic processes. These enzymes' levels mostly are not detectable, and increase in response to transcriptional regulators [3,4]. MMP-9 (Gelatinase B) is up-regulated in neurological injuries such as cerebral ischemia, BBB disruption, edema formation, and hemorrhagic transformation [5-8]. Different explanations provided to clarify relation of this enzyme and neurotoxicity [9-11]. In particular MMP-9 level rises in acute neurological injuries, so this enzyme proposed to be closely related to neurological impairments [3,12,13]. On the other hand,

* Correspondence: khgholami@tums.ac.ir
[1]Department of Clinical Pharmacy, Faculty of Pharmacy, Tehran University of Medical Sciences, Tehran, Iran
Full list of author information is available at the end of the article

blockade of MMP-9 activity have shown to be neuroprotective, and appropriate for the treatment of acute brain injuries [14-16]. Experimental studies suggest that preoperative inhibition of MMP-9 reduce brain injuries following neurosurgical procedures [1,2].

Statins not only lower cholesterol effectively [17] but also have other properties called "pleiotropic effects." Several clinical trials have indicated that statins suppress inflammatory reactions, recover neurological injuries, decrease the incidence of ischemic stroke, improve endothelial function, inhibit platelet activation, control vasospasm following subarachnoid hemorrhage, have neuroprotective activity in spinal cord injury, and prevent progression of Alzheimer's disease [18-30]. There are published documents claiming that statins decrease MMP-9 levels [30-32]. Many of these evidences are related to atorvastatin, a potent member of this family. This study was designed to evaluate atorvastatin effects on plasma MMP-9 concentration in neurosurgical- induced brain injuries after glial tumor resection. To minimize confounding factors Patients with gliomas grade 1, 2 and 3 which pathologically do not increase MMP-9 plasma levels substantially were entered the study and patients with Glioblastomamultiforme (GBM) were excluded.

Methods

This is a randomized, double blind, placebo-controlled prospective clinical trial performed in neurosurgery ward of a tertiary care Hospital from March 2011 to December 2012. The protocol was approved by the ethics committee of Tehran University of Medical Sciences (TUMS). This clinical trial was registered at Iranian Registry of Clinical Trial (IRCT) with the registration ID of "IRCT201203039196N1". For detecting any significant changes of MMP-9 concentration as main endpoint a sample size was calculated to be 21 patients at each group. Standard deviation for plasma MMP9 in human was supposed 23 ng/ml and 20 ng/ml was accepted as significant rise in MMP9 level, with $\alpha = 0.05$ and $ß = 0.20$. [n = 2(Z1- α/2+ Z1-β)2 S2/d2, i.e. n = 2(1.96 + 0.84)2 × 232/202, n = 21] Patients undergoing elective surgery as therapeutic approach for tumor resection with diagnosis of glial tumor based on radiographic findings were included in this study. Patients excluded from the study with any atorvastatin contraindications such as, atorvastatin sensitivity, active hepatic disease, pregnancy and lactation; elevated liver enzymes; history of serious adverse reaction induced by atorvastatin; severe renal or hepatic failure; concurrent infectious disease; use of atorvastatin or other statins before the study; pathology report of other type of tumors instead of glioma grade 1,2 and 3; serious interaction between patients medications and atorvastatin; MAP < 70 mmHg; Na < 130 mEq/L; Hematocrit < 28%.

After obtaining informed consent, using permuted-block randomization patients were randomly assigned to atorvastatin or placebo group. Patients received atorvastatin or placebo 40 mg oral tablets, twice daily (totally 80 mg) for 3 weeks, from one week before to 2 weeks after surgery. Standard therapeutic regimen and supportive care, such as antibiotic prophylaxis, seizure prophylaxis, fluid therapy, and gastro intestinal ulcer prophylaxis have been used for both groups. This standard therapeutic regimen was including cefazolin as antibiotic prophylaxis, phenytoin for seizure prophylaxis, appropriate fluid therapy with normal saline, ranitidine as gastrointestinal ulcer prophylaxis, and dexamethasone for controlling brain edema after surgery.

At the beginning of the study, patients' demographic data such as age, sex, weight, comorbidity (having any concurrent disease other than glial tumor), history of hypertension, drug history, and neurological exam were collected on pre-designed questionnaires. Laboratory data recorded at baseline, were as follow: Fasting blood sugar (FBS), creatinin (Cr), blood urea nitrogen (BUN), white blood cell count (WBC count), hemoglobin, erythrocyte sedimentation rate (ESR), C-reactive protein (CRP), liver function tests (LFTs), lipid profile (including total cholesterol, LDL Cholesterol, HDL Cholesterol, and triglycerides). For detection of plasma MMP-9 concentration blood samples collected 4 times from each patient: immediately before starting atorvastatin or placebo, immediately before surgery, 24 hours and two weeks after the surgery. The plasma MMP-9 measured by enzyme-linked immunosorbent assay (ELISA) kits, Quantikine®, manufactured by R&D Systems, United States of America. Based on the kit catalog recommendations blood samples carried with heparinized tubes on ice. To separate plasma, blood centrifuged for 15 minutes at 1000 × g within 30 minutes of collection. Following the above an additional centrifugation step of the plasma at 10,000 × g for 10 minutes at 2 - 8°C performed for complete platelet removal, then all samples stored at −80°C till the assay day. This kit uses the quantitative sandwich enzyme immunoassay technique to assay MMP-9 levels. A monoclonal antibody specific for MMP-9 has been pre-coated on a microplate. All Standard samples and study samples are pipetted into the wells, and MMP-9 is bound by the immobilized antibody. Following washing away unbound substances, an enzyme-linked polyclonal antibody specific for MMP-9 is added to the wells. After a wash to eliminate unbound antibody-enzyme reagent, a substrate solution is added to the wells and color develops in proportion to the quantity of MMP-9 bound in the primary step. The color expansion is stopped and the intensity of the color is measured.

Clinical outcome were assessed with Karnofsky performance score at the baseline (one week before surgery) and 2 months after the surgery by the same examiner. Type and grade of tumors recorded after pathology report. Hospital stay defined as number of nights patient spent at the hospital. Our patients were closely observed for atorvastatin adverse effects, by interviewing patients during hospitalization and also after discharge in the clinic. Baseline and LFTs was measured in all patients and recheck CPK in any patient with symptoms suggestive of myopathy and also repeat transaminase levels when clinically indicated thereafter was about to be done. High rate reported adverse reactions such as diarrhea, arthralgia, limb pain, myalgia, muscle spasms, musculoskeletal pain, insomnia, nausea, and dyspepsia was asked from each patient specifically.

Statistical analyses were executed with the Statistical Package for Social Sciences (SPSS version 17; SPSS Inc., Chicago, IL, USA) and significance level was defined as p-value less than 0.05. The normal distribution of quantitative data was assessed with one sample Kolmogorov-Smirnov test. Data with a normal distribution were expressed as means ± standard deviations (SDs) and student *t*-test as well as paired *t*-test was used to compare quantitative variables between or within groups, respectively. The Mann–Whitney *U* test and Wilcoxon test were applied to compare non-normally distributed data (expressed as median (inter quartile range) to assess differences between and within groups, respectively. Regarding qualitative variables (categorical data), the chi-square or Fisher's exact test were performed.

Results

Forty- two patients, (25 males and 17 females) randomly assigned to 21 in atorvastatin group and 21 in placebo group. Patients' demographic data is presented in Table 1.

Patients mean ± SD age were 53.62 ± 15 years for atorvastatin group, and 40.43 ± 13.09 years in placebo group (p = 0.006, 95% CI: - 22.31- -4.08).

There were no statistically significant difference in regard to baseline parameters such as sex, weight, comorbidity (11 patients with hypertension [26%], 5 patients with ischemic heart disease [12%], 2 patients with gastrointestinal diseases [4.7%], one with lumbar herniated disc [2.4%], a patient with inherited neurofibromyalgia[2.4%], a patient with cataract [2.4%], and one patient with glaucoma [2.4%]), hypertension, concurrent drug therapy, and laboratory data such as FBS, Cr, BUN, WBC count, ESR, CRP (Table 1). The drug history of each patient obtained carefully, and there was no significant difference among the groups regarding medications. Considering drugs that may affect level of MMP-9 just 6 (3 patients in atorvastatin and 3 in placebo group) patients took low doses of aspirin (81 mg) to suppress platelet function. Dexamethasone as a part of standard post-operative protocol administered to all of the patients, 8 mg three times daily.

There were significant differences between baseline lipid profile (total cholesterol (p = 0.006), LDL Cholesterol (p = 0.009), and triglycerides (p = 0.04)) of the study groups. Lipid levels were higher in atorvastatin group; however, in both groups patients were not categorized as hyperlipidemic (Table 1).

Baseline plasma MMP-9 concentration, Karnofsky performance score, type of tumor, and grade of tumor among the groups were not significantly different (Table 1). Pathologic reports indicated grade 1, 2, 3 of glial tumor including, ependymoma grade 1 and 2, pilomyxoid astrocytoma, grade 2 astrocytoma, oligodendroglioma, ganglioglioma, anaplastic astrocytoma, and anaplastic oligodendroglioma.

Comparison of Karnofsky performance scale before and 2 months after surgery showed no significant difference among the groups (p = 0.07), however by further exploration of patients leading to exclusion of just one patient as outlier, significant difference showed up (p = 0.03). Atorvastatin group showed significantly better improvement of Karnofsky performance scale after surgery (11.43 ± 10.62 vs. 4.00 ± 8.21).

MMP-9 plasma level changes, immediately before surgery and 24 hours after surgery was not significantly different among the groups (p = 0.38).

In within group statistical analysis Karnofsky performance score showed significant increase in both atorvastatin (P = 0.001) and placebo (P = 0.03) groups. However, as it is depicted in Table 2 more progression was seen in atorvastatin group. MMP-9 plasma concentration levels increased significantly 24 hours after surgery in placebo group (P = 0.02). Nevertheless, there was no significant rise in MMP-9 levels in the atorvastatin group (P = 0.42). Comparison of MMP-9 plasma levels before surgery and 2 weeks after surgery revealed no significant changes in any of the groups, however there were an increasing trend in the placebo group and a decreasing trend in the atorvastatin group (Table 2).

Comparison of MMP -9 plasma level changes just before surgery with 2 weeks after surgery demonstrated significant difference among the groups (p = 0.048). Increase in MMP-9 levels 2 weeks after surgery was less in atorvastatin group. Atorvastatin and placebo groups MMP-9 plasma level changes between the first week of drug therapy and before surgery (1st and 2nd measurements), and changes between 3rd and 4th measurements indicated no significant difference. Likewise, comparison of ESR and CRP measurements before and after surgery did not indicate any significance in response to atorvastatin treatment.

Length of hospital stay was slightly in favor of atorvastatin group, but not to a significant degree (8.52 ± 6.77 days for drug group, and 11.29 ± 11.50 days for placebo group). There was no significant relation between

Table 1 Distribution of the baseline demographic and medical characteristics of patients in atorvastatin and placebo groups

Parameter	Atorvastatin group	Placebo group	P value
Sex			0.12
Male	15	10	
Female	6	11	
Age	53.62 ± 15	40.43 ± 13.09	0.006(95% CI: - 22.31- -4.08)
Weight	75.95 ± 12.35	72.43 ± 16.63	0.44(95% CI: - 12.66- 5.61)
Comorbidity	14	8	0.06
Hypertension	8	3	0.08
Concurrent drug therapy	14	8	0.06
FBS	94.57 ± 17.72	94.43 ± 24.16	0.98(95% CI: -13.36 – 13.07)
Cr	0.93 ± 0.19	0.81 ± 0.15	0.03 (95% CI: -0.23 – -0.01)
BUN	19.90 ± 6.36	15.48 ± 5.44	0.02(95% CI: -8.12 – -074)
WBC count	7400.48 ± 2857.89	7968.57 ± 379.129	0.98
ESR	20.24 ± 8.54	23.00 ± 10.29	0.35(95% CI: -3.13 – 8.66)
CRP	10.52 ± 10.96	11.62 ± 10.28	0.50
Total cholesterol	198.86 ± 33.45	173.52 ± 31.88	0.006
LDL cholesterol	129.62 ± 30.69	107.76 ± 31.73	0.009
Triglycerides	153.14 ± 50.58	173.52 ± 31.88	0.04
Plasma MMP-9 concentration	256.24 ± 279.81	130.95 ± 78.50	0.33
Karnofsky performance scale	82.38 ± 17.29	76.67 ± 19.32	0.25
Grade of tumor			0.80
Grade 1	4	3	
Grade 2	15	15	
Grade 3	2	3	
Type of tumor			0.73
Ependymoma grade 1	0	1	
Ependymoma grade 2	4	2	
Pilomyxoid astrocytoma	0	2	
Astrocytoma grade 2	5	7	
Oligodendroglioma	3	4	
Ganglioglioma	3	0	
Anaplastic astrocytoma	2	1	
Anaplastic oligodendroglioma	0	2	

age and Karnofsky performance score, MMP9 level changes, or hospital stay in any of the groups. BUN and Cr level changes were not significantly different between two groups. No adverse drug reaction reported by atorvastatin group.

Discussion

Neurosurgical procedures can induce serious neurological injuries [1,2]. Different medications such as diuretics, osmotic agents, and corticosteroids are suggested to decrease ameliorating brain edema induced by operation,

Table 2 Mean ± SD of outcome indicators in atorvastatin (drug) and placebo group

Variable	Plasma MMP-9 concentration before surgery	Plasma MMP-9 concentration 24 hours after surgery	Plasma MMP-9 concentration 2 weeks after surgery	Karnofsky performance scale before surgery	Karnofsky performance scale 2 months after surgery
Drug group	190.14 ± 197.74	236.38 ±225.08	164.95 ± 126.68	82.38 ± 17.29	93.81 ± 9.73
Placebo group	130.19 ± 83.04	184.81 ± 107.04	180.81 ± 115.93	76.67 ± 19.32	82.86 ± 14.88

but there is no clinical study in this regard [33]. Immunohistochemical evidences specified that MMP-9 increases surrounding surgical induced brain injury areas [2]. Two experimental studies have demonstrated that MMP inhibitors preserve the BBB, attenuate brain edema, and act as a neuroprotectant after brain surgery [1,2].

There is some evidence that suggesting statins decrease MMP-9 levels [30-32]. Various retrospective and prospective clinical trials, meta-analysis, and researches evaluated pleiotropic effects of statins on surgical outcome. In cardiac, vascular, or non cardiovascular operations, irrespective to the type of surgery, positive effects and reduction of undesirable postoperative outcomes, such as mortality, morbidity, length of hospital and ICU stay have been reported fallowing statin therapy [34-38]. Neuro-protective effects of statins were established in many studies [19-30].

In this prospective, randomized, double blind, controlled trial, 42 patients underwent glial tumor surgery, atorvastatin 40 mg or placebo used two times daily. Since most of the studies use full dose of statins to evaluate surgical induced injuries, 80 mg atorvastatin as a full dose is used in this study. Results demonstrated significant reduction in MMP-9 plasma level in atorvastatin patients after two weeks. Regarding clinical endpoint (Karnofsky performance scale at 2 months after surgery), better outcome observed in atorvastatin group. Length of hospital stay was less in patients who had received atorvastatin, but not to a statistical significant degree.

Plasma MMP9 changes followed the anticipated pattern. No significant change observed in the baseline measurement and second measurement (immediately before surgery), since there was no neuronal injury happened before surgery. Plasma MMP9 increased 24 hours after surgery as expected confirming the hypothesis of MMP9 surge after surgery. There was decrease in the MMP9 plasma concentration 2 weeks after surgery indicating improvement in patients. Between groups, statistical analyses demonstrated that atorvastatin group had significantly more reduction in MMP9 level after two weeks in comparison with placebo.

Within group statistical analyses revealed that atorvastatin diminished MMP-9 peak 24 hours after surgery. This outcome improvement was also confirmed by better neurological outcome as assessed with Karnofsky performance score in atorvastatin group. Despite no significant change in MMP-9 plasma concentration 2 weeks after surgery in within group statistical analyses, mean level increased in placebo group and decreased in atorvastatin group. All these findings indicate beneficial effects of atorvastatin in these patients.

Anti-inflammatory effects and MMP9 suppression appear to be irrelevant to concomitant medications. Although age of two patient groups was significantly different, there was no significant relation between age and outcome variables (i.e. karnofsky performance score, MMP9 level changes, or hospital stay).

Atorvastatin administration was well tolerated during the study period. No adverse drug reaction detected same as other studies on statins [37,38]. Acute kidney injuries were recently reported with high doses of statins [39-42]; therefore renal laboratory values were carefully monitored in this study. There were no significant changes in renal laboratory values between two groups. There is even a retrospective cohort of 98,939 patients who underwent various operations including; major open abdominal, cardiac, thoracic, or vascular procedure between 2000 and 2010 claims that statin use before surgery reduce risk of postoperative acute kidney injury [42]. Preoperative statin therapy decreased the need for postoperative renal replacement therapy [34].

Study had some limitations due to complexity of neurologic, physiologic and pathologic of human brain. Due to diversity of functioning regions of brain each glioma can cause different symptoms and debilities in different functioning parts of human brain within and or between different groups of patients pre and postoperatively. Due to complexity of circuits of brain (mostly unknown) different people suffer from different disabilities even when the glioma is operated on, in same area of brain; different surgical approaches caused different complications that could have been misinterpreted as effect of drug while being merely surgical.

Conclusion

Pre-operative atorvastatin administration resulted in reduction of MMP-9 level 2 weeks postoperatively and improvement of Karnofsky performance scale 2 month after surgery. Larger trials, longer duration of statin therapy, retrospective analysis of neurosurgical procedures in patients with long term statins use, could be helpful for decisive evidence.

Competing interests

All authors declare that they have no competing interests.

Authors' contributions

All authors participated in study design. KG and AK wrote the study protocol, and supervised all the stages of the research. KG managed supplying drug and placebo. AK performed surgeries. NM as a clinical pharmacist was involved in every steps of the project including literature review, writing the proposal, performing randomization and keeping it secret, collecting demographic data, design and filling the questionnaire, analyzing blood samples and providing article draft. SN and SA did neurological physical examination of patients, involved in blood sample collection, and assessed Karnofsky performance score. JS did all statistical analyses. MM and MJ consulted us in different stages of the project. KG, AK, JS, SA, and SN edited the draft. All authors read and approved the final manuscript.

Acknowledgements

We would like to thank Tehran University of Medical Sciences for providing the research fund. We also gratefully appreciate all attendants, residents, nurses and staffs of the neurosurgery ward at Shariati hospital for their supports in this project.

Author details
[1]Department of Clinical Pharmacy, Faculty of Pharmacy, Tehran University of Medical Sciences, Tehran, Iran. [2]Department of Neurosurgery, Tehran University of Medical Sciences, Tehran, Iran. [3]Department of Clinical Pharmacy, Shahid Beheshti University of Medical Sciences, Tehran, Iran.

References

1. Jadhav V, Yamaguchi M, Obenaus A, Zhang JH: **Matrix metalloproteinase inhibition attenuates brain edema after surgical brain injury.** *Acta Neurochir Suppl* 2005, **105**:357–361.
2. Jadhav V, Yamaguchi M, Obenaus A, Zhang JH: **Matrix metalloproteinase inhibition attenuates brain edema in an *in vivo* model of surgically-induced brain injury.** *Neurosurg* 2007, **61**:1067–1076.
3. Yong VW, Agrawal SM, Stirling DP: **Targeting MMPs in acute and chronic neurological conditions.** *Neurother* 2007, **4**:580–589.
4. Liu W, Hendren J, Qin XJ, Shen J, Liu KJ: **Normobarichyperoxia attenuates early blood–brain barrier disruption by inhibiting MMP-9-mediated occludin degradation in focal cerebral ischemia.** *J Neurochem* 2009, **108**:811–820.
5. Rosenberg GA, Estrada EY, Dencoff JE: **Matrix metalloproteinases and TIMPs are associated with blood–brain barrier opening after reperfusion in rat brain.** *Stroke* 1998, **29**:2189–2195.
6. Noble LJ, Donovan F, Igarashi T, Goussev S, Werb Z: **Matrix metalloproteinases limit functional recovery after spinal cord injury by modulation of early vascular events.** *J Neurosci* 2002, **22**:7526–7535.
7. Pfefferkorn T, Rosenberg GA: **Closure of the blood–brain barrier by matrix metalloproteinase inhibition reduces rtPA-mediated mortality in cerebral ischemia with delayed reperfusion.** *Stroke* 2003, **34**:2025–2030.
8. Sumii T, Lo EH: **Involvement of matrix metalloproteinase in thrombolysis-associated hemorrhagic transformation after embolic focal ischemia in rats.** *Stroke* 2002, **33**:831–836.
9. Gu Z, Kaul M, Yan B, Kridel SJ, Cui J, Strongin A, Smith JW, Liddington RC, Lipton SA: **Snitrosylation of matrix metalloproteinases: signaling pathway to neuronal cell death.** *Science* 2002, **297**:1186–1190.
10. Xue M, Hollenberg M, Yong VW: **Combination of thrombin and matrix metalloproteinase-9 exacerbates neurotoxicity in cell culture and intracerebral hemorrhage in mice.** *J Neurosci* 2006, **26**:10281–10291.
11. Van den Steen PE, Proost P, Wuyts A, Van Damme J, Opdenakker G: **Neutrophil gelatinase B potentiates interleukin-8 tenfold by aminoterminal processing, whereas it degrades CTAP-III, PF-4, and GRO-alpha and leaves RANTES and MCP-2 intact.** *Blood* 2000, **96**:2673–2681.
12. Alvarez-Sabin J, Delgado P, Abilleira S, Molina CA, Arenillas J, Ribó M, Santamarina E, Quintana M, Monasterio J, Montaner J: **Temporal profile of matrix metalloproteinases and their inhibitors after spontaneous intracerebral hemorrhage relationship to clinical and radiological outcome.** *Stroke* 2004, **35**:1316–1322.
13. Abilleira S, Montaner J, Molina CA, Monasterio J, Castillo J, Alvarez-Sabı'n J: **Matrix metalloproteinase concentration after spontaneous intracerebral hemorrhage.** *J Neurosurg* 2003, **99**:65–70.
14. Wang J, Tsirka SE: **Neuroprotection by inhibition of matrix metalloproteinases in a mouse model of intracerebralhaemorrhage.** *Brain* 2005, **128**:1622–1633.
15. Rosenberg GA, Navratil M: **Metalloproteinase inhibition blocks edema in intracerebral hemorrhage in the rat.** *Neurol* 1997, **48**:921–926.
16. Rosenberg GA, Kornfeld M, Estrada E, Kelley RO, Liotta LA, Stetler-Stevenson WG: **TIMP-2 reduces proteolytic opening of blood–brain barrier by type IV collagenase.** *Brain Res* 1992, **576**:203–207.
17. Gotto AM: **Management of dyslipidemia.** *Am J Med* 2002, **112**(Suppl 1):10–18.
18. Chopp M, Zhang ZG, Jiang Q: **Neurogenesis, angiogenesis, and MRI indices of functional recovery from stroke.** *Stroke* 2007, **38**:827–831.
19. Khoshnevisan A, Mardani A, Kamali S: **An overview of pharmacological approaches for management and repair of spinal cord injuries.** *Iran J Psychiatry* 2010, **5**:119–127.
20. Chen J, Chopp M: **Neurorestorative Treatment of Stroke: Cell and Pharmacological Approaches.** *NeuroRx* 2006, **3**:466–473.
21. Chen J, Zhang ZG, Li Y, Wang Y, Wang L, Jiang H, Zhang C, Lu M, Katakowski M, Feldkamp CS, Chopp M: **Statins induce angiogenesis, neurogenesis, and synaptogenesis after stroke.** *Ann Neurol* 2003, **53**:743–751.
22. Endres M, Laufs U, Huang Z, Nakamura T, Huang P, Moskowitz MA, Liao JK: **Stroke protection by 3-hydroxy- 3-methylglutaryl (HMG)-CoA reductase inhibitors mediated by endothelial nitric oxide synthase.** *ProcNatl AcadSci U S A* 1998, **95**:8880–8885.
23. Laufs U, Gertz K, Dirnagl U, Bohm M, Nickenig G, Endres M: **Rosuvastatin, a new HMG-CoA reductase inhibitor, upregulates endothelial nitric oxide synthase and protects from ischemic stroke in mice.** *Brain Res* 2002, **942**:23–30.
24. Aslanyan S, Weir CJ, McInnes GT, Reid JL, Walters MR, Lees KR: **Statin administration prior to ischaemic stroke onset and survival: exploratory evidence from matched treatment-control study.** *Eur J Neurol* 2005, **12**:493–498.
25. Elkind MS, Flint AC, Sciacca RR, Sacco RL: **Lipid-lowering agent use at ischemic stroke onset is associated with decreased mortality.** *Neurol* 2005, **65**:253–258.
26. McGirt MJ, Garces Ambrossi GL, Huang J, Tamargo RJ: **Simvastatin for the prevention of symptomatic cerebral vasospasm following aneurysmal subarachnoid hemorrhage: a single-institution prospective cohort study.** *J Neurosurg* 2009, **110**:968–674.
27. Miida T, Takahashi A, Ikeuchi T: **Prevention of stroke and dementia by statin therapy: experimental and clinical evidence of their pleiotropic effects.** *PharmacolTher* 2007, **113**:378–393.
28. Amarenco P, Bogousslavsky J, Callahan AS, Goldstein L, Hennerici M, Sillsen H, Welch MA, Zivin J: **Design and baseline characteristics of the stroke prevention by aggressive reduction in cholesterol levels (SPARCL) study.** *Cerebrovasc Dis* 2003, **16**:389–395.
29. Chen J, Zacharek A, Li A, Zhang C, Ding J, Roberts C, Lu M, Kapke A, Chopp M: **Vascular endothelial growth factor mediates atorvastatin-induced mammalian achaete-scute homologue-1 gene expression and neuronal differentiation after stroke in retired breeder rats.** *Neurosci* 2006, **141**:737–744.
30. Kwak BR, Mulhaupt F, Mach F: **Atherosclerosis: anti-inflammatory and immunomodulatory activities of statins.** *Autoimmun Rev* 2003, **2**:332–338.
31. Corsini A, Bellosta S, Baetta R, Fumagalli R, Paoletti R, Bernini F: **New insights into the pharmacodynamic and pharmacokinetic properties of statins.** *PharmacolTher* 1999, **84**:413–428.
32. Bellosta S, Via D, Canavesi M, Pfister P, Fumagalli R, Paoletti R, Bernini F: **HMG-CoA reductase inhibitors reduce MMP-9 secretion by macrophages.** *Arterioscler Thromb Vasc Biol* 1998, **18**:1671–1678.
33. Menon D: **Critical care medicine: management of raised intracranial pressure.** In *Oxford textbook of medicine.* Volume 24th edition. Edited by Warrell DA, Cox TM, Firth JD. New York: Oxford University Press; 2003:1256.
34. Singh Singh I, Rajagopalan S, Srinivasan A, Achuthan S, Dhamija P, Hota D, Chakrabarti A: **Preoperative statin therapy is associated with lower requirement of renal replacement therapy in patients undergoing cardiac surgery: a meta-analysis of observational studies.** *Int Cardiov Thorac Surg* 2013, **17**:345–352.
35. Hindler K, Shaw AD, Samuels J, Fulton S, Collard CD, Riedel B: **Improved postoperative outcomes associated with preoperative statin therapy.** *Anesthesiol* 2006, **105**:1260–1272.
36. Chopra V, Wesorick DH, Sussman JB, Greene T, Rogers M, Froehlich JB, Eagle KA, Saint S: **Effect of perioperative statins on death, myocardial infarction, atrial fibrillation, and length of stay: a systematic review and meta-analysis.** *Arch Surg* 2012, **147**:181–189.
37. Liakopoulos OJ, Kuhn EW, Slottosch I, Wassmer G, Wahlers T: **Preoperative statin therapy for patients undergoing cardiac surgery.** *Cochrane Database Syst Rev* 2012, **4**:CD008493.
38. Sanders RD, Nicholson A, Lewis SR, Smith AF, Alderson P: **Perioperative statin therapy for improving outcomes during and after noncardiac vascular surgery.** *Cochrane Database Syst Rev* 2013, **3**(7):CD009971.
39. Sarma A, Cannon CP, Wiviott SD, Sabatine MS, Pfeffer MA, Hoffman EB, Guo J: **The incidence of kidney injury for patients treated with intensive versus less potent statin therapy after an acute coronary syndrome [abstract].** *Circulation* 2013, **128**:00–00. 10.1161/CIR.0b013e31829ecc16.
40. Carney EF: **Acute kidney injury: high-potency statin therapy and risk of acute kidney injury.** *Nat Rev Nephrol* 2013, **9**:309. 10.1038/nrneph.2013.68.

41. Dormuth CR, Hemmelgarn BR, Paterson JM, James MT, Teare GF, Raymond CB, Lafrance J-P, Levy A, Garg AX, Ernst P: **Use of high potency statins and rates of admission for acute kidney injury: multicenter, retrospective observational analysis of administrative databases.** *BMJ* 2013, **346**. http://dx.doi.org/10.1136/bmj.f880.
42. Brunelli SM, Waikar SS, Bateman BT, Chang TI, Lii J, Garg AX, Winkelmayer WC, Choudhry NK: **Preoperative statin use and postoperative acute kidney injury.** *Am J Med* 2012, **125:**1195–1204.

Effect of *Linum usitatissimum* L. (linseed) oil on mild and moderate carpal tunnel syndrome: a randomized, double-blind, placebo-controlled clinical trial

Mohammad Hashem Hashempur[1,2], Kaynoosh Homayouni[3,4], Alireza Ashraf[5,3*], Alireza Salehi[1], Mohsen Taghizadeh[6] and Mojtaba Heydari[2]

Abstract

Background: Carpal tunnel syndrome is known as the most common entrapment neuropathy. Conservative treatments cannot reduce the symptomatic severity satisfactorily; therefore, effectiveness of *Linum usitatissimum* L. (linseed) oil on carpal tunnel syndrome, as a complementary treatment, was evaluated in the current study. Linseed oil is a well-known preparation in Iranian traditional medicine and its analgesic, anti-inflammatory and anti-oxidative effects have been shown in previous studies.

Methods: A randomized, double-blind, placebo-controlled clinical trial was conducted. One hundred patients (155 hands) with idiopathic mild to moderate carpal tunnel syndrome aged between 18 and 65 years old were randomized in two parallel groups. These two groups were treated during 4 weeks with topical placebo and linseed oil. In addition, a night wrist splint was prescribed for both groups. Symptomatic severity and functional status were measured using Boston Carpal Tunnel Questionnaire. In addition, median sensory nerve conduction velocity, motor distal latency, sensory distal latency and compound latency as electrodiagnostic parameters were measured at baseline and after the intervention period.

Results: After the intervention, significant improvement was observed regarding Boston Carpal Tunnel Questionnaire symptomatic severity and functional status mean differences (p <0.001) in the linseed oil group compared with those in the placebo group. Also, regarding the mean differences of both groups, significant improvement of nerve conduction velocity of the median nerve was seen in the linseed oil group by a value of 2.38 m/sec ($p < 0.05$). However, motor distal latency and sensory distal latency of the median nerve showed no between-group significant changes ($p = 0.14$ for both items). Finally, compound latency was improved slightly in the case group, comparing mean differences between the groups (p <0.05). No significant adverse events were reported from using linseed oil.

Conclusions: It seems that linseed oil could be effective in the management of mild and moderate carpal tunnel syndrome, especially in improving the severity of symptoms and functional status. In addition, its effect on electerodiagnostic parameters, especially on the nerve conduction velocity, can be considered as a valuable point.

Keywords: Carpal tunnel syndrome, *Linum usitatissimum*, Linseed oil, Iranian traditional medicine, Randomized controlled trial, Herbal medicine, Complementary therapies

* Correspondence: sbahar7@gmail.com
[5]Shiraz Burn Research Center, Shiraz University of Medical Sciences, Shiraz, Iran
[3]Department of Physical Medicine and Rehabilitation, Shiraz University of Medical Sciences, Shiraz, Iran
Full list of author information is available at the end of the article

Background

Carpal tunnel syndrome (CTS), a condition in which the median nerve compression occurs, is known as the most common entrapment neuropathy [1]. Various treatment options, as surgical and non-surgical, have been suggested for CTS. Surgery is usually considered for patients with an experience of conservative treatment failure and those who have severe CTS [2,3], while non-surgical treatments are usually prescribed as an initial option for the patients who do not have any evidence of denervation in electromyography, cannot undergo surgery, or suffer from non-constant symptoms of mild to moderate CTS [4,5]. Standard non-surgical treatments vary from exercise and activity modification to wrist splinting (as the most frequently reported treatment [6]), use of oral medications like NSAIDs and corticosteroids, and even locally injected steroids [7,8]. However, conservative treatments cannot reduce symptomatic severity satisfactorily [9-11]; therefore, new conservative treatments are needed to be evaluated in randomized controlled trials.

Nowadays, complementary and alternative medicine (CAM) is welcomed by general population, governments and World Health Organization. Easy accessibility, lower costs and origination of them from nature are the main causes of this worldwide popularity [12]. Therefore, CAM treatments can play an important role as new conservative treatments for CTS.

Linum usitatissimum L. (from the family Linaceae), commonly known as flax or linseed, is a herb that is native to Europe, Asia and Mediterranean regions [13]. Linseed oil or flaxseed oil is obtained from its dried ripe seeds. In addition to edible uses of this oil, it is known as an anti-inflammatory [14,15] antioxidant [16,17] and analgesic [18] oil. Therefore, due to the mentioned beneficial properties, it is used in several studies on a variety of subjects such as arthritis [15], dermatologic complaints [19], breast cancer [20] and even keratoconjunctivitis [21].

The topical use of linseed oil has been approved for a variety of skin disorders [22]. For instance, the Brazilian national pharmacopoeia has approved its topical administration in cases with pruritus, and in patients of burn [13]. In addition, some studies examined the topical usage of this compound in animal model of skin wound healing, and in the prevention of peri-ileostomy skin excoriation. No toxicity was reported in such studies [23].

Linseed oil could play an anti-inflammatory role when used by different routes of administration in animal models. In fact, its inhibition on prostaglandin E_2, leukotriene B_4, histamine and bradykinin can make it a potent anti-inflammatory agent against distinct phases of inflammation, comparable with standard aspirin [24]. In addition, it seems that analgesic activity of linseed oil is peripherally mediated [18]. Analgesic activity of linseed oil may be due to a combination of its inhibitory effect of prostaglandin, histamine, bradykinin and acetylcholine [25].

In addition, linseed oil is a well-known and frequently-used medicine in Iranian traditional medicine (ITM). According to the most famous and reliable ITM books, i.e. Avicenna's Canon of Medicine and Liber Continens of Rhazes, linseed oil can be used as an analgesic and anti-fibrosis drug [26,27].

Therefore, according to ITM concepts and some unpublished experiences by experts about potential effect of linseed oil on CTS and also supporting data about some properties of linseed oil (e.g. analgesic, antioxidant and anti-inflammatory), we hypothesized its possible effect for CTS. Therefore, the current study aimed to assess the effectiveness of topical flaxseed oil in patients with mild and moderate CTS.

Materials and methods

Study design

The study was designed as a two-arm, randomized, placebo-controlled, double- blind clinical trial using a parallel design.

Ethical considerations

The study protocol was in compliance with the Declaration of Helsinki (1989 revision) and approved by the Local Medical Ethics Committee of Shiraz University of Medical Sciences (SUMS) with reference number: CT-92-6709. The trial was registered in Iranian Registry of Clinical Trials (registration ID: IRCT2012103111341N1). A written informed consent was signed by all of the enrolled participants.

Preparation of test drug, placebo and wrist splint

Seeds of the test drug were purchased from the local market and authenticated by a botanist at Kashan University of Medical Sciences. A voucher specimen was preserved for future reference.

The seeds were coarsely ground in an environment of mild heat, and then cold-pressed (35°C). The extracted oil was subjected to gas chromatographic (GC) analysis. The findings revealed the presence of major components as linolenic acid (54.2%), oleic acid (20.39%), linoleic acid (12.26%), palmitic acid (5.99%), and stearic acid (5.7%). Nitrogen purging was carried out to avoid oxidation. In addition, the bottles had no head space (the oil was filled to the bottle brim).

Pharmaceutical graded paraffin was considered as the placebo. In addition, standard coloring agent in a little amount and standard range was used to make paraffin's color similar to that of the linseed oil.

A wrist splint (Dr. K. H.®) immobilized the wrist in an extension position (external angle: 20° and internal angle: 5°). The splint was made of 5-mm medical foam, lined internally with fabric and externally with thin leather. In addition, it had three adjustable Velcro fastenings on its dorsal side (Figure 1).

Inclusion and exclusion criteria

Patients (from the Outpatient Clinic of Shahid Faghihi Hospital, an academic teaching center, affiliated with SUMS) with suspected CTS (according to history and physical examination) were selected after electrophysiologic confirmation study.

Detailed inclusion and exclusion criteria are shown in Table 1. The eligibility criteria included briefly: patients of both sexes aged between 18 and 65 years old, with idiopathic mild and moderate CTS. Some of the most important exclusion criteria were: coexisting serious illness, rheumatoid arthritis, CTS related to systemic diseases and pregnancy. In addition, the patients were excluded if they had previous surgery for CTS or intracarpal steroid injections.

Electrodiagnosis

The electrophysiologic assessments were performed by a "MEDLEC SYNERGY VIASIS" electromyography device with two 6 mm felt tips bar electrodes as the stimulators and recorders (diameter of pads 23 mm apart). Median distal motor latency was measured by a bipolar stimulating electrode at the wrist and a bipolar surface-recording located on the abductor pollicis brevis muscle (8 cm from stimulus electrodes at the wrist). Antidromic sensory nerve action potentials evoked at the wrist were recorded from the middle finger. Standard distances (7 cm from recorder, at mid palm and 14 cm from recorder at wrist) were kept between the stimulator and recorder electrodes. For recording the compound nerve action potential, stimulation at mid palm and recording at wrist (7 cm apart) was performed. In addition, using a concentric needle electrode, electromyography was performed on the abductor pollicis brevis muscle. We defined denervation as sustained, abnormal spontaneous activity. This ranged from 0 to 4+, in the form of positive waves or fibrillations. The skin temperature during all of the electrodiagnostic studies was at least 31°C and all of the assessments were carried out in a similar constant room temperature between 23°C and 25°C. In addition, due to the possibility of diurnal variation in clinical and electrophysiologic assessments [28], all of the patients were assessed at the follow up visit at a similar time of the day as the first session. In addition, the patients were assessed on their visits by the same authors (K.H and A.A) who performed clinical examinations and electrodiagnostic assessments and were blinded about each patient's allocation.

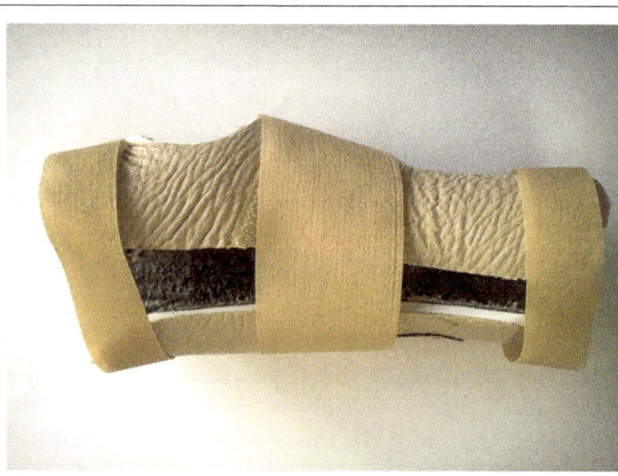

Figure 1 A photograph of fabricated wrist splint that was prescribed for all of the participants (dorsal view).

Intervention

Splint

All of the patients were prescribed to use the wrist splint during the study period. In fact, the test drug and placebo were added to this standard treatment. The wrist splint prescription was night-only because of symptoms usually worsening at night, in addition to obtaining a higher compliance, considering the patient's concern about splint's interference with his/her daily activities.

Placebo and test drug

Both of the drug and placebo were prescribed to be used in the morning and evening time for a period of 4 weeks, 5 drops per use, topically on the palmar wrist territory. The patients were advised not to massage the mentioned zone.

Outcome assessment

Boston Carpal Tunnel Questionnaire (BCTQ), as a self-administered, validated measurement, was the primary outcome measure. The BCTQ assesses symptom severity score (BCTQ SYMPT) and functional status score (BCTQ FUNCT). These scores are evaluated by an eleven-item scale and an eight-item scale, respectively [29]. The items of each scale consist of multiple-choice responses from 1 (as the mildest) to 5 (as the most severe). The BCTQ SYMPT and FUNCT are calculated as the mean of the scores for the individual items.

We used the Persian version of BCTQ that was validated previously, showing to have a reasonable reliability, sensitivity and internal consistency [30].

Secondary outcome measures were median nerve sensory distal latency (SDL), sensory nerve conduction velocity (NCV), motor distal latency (MDL) and compound latency (CL).

At the beginning of the enrollment and after 4 weeks of intervention, the data related to both primary and

Table 1 Inclusion and exclusion criteria

Inclusion criteria	Patients of both sexes aged between 18 and 65 years old willing to sign the informed consent form
	Clinical symptoms and signs of CTS (at least 2 symptoms or 1 sign plus 1 symptom[37]), including:
	- Pain
	- Paraesthesia
	- Hypoesthesia
	- Numbness
	- Tingling
	- Positive Phalen test
	- Positive Tinnel test
	Electrodiagnostic evidence of mild and moderate idiopathic CTS, including:
	• SDL > 3.7 m Sec
	• SNCV < 40 m/Sec
	• MDL > 4.2 m Sec
	• CL > 2.4 m Sec
Exclusion criteria	Positive history of hypersensitivity to linseed oil
	Inability of data gathering forms completion (such as cognitive impairment or language problem)
	Patients with severe CTS, clinical and electrodiagnostic evidence including (if any of these evidences was found):
	– Thenar atrophy
	–Fibrillation potentials or reinnervation on needle EMG of APB muscle
	–Electrophisiologic study:
	• SDL > 5.3 m Sec OR Absent
	• SNCV < 28 m/Sec
	• MDL > 6.5 m Sec OR Absent
	• CL > 3.2 m Sec
	Coexisting cervical radiculopathies, brachial plexopathies or more proximal median mononeuropathies
	Clinical and electrophysiological signs of polyneuropathy
	Rheumatologic diseases, like RA, systemic sclerosis, SLE and amyloidosis
	Endocrinologic diseases, such as DM and hypothyroidism
	Conditions that can mimic CTS such as multiple sclerosis
	Pregnancy
	Coexisting serious illness, such as renal and heart failure
	Recent or ongoing inevitable use of corticosteroids or analgesics
	Previous surgery for CTS
	Intra-articular injection within the previous 6 months
	Positive history of severe trauma or fracture of wrist bones

SDL: sensory distal latency; SNCV: sensory nerve conduction velocity; MDL: motor distal latency; CL: compound latency; EMG: electromyography; APB: abductor policis brevis; RA: rheumatoid arthritis; SLE: systemic lupus erythematosus; DM: diabetes mellitus.

secondary outcome measures were obtained and recorded on the patient's data form. We excluded the patients who had recent or ongoing inevitable use of corticosteroids or analgesics; however, the included patients were asked to record their use of analgesics as the rescue drug.

Randomization, blinding and concealment of allocation

The eligible patients were randomly allocated to two parallel groups, the drug and placebo groups, by the secretary of the clinic. She was trained and instructed to use a block-randomization list (non-stratified, with the same block lengths, generated by computer) sequentially. In the case of patients affected by CTS bilaterally, both wrists were allocated to the same intervention (i.e. drug or placebo). The physicians, researchers, and statisticians were blind to the allocation of patients. Moreover, due to the same shape and size of the drug and placebo containers and similarity in color, the patients were blind to their allocation.

Statistical analysis

The intention-to-treat population used in all of the analyses included all randomized patients who completed their follow up, whether adhering completely to the clinical trial protocol or not.

Demographic and clinical characteristics of the participants were shown as the mean ± standard deviation (SD) for continuous variables. Differences of pre- and post-treatment were reported as mean and 95% confidence intervals.

Normality for continuous variables was checked using Kolmogorov-Smirnov test. Data were analyzed using Chi-square test, independent and paired samples t-test, and Mann–Whitney test. *P* values less than 0.05 were considered statistically significant.

Results

The first enrollment was done in October 2013 and the last patient's follow-up was completed in January 2014. A total of 119 patients (183 hands) were assessed for eligibility, and finally 100 patients (155 hands) who were eligible and gave their written informed consent were randomly assigned to drug and placebo groups (79 and 76 hands for placebo and drug, respectively). Sixty four hands in the linseed oil group and 68 hands in the placebo group completed the study. Detailed description of the patients' enrolment, randomization and outcomes are outlined in Figure 2.

The baseline demographic and clinical characteristics of the patients are shown in Table 2. No significant differences with regard to age, gender, duration of symptoms and BMI were observed between two arms. Additionally,

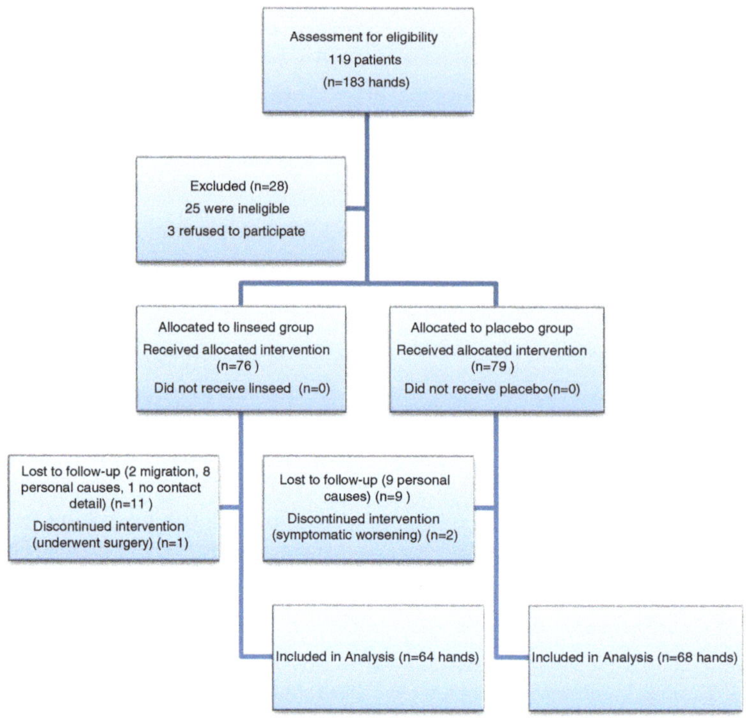

Figure 2 The trail flowchart.

baseline measures for all of the outcome assessments were similar in both groups.

The patients were asked about their adherence to the study protocol at the follow-up visit. In the linseed oil group, only 3 patients reported some missing doses of oil and 2 patients had not used the splint as it was prescribed. In addition, in the placebo group 4 and 2 patients reported some forgotten doses of oil and inappropriate use of splint, respectively. However, all of them were analyzed in the predetermined groups. Additionally, according to the patients' report, no rescue drug was used by them in each group.

Table 3 shows a full description of each outcome measurement changes, considering before and after trial, as well as mean differences in each group. Comparison of the mean differences between the groups showed a significant improvement in BCTQ SYMPT and FUNCT of the linseed oil group, after a 4 week period of

Table 2 Baseline demographic and clinical characteristics of participants in the two groups of linseed oil and placebo

Variable	Placebo group (n = 79)	Linseed oil group (n = 76)	*p* value	Statistical test
Age (years), Mean(±SD)	45.01(±8.71)	42.95(±10.63)	0.227	t-test
Male/female (n)	4/64	10/54	0.069	Chi-Square
Duration(months), Mean(±SD)	13.66(±13.45)	13.56(±13.78)	0.912	Mann-Whitney
BMI (kg/m^2), Mean(±SD)	27.03(±3.25)	25.99(±5.22)	0.173	t-test
BCTQ SYMPT (pts), Mean(±SD)	2.75(±0.62)	2.74(±0.75)	0.921	t-test
BCTQ FUNCT (pts), Mean(±SD)	2.41(±0.74)	2.61(±0.71)	0.120	t-test
Median NCV (m/sec), Mean(±SD)	36.27(±4.29)	35.54(±3.81)	0.303	t-test
Median MDL (msec), Mean(±SD)	4.16(±0.20)	4.20(±0.34)	0.384	t-test
Median CL (msec), Mean(±SD)	2.533(±0.17)	2.52(±0.14)	0.872	t-test
Median SDL (msec), Mean(±SD)	3.99(±0.26)	3.95(±0.43)	0.519	t-test

SD: standard deviation, BMI: body mass index, BCTQ: Boston Carpal Tunnel Questionnaire, SYMPT: symptom severity, FUNCT: functional status, pts: points, NCV: nerve conduction velocity, MDL: motor distal latency, CL: compound latency, SDL: sensory distal latency.

Table 3 Changes in BCTQ symptoms, BCTQ function and electrophysiologic measurements, comparing mean values before and after trial within groups, and mean differences between groups

	Study groups	Before (Mean ± SD)	After (Mean ± SD)	*p*-value	Statistical test	Mean difference	*p*-value	Statistical test
BCTQ SYMPT	Linseed oil	2.74 ± 0.75	1.90 ± 0.54	<0.0001	Paired t-test	0.83 ± 0.59 (CI 95% 0.69–0.99)	<0.001	Independent t-test
	Placebo	2.75 ± 0.62	2.59 ± 0.75	<0.0001	Paired t-test	0.16 ± 0.48 (CI95% 0.05–0.28)		
BCTQ FUNCT	Linseed oil	2.61 ± 0.71	2.17 ± 0.71	<0.0001	Paired t-test	0.44 ± 0.5 (CI 95% 0.32–0.56)	<0.001	Independent t-test
	Placebo	2.41 ± 0.74	2.59 ± 0.80	0.024	Paired t-test	- 0.18 ± 0.5 (CI 95% -0.31- -0.07)		
Median NCV	Linseed oil	35.54 ± 3.81	37.92 ± 6.23	0.007	Paired t-test	2.38 ± 6.78 (CI 95% 0.72–4.04)	0.034	Independent t-test
	Placebo	36.27 ± 4.29	36.22 ± 6.07	0.57	Paired t-test	0.04 ± 6.21 (CI 95% -1.52–1.43)		
Median MDL	Linseed oil	4.20 ± 0.34	4.06 ± 0.33	<0.0001	Paired t-test	0.14 ± 0.29 (CI 95% 0.07–0.21)	0.140	Independent t-test
	Placebo	4.16 ± 0.20	4.10 ± 0.35	<0.0001	Paired t-test	0.06 ± 0.32 (CI 95% -0.02–0.14)		
Median CL	Linseed oil	2.52 ± 0.14	2.43 ± 0.23	0.004	Paired t-test	0.09 ± 0.21 (CI 95% 0.03–0.15)	0.044	Independent t-test
	Placebo	2.53 ± 0.17	2.54 ± 0.32	0.145	Paired t-test	−0.008 ± 0.28 (CI 95% -0.08–0.06)		
Median SDL	Linseed oil	3.95 ± 0.43	3.82 ± 0.34	0.032	Paired t-test	0.12 ± 0.45 (CI 95% 0.01–0.24)	0.144	Independent t-test
	Placebo	3.99 ± 0.26	3.97 ± 0.36	0.053	Paired t-test	0.02 ± 0.36 (CI 95% -0.07–0.11)		

SD: standard deviation, BCTQ: Boston Carpal Tunnel Questionnaire, SYMPT: symptom severity, FUNCT: functional status, NCV: nerve conduction velocity, MDL: motor distal latency, CL: compound latency, SDL: sensory distal latency, CI 95%: 95%confidence interval

treatment (p <0.001). Mean differences of these measures were 0.83 (CI 95% 0.69 – 0.99) and 0.44 (CI 95% 0.32 – 0.56), respectively.

In addition, regarding mean differences of both groups, a significant improvement of NCV of the median nerve was seen in the linseed oil group by a difference of 2.38 m/sec (CI 95% 0.72 – 4.04, $p = 0.034$). However, mean differences of the median nerve's MDL and SDL in the linseed oil group showed no significant differences as compared with the placebo group ($p = 0.14$ for both items). Finally, comparison of the mean differences between the groups revealed a slight improvement in the CL of the linseed oil group (CI 95% 0.03 – 0.15, $p = 0.044$).

Safety and tolerability

The patients in both groups were asked about positive history of dermal reactions to any topical products and if it was positive, they were instructed to test the prescribed oil on their arm for the first use.

Linseed oil was well tolerated by patients. No serious adverse effects, neither local nor systemic, were reported in the treated group. Likewise, no additional neuropathy or local neural injury was noted in electrophysiologic tests on the follow-up visit.

Discussion

To the best of our knowledge, the present study is the first research to evaluate the effects of linseed oil on CTS. However, this herbal preparation has an ancient history of administration for different disorders, dating back to more than 10 centuries ago in ITM [22,23]. Linseed oil is a rich source of α-linolenic acid that has been proved to possess noticeable anti-inflammatory activity [31]. In addition, further studies have confirmed its anti-inflammatory [14,15], antioxidant [16,17], and analgesic [18] properties.

Different mechanisms for its anti-inflammatory effects are explained. The linseed oil inhibits prostaglandin E_2, leukotriene B_4, histamine and bradykinin-induced inflammation. The oil also inhibits arachidonic acid-induced inflammation. It shows inhibition of both cyclooxygenase and lipoxygenase pathways of arachidonate metabolism [18]. Similar to other multiple herbal formulations, anesthetic properties of topical use of linseed is also shown in animal models [32]. According to the important role of inflammatory and oxidative processes in the pathophysiology of CTS [33,34], its significant effect on improving symptomatic and functional status of our patients, and slightly but statistically significant improving effect on NCV and CL can be explained partially.

Although no previous study on the efficacy of linseed oil on CTS was found, some studies evaluated other herbal preparations in the management of CTS. In a study by Zhang et al. on the efficacy of Chinese herbal therapy on CTS comparing with two other groups, 22 patients who received this therapy had a superior benefit on their visual analogue scale (VAS) score than the splint group and no significant changes of electromyography was shown [35]. Our results are in compliance with symptomatic relief of their patients with a common aspect about the presence of oleic and linoleic acid in some of these used herbs. However, this study was not blind and had a small sample size. Furthermore, they did not assess the effects of a specific herb with determined constituents and they used an uncommon drug delivery system (steaming and washing). Also, Branco et al. published an open protocol study in which CTS patients, who experienced standard treatments failure, were treated by a two-stage protocol. They were treated primarily with a specific laser acupuncture and microamps transcutaneous electrical nerve stimulation and secondarily with herbal formulas and supplements in a case-by-case manner [36]. Similar to our trial, this small size study (only 36 patients) showed a significant effect on symptomatic improvement (91.6%). However, the complexity of their management can result in practical difficulties during usage.

Another notable study, which was conducted by Eftekharsadat et al. on two groups of 30 patients, evaluated the efficacy of topical *Eremostachys laciniata* on CTS. This medicinal herb has been shown to have anti-inflammatory and antioxidant properties, like linseed oil. They showed significant improvement on palmar prehension and VAS of pain, compared with placebo. However, this plant had a local popularity, and no significant effect on electrodiagnostic criterion was reported [37].

There is also a case-series carried out by Jung et al. that assessed the usefulness of Jackyakamcho-tang on muscle spasm and pain on 81 patients complaining about these symptoms. The usefulness was reported as 72.8% for treating CTS (where only 11 CTS patients had been included). But, unlike the safety of linseed oil, they reported adverse effects in 11.1% of the total patients, 3.7% of which were severe [38].

In regard of the topical treatment for CTS, few studies were found. Of those, Jazayeri et al. published a clinical trial evaluating EMLA cream which had some beneficial effects [39]. However, this trial was not blind and EMLA cream was not as cheap and available as linseed oil.

According to ITM, patient's temperament can affect some herbal medicine effects [40]. Therefore, as a minor assessment we evaluated the participant's temperament. However, no relationship was found between the participant's temperament and outcome measures. It could be explained in some ways. The used questionnaire was not designed for our target population [41] and the drug effects are possibly independent of the patient's temperament.

Linseed oil has some important advantages as feasibility of use as a topical drug and no disturbance of ordinary daily activities (comparable with treatments such as wrist splint), conservative and noninvasive nature (regarding some invasive options such as surgery), price of the oil (1 $ for a 40 cc bottle that is adequate for a one month use), worldwide availability, and its acceptable and significant effects, especially on symptomatic and functional status and even on some electrodiagnostic parameters.

Study limitations

Here we should highlight some limitations that we have faced with in this trial. First, insufficient number of male participants (only about 10.5% of our patients), which can affect the generalizability of our findings. In fact, according to previous epidemiologic studies, about 30% of CTS encounters were attributable to males [42]. Indeed, this is a common problem in several trials on CTS, even with male samples as small as 0-10% [43-45].

Second, as regards to reliable and valid assessment by BCTQ about subjective functional status of patients, objective functional outcome measures such as dynamometer findings could offer more reliable results.

The other important issue is to determine the transdermal penetration of the linseed oil. In this respect, the measurement of transdermal permeation of the oil and its consequent absorption into the systemic circulation can be the subject of the future studies.

And finally, the short term follow-up is another limitation. However, this is partially related to our aim as evaluation of efficacy and safety of topical linseed oil as a new complementary treatment for the management of CTS. It is also considerable that herbal medicaments might show delayed pharmacological activity. Thus, long term assessment possibly leads to better results. On the other side, unwanted effects may also be revealed in long term evaluation.

Conclusion

It seems that linseed oil could be effective as an adjunctive therapy in the management of mild and moderate CTS, especially in improving the severity of symptoms and functional status. In addition, its effect on electerodiagnostic parameters, especially on NCV, can be considered as a valuable point.

It is, therefore, suggested that further trials of longer follow-up and larger sample size, including appropriate male/female ratio and objective functional status outcome measures are needed to confirm the value of linseed oil as a good choice for CTS and for evaluation of the involved mechanisms. Moreover, other easily applicable pharmaceutical dosage forms (such as ointment, cream, gel and patch form) can be considered in future studies.

Abbreviations

CTS: Carpal tunnel syndrome; ITM: Iranian traditional medicine; BCTQ: Boston carpal tunnel questionnaire; NCV: Nerve conduction velocity; MDL: Motor distal latency; SDL: Sensory distal latency; CL: Compound latency; CAM: Complementary and alternative medicine; BMI: Body mass index; SUMS: Shiraz University of Medical Sciences; GC: Gas chromatography; SYMPT: Symptom severity; FUNCT: Functional status; SD: Standard deviation; VAS: Visual analogue scale.

Competing interests

The authors declare no competing interests.

Authors' contributions

MHH has made substantial contributions in conception, designing, acquisition of data and drafted the manuscript. KH had contribution in designing and preformed electrodiagnostic assessments. AA had contribution in designing, preformed electrodiagnostic assessments and revised the manuscript critically for important intellectual content. AS had contribution in designing and analyzing of data. MT produced the linseed oil and performed its standardization. MH had contribution in conception and designing and revised the manuscript critically for important intellectual content. All authors read and approved the final manuscript.

Acknowledgments

This study was a part of a PhD thesis by Dr. Mohammad Hashem Hashempur that was supported by Shiraz University of Medical Sciences (grant number: 92-6709). The authors would like to thank the Vice Chancellery of Technology and Research of the University, all the study participants for their participation, the University's Research Consultation Center for editing the final manuscript.

Author details

[1]Research Center for Traditional Medicine and History of Medicine, Shiraz University of Medical Sciences, Shiraz, Iran. [2]Essence of Parsiyan Wisdom Institute, Traditional Medicine and Medicinal Plant Incubator, Shiraz University of Medical Sciences, Shiraz, Iran. [3]Department of Physical Medicine and Rehabilitation, Shiraz University of Medical Sciences, Shiraz, Iran. [4]Shiraz Geriatric Research Center, Shiraz University of Medical Sciences, Shiraz, Iran. [5]Shiraz Burn Research Center, Shiraz University of Medical Sciences, Shiraz, Iran. [6]Research Center for Biochemistry and Nutrition in Metabolic Disease, Kashan University of Medical Sciences, Kashan, Iran.

References

1. Ashraf A, Daghaghzadeh A, Naseri M, Nasiri A, Fakheri M: **A study of interpolation method in diagnosis of carpal tunnel syndrome.** *Ann Indian Acad Neurol* 2013, **16**:623–626.
2. Bleecker ML: **Splinting vs surgery for carpal tunnel syndrome.** *JAMA* 2003, **289**:420.
3. Di Geronimo G, Caccese AF, Caruso L, Soldati A, Passaretti U: **Treatment of carpal tunnel syndrome with alpha-lipoic acid.** *Eur Rev Med Pharmacol Sci* 2009, **13**:133–139.
4. Page MJ, Massy-Westropp N, O'Connor D, Pitt V: **Splinting for carpal tunnel syndrome.** *Cochrane Database Syst Rev* 2012, **7**:CD010003.
5. Ashraf A, Moghtaderi A, Yazdani A, Mirshams S: **Evaluation of effectiveness of local insulin injection in none insulin dependent diabetic patient with carpal tunnel syndrome.** *Electromyogr Clin Neurophysiol* 2008, **49**:161–166.
6. Miller RS, Iverson DC, Fried RA, Green LA, Nutting PA: **Carpal tunnel syndrome in primary care: a report from ASPN. Ambulatory Sentinel Practice Network.** *J Fam Pract* 1994, **38**:337–344.
7. Bland JD: **Carpal tunnel syndrome.** *BMJ* 2007, **335**:343–346.
8. Piazzini DB, Aprile I, Ferrara PE, Bertolini C, Tonali P, Maggi L, Rabini A, Piantelli S, Padua L: **A systematic review of conservative treatment of carpal tunnel syndrome.** *Clin Rehabil* 2007, **21**:299–314.
9. Marshall S, Tardif G, Ashworth N: **Local corticosteroid injection for carpal tunnel syndrome.** *Cochrane Database Syst Rev* 2002, **4**:CD001554.
10. O'Connor D, Marshall S, Massy-Westropp N: **Non-surgical treatment (other than steroid injection) for carpal tunnel syndrome.** *Cochrane Database Syst Rev* 2003, **1**:CD003219.
11. Scholten RJ, Mink van der Molen A, Uitdehaag BM, Bouter LM, de Vet HC: **Surgical treatment options for carpal tunnel syndrome.** *Cochrane Database Syst Rev* 2007, **4**:CD003905.
12. World Health Organization: *WHO traditional medicines strategy 2002–2005.* Geneva: World Health Organization; 2002.
13. de Souza FE, de Aquino CM, de Medeiros PL, Evencio LB, da Silva Goes AJ, de Souza Maia MB: **Effect of a Semisolid Formulation of Linum usitatissimum L (Linseed) Oil on the Repair of Skin Wounds.** *Evid Based Complement Alternat Med* 2012, **2012**:270752.
14. Kaithwas G, Majumdar DK: **Therapeutic effect of linum usitatissimum (flaxseed/linseed) fixed oil on acute and chronic arthritic models in albino rats.** *Inflammopharmacology* 2010, **18**:127–136.
15. Singh S, Nair V, Gupta YK: **Linseed oil: an investigation of its antiarthritic activity in experimental models.** *Phytother Res* 2012, **26**:246–252.
16. Shahidi F: **Antioxidant factors in plant foods and selected oilseeds.** *Biofactors* 2000, **13**:179–185.
17. Kinniry P, Amrani Y, Vachani A, Solomides CC, Arguiri E, Workman A, Carter J, Christofidou-Solomidou M: **Dietary flaxseed supplementation ameliorates inflammation and oxidative tissue damage in experimental models of acute lung injury in mice.** *J Nutr* 2006, **136**:1545–1551.
18. Kaithwas G, Mukherjee A, Chaurasia AK, Majumdar DK: **Anti-inflammatory, analgesic and antipyretic activities of Linum usitatissimum L. (flaxseed/linseed) fixed oil.** *Indian J Exp Biol* 2011, **49**:932–938.
19. Rahman M, Alam K, Ahmad MZ, Gupta G, Afzal M, Akhter S, Kazmi I, Jyoti, Ahmad FJ, Anwar F: **Classical to current approach for treatment of psoriasis: a review.** *Endocr Metab Immune Disord Drug Targets* 2012, **12**:287–302.
20. Thompson LU, Chen JM, Li T, Strasser-Weippl K, Goss PE: **Dietary flaxseed alters tumor biological markers in postmenopausal breast cancer.** *Clin Cancer Res* 2005, **11**:3828–3835.
21. Neves ML, Yamasaki L, Sanches Ode C, Do Amaral MS, Stevanin H, Giuffrida R, Candido ER, Goes JE, Zulim LF, Schweigert A, Fukui RM, Meirelles CC, Sasaki CA, Andrade SF: **Use of linseed oil to treat experimentally induced keratoconjunctivitis sicca in rabbits.** *J Ophthalmic Inflamm Infect* 2013, **3**:4.
22. 2559: In *Martindale: The Complete Drug Reference: Supplementary Drugs and Other Substances*, Volume 3. 37th edition. Edited by Sweetman SC. London: Pharmaceutical Press; 2011:2559.
23. Saxena S, Suryawanshi S, Somashekar U, Sharma D: **Use of linseed oil in preventing peri-ileostomy skin excoriation.** *Indian J Gastroenterol* 2009, **28**:190–191.
24. Kaithwas G, Majumdar DK: **Effect of L. usitatissimum (flaxseed/linseed) fixed oil against distinct phases of inflammation.** *ISRN Inflamm* 2013, **2013**:735158.
25. Kaithwas G, Majumdar DK: **Evaluation of antiulcer and antisecretory potential of Linum usitatissimum fixed oil and possible mechanism of action.** *Inflammopharmacology* 2010, **18**:137–145.
26. Ibn-e-sina (Avicenna Husain): *Al-Qanun fit-tib [The Canon of Medicine], (research of ebrahim shamsedine).* Beirut, Lebanon: Alaalami Beirut library Press; 2005 [in Arabic].
27. Razi Mohammad ibn-e-Zakarya: *Alhavi al-kabir [Liber Continens].* Tehran: The Institute for Medical History- Islamic and Complementary Medicine, Tehran University of Medical Sciences; 2010. in Arabic.
28. Sozay S, Sarfakoglu AB, Ayas S, Cetin N: **Diurnal variation in clinical and electrophysiologic parameters associated with carpal tunnel syndrome.** *Am J Phys Med Rehabil* 2011, **90**:731–737.
29. Levine DW, Simmons BP, Koris MJ, Daltroy LH, Hohl GG, Fossel AH, Katz JN: **A self-administered questionnaire for the assessment of severity of symptoms and functional status in carpal tunnel syndrome.** *J Bone Joint Surg Am* 1993, **75**:1585–1592.
30. Afshar A, Yekta Z, Etemadi A, Mirzatoloee F: **Outcome measurement questionnaires for carpal tunnel syndrome.** *Iranian Orthopaedic Surg* 2005, **3**:46–50.
31. Nykter M, Kymäläinen H-R, Gates F, Sjöberg A-M: **Quality characteristics of edible linseed oil.** *Agric Food Sci* 2006, **15**:402–413.
32. Heydari M, Shams M, Homayouni K, Borhani-Haghighi A, Salehi A, Hashempur MH: **An option for painful diabetic neuropathy with simultaneous 'antioxidative' and 'anesthetic' properties: topical citrullus colocynthis.** *J Exp Integr Med* 2014, **4**:9–12.
33. Kim JK, Koh YD, Kim JS, Hann HJ, Kim MJ: **Oxidative stress in subsynovial connective tissue of idiopathic carpal tunnel syndrome.** *J Orthop Res* 2010, **28**:1463–1468.
34. Werner RA, Andary M: **Carpal tunnel syndrome: pathophysiology and clinical neurophysiology.** *Clin Neurophysiol* 2002, **113**:1373–1381.
35. Zhang CY, Wang YX: **Observation on therapeutic effects of acupuncture combined with TDP irradiation and chinese herbal steaming and washing therapy for treatment of carpal tunnel syndrome in early stage.** *Zhongguo Zhen Jiu* 2009, **29**:708–710.
36. Branco K, Naeser MA: **Carpal tunnel syndrome: clinical outcome after low-level laser acupuncture, microamps transcutaneous electrical nerve stimulation, and other alternative therapies–an open protocol study.** *J Altern Complement Med* 1999, **5**:5–26.
37. Eftekharsadat B, Kazem Shakouri S, Shimia M, Rahbar M, Ghojazadeh M, Reza Rashidi M, Hadi Faraji M: **Effect of E. laciniata (L) ointment on mild and moderate carpal tunnel syndrome: a double-blind, randomized clinical trial.** *Phytother Res* 2011, **25**:290–295.
38. Jung WS, Moon SK, Park SU, Ko CN, Cho KH: **Clinical assessment of usefulness, effectiveness and safety of jackyakamcho-tang**

(shaoyaogancao-tang) on muscle spasm and pain: a case series. *Am J Chin Med* 2004, **32**:611–620.

39. Moghtaderi A, Jazayeri S, Azizi S: **EMLA cream for carpal tunnel syndrome: how it compares with steroid injection.** *Electromyogr Clin Neurophysiol* 2008, **49**:287–289.
40. Mokaberinejad R, Zafarghandi N, Bioos S, Dabaghian FH, Naseri M, Kamalinejad M, Amin G, Ghobadi A, Tansaz M, Akhbari A, Hamiditabar M: **Mentha longifolia syrup in secondary amenorrhea: a double-blind, placebo-controlled, randomized trials.** *Daru* 2012, **20**:97.
41. Mojahedi M, Naseri M, Majdzadeh R, Keshavarz M, Ebadini M, Nazem E, Isfeedvajani M: **Reliability and validity assessment of Mizaj questionnaire: a novel self-report scale in Iranian traditional medicine.** *Iran Red Crescent Med J.* in press.
42. Charles J, Fahridin S, Britt H: **Carpal tunnel syndrome.** *Aust Fam Physician* 2009, **38**:665.
43. Bye R, Hajiaqai B, Frorough B: **Comparison between efficacy of manu splint and cock-up splint in carpal tunnel syndrome treatment.** *J Babol Univ Med Sci* 2011, **13**:51–57.
44. Çeliker R, Arslan S, Inanc F: **Corticosteroid injection vs. nonsteroidal antiinflammatory drug and splinting in carpal tunnel syndrome.** *Am J Phys Med Rehabil* 2002, **81**:182–186.
45. Kumnerddee W, Kaewtong A: **Efficacy of acupuncture versus night splinting for carpal tunnel syndrome: a randomized clinical trial.** *J Med Assoc Thai* 2010, **93**:1463–1469.

4

The effect of piperine on midazolam plasma concentration in healthy volunteers, a research on the CYP3A-involving metabolism

Mohammad Mahdi Rezaee[1], Sohrab Kazemi[1,3], Mohammad Taghi Kazemi[1], Saeed Gharooee[1], Elham Yazdani[1], Hoda Gharooee[1], Mohammad Reza Shiran[2] and Ali Akbar Moghadamnia[1,3*]

Abstract

Some studies showed that piperine (the alkaloid of *piper nigrum*) can change the activities of microsomal enzymes. Midazolam concentration is applied as a probe to determine the CYP3A enzyme activity. This study was done to determine piperine pretreatment role on midazolam plasma concentration.

Twenty healthy volunteers (14 men and 6 women) received oral dose of piperine (15 mg) or placebo for three days as pretreatment and midazolam (10 mg) on fourth day of study and the blood samples were taken at 0.5, 2.5 and 5 h after midazolam administration. The midazolam plasma levels were assayed using HPLC method (C18 analytical column, 75:25 methanol:water as mobile phase, UV detector at 242 nm wavelength and diazepam as internal standard). Data were fit in a "one-compartment PK model" using *P-Pharm 1.5* software and analyzed under statistical tests. The mean ±SD of the age and body mass index were 24.3 ± 1.83 years (range: 21–28 years) and 23.46± 2.85, respectively. The duration of sedation in piperine receiving group was greater that the placebo group (188±59 *vs.* 102±43 min, p<0.0001). Half-life and clearance of midazolam were higher in piperine pretreatment group compared to placebo [1.88±0.03 *vs.* 1.71± 0.04 h (p<0.0001) and 33.62 ± 0.4 *vs.* 37.09 ± 1.07 ml/min (p<0.0001), respectively]. According to the results, piperine can significantly increases half-life and decreases clearance of midazolam compared to placebo. It is suggested that piperine can demonstrate those effects by inhibition CYP3A4 enzyme activity in liver microsomal system.

Keywords: Piperine, Midazolam, CYP3A, Clearance, Half-life, Microsomal hepatic metabolism, HPLC

Introduction

Some specific substances of food products and additives can manipulate drugs disposition and fate in body through mechanisms that make changes their plasma concentration [1-3]. These changes will exert as inducers or inhibitors of hepatic microsomal enzymes or transporters [1,3-5]. Black pepper (piper nigrum) has been used widely throughout the world. It has been shown that pepper can change metabolism of some drugs in those that take foods containing high pepper [6]. Piperine is an isolated alkaloid of black pepper [7] that belongs to capsaicin like family [8]. Animal studies have previously demonstrated that piperine inhibits several enzymatic pathways involving P450, as well as phase II metabolism [9,10].

Grilled meat using wood charcoal, smoked meats, foods containing cruciferous vegetables, and some medicinal plants can induce several microsomal and transporter enzymes and decrease plasma concentration of xenobiotics, such as cyclosporine A and anti-HIV protease inhibitors [11]. Other drugs, such as verapamil induces CYP3A4 and increases transport of p-glycoproteine precursor [11]. On the other hand, some foods such as grape fruit can increase plasma concentration of felodipine, nitrondipine, secoanavir and cyclosporine A by inhibiting of CYP3A [12,13]. It has been suggested that pretreatment piperine in mice, may result in increasing plasma concentration of theophylline [9,14]. This similar effect of piperine on plasma level of theophylline, rifampine, phenytoin and

* Correspondence: moghadamnia@yahoo.com
[1]Department of Pharmacology, Babol University of Medical Sciences, Babol, Iran
[3]Cellular and Molecular Biology Research Centre, Babol University of Medical Sciences, Babol, Iran
Full list of author information is available at the end of the article

propranolol has been observed in human studies [15]. It has been reported that administration of 1 g of black pepper as a single dose, may increase time-concentration area under the curve (AUC) of phenytoin more than two times compared to placebo.

CYP3A enzymes are the most important enzymatic group that involve in drug metabolism. More than 50% of microsomal enzymes are made up of CYP3A and about 60% of drugs used in treatment (e.g. calcium channel blockers, corticosteroids, sex hormones, macrolide antibiotics, benzodiazepines and immunosuppressant drug cyclosporine) are metabolized by CYP3A [16]. Plasma concentration of some drugs such as midazolam and caffeine can serve as a probe of the enzyme activity [17,18]. Midazolam is a short acting sedative bezodiazepins that is mainly metabolized by CYP3A4 [7]. Determination of plasma concentration of midazolam can help to assess the activity level of CYP3A4 [6].

Based on the mentioned effect of piperine and the important role of CYP3A in drug metabolism, this study was designed to investigate the effect of three days pretreatment of low dose piperine on midazolam plasma concentration in healthy volunteers.

Materials and methods

This study has been approved by ethics committee of Babol University of Medical Sciences (Babol, Iran) and recorded in IRCT (Iranian registry of clinical trials) data bank with registration number:IRCT201203129271N1. All healthy volunteers were given information of the aims of the study, methods and possible outcomes of the treatment so that they could understand the main objective of the investigation. All selected participants signed a written informative consent form and then they were entered into the study. Although, neither midazolam nor piperine have serious side effects at lower doses, all participants were allowed to leave the study at any time of the follow up when they developed considerable complications.

Type of study

This was a cross-over controlled study on two groups (n=10) of healthy volunteers. A one-month period was considered as wash out time between two trials. Based on previous reports in 100 healthy volunteers of Mazandaran province (Northern Iran) to find out the CYP3A activity and recorded moderate activity in this sample size of the population [17,18], all participants were selected from Babol, one of the big cities of the province. After providing adequate information to the subjects, eligible healthy volunteers will be enrolled in the study. Inclusion criteria: being healthy; age ranging 18 to 35; normal diet; not receiving microsomal enzyme inhibitor or inducer agents for at least 7 days before the study; not using black pepper for at least 7 days before the study. Exclusion criteria: age being below 18 and above 35; smocking; pregnancy; metabolic disorders; high pepper diet, receiving enzyme inhibitors or inducers.

Drugs & chemicals

Midazolam (Exir Lorestan, Iran), EDTA (Sigma Chemical Co. USA), piperine (Merck, Germany), n-hexan, HPLC grade methanol, isoamyl alcohol and HCl (Merck, Germany) and deionized water were used. Standard form of midazolam and diazepam as base (used as internal standard) were prepared from Dr. Abidi Pharmaceuitical Company (Tehran, Iran).

Devices

Centrifuge (Clements 2000, Australia) and HPLC [(Knauer, Germany); column Eurospher 100–5 C18 of silica gel, dimension: 250 × 4.6 mm with pre-column, UV detector, EZchrom Elite software] were used.

Steps

All participants received adequate description about the setting, treatment schedule and outcome of drug administration. Then they recorded their personal information including age, sex, height, weight, general health situation, and history of drug use, food sensitivity, smoking, occupation, education and consent to the study in a special form.

Drug administration and sampling

Healthy volunteers regardless of gender were randomly divided into two control and piperine receiving groups (n=20 per group). The subject received placebo or piperine (1 capsule 15 mg of piperine daily for 3 days before midazolam) and midazolam (10 mg as an oral single dose) on fourth day of the study. Total period of the study is 4 days. Blood samples (maximum 10 ml) were taken at 0.5, 2.5 and 5 hour after midazolam administration. After a month as a wash out period, the treatment program was exchanged between placebo and piperine groups and all steps were done as same as the previous.

Blood samples preparation

Blood samples were transferred into labeled tubes containing Ca-EDTA and shake gently to mix Ca-EDTA with blood for preventing of coagulation.The samples were centrifuged at 3500 ×g for 15 min and supernatant plasma layer transferred into a blank tube. Until the assay of midazolam or diazepam concentration, the plasma samples were kept at −20°C.

HPLC assay

For measurement of the drugs concentration, plasma samples were removed from the freezer condition and left in the laboratory to convert from frozen into a liquid sample. Then 0.5 ml of thawed plasma sample was transferred into a capped falcon tube. In the next step, 100 micl of 1 M NaOH and 100 micl isoamyl alcohol were added. After a gently shaking, 4.5 ml of n-hexan was added and shake for 1 minute. The final solutions were centrifuged at 300 ×g for 5 min. After this step, 4.2 ml of supernatant was drawn and transferred into a plastic tube and 100 miclof 0.05 M HCl was added to the solution and centrifuged similar as the previous. Then the supernatant (organic layer) was discarded and the remaining was directly injected into the HPLC.

HPLC analysis

The separation was carried out at ambient temperature using a single-column isocratic reverse-phase method. The mobile phase consisted of 75% methanol and 25% water. Flow rate was set at 0.8 ml/min. The extracts were detected by UV detector at 242 nm wavelength. Twenty micl of the aqueous layer of final extract was injected into the HPLC using a Hamilton's syringe. The injection was repeated 3 times for each sample. Peaks area and height were considered for midazolam and diazepam detection and used for calculation of the drugs concentration in the final plasma extract.

Standard preparations

A working solution containing 10 micg of midazolam in 1 mL of mobile phase was prepared. Six standard solutions of different concentrations of midazolam (20, 50, 75, 100, 150 and 200 ng/ml) were prepared. Then 20 micl of 25 ng/ml of diazepam solution as internal standard as added to each standard concentration of midazolam.

Data handling and analysis

Data were analyzed in two steps. The first; personal information of the participants and data of drugs assay were handled using Excel software. Calibration curves were plotted based on peak area and/or height ratio of midazolam to diazepam.

The slope, intercept and R^2coefficient were calculated. Coefficient variation (CV) for this analysis was 3.8%.

The second; pharmacokinetic (PK) parameters such as absorption rate constant (Ka), clearance, half-life and volume of distribution of midazolam in the placebo and piperine groups were calculated based on assumed one-compartment kinetics using *P-Pharm* software.

Based on non-parametric distribution, data of three concentrations by time were analyzed using Friedman test. Wilcoxon U-test was used for the results of clearance, volume of distribution and half-life of midazolam in piperine group compared to placebo. The difference of the PK parameters between two groups was considered statistically significant at p<0.05.

Table 1 Comparison of the mean (±SD) of onset and duration of sedative effect and frequency of sedation and amnesia following midazolam administration in placebo and piperine pretreatment groups (n=20)

	Onset of drug effect (min)	End of drug effect (min)	Sedation	Amnesia
Placebo	11.25 (±4.5)	102 (±43)	16	4
Piperine	11.75 (±4.9)	188 (±59)	20	**7**
p value	NS*	0.0001	NS	NS

*NS: non-significant.

Results

The age range of the participants was from 21 to 28 year (24.3±1.83). Six subjects were female and 14 were male (mean±SD of age: males: 25±1.26, females: 22.66±1.86). All participants were healthy volunteer and selected from Mazandaran province. The subjects' weight ranged from 49 to 101 kg (68.05±2.85). Their average (±SD) BMI was 23.46 (±2.85).

Clinical features

All the subjects experienced sedation and mild hypnosis following midazolam administration. This situation was transient and they've got improvement during next 4 hours after administration of midazolam. In some subjects, severe sedation and dizziness were observed in placebo and piperine groups (30% and 55%, respectively). The mean duration of the sedation in piperine receiving group was greater than placebo (188±59 *vs.* 102±43 min, p<0.0001) (Table 1).

Duration of midazolam sedative effect in piperine pretreatment group in the females was greater than the males when compared to placebo (p=0.027 and p<0.001) (Figure 1). Seven subjects of piperine group showed predominant amnesia but only 4 subjects were amnesic in placebo group. One subject of piperine group showed

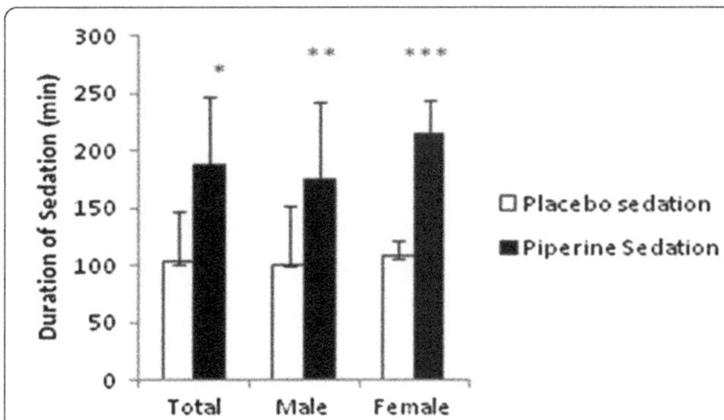

Figure 1 Comparison of duration of sedation (min) after midazolam (10 mg, p.o.) in placebo and piperine pretreatment (15 mg p.o. in three sequential days before midazolam) groups. Total data and data by sex are shown for 20 subjects. Sedation in piperine pretreatment group is greater than placebo group (*p<0.001, **p<0.01, ***p<0.0001).

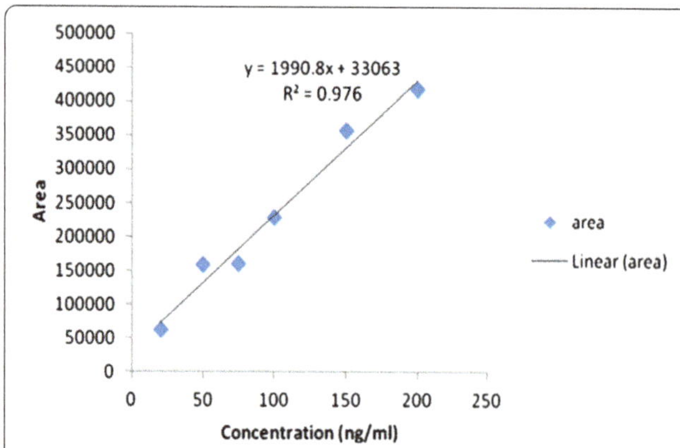

Figure 2 Peak area ratios (midazolam/diazepam)-concentration curve of six different concentrations (ng/ml) of midazolam containing equal diazepam (25 ng/ml) as internal standard.

hiccup when receiving midazolam that was disappeared during first hours after drug administration. The supine position was recommended for participants suffering from severe dizziness and possible hypotension.

Standard curve

Six concentrations (20, 50, 75, 100, 150 and 200 ng/ml) as standard solution of midazolam were prepared. Equal volume of diazepam solution (25 ng/ml) as internal standard was spiked on each concentration of midazolam. Based on peak area ratios of different concentration of midazolam on diazepam, the standard curve was obtained (Figure 2). The linearity (R^2) constant and the line equation are shown in the Figure 2.

The chromatograms of standard midazolam (50 ng/ml) and diazepam (25 ng/ml) are shown in Figure 3. Diazepam was used as internal standard.

The comparison of primary data of drug concentrations showed a significant different between placebo and piperine pretreatment groups at 2.5 and 5 hours after midazolam (p=0.015 and p=0.002, respectively). Analysis of intra-group variation of concentration by time showed a significant profile (p=0.03). There was no significant difference in $AUC_{0\text{-}5}$ of placebo compared to piperine pretreatment group (411.1± 235.4 *vs.* 495, 9 ± 273, respectively).Pharmacokinetics parameters were estimated in an assumed one-compartment model using *P-Pharm* software. For comparing final estimation, non-parametric paired Wilcoxon U-test was applied.

All PK parameters except of Vd, in piperine pretreated subjects has demonstrated a significant difference compared to placebo (p<000.1). Half-life of midazolam in piperine pretreatment group is considerably greater than in placebo (Table 2). For this reason, it could be said that piperine may decrease metabolism of midazolam.

After modeling with input of initial data assumption (Cl= 40 ml/min, Vd=80 L, Ka=1, F=1), concentration-time curves were plotted. Individual Bayesian fits of concentration (ng/ml) of midazolam by time (h) profile placebo and piperine pretreatment are shown in Figure 4.

The population plasma midazolam concentrations time curves in placebo (A) and piperine (B) treatment groups are shown in Figure 4. Based on the figure (A), one subject showed an out of range concentration at the time of 2.5 h. It is considered that the maximum concentration in placebo group occurred at 1.5 h after midazolam administration.

Discussion

This investigation showed 3 days piperine pretreatment can significant increase elimination half-life (t1/2) and decrease clearance of midazolam when compared to control. Our results can demonstrate a possible relation between midazolam concentration and CYP3A activity.

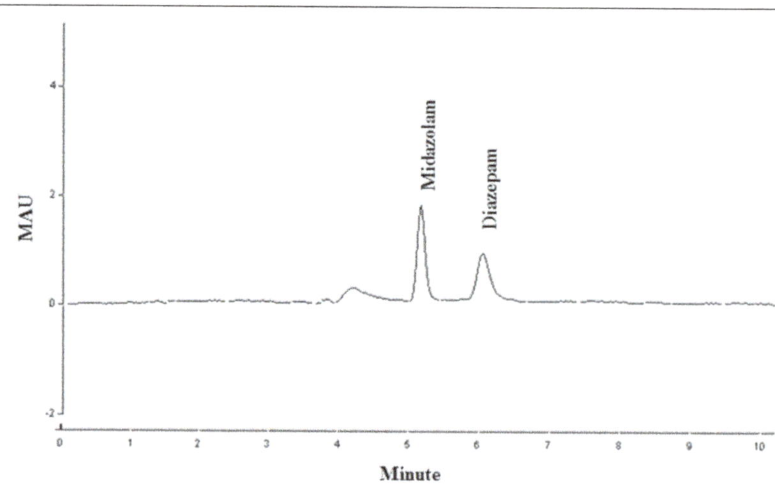

Figure 3 Chromatograms of midazolam standard concentration (50 ng/ml) and diazepam (25 ng/ml).

Table 2 Comparison of pharmacokinetics (PK) data of midazolam in placebo and piperine pretreatment groups

Group	Clearance	Volume	Kel†	T1/2‡
Placebo (n=20)				
Mean	37.09	91.44	0.41	1.71*
Min	34.27	87.63	0.390	1.63
Max	38.48	93.03	0.42	1.78
S.D.	1.07	1.54	0.01	0.04
Fold	1.12	1.06	1.1	1.1
C.V.	2.89	1.69	2.62	2.61
Piperine (n=20)				
Mean	33.62	91.43	0.37	1.88
Min	32.63	84.45	0.35	1.86
Max	34.02	92.35	0.37	1.96
S.D.	0.4	1.7	0.01	0.03
Fold	1.04	1.09	1.05	1.05
C.V.	1.2	1.86	1.29	1.33

†Elimination rate constant.
‡Half- life.
*$p<0.0001$ (with piperine group).

This enzyme has an important role in microsomal drug metabolisms. Thirty percent of cytochrome P450 enzymes of liver are made of CY3A4 [19]. It has been estimated that CYP3A4 is responsible for 50 percent of the metabolism of all drugs that being eliminated via hepatic microsomal enzymatic system [20,21]. In addition to having an active role in hepatic metabolism of drugs, CYP3A4 is sufficiently active in the small intestine [22,23]. CYP3A4 is active in the metabolism of lipophilic substrates such as fentanyl, alfentanil, oxycodone, and methadone [24-28]. CYP3A4 inhibitors that have been well studied include: azole antifungal agents and a number of the macrolide antibodies [29]. There are clinically important examples such as midazolam, alprozolam, atorvastatin, simvastatin, felodipine, nifedipine, and cyclosporine that are affected by this system [29]. Among the CYP3A substrates, midazolam has been introduced as a predominant substrate of CYP3A4 and CYP3A5 [29]. The metabolism of intravenous midazolam can reflect to the rate of hepatic CYP3A activity but when it is administered by mouth, the metabolism can demonstrate both liver and enteral origin of CYP3A [22,23]. Any changes in CYP3A enzymatic pathway, may affect midazolam metabolism. CYP3A activity can be affected by different factors such as genetics, nutritional, environmental, and hormonal and disease conditions. These variations in CYP3A activity may create some problems in dosing of the drugs those are metabolized by this enzymatic system. These variations may increase drug interaction episodes and cause side effects to the patients. More than 50% of drugs that are eliminated by liver microsomal enzymes are metabolized by CYP3A system [20,21].

In the present study piperine the main alkaloid of black pepper [7], could significantly prolong life time of midazolam in body. This may increase the pharmacologic activity and can induce and prolong sedative-hypnotic properties of the drug. These effects of piperine may be the result of inhibition of CYP3A4 activity. Previous animal studies have demonstrated that piperine inhibits several CYP450 mediated pathways [30]. Piperine is a selective non-competitive inhibitor of CYP3A but has lower activity on the other microsomal enzymes. It can inhibit activity UDP-glucuronosyl transferase as well [31,32]. Pretreatment of piperine in mice induced higher plasma levels of theophylline, rifampin, phenytoin and propranolol and Q10-CoA compared to control [33,34]. Such an effect has been reported in a previous clinical study [15]. It has been reported that a single dose of 1 g of black pepper can increase the AUC (area under the curve of plasma concentration-time) of phenytoin [14]. In the present study piperine was given in low dose and seems that in this dose, it can change important PK parameters such as clearance and t/12 of midazolam. It

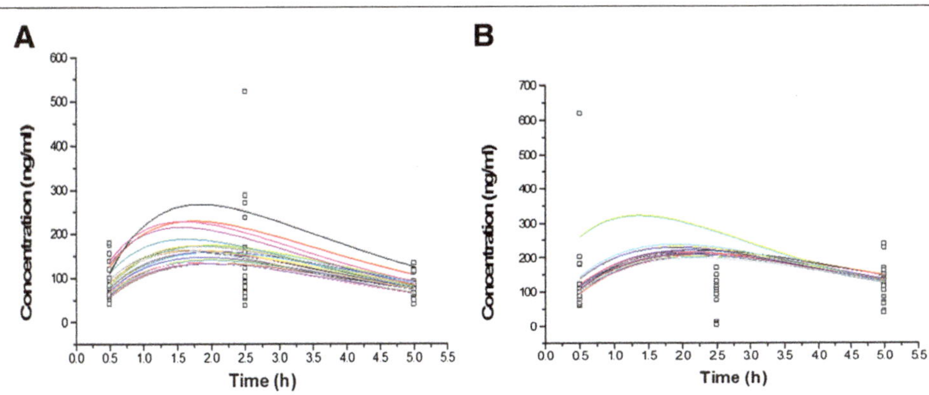

Figure 4 Bayesian predicted (thin line) and observed (symbols) plasma midazolam concentrations in placebo (A) and piperine (B) receiving groups. Note the different scales of concentrations in the figures.

means that piperine's direct effect on midazolam elimination is not assumed and it can increase the half-life of midazolam via inhibition of its hepatic microsomal elimination. This may increase duration and severity of side effects of subject drugs (substrate of CYP3A) following their elevated plasma levels. As we already showed the midazolam side effects in piperine pretreated subjects were considerable compared to placebo. The inhibition or induction of enteral CYP3A4 and p-glycoprotein can mediate considerable drug interactions. These of interactions may be due to a considerable variation in drug action from no effect to toxic effect of drugs [35-38].

The genes of CYP3A4 and p-glycoprotein are expressed in enterocytes and the bioavailability of many drugs such as cyclosporine A, midazolam, verapamil, HIV protease inhibitors and digoxin could be affected by the enzyme and transporter [11,36,38-40]. Metabolism of midazolam when prescribed intravenously shows the activity of hepatic CYP3A, but when it is prescribed orally, it can show the activity of both hepatic and intestinal CYP3A [41,42]. After oxidative metabolism, midazolam changes into one of its main metabolites, hydroxide midazolam, in liver, and is mediated in an exceptional rout by CYP3A isoforms [43,44]. Piperine inhibits p-glycoprotein and CYP3A activity. Since, these proteins become expressed in enterocytes and hepatocytes; they have an effective role in first-pass metabolism of subject drugs. Piperine content of nutritional regimen can change the levels of p-glycoprotein and CYP3A substrates in blood when those administered by mouth [45]. However more researches are needed to prove intestinal or hepatic effects of piperine, especially to justify their mechanism in the present study. In this investigation duration of sedation and possible hypnosis action of midazolam in females was longer than the males. This may be to the result from higher plasma level of midazolam after piperine pretreatment in female subjects. Perhaps, it is concluded that sex may be an important factor to obtaining plasma concentration of midazolam. This may be due to higher activity of CYP3A4 in female at normal condition compared to male [46-49]. In a previous phenotyping study by the authors, similar results by sex variability on CYP3A activity has been reported [17]. For this reason more clinical effects are expected in females if the enzyme becomes inhibited.

Conclusion

Individual PK variations can significantly determine CYP3A activity in general population. This may predispose patients to demonstrate unexpected drug manifestations compared to normal subjects. According to the present investigation, piperine may inhibit CYP3A4 activity and increase the level of midazolam as a substrate of the enzyme.

Competing interests

The authors declared that they have no competing interests.

Authors' contributions

MMR: data collection and executive affairs; SK: laboratory works and review literature searching; MTK: lab tests and data collection; SGh: HPLC model setting; EY and HGh: data collection; MRS: study design and modeling; AAM: study design, to register study in IRCT, data handling and statistical analysis, manuscript writing and correction. All authors read and approved the final manuscript.

Acknowledgements

Authors wish with to give their special thanks to Dr. Amin Rostami, professor of the University of Manchester (UK) for his co-operation to hand *P-Pharm* software, Dr. Roueini, professor of Tehran University of Medical Sciences and Dr. Abidi Pharmaceutical Company for their co-operation to kindly provide standards midazolam and diazepam and Mrs. Hashemi and Dr. Aliasghar Sefidgar for their technical efforts and finally all the participants. This investigation (*project No: 8827910*) has been financially supported by Research Affairs division of Babol University of Medical Sciences.

Author details

[1]Department of Pharmacology, Babol University of Medical Sciences, Babol, Iran. [2]Department of Pharmacology, Mazandaran University of Medical Sciences, Sari, Iran. [3]Cellular and Molecular Biology Research Centre, Babol University of Medical Sciences, Babol, Iran.

References

1. Evans AM: **Influence of dietary components on the gastrointestinal metabolism and transport of drugs.** *Ther Drug Monit* 2000, **22**:131–136.
2. Wilkinson GR: **The effects of diet, aging and disease-states on presystemic elimination and oral drug bioavailability in humans.** *Adv Drug Deliv Rev* 1997, **27**:129–159.
3. Walter-Sack I, Klotz U: **Influence of diet and nutritional status on drug metabolism.** *Clin Pharmacokinet* 1996, **31**:47–64.
4. Ayrton A, Morgan P: **Role of transport proteins in drug absorption, distribution and excretion.** *Xenobiotica* 2001, **31**:469–497.
5. Wilkinson GR: **Cytochrome P4503A (CYP3A) metabolism: prediction of in vivo activity in humans.** *J Pharmacokinet Biopharm* 1996, **24**:475–490.
6. Lauterburg BH, Velez ME: **Glutathione deficiency in alcoholics: risk factor for paracetamol hepatotoxicity.** *Gut* 1988, **29**:1153–1157.
7. Durgaprasad S, Pai CG, Vasanthkumar, Alvres JF, Namitha S: **A pilot study of the antioxidant effect of curcumin in tropical pancreatitis.** *Indian J Med Res* 2005, **122**:315–318.
8. Kapelyukh Y, Paine MJ, Marechal JD, Sutcliffe MJ, Wolf CR, Roberts GC: **Multiple substrate binding by cytochrome P450 3A4: estimation of the number of bound substrate molecules.** *Drug Metab Dispos* 2008, **36**:2136–2144.
9. Atal CK, Zutshi U, Rao PG: **Scientific evidence on the role of Ayurvedic herbals on bioavailability of drugs.** *J Ethnopharmacol* 1981, **4**:229–232.
10. Singh J, Dubey RK, Atal CK: **Piperine-mediated inhibition of glucuronidation activity in isolated epithelial cells of the guinea-pig small intestine: evidence that piperine lowers the endogeneous UDP-glucuronic acid content.** *J Pharmacol Exp Ther* 1986, **236**:488–493.
11. Darbar D, Fromm MF, Dell'Orto S, Kim RB, Kroemer HK, Eichelbaum M, Roden DM: **Modulation by dietary salt of verapamil disposition in humans.** *Circulation* 1998, **98**:2702–2708.
12. Bailey DG, Malcolm J, Arnold O, Spence JD: **Grapefruit juice-drug interactions.** *Br J Clin Pharmacol* 1998, **46**:101–110.
13. Kane GC, Lipsky JJ: **Drug-grapefruit juice interactions.** *Mayo Clin Proc* 2000, **75**:933–942.
14. Velpandian T, Jasuja R, Bhardwaj RK, Jaiswal J, Gupta SK: **Piperine in food: interference in the pharmacokinetics of phenytoin.** *Eur J Drug Metab Pharmacokinet* 2001, **26**:241–247.
15. Zutshi RK, Singh R, Zutshi U, Johri RK, Atal CK: **Influence of piperine on rifampicin blood levels in patients of pulmonary tuberculosis.** *J Assoc Physicians India* 1985, **33**:223–224.

16. Kreek MJ, Garfield JW, Gutjahr CL, Giusti LM: **Rifampin-induced methadone withdrawal.** *N Engl J Med* 1976, **294:**1104–1106.
17. Shiran MR, Gharooee Ahangar S, Rostamkolaee S, Sefidgar SAA, Baradaran M, Hashemi M, Baleghi M, *et al*: **Phenotyping of CYP3A by oral midazolam in healthy mazandarani volunteers.** *J Babol Univ Med SCI* 2011, **13:**19–25.
18. Rostamkolaee S, Gharooee Ahangar S, Kazemi M, Shiran MR, Moghadamnia AA: **Determination of CYP1A1 phenotype in a sample of healthy volunteers.** *J Babol Univ Med SCI* 2011, **14:**25–32.
19. Shimada T, Yamazaki H, Mimura M, Inui Y, Guengerich FP: **Interindividual variations in human liver cytochrome P-450 enzymes involved in the oxidation of drugs, carcinogens and toxic chemicals: studies with liver microsomes of 30 Japanese and 30 Caucasians.** *J Pharmacol Exp Ther* 1994, **270:**414–423.
20. Johnson WW: **Cytochrome P450 inactivation by pharmaceuticals and phytochemicals: therapeutic relevance.** *Drug Metab Rev* 2008, **40:**101–147.
21. Guengerich FP: **Mechanisms of cytochrome P450 substrate oxidation: MiniReview.** *J Biochem Mol Toxicol* 2007, **21:**163–168.
22. Kato M: **Intestinal first-pass metabolism of CYP3A4 substrates.** *Drug Metab Pharmacokinet* 2008, **23:**87–94.
23. Paine MF, Hart HL, Ludington SS, Haining RL, Rettie AE, Zeldin DC: **The human intestinal cytochrome P450 "pie".** *Drug Metab Dispos* 2006, **34:**880–886.
24. Feierman DE, Lasker JM: **Metabolism of fentanyl, a synthetic opioid analgesic, by human liver microsomes. Role of CYP3A4.** *Drug Metab Dispos* 1996, **24:**932–939.
25. Ferrari A, Coccia CP, Bertolini A, Sternieri E: **Methadone–metabolism, pharmacokinetics and interactions.** *Pharmacol Res* 2004, **50:**551–559.
26. Lalovic B, Phillips B, Risler LL, Howald W, Shen DD: **Quantitative contribution of CYP2D6 and CYP3A to oxycodone metabolism in human liver and intestinal microsomes.** *Drug Metab Dispos* 2004, **32:**447–454.
27. Klees TM, Sheffels P, Dale O, Kharasch ED: **Metabolism of alfentanil by cytochrome p4503a (cyp3a) enzymes.** *Drug Metab Dispos* 2005, **33:**303–311.
28. Trescot AM, Datta S, Lee M, Hansen H: **Opioid pharmacology.** *Pain Physician* 2008, **11:**S133–S153.
29. Pelkonen O, Turpeinen M, Hakkola J, Honkakoski P, Hukkanen J, Raunio H: **Inhibition and induction of human cytochrome P450 enzymes: current status.** *Arch Toxicol* 2008, **82:**667–715.
30. Volak LP, Ghirmai S, Cashman JR, Court MH: **Curcuminoids inhibit multiple human cytochromes P450, UDP-glucuronosyltransferase, and sulfotransferase enzymes, whereas piperine is a relatively selective CYP3A4 inhibitor.** *Drug Metab Dispos* 2008, **36:**1594–1605.
31. Atal CK, Dubey RK, Singh J: **Biochemical basis of enhanced drug bioavailability by piperine: evidence that piperine is a potent inhibitor of drug metabolism.** *J Pharmacol Exp Ther* 1985, **232:**258–262.
32. Reen RK, Singh J: **In vitro and in vivo inhibition of pulmonary cytochrome P450 activities by piperine, a major ingredient of piper species.** *Indian J Exp Biol* 1991, **29:**568–573.
33. Bano G, Raina RK, Zutshi U, Bedi KL, Johri RK, Sharma SC: **Effect of piperine on bioavailability and pharmacokinetics of propranolol and theophylline in healthy volunteers.** *Eur J Clin Pharmacol* 1991, **41:**615–617.
34. Pattanaik S, Hota D, Prabhakar S, Kharbanda P, Pandhi P: **Effect of piperine on the steady-state pharmacokinetics of phenytoin in patients with epilepsy.** *Phytother Res* 2006, **20:**683–686.
35. Fromm MF, Kim RB, Stein CM, Wilkinson GR, Roden DM: **Inhibition of P-glycoprotein-mediated drug transport: a unifying mechanism to explain the interaction between digoxin and quinidine [seecomments].** *Circulation* 1999, **99:**552–557.
36. Greiner B, Eichelbaum M, Fritz P, Kreichgauer HP, von Richter O, Zundler J, Kroemer HK: **The role of intestinal P-glycoprotein in the interaction of digoxin and rifampin.** *J Clin Invest* 1999, **104:**147–153.
37. Thummel KE, O'Shea D, Paine MF, Shen DD, Kunze KL, Perkins JD, Wilkinson GR: **Oral first-pass elimination of midazolam involves both gastrointestinal and hepatic CYP3A-mediated metabolism.** *Clin Pharmacol Ther* 1996, **59:**491–502.
38. Westphal K, Weinbrenner A, Zschiesche M, Franke G, Knoke M, Oertel R, Fritz P, *et al*: **Induction of P-glycoprotein by rifampin increases intestinal secretion of talinolol in human beings: a new type of drug/drug interaction.** *Clin Pharmacol Ther* 2000, **68:**345–355.
39. Fromm MF, Busse D, Kroemer HK, Eichelbaum M: **Differential induction of prehepatic and hepatic metabolism of verapamil by rifampin.** *Hepatology* 1996, **24:**796–801.
40. Kim RB, Fromm MF, Wandel C, Leake B, Wood AJ, Roden DM, Wilkinson GR: **The drug transporter P-glycoprotein limits oral absorption and brain entry of HIV-1 protease inhibitors.** *J Clin Invest* 1998, **101:**289–294.
41. Paine MF, Shen DD, Kunze KL, Perkins JD, Marsh CL, McVicar JP, Barr DM, *et al*: **First-pass metabolism of midazolam by the human intestine.** *Clin Pharmacol Ther* 1996, **60:**14–24.
42. Wandel C, Bocker RH, Bohrer H, de Vries JX, Hofmann W, Walter K, Kleingeist B, *et al*: **Relationship between hepatic cytochrome P450 3A content and activity and the disposition of midazolam administered orally.** *Drug Metab Dispos* 1998, **26:**110–114.
43. Kronbach T, Mathys D, Umeno M, Gonzalez FJ, Meyer UA: **Oxidation of midazolam and triazolam by human liver cytochrome P450IIIA4.** *Mol Pharmacol* 1989, **36:**89–96.
44. Ghosal A, Satoh H, Thomas PE, Bush E, Moore D: **Inhibition and kinetics of cytochrome P4503A activity in microsomes from rat, human, and cdna-expressed human cytochrome P450.** *Drug Metab Dispos* 1996, **24:**940–947.
45. Bhardwaj RK, Glaeser H, Becquemont L, Klotz U, Gupta SK, Fromm MF: **Piperine, a major constituent of black pepper, inhibits human P-glycoprotein and CYP3A4.** *J Pharmacol Exp Ther* 2002, **302:**645–650.
46. Gleiter CH, Gundert-Remy U: **Gender differences in pharmacokinetics.** *Eur J Drug Metab Pharmacokinet* 1996, **21:**123–128.
47. Miao J, Jin Y, Marunde RL, Kim S, Quinney S, Radovich M, Li L, *et al*: **Association of genotypes of the CYP3A cluster with midazolam disposition in vivo.** *Pharmacogenomics J* 2009, **9:**319–326.
48. Tanaka E: **Gender-related differences in pharmacokinetics and their clinical significance.** *J Clin Pharm Ther* 1999, **24:**339–346.
49. Harris RZ, Benet LZ, Schwartz JB: **Gender effects in pharmacokinetics and pharmacodynamics.** *Drugs* 1995, **50:**222–239.

5

Computational investigation of inhibitory mechanism of flavonoids as bovine serum albumin anti-glycation agents

Anahita Johari[1,2], Ali Akbar Moosavi-Movahedi[2] and Massoud Amanlou[1*]

Abstract

Background: Glycation of serum albumin and its consequence products were considered as an important factor in drug distribution and diabetic complications, therefore finding the glycation inhibitors and their inhibitory mechanisms became a valuable field of study. In this work, bovine serum albumin (BSA) became a subject as a model protein for analyzing the inhibitory mechanism of flavonoids, known as natural BSA glycation inhibitors in the early stage of glycation.

Methods: Firstly, for theoretical study, the three-dimensional model of BSA structure was generated by homology modeling and refined through molecular dynamic simulation. Secondly, several validation methods (statistical assessment methods and also neural network methods) by simultaneous docking study were employed for insurance about accuracy of our simulation. Then docking studies were performed for visualizing the relation between flavonoids' binding sites and BSA glycation sites besides, the correlation analyzes between calculated binding energy and reported experimental inhibitory IC_{50} values of the flavonoids set, was considered to explore their molecular inhibitory mechanism.

Results: The quality assessment methods and simultaneous docking studies on interaction of quercetin (as the most studied flavonoids) with BSA and Human serum albumin (HAS), confirm the accuracy of simulation and the second stage of docking results which were in close agreement with experimental observations, suggest that the potential residues in flavonoids binding sites (which were place neighbor of tryptophan 212 within 5Å) cannot be considered as one of glycation sites.

Conclusions: Based on the results, flavonoids don't participate in inhibitory interference mechanism, and also, the differentiation between complexes of flavonoids with BSA and HSA could destroy the speculation of using them as an exchangeable model protein in study of serum albumin and flavonoids interactions.

Keywords: Homology modeling, Molecular dynamics simulation, Correlation analyzes, Glycation sites, Flavonoids, BSA

Background

Diabetes is considered as one of the main threat to human health, according to WHO report, it is predicted that diabetes will exceed to 300 million in the years of 2025. Diabetes has a devastating effect on almost every organ in body. The hyperglycemia in diabetic conditions causes non-enzymatic glycation of proteins [1]. This reaction initiates the formation of reversible Schiff base between glucose and ε-amino group of lysine residues in proteins which by consequent intermolecular rearrangements leading to a formation of ketamine adduct. Then, the potent precursors of protein cross-linkers such as glucosone, 5-hydroxymethyl-2-furaldehyde, and 3-deoxyglucosone are formed due to the initial reaction. Next, those intermediates are oxidized, and cross linked, and fluorescent heterogeneous group of protein-bound moieties (called advanced glycated end products or AGEs) are detected in the last stage of glycation [2,3]. With body of evidence, formation and accumulation of advanced glycation products can be considered as a major factor

* Correspondence: amanlou@tums.ac.ir
[1]Department of Medicinal Chemistry, Faculty of Pharmacy and Pharmaceutical Sciences Research Center, Tehran University of Medical Sciences, Tehran, Iran
Full list of author information is available at the end of the article

in development of diabetic complication, Alzheimer's disease, and normal aging process. Therefore, the considerable efforts have been made to propose and discover inhibitors of glycation for therapeutic application in treatment of diseases that advanced glycation end product could be responsible for their pathogenesis [4].

Serum albumin is the most abundant protein in body which has a tremendous interest for binding to various natural or synthetic small-molecules such as glucose and related compounds. In diabetic condition, serum albumin undergoes glycation [5]. This character, continually expose serum albumin to altering factors which can participate in serum albumin modifications and biological compound formation that can be considered as a causative agent for some diseases [6]. Among the wide variety of interaction, the none-enzymatic interaction of serum albumin with glucose is one of the most important underlying modification factors, which are in associated with various alterations of albumin's structure and functions [7,8].

Among the glycation inhibitors' which were examined on bovine serum albumin (BSA) as a model protein, specific considerations were given to dietary natural products such as several phenolic compounds [9,10]. Researches on a limited number of flavonoids compounds indicated their ability to prevention both stage of glycation reaction [7]. In the late stage, the inhibition mechanisms of flavonoids are that, they may act as a both metal chelator and radical scavenger [11,12]. However, the inhibitory mechanism of flavonoids in the early stage completely remains unclear [7]. For some anti-glycation agent such as α-lipoate or non-steroidal anti-inflammatory drugs such as diclofenac and aspirin, hydrophobic hindrance or binding near the glycation site was considered as possible mechanism of anti-glycation activity [9,13]. Although we have no evidence that flavonoids react with the glycation site [7], in the present study, the attentions are drawn to binding behavior of flavonoids to clarifying the inhibition mechanism of them for the early stage of glycation.

Since, docking simulation results can be used to understanding the molecular interaction and analyze biological presses, rapidly and efficiently [2], in the present study, we explored the series of flavonoids' binding behavior with BSA through docking studies.

However, in the case of BSA which was considered here as a model protein (such as studies mentioned above by Morimitsu, Y., et al. and Matsuda, H., et al. [3,12]). When this study was started nobody has succeeded in obtaining crystals of intact BSA [14]. However, simultaneous with our study the importance of this protein draws the other researchers' attention to solving the tertiary structure of BSA. However, the new crystals also haven't been at high resolution (<2 Å resolution limit) [15], which can be satisfactory resolution for using in docking simulation. In this study, simulation, homology modeling was employed. While, it is generally recognized that homology modeling of proteins could be considered as accurate methods for 3D structure prediction while a model and related template sharing high sequence identity [16,17].

In present work, the model was refined with energy minimization and molecular dynamic simulation. Then, different assessment tools were adapted for checking the proper folding of constructed BSA 3D structure.

Consequently, by docking methods the validity of the model protein was examined and for getting better insight into the flavonoids' inhibitory mechanism. Firstly, the predicted binding affinity and reported IC_{50} [12] was subjected to correlation analyzes and secondly, the flavonoids binding location was studied for tracing the relation among participated amino acids in the flavonoids' binding site with ones proposed as the glycation site of BSA [18].

In addition, according to docking results, the comparison is made between obtained 3D structure of BSA and crystallographic structure of HSA for understanding their specificity in flavonoids binding location and the verification of using BSA and HSA as an exchangeable mode protein for the same case of investigation.

Methods

Amino acid sequence alignment and homology modeling of bovine serum albumin

In the first step, Amino acid sequence of BSA (UniProt ID: P02769) was retrieved from Swiss-Prot (http://www.uniprot.org/uniprot). And then, Blastp matrix blosum62 against PDB database was used to find out the best homologous structure with a known 3D structure, for applying as a template in homology modeling. Finally, among the HSA structures, the structure with a highest resolution at 1.9 Å [19] that belong to HSA (PDB ID: 1N5U) was adopted as the final target.

Sequence alignment was generated using 2d alignment function of MODELLER 9v8 program (www.salilab.org/modeller). Align 2d is based on a dynamic programming algorithm, considering the template structural information for constructing an alignment, this advantages is more significant as the similarity between the sequences decrease and the number of gaps increase [20]. After alignment, the 3D structure of fifty models were calculated completely automatically with MODELLER 9v8 [21].

Refinement of homology model by minimization and MD simulation

Molecular dynamic simulation were carried out using the parallel version of GROMACS 4.5.3 [22] In the AMBER99SB force field [23] to monitor stability and conformation of the selected model. The starting coordinates were taken from the best model that was retrieved from MODELLER and for prediction of non-standard ionization state of residues PROPKA 2.0 was applied [24]. Among the whole residues that may be adapted standard ionization state, lysine 219 was deprotonated and six histidine residues (histidine 16, histidine 37, histidine 143, histidine 239, histidine 335, and histidine 332) were completely protonated.

After assigning charge state, the protein was put into a suitable sized simulation cubic box and immersed in 41760 simple point charges (SPC) water model. Then, appropriate number of Na^+ ions were added to neutralize the charge of the system. The first energy minimization, which targeted water molecules and ions alone while configuration of protein was kept, fixed, followed by 20 ps MD simulation which again, the protein was kept fixed and the water molecules and ions were allowed to evolve. The second minimization step began with 1000 steepest descent and conjugate gradient of 9000 steps afterward. For equilibrating further the system v-rescale thermostat [25] was applied by using coupling constant (τ_t) of 0.1 ps to keep the system at the constant temperature in 100 ps at 100 K and 200 K respectively. While the pressure of the system maintained at 1 atm by using the Berendsen weak coupling algorithm [26] with coupling constant (τ_p) of 0.5 ps. For obtaining the stable system at 300 K and 1 atm, the same aforementioned parameters were determined for heating the system.

In this simulation, the non-bonded interactions were calculated by applying a 14 Å cut off and periodic boundary conditions were also applied in all directions. The Electrostatic interactions were calculated using the Particle Mesh Ewald (PME) [27]. During simulation, the frame was stored at every 1.000 ps.

Subsequently, all the analysis was performed by taking advantage of Gromacs tools and the structure which was retrieved after system stabilization was subject to evaluate the protein geometry.

Assessment of the homology model

To verify the quality of the model after molecular dynamic refinement, using different tools, which include: PRoQ, as a neural network based predictor [28], verify 3D, which analyzes the compatibility of an atomic model (3D) with its own amino acid sequence (1D) [29], PROSA program, which evaluate the energy of using a distance based pair potential [30] as well PROCHECK for checking the detailed stereochemical properties [31].

Docking analysis

Autodock 4.0 [32] was used for docking studies and for adding charges and active torsions to the ligands and assign Kollman charges to protein AutoDockTools (ADT) was employed. The rectangular lattice (100 × 100 × 100) with points separated by 0.375 Å was built by AutoGrid that was superposed on subdomin IIA of serum albumin (proposed as a primarily binding site of flavonoids) [33]. The Lamarckian genetic algorithm (LGA) was used with 100 runs for docking simulation, while an initial population size of 100, and the maximum number of 2500000 energy evaluations. All other parameters were set to default values, and the results were ranked according to Autodock scoring function and the final conformation of each structure was selected based on the highest dock score.

The chemical structures of interested flavonoids were optimized at MM+ level of molecular mechanic methods using HYPERCHEM software program (version 8.0.3 Hypercube, Inc) [34]. The geometry optimization was preceded by Polak-Ribiere algorithm to reach the 0.01 root mean square gradient. Then all these refinement structures were subject to docking simulations.

MD simulation after docking

All MD simulations were performed using the Gromacs 4.5.3 program together with the 43a2 force field [35-37] for each simulation to study the complex of BSA-quercetin, while the topology of quercetin was generated by the PRODRG 2.5 beta server [38].

Then, the protein was solvated by simple point charge water molecule in the cubic box with minimal distance of protein from its wall being 1.0 nm and the system was neutralized by adding appropriate counter ions. After performing energy minimization of the entire system, it was equilibrated under NVT ensemble for 100 ps and the periodic boundary conditions were used in tree-coordinate direction, whereas, position restrains were placed on ligand using force restraint of 1000 kcal/mol. NVT equilibration is followed by isothermal–isobaric (NPT) which was performed for 100 ps. The pressure of the system was regulated by Berendsen barostat with a relaxation time (τp) of 2.0 ps. The position restraints and simulation parameter which was applied in the NPT ensemble was the same as the ones which have been used during NPT equilibration. After convergence had been reached, the protein-ligand and water-ions groups were coupled in separate temperature baths, and v-rescale thermostat was used to keep the temperature constant at 300 k during the 2 ns simulation. Lennard-Jones interactions were calculated within a cut-off distance of 1.0 nm, and electrostatic interactions were treated with the particle mesh Ewald's method. Ultimately, from 2 ns MD simulation, the structure with low RMSD value was selected for analyzing the local conformational changes of BSA- quercetin complex.

Computational resources

The computational studies were performed on computer cluster 4 HP Prolient ML370-G5 Tower servers equipped with 2 Quad Core Intel Xeon processors E5355, 2.66 GHz and 4GB of RAM on a Linux platform.

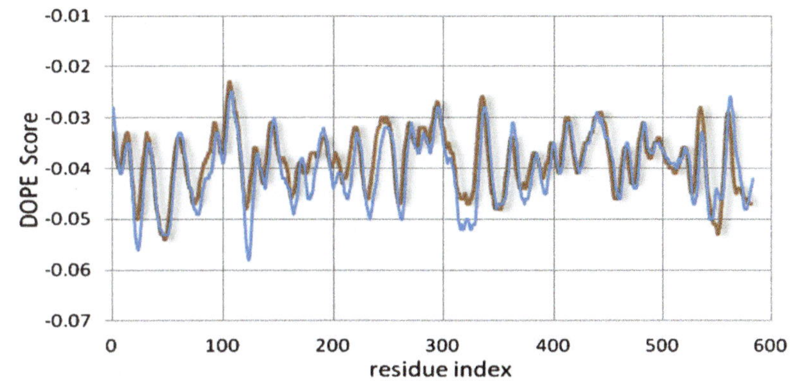

Figure 1 Analysis of DOPE score profile (obtained from Modeller). The Blue line indicates, energy profile of HSA (PDB ID: 1N5U) which used as a model and the red line indicates energy profile of target, which constructed by Modeller.

Results

Sequence alignment and modeling building

Based on the highest similarity and the lowest D-value, human serum albumin (HSA) can be considered the best homologues structure for BSA. The Sequence alignment of BSA (UniProt ID: P02769) and HSA (UniProt ID: P02768) which was generated by ClustalX program shows 76% identity between them [39]. The precursor proteins of BSA and HSA have 603 and 607 amino acid in length, respectively. Though all the crystallographic structures of HSA which were reported, only consist of 583 amino acids. This can be referred to the fact that during a secretion and maturation process of serum albumins, the 25 N-terminal amino acids were cleaved [40]. Therefore, the 25 N –terminal amino acids, which are placed out of the chain, were separated from the HSA amino acids sequence and the rest of them used as a target for homology modeling.

After alignment, the 3D structure of fifty models was calculated completely automatically with modeler 9v8. In this process, the population of the constructed model was increased for improving the DOPE energy assessment

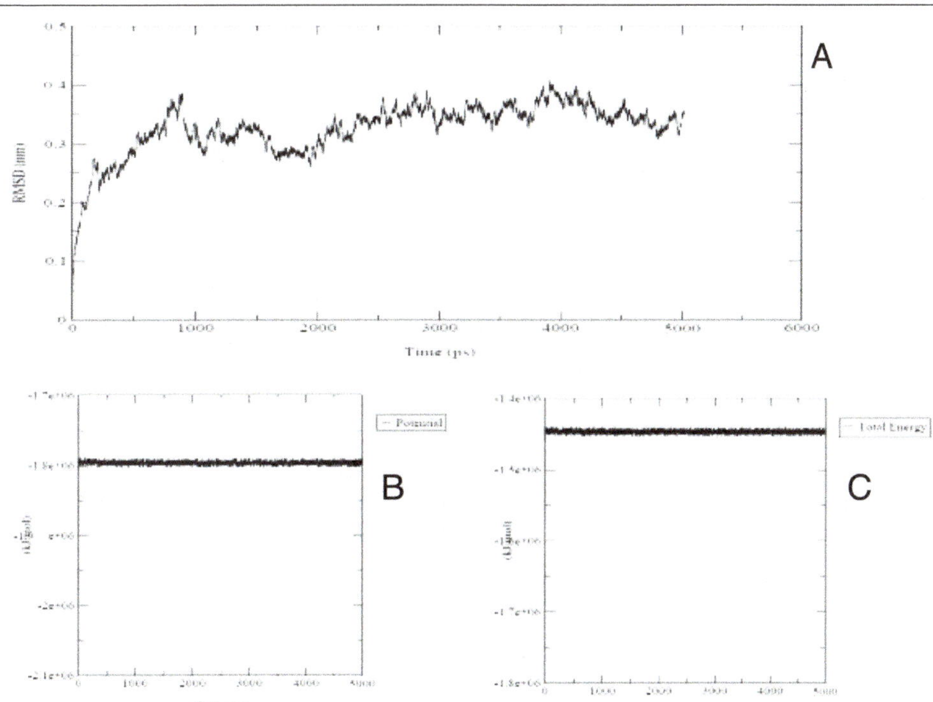

Figure 2 Analysis of a molecular dynamics simulation trajectory during 5ns generated by Gromacs. (A) The backbone root mean square deviation (RMSD) plot of the model, during 5ns simulation. **(B)** The variation of potential around constant value. **(C)** The fluctuation of total energy.

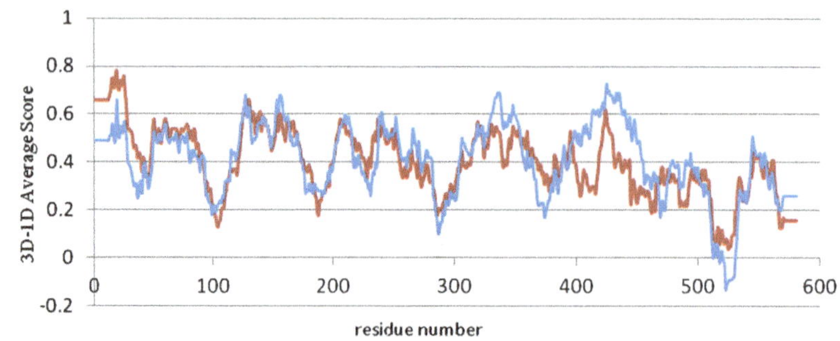

Figure 3 The Verify-3D analysis is shown for all residues. The blue line belongs to molecular structure after MD, and red one belongs to model that constructed by the Modeller. The refinement model after MD was validated by positive scores of Verify-3D.

and MODELLER objective function calculation and then the best model was selected based on the lowest DOPE score. Next, for gave an idea about the quality of input alignment the DOPE score profile (Figure 1) was calculated with "assess_dope" function of MODELLER. It can be seen in Figure 1, that in the whole range of residues, the DOPE score of both proteins converges and the results aren't showing any problematic regions.

Analysis the trajectory of the molecular dynamics simulation

During 5 ns MD simulation, the system was analyzed for its stability. The deviation plot of potential, and root mean square deviation (Figure 2) were derived from the respective trajectory by Gromacs software output. The low degree of RMSD fluctuation during last 2 ns indicates that the system tends to be converging and therefore, it is become stable. According to what illustrated in Figure 2, the total energy of the complex was observed within the range from −1.4 to −1.5 kJ/mol, which can be a reasonable value.

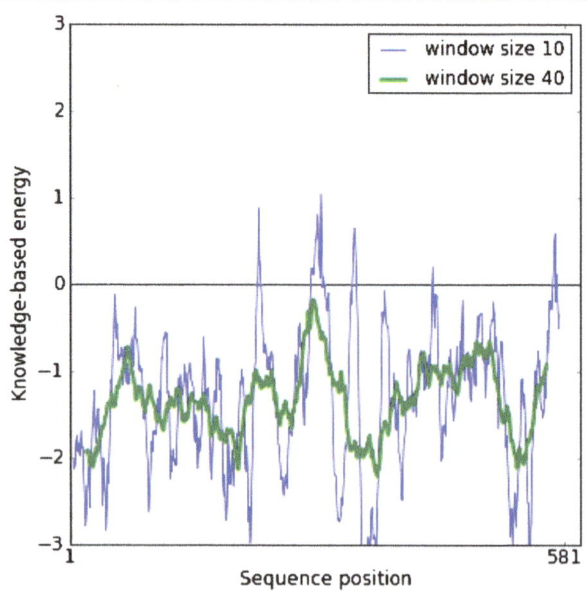

Figure 4 Energy plot from ProSA program, all residues have negative ProSA energies which confirms the reliability of the model.

Assess the validity of generated model after MD

In present work two statistical approaches such as verify3D and PROSA confirm a reliability of the constructed model.

In the first approach, the Verify 3D profile (Figure 3) represents that 3D-1D average score of the most residues in the model proteins both before and after MD, given a score over 0.2 except the ones rage 514–532. In the model protein that refined after MD, the whole residues have a positive score, whereas in the model that constructed by the modeler the amino acids in the range of 518–530 have a negative score. Therefore, based on these results, the sign of model folding improvement after molecular dynamic simulation is traceable.

The second statistical assessment method was processed with ProSA program. The Normalized Z-score calculation indicates standard deviation value is found in the range of native conformation of crystallographic structure and also according to Figure 4, ProSA score, which was calculated interaction energy per residues, has a negative score across the most of the residues' length.

After performing those earlier methodologies based on statistical approaches (Verify3D, ProSA), the PRoQ was applied to compare the validity of the model before and after MD simulation. This program is based on a neural

Table 1 Ramachandran plot statistics

% residues in most favored regions	90.8%
% residues in additional allowed regions	8.8%
% residues in generously allowed regions	0.4%
% residues in disallowed regions	0.0%
% Num. of non-glycine and non-proline residues	100.0%

Table 2 Main chain parameters plot statistics

Stereochemical parameter	No. of data pts	Parameter value	Comparison values Typical value	Comparison values Band width	No. of band widths from mean	
%-tage residues in A,B,L	535	90.8	84.9	10.0	0.6	Inside
Omega angle Std. dev.	380	7.0	6.0	3.0	0.3	Inside
Bad contacts/100 residues	0	0.0	3.3	10.0	−0.3	Inside
Zeta angle Std. dev.	565	1.3	3.1	1.6	−1.1	Better
H-bond energy Std. dev.	400	0.7	0.8	0.2	0.5	Inside
Overall G-factor	581	0.0	−0.3	0.3	1.0	Better

network that by considering the Wallner and Elofsson's study it is indeed superior to statistics-based methods [41]. In this method two quality measures are predicted, LG score and MaxSub score. Based on their range of qualities; predicted LG score and MaxSub score of the model after MD is 4.14 (which is within the range of a 'extremely good') and 0.45(which are within the range of 'good'), while values of 2.915 and 0.304 were obtained for LG score and MaxSub score, respectively in the model before MD simulation. These scores indicate the refinement of the model after MD simulation.

Ultimately, the validity of the model was evaluated by PROCHECK, and stereochemical properties of protein structure were listed in Tables 1 and 2 [31,42]. In the Figure 5, phi and psi distribution of Ramachandran plot indicate that 100% of residues were present in favored and allowed regions, which confirm that the structure is comparable with good homology model [43]. Also the main chain parameters which consist of six properties plotted are all well within the established limit of reliable structures (Table 2).

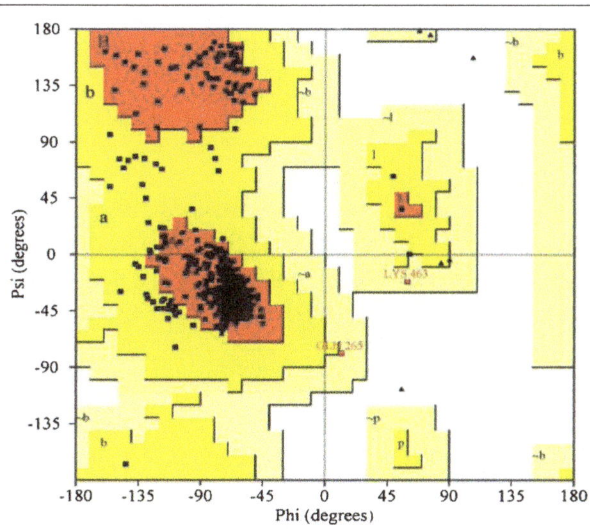

Figure 5 Ramachandran plot for 3D structural model of bovine serum albumin.

In brief, according to all applied evaluated methods, it can be concluded that obtained 3.D structural model has an acceptable geometry for further study by docking approach.

Docking studies

With the interest of comparability of docking result with experimental data (which studied the interaction among flavonoids and BSA), and also shedding the light at an ambiguous point of experimental observation in molecular level, with respect to Dufour and Dangles work [33] one stage of docking simulation was designed. Therefore, the binding interaction of quercetin (as the most studied flavonoid) and warfarin (as a site marker of subdomain IIA HSA) was subject to docking simulation.

First of all, in this process, the accuracy of applied docking protocol was examined. So, warfarin as a probe of HSA (whose high affinity binding site was known as a subdomain IIA) was docked into HSA (PDB ID: 1H9Z), which co-crystallized with it. Docking results demonstrates that the warfarin docks back into the experimental binding location which was retrieved based on the crystallographic study (Figure 6).Therefore; this protocol was confirmed and consequently, applied in docking simulation for complexes of quercetin with HSA and BSA.

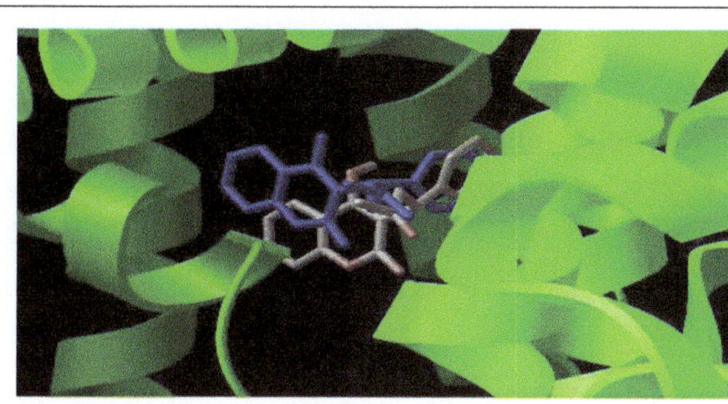

Figure 6 The docking conformation and location of warfarin on the Human serum albumin (PDB ID: 1H9Z). The conformation of warfarin after docking indicates with DG colored sketch (David Goodsell's scheme) and what was retrieved from the crystallographic study indicate as a blue sketch.

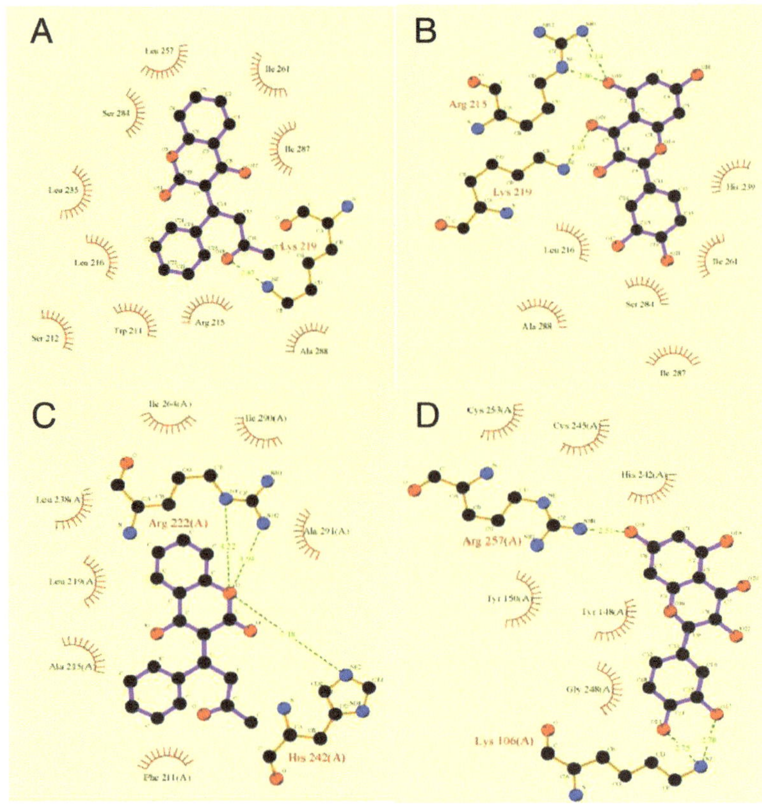

Figure 7 The structure of bovine serum albumin complexes with warfarin and quercetin (A, B), consequently (C) The structure of human serum albumin complexes with warfarin and quercetin, (D) was analyzed using the Ligplot 4.22 program. The hydrogen bonds are shown as dash lines and hydrophobic contacts are indicated with half-moon.

For analyzing the specific contact and indicating the participated amino acids in biding sites the Ligplot program was employed [44]. It is indicated in Figure 7, That in the binding site of bovine serum albumin, serine 284, isoleucine 261 and 287, alanine 288 involve in hydrophobic interaction with quercetin and warfarin, and also arginine 219 contribute in a hydrogen bond with both, this means that in the case of BSA, the warfarin and quercetin binding sites completely overlap, while these ligands are bonded in different location in HSA.

The Dufour and Dangles fluorescence spectroscopy study had shown that fluorescence of BSA-quercetin complex (protein/marker molar ratio of 1) is affected by constant concentration of warfarin (site marker of subdomain IIA),

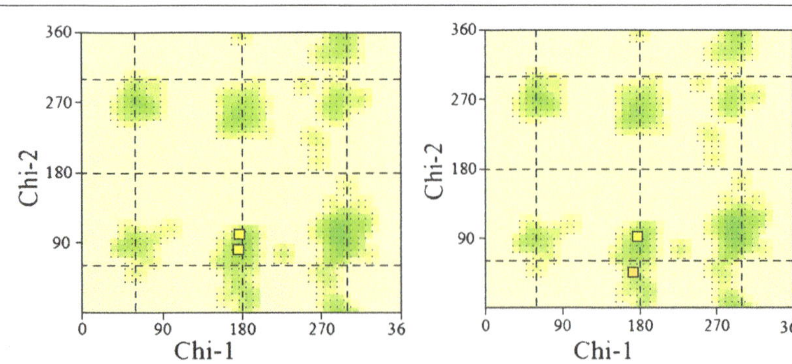

Figure 8 The χ_1/χ_2 plots are obtained from PROCHECK program. Each square represents one residue. The color coding of the squares is corresponding the range of yellow to red which is reflects the degree to which the orientation is favored; therefore, yellow indicate the residue is in a favored and red indicate the residue is an unflavored region. Two tryptophan of bovine serum albumin was indicated in both plots. The left plot indicate χ_1/χ_2 coordinate of tryptophans before MD (Left). The right plot indicates the χ_1/χ_2 coordinates of tryptophans after MD (Right). How it is shown, trp 134 remains constant while the χ_1/χ_2 coordinates of trp 212 is changed and located in unflavored region.

but fluorescence of HSA-quercetin complex is independent of warfarin presence [33].

For better understanding of the relation between experimental observations and what was retrieved from docking calculations. The more investigations were taken to visualization the effect of BSA-flavonoids interaction on local conformational changes, which leads to fluorescence quenching.

First notable issue which was considered is that the amino acids lining in the common binding site of quercetin and warfarin, are neighbors of tryptophan 212 within 5Å. This is important because the intrinsic fluorescence of BSA with excitation at 295 nm is due to the tryptophan residues (BSA has two tryptophan, tryptophan 212 and tryptophan 134) and quercetin actually promoted a strong quenching of the tryptophan emission at 340 nm

Table 3 The free energy of binding between, 12 Flavones, 12 Flavonols, 3 Flavanones, 2 Flavan-3-ols and bovine serum albumin obtained from docking study, and their AGEs inhibitions' IC_{50} (in regard to Matsuda, H., et al. [12])

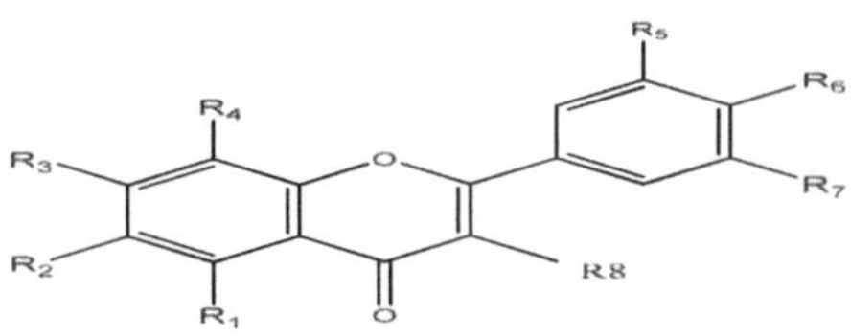

Num	Name	R^1	R^2	R^3	R^4	R^5	R^6	R^7	R^8	ΔG (Kcal/mol)	AGEs inhibition IC_{50} (% in 200 μM)
1	Flavone	H	H	H	H	H	H	H	H	−7.09	5%
2	7-Hydroxyflavone	H	H	OH	H	H	H	H	H	−6.96	27%
3	Chrysin	OH	H	OH	H	H	H	H	H	−7.56	43%
4	4,7-Dihydroxyflavone	H	H	OH	H	H	OH	H	H	−7.0	44%
5	3,4,7-Trihydroxyflavone	H	H	OH	H	OH	OH	H	H	−7.53	44%
6	Apigenin	OH	H	OH	H	H	OH	H	H	−7.52	53%
7	Luteolin	OH	H	OH	H	OH	OH	H	H	−7.53	64%
8	Diosmetin	OH	H	OH	H	OH	OCH_3	H	H	−7.05	27%
9	Pilloin	OH	H	OCH_3	H	OH	OCH_3	H	H	−7.9	29%
10	10 F	OH	H	OCH_3	H	OCH_3	OCH_3	H	H	−7.0	29%
11	Wogonin	OH	H	OH	OCH_3	H	H	H	H	−7.03	50%
12	Baicalin	OH	OH	OH	H	H	H	H	H	−7.75	79%
13	3-Hydroxyflavone	H	H	H	H	H	H	H	OH	−7.1	3%
14	Kaempferol	OH	H	OH	H	H	OH	H	OH	−7.47	46%
15	Quercetin	OH	H	OH	H	OH	OH	H	OH	−7.67	57%
16	Rhamnetin	OH	H	OCH_3	H	OH	OH	H	OH	−7.57	55%
17	Tamarixetin	OH	H	OH	H	OH	OCH_3	H	OH	−7.89	45%
18	F18	OH	H	OCH_3	H	OH	OH	H	OCH_3	−7.4	57%
19	Ombuine	OH	H	OCH_3	H	OH	OCH_3	H	OH	−7.66	27%
20	Ayanin	OH	H	OCH_3	H	OH	OCH_3	H	OCH_3	−7.66	40%
21	21 F	OH	H	OCH_3	H	OCH_3	OCH_3	H	OH	−7.69	13%
22	Myricetin	H	H	H	H	H	H	H	OH	−7.48	61%
23	Mearnsetin	H	H	H	H	H	CH3	H	OH	−7.51	10%
24	24 F	H	H	CH_3	H	H	H	H	OH	- 7.81	42%
25	Liquiritigenin	H	H	OH	H	H	OH	H	H	−7.16	40%
26	26 F	H	H	OCH_3	H	H	OH	H	H	−6.74	44%
27	Eriodictyol	OH	H	OH	H	OH	OH	H	H	−7.46	46%
28	(+)-Catechin	OH	H	OH	H	OH	OH	H	β-OH	−7.74	69%
29	(−)-Epigallocatechin	OH	H	OH	H	OH	OH	OH	α-OH	−7.06	4%

[33]. These observations lead to further study of checking the tryptophan flexibility after interaction between the quercetin and BSA complex.

So, the complex of BSA model and quercetin (best conformation after docking) was subjected to molecular dynamic simulation for 2 ns. After the stability of the system, for describing the side chain conformational changes the dihedral angles of our interested aromatic residue, χ_1 / χ_2 plot was provided by PROCHECK program [31]. The results represent the significant shuffling between side-chain conformations of tryptophan 212 before and after the refinement of BSA-quercetin complex with molecular dynamic simulation. Figure 8 indicates that the BSA residues which were involved in interaction with quercetin, pushing the tryptophan 212 side chain conformations to unflavored regions.

Discussion

In present work, based on docking calculation and molecular dynamic simulation, the detailed understanding was obtained about the interaction of quercetin (as a typical flavonoids) and BSA, which is in consistence with previous experimental data [33]. In addition, these calculations in molecular levels demonstrate its ability to providing the interpretation for experimental observation.

The first-stage docking results confirm on one hand the reliability of obtained 3D structural model, and on the other hand, by showing the significant specificity between high homologous BSA and HSA proteins, indicate the necessity of constructing BSA model's for analyzing the interaction flavonoids with it.

According to visualization of the predicted binding site of quercetin, any interventions are not observed between the quercetin binding site and reported glycation site of BSA [18]. However, for the more reliable conclusion, a number of flavonoids which introduced as an inhibitor of BSA glycation [3,12] were employed for the further docking studies.

By the speculation that the radical scavenging activity in physiological condition could inhibit oxidative fragmentation of Amadori rearrangement product and subsequently prevented the AGEs formation, the number of flavonoids was studied to find a correlation between the experimental anti glycation activity and radical scavenging activity of them [12]. In the present investigation with respect to their works, interested flavonoids was selected and by considering an interference reaction in the glycation site as the possible inhibitory mechanism [9,45,46], the theoretical binding energies of flavonoids in the complex with BSA were calculated by docking methods(calculated free energy of binding were listed in Tables 3 and 4). Then, analytical methods were performed by SPSS software (version 15). The correlation analyzes between the experimental activity (IC_{50}) and predicted binding energy reveal that there is no significant correlation between these values ($p > 0.3$).

Besides the statistical analyzes, the AutoDockTools (ADT) was used for visualization the relationship between the predicted flavonoids' binding site and the reported glycation site on BSA. Interestingly, despite the structural differentiations which exist among these flavonoids, the most likely conformation of each one of them, were placed in the same binding site (consist of lysine 219, arginine 215, isoleucine 287, and serine 284) (Figure 9) which can't be considered as any glycation sites of BSA (in respect to aforementioned Hinton and Ames study). Therefore, by considering these results, maybe it can be concluded that the hydrophobic hindrances in the glycation site can't be considered as an inhibitory mechanism for flavonoids.

Conclusion

In previous experimental studies, the high homology between BSA and HSA has invoked speculation that they have a similar structure and so share similar capability in some of their properties like ligands binding [45]. However, simulating the quercetin (as the most studied flavonoids) interactions with both BSA and HSA show significant differences between them, which confirms our speculation about the necessity of providing the affordable BSA 3D structural model for analyzing its specific

Table 4 The free energy of binding between 3 isoflavones and bovine Serum albumin obtained from docking study, and their AGEs inhibitions' IC_{50}

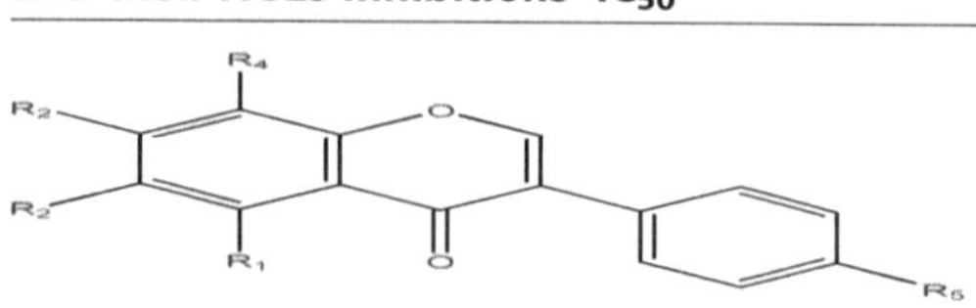

Num.	Name	R[1]	R[2]	R[3]	R[4]	R[5]	ΔG (Kcal/mol)	AGEs inhibition IC_{50} (% in 200 μM)
30	Daidzein	H	H	OH	H	OH	−7.05	33%
31	Genistein	OH	H	OH	H	OH	−6.44	34%
32	Biochanin A	OH	H	OH	H	OCH_3	−7.68	36%

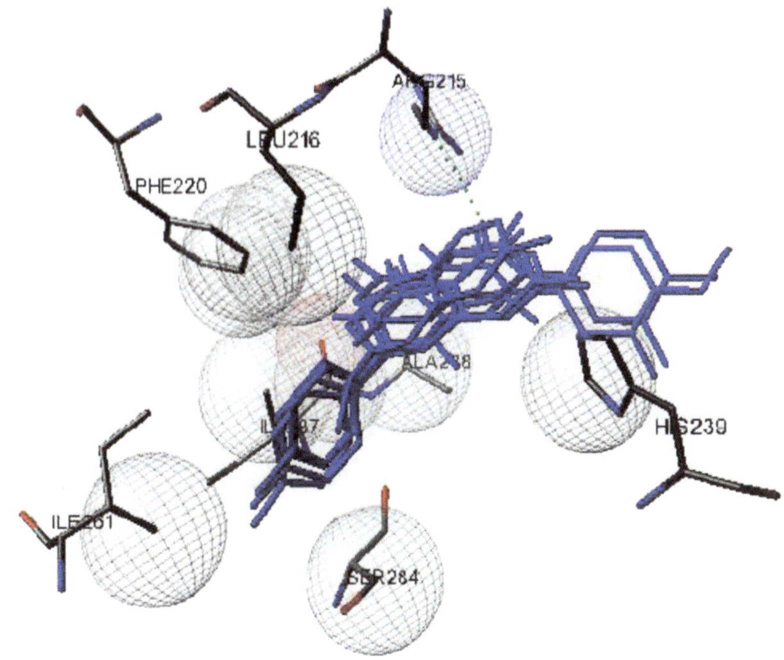

Figure 9 The superimposition of docked complex. The most likely conformation of representative flavonoids of under study groups (Flavones, flavonols, flavanones, flavan-3-ols, isoflavones), is represented in their binding site.

binding location and binding affinity for our interested ligands.

Interestingly, in the present study, the consistency between docking results and experimental data not only indicate the validity of our simulation but also become helpful in interpreting about experimental observation in molecular levels [33].

Thus different aspect of results was considered, on one hand the visualization of quercetin binding site leads to find the relationship between the binding site residues and tryptophan 212, and also by employing the MD simulation it is revealed that participated residues in flavonoids interaction site affect on tryptophan local conformational change, which at last is observed as fluorescence quenching.

On the other hand, according to our obtained results, the possibility of relation between the flavonoids binding site and glycation sites was investigated, while the correlation analyzes was adopted between binding affinity of flavonoids to BSA and IC_{50} of AGE inhibition. How was mentioned before based on the results, the flavonoids can't be considered as an intervention agent for glycation site and therefore, the possibility of this inhibitory mechanism is unacceptable in the case of flavonoids.

Ultimately, the other interesting outcome of this study is laid beneath the final examination. Coincident with our study the crystallographic structure of bovine serum albumin was determined [15]. Therefore, the comparison has been made between our calculated 3D structural models of BSA with the reported model which retrieved from crystallographic technique to get insight into their distinctive difference. These two structures were superimposed with Swiss PDB viewer software (Figure 10) [47]. And strong correlation (RMSD: 1.9) between them shades a light in the hypothesis that applied methods in this study are accurate and reliable.

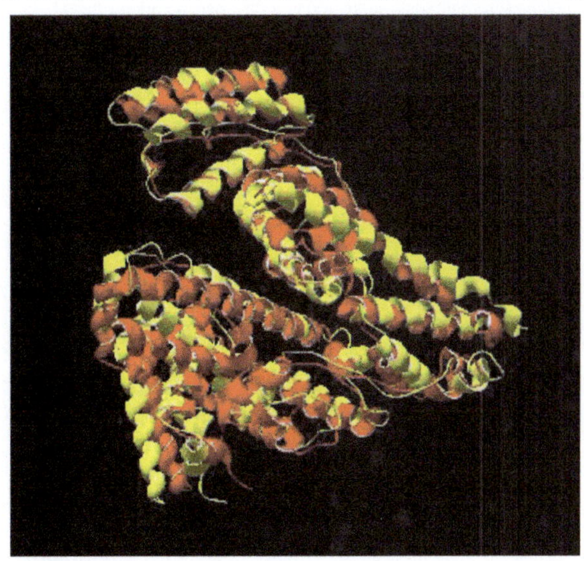

Figure 10 The superimposition between crystallographic structure of bovine serum albumin (PDB ID: 4F5S) (orange) and calculated 3D structure model (yellow), obtained with Swiss PDB viewer software.

Competing interests

The authors declare that they have no competing interests.

Authors' contributions

All authors contributed to the concept and design of study. AJ and MA performed all computational experiments and analyzed the data. MA is responsible for the study registration, financial and administrative support. AJ, MA and AAMM wrote the manuscript and all authors read and approved the final manuscript.

Acknowledgements

This work was financially supported by grants from Research Council of Tehran University of Medical Science and UNESCO Chair on Interdisciplinary Research in Diabetes, University of Tehran, Iran.

Author details

[1]Department of Medicinal Chemistry, Faculty of Pharmacy and Pharmaceutical Sciences Research Center, Tehran University of Medical Sciences, Tehran, Iran. [2]Institute of Biochemistry and Biophysics, University of Tehran, Tehran, Iran.

References

1. Nawale RB, Mourya VK, Bhise SB: **Non-enzymatic glycation of proteins: a cause for complications in diabetes.** *Indian J Biochem Biophys* 2006, **43**:337–344.
2. Iberg N, Fluckiger R: **Nonenzymatic glycosylation of albumin in vivo. identification of multiple glycosylated sites.** *J Biol Chem* 1986, **261**:13542–13545.
3. Morimitsu Y, Yoshida K, Esaki S, Hirota A: **Protein glycation inhibitors from thyme (*Thymus vulgaris*).** *Biosci Biotechnol Biochem* 1995, **59**:2018–2021.
4. Rahbar S, Figarola JL: **Novel inhibitors of advanced glycation endproducts.** *Arch Biochem Biophys* 2003, **419**:63–79.
5. Deeb O, Rosales-Hernández MC, Gómez-Castro C, Garduño-Juárez R, Correa-Basurto J: **Exploration of human serum albumin binding sites by docking and molecular dynamics flexible ligand–protein interactions.** *Biopolymers* 2010, **93**:161–170.
6. Cŕdova J, Ryan JD, Boonyaratanakornkit BB, Clark DS: **Esterase activity of bovine serum albumin up to 160°C: a new benchmark for biocatalysis.** *Enzyme Microb Techno* 2008, **42**:278–283.
7. Rondeau P, Bourdon E: **The glycation of albumin: structural and functional impacts.** *Biochimie* 2011, **93**:645–658.
8. Bousova I, Vukasovic D, Juretic D, Palicka V, Drsata J: **Enzyme activity and AGE formation in a model of AST glycoxidation by D-fructose in vitro.** *Acta Pharm* 2005, **55**:107–114.
9. Kawabata T, Packer L: **[alpha]-lipoate can protect against glycation of serum albumin, but not low-density lipoprotein.** *Biochem Biophys Res Commun* 1994, **203**:99–104.
10. Gutiérrez RMP, Diaz SL, Reyese IC, Gonzalez AMN: **Anti-glycation effect of spices and chilies uses in traditional mexican cuisine.** *J Nat Prod* 2010, **3**:95–102.
11. Bors W, Heller W, Michel C, Saran M: **Flavonoids as antioxidants: determination of radical-scavenging efficiencies.** *Methods Enzymol* 1990, **186**:343–355.
12. Matsuda H, Wang T, Managi H, Yoshikawa M: **Structural requirements of flavonoids for inhibition of protein glycation and radical scavenging activities.** *Bioorg Med Chem* 2003, **11**:5317–5323.
13. Van Boekel MA, van den Bergh PJ, Honders HJ: **Glycation of human serum albumin: inhibition by Diclofenac.** *Biochim Biophys Acta* 1992, **1120**:201–204.
14. Tai HC: *X-ray Crystallographic Studies of Bovine Serum Albumin and Helicobacter Pylori Thioredoxin-2.* Saskatoon, Canada: Thesis, University of Saskatchewan; 2004.
15. Bujacz A: **Structures of bovine, equine and leporine serum albumin.** *Acta Crystallogr Sect D Biol Crystallogr* 2012, **68**:1278–1289.
16. Ginalski K: **Comparative modeling for protein structure prediction.** *Curr Opin Struct Biol* 2006, **16**:172–177.
17. Azizian H, Bahrami H, Pasalar P, Amanlou M: **Molecular modeling of Helicobacter pylori arginase and the inhibitor coordination interactions.** *J Mol Graph Model* 2010, **28**:626–635.
18. Hinton DJS, Ames JM: **Site specificity of glycation and carboxymethylation of bovine serum albumin by fructose.** *Amino Acids* 2006, **30**:425–434.
19. Wardell M, Wang Z, Ho JX, Robert J, Ruker F, Ruble J, Carter DC: **The atomic structure of human methemalbumin at 1.9 A.** *Biochem Biophys Res Commun* 2002, **291**:813–819.
20. Sali A, Blundell TL: **Comparative protein modelling by satisfaction of spatial restraints.** *J Mol Biol* 1993, **234**:779–815.
21. Laurie AT, Jackson RM: **Q-SiteFinder: an energy-based method for the prediction of protein-ligand binding sites.** *Bioinformatics* 2005, **21**:1908–1916.
22. Hess B, Kutzner C, van der Spoel D, Lindahl E: **GROMACS 4: algorithms for highly efficient, load-balanced, and scalable molecular simulation.** *J Chem Theory Comput* 2008, **4**:435–447.
23. Hornak V, Abel R, Okur A, Strockbine B, Roitberg A, Simmerling C: **Comparison of multiple Amber force fields and development of improved protein backbone parameters.** *Proteins* 2006, **65**:712–725.
24. Bas DC, Rogers DM, Jensen JH: **Very fast prediction and rationalization of pKa values for protein–ligand complexes.** *Proteins Struct Funct Bioinf* 2008, **73**:765–783.
25. Bussi G, Donadio D, Parrinello M: **Canonical sampling through velocity rescaling.** *J Chem Phys* 2007, **126**:014101.
26. Berendsen H, Postma J, van Gunsteren W, DiNola A, Haak J: **Molecular dynamics with coupling to an external bath.** *J Chem Phys* 1984, **81**:3684–3690.
27. Essmann U, Perera L, Berkowitz ML, Darden T, Lee H, Pedersen LG: **A smooth particle mesh ewald method.** *J Chem Phys* 1995, **103**:8577–8593.
28. Wallner B, Elofsson A: **Can correct protein models be identified?** *Protein Sci* 2003, **12**:1073–1086.
29. Luthy R, Bowie JU, Eisenberg D: **Assessment of protein models with three-dimensional profiles.** *Nature* 1992, **356**:83–85.
30. Wiederstein M, Sippl MJ: **ProSA-web: interactive web service for the recognition of errors in three-dimensional structures of proteins.** *Nucleic Acids Res* 2007, **35**:W407–W410.
31. Laskowski RA, MacArthur MW, Moss DS, Thornton JM: **PROCHECK: a program to check the stereochemical quality of protein structures.** *J Appl Crystallogr* 1993, **26**:283–291.
32. Morris GM, Goodsell DS, Halliday RS, Huey R, Hart WE, Belew RK, Olson AJ: **Automated docking using a Lamarckian genetic algorithm and an empirical binding free energy function.** *J Comput Chem* 1998, **19**:1639–1662.
33. Dufour C, Dangles O: **Flavonoid-serum albumin complexation: determination of binding constants and binding sites by fluorescence spectroscopy.** *Biochim Biophys Acta* 2005, **1721**:164–173.
34. Froimowitz M: **HyperChem: a software package for computational chemistry and molecular modeling.** *Biotechniques* 1993, **14**:1010–1013.
35. Bekker H, Berendsen H, Dijkstra E, Achterop S, van Drunen R: **Gromacs method of virial calculation using a single sum.** In *Physics Computing.* 1993:257–26.
36. Lindahl E, Hess B, van der Spoel D: **GROMACS 3.0: a package for molecular simulation and trajectory analysis.** *J Mol Mod* 2001, **7**:306–317.
37. Berendsen H, van der Spoel D, van Drunen R: **GROMACS: a message-passing parallel molecular dynamics implementation.** *Comp Phys Comm* 1995, **91**:43–56.
38. Schuttelkopf AW, Van Aalten DM: **PRODRG: a tool for high-throughput crystallography of protein-ligand complexes.** *Acta Crystallogr Sect D Biol Crystallogr* 2004, **60**:1355–1363.
39. Thompson JD, Gibson TJ, Plewniak F, Jeanmougin F, Higgins DG: **The CLUSTAL_X windows interface: flexible strategies for multiple sequence alignment aided by quality analysis tools.** *Nucleic Acids Res* 1997, **25**:4876–4882.
40. Hirayama K, Akashi S, Furuya M, Fukuhara K: **Rapid confirmation and revision of the primary structure of bovine serum albumin by ESIMS and Frit-FAB LC/MS.** *Biochem Biophys Res Commun* 1990, **14**:639–646.
41. Fasnacht M, Zhu J, Honig B: **Local quality assessment in homology models using statistical potentials and support vector machines.** *Protein Sci* 2007, **16**:1557–1568.
42. Sakkiah S, Thangapandian S, John S, Lee KW: **Identification of critical chemical features for Aurora kinase-B inhibitors using Hip-Hop, virtual screening and molecular docking.** *J Mol Struct* 2011, **985**:14–26.

43. Xu Y, Colletier JP, Weik M, Jiang H, Moult J, Silman I, Sussman JL: **Flexibility of aromatic residues in the active-site gorge of acetylcholinesterase: X-ray versus molecular dynamics.** *Biophys J* 2008, **95**:2500–2511.
44. Wallace AC, Laskowski RA, Thornton JM: **L{IGPLOT}: a program to generate schematic diagrams of protein-ligand interactions.** *Protein Eng* 1995, **8**:127–134.
45. Hosseinzadeh R, Maleki R, Matin AA: **Interaction of diclofenac with bovine serum albumin investigated by diclofenac-selective electrode.** *Acta Chim Slov* 2007, **54**:126–130.
46. Hamilton JA1, Era S, Bhamidipati SP, Reed RG: **Locations of the three primary binding sites for long-chain fatty acids on bovine serum albumin.** *Proc Natl Acad Sci* 1991, **88**:2051–2054.
47. Guex N, Peitsch MC: **SWISS-MODEL and the Swiss-Pdb viewer: an environment for comparative protein modeling.** *Electrophoresis* 1997, **18**:2714–2723.

6

Osteogenic potential of *punica granatum* through matrix mineralization, cell cycle progression and runx2 gene expression in primary rat osteoblasts

Sahabjada Siddiqui and Mohammad Arshad*

Abstract

Background: Osteoporosis is one of the prevalent diseases in ageing populations. Due to side effects of many chemotherapeutic agents, there is always a need to search for herbal products to treat the disorder. *Punica granatum* (PG) represent a potent fruit-bearing medicinal herb which exerted valuable anti-osteoporotic activities. The present study was carried out to validate the *in vitro* osteogenic effects of the PG seed extract in primary calvarial osteoblast cultures harvested from neonatal rats.

Methods: The ethanolic extract of PG was subjected to evaluate cell proliferation, regeneration, mineralization and formation of collagen matrix using MTT, alkaline phosphatase, Alizarin Red-S staining and Sirius Red dye, respectively. Cell cycle progression and osteogenic gene Runx2 expression were carried out by flow cytometry and real time PCR, respectively.

Results: Exposure of different concentrations (10–100 μg/ml) of the extract on osteoblastic cells showed characteristic morphological changes and increment in cell number. A significant growth in cell proliferation, ALP activity, collagen contents and matrix mineralization of osteoblasts in a dose dependent manner ($p < 0.05$), suggested that PG has a stimulatory effect on osteoblastic bone formation or potential activity against osteoporosis. In addition, PG extract also enhanced DNA content in S phase of cell cycle and Runx2 gene expression level in osteoblasts.

Conclusion: The data clearly indicated that PG promoting bone cell proliferation and differentiation in primary osteoblasts might be due to elevating the osteogenic gene Runx2 expression. The present study provides an evidence for PG could be a promising herbal medicinal candidate that able to develop drugs for osteoporosis.

Keywords: Cell cycle, Osteoblast, Osteogenesis, *Punica granatum*, Runx2

Introduction

Osteoporosis is a metabolic bone disorders that afflicts about 200 million people worldwide. It is mainly prevalent in women (approximately 80%) and also older men [1]. The bone remodeling process is the alternative of this severe concern, and it's dependable for repair of damage or formation and resorption of bones to maintain the integrity of the skeleton. However, any abnormalities in remodeling that lead to fracture in the bones and osteoporosis.

Recently, several conventional and antiresorptive drugs are used to reduce fracture risk in osteoporosis including hormone replacement therapy (HRT), bisphosphonates, selective estrogen receptor modulators (SERMs) and calcitonin [2]. However, these drugs and therapy have multiple side effects, which causes heart related issues, headache, dizziness, anorexia, cramping of legs and gastrointestinal related problem, particularly pain in stomach and heartburn [3]. The research still continues for the enhancement of such benefit to lower risk involved in human beings.

Anabolic or osteogenic therapies are preferred for pharmacological development to treat osteoporosis [4]. Parathyroid hormone (PTH 1–34) only anabolic agent for the treatment of postmenopausal osteoporosis that is also recommended by the FDA (Food and Drug Administration) which regulates the formation of bones by enhancing the cell proliferation of the osteoblastic lineage or inducing differentiation of osteoblast progenitor cells.

* Correspondence: molendolab@gmail.com
Molecular Endocrinology Laboratory, Department of Zoology, University of Lucknow, Lucknow 226007, India

Whilst, this therapy is also related to an increased risk of cancer, such as osteosarcoma [5,6].

In the recent time, several medicinal plants are used for health care treatments and management especially bone related diseases. Although compared with other drug treatments, herbal products create no/little side effects. *Punica granatum* (Pomegranate, PG) is one of the most potent fruit-bearing medicinal herbs widely distributed throughout the Mediterranean region of southern Europe, northern Africa and tropical Africa, Indian subcontinent, Central Asia and the drier parts of South-East Asia. PG seeds contain punicic acid, ellagic acid, steroidal estrogen and non-steroidal phytoestrogens, including comesten, coumoestrol and isoflavones genistein, daidzein and ascorbic acids. PG also contains estrogenic compound such as luteolin, quercetin, kaempferol, estrone and estradiol, which are responsible for bone formation and also inhibit the resorption process [7-12]. A non-isoflavone phytoestrogenic compounds such as quercetin, rutin, apigenin and coumestrol has also been reported in various legumes [13]. A crude PG extract and its seed oil enhance bone healing properties and prevent loss of bones because of the proliferation of osteoblast, inhibition of osteoclast cell and also decrease the inflammation. [14,15]. Recently, PG has been also utilized to inhibit acetyl cholinesterase activity as a new source for management of Alzheimer's disease [16].

Osteoblast differentiation and proliferation mediated by different growth factors such as bone morphogenetic proteins (BMPs), transforming growth factor beta (TGFβ) and core-binding factor alpha1 (Cbfα1) are known to be targeted the osteogenic Runt-related transcription factor2 (Runx2) gene [17]. Runx2 is the key transcription factor initiating and regulating the early osteogenesis and late mineralization of bone. Furthermore, Runx2 triggers the expression of major bone matrix genes during the early stages of osteoblast differentiation [18].

There is no evidence regarding the investigation of the PG seed extract on bone cell proliferation, differentiation, and collagen matrix formation in primary culture of osteoblasts. The present study also described the matrix mineralization activity along with osteogenic gene Runx2 expression by real time PCR and DNA content analysis in the S phase of the cell cycle in osteoblastic cells. The findings suggested that PG may be a potent osteogenic herbal drug that induces bone cells proliferation and regeneration following increased DNA contents and Runx2 gene expression which provide future prospects in the development of anti-osteoporotic drugs and therapy.

Materials and methods

Reagents and chemicals

Alpha modified minimum essential medium (α-MEM), fetal bovine serum (FBS), MTT (3-(4,5-dimethylthiazol-2-yl) -2,5-diphenyltetrazolium bromide) dye, *p*-nitrophenyl phosphate (pNPP), naphthol ASMX phosphate, fast blue BB salt, ascorbic acid and Sirius Red dye were purchased from Himedia, India. β-glycerophosphate, Ribonuclease (RNase) A and propidium iodide (PI) were purchased from Sigma-Aldrich, USA. RNAiso Plus reagent was procured from Takara, India. cDNA synthesis kit was purchased from Thermo Scientific, USA and SYBER green kit from Roche, USA. All the reagents used were of high purity grade.

Plant materials and extraction

The fresh cultivated PG plant was collected from nearby University of Lucknow, Lucknow, India. Plant materials were identified and authenticated from Department of Pharmacognosy, Faculty of Pharmacy, Integral University, Lucknow. A reference specimen (voucher No. IU/PHAR/HRB/14/08) has been deposited in the herbarium of Faculty of Pharmacy, Integral University, Lucknow. Seed parts of collecting plant were air dried in the shade and crushed to a powder in a mechanical grinder. The 95% ethanolic extract of PG was prepared with the help of Soxhlet apparatus (Borosil Glass Works Limited, India) at 60°C and Whatman No. 1 filter paper was used to obtain filtrate of extract. The filtrate was concentrated in vacuum at 40°C using a rotary evaporator (BUCHI Rotavapor R-205, Switzerland).

Primary culture of osteoblasts

Osteoblastic cells were isolated from neonatal rat pups calvaria using sequential digestion with slight modification [19]. Briefly, calvaria were dissected from four to five neonatal (1–2 days old) rat pups. After removal of sutures and adherent mesenchymal tissues, calvaria were subjected to five sequential (10–15 min) digestions at 37°C in shaking water bath at 120 rpm containing each of 0.1% dispase and collagenase type II enzymes. Supernatants were pooled from the second to fifth digestions in a tube containing 800 μl FBS. Cells were re-suspended in α-MEM containing 10% FBS with 1% penicillin/streptomycin solution and transfer in T-25 cm^2 culture flasks. The flasks were incubated at 37°C with 5% CO_2 in CO_2 incubator (Excella ECO-170, New Brunswick). The study was approved by the Institutional Animal Ethics Committee of Azad Institute of Pharmacy and Research, Lucknow (Ref. No.: AIPR/2013-14/1398).

Cell proliferation

The proliferative effect of PG extract was determined using MTT assay with some modification [20]. Calvarial osteoblasts were suspended in α-MEM medium and plated at a density of 2×10^3 cells/well in a 96 wells plate. After overnight incubation, the medium was replaced with a medium containing PG extract solution prepared in media with different concentrations (0, 10, 25, 50 and 100 μg/ml) in triplicate for 48 h. 17β-estradiol (E2) at the concentration of 1 nM was used as a positive control. After exposure period, 10 μl of 5 mg/ml MTT solution was added to each wells and further incubated at 37°C. After 4 h, medium was discarded and 100 μl of dimethyl sulphoxide (DMSO) was added to solubilise the dark blue formazan crystals at 37°C for 10 min. Absorbance was recorded at 540 nm with microplate reader (BIORAD-680, USA) and the percentage viable cells were calculated using the formula:

$$\%\text{Cell viability} = [(\text{OD of treated}) / (\text{OD of control})] \times 100$$

The cellular morphology was also observed in other sets of PG treatment under trinocular inverted phase contrast microscopy (Nikon ECLIPSE T*i*-S, Japan).

Alkaline phosphatase (ALP) activity

ALP assay is based on the hydrolysis of pNPP by ALP into a yellow colored product at alkaline pH. ALP activity of osteoblasts was determined with a slight modification [21]. A 100 μl of cell suspension containing 2×10^3cells /well was seeded in 96-well plates using α-MEM supplemented with 10% FBS, 10 mM β-glycerophosphate, 50 μg/ml ascorbic acid and 1% penicillin/streptomycin (osteoblast differentiation medium) and treated with different concentrations (10–100 μg/ml) of the extract for 48 h. E2 at the concentration of 1 nM was used as a positive control. After completion of incubation period, osteoblast cultures were fixed in 4% paraformaldehyde and stained with a solution containing 0.1 mg/ml naphthol ASMX phosphate, 0.5% N, N- dimethylformamide, 2 mM MgCl2, and 0.6 mg/ml of fast blue BB salt in 0.1 mM Tris–HCl (pH 8.5) for 20 min. The formation of color was examined and images were taken under an inverted phase contrast microscope. For the quantitative estimation of ALP, the plate was fixed and kept in −70°C for 20 min, and then brought to 37°C for freeze fracture. Next, 50 μl of chilled *p*-nitrophenyl phosphate (pNPP) substrate was added to each wells and incubated at 37°C for 30 min for color development. The absorbance was measured at 405 nM using an ELISA reader.

Assessment of collagen deposition

Sirius Red is an anionic dye that binds strongly to collagen molecules. Collagen deposition was quantified using Sirius Red dye following slightly modification [22]. Treated cells were washed with PBS and dried at 37°C in 96-wells plate for overnight incubation and then stained with 20 μl of Sirius Red dye (0.1% in saturated picric acid) for 1 h with mild shaking. Sirius Red dye solution (pH 3.5) was prepared in saturated aqueous picric acid (1.3% in H_2O) at a concentration of 0.1 mg/ml. The stained cell layers were extensively washed with 0.01 N HCl to remove all non-bounded dye. After rinsing, photographs were taken under inverted phase contrast microscope. For quantitative analysis, the stained cells were dissolved in 0.2 ml 0.1 N NaOH at shaker for 30 min. Next, absorbance was measured colorimetrically at 550 nm against 0.1 N NaOH serve as a blank.

Mineralization assay

Alizarin Red S, an anthraquinone derivative, was used to identify calcium content in osteoblasts according to a method reported previously [23]. Approximately, 2×10^4 cells/well were seeded in 12-wells culture plate in osteoblast differentiation medium with 10^{-7} M dexamethasone. Cells were treated with PG extract at various concentrations (10–100 μg/ml) for 21 days and the medium was changed every alternate day. At the end of the experiment, cells were washed with PBS and fixed with 4% paraformaldehyde in PBS for 15 min. The fixed cells were stained with 40 mM Alizarin Red-S (pH 4.5) for 30 min followed by washing with distilled water. Calcified nodules appearing as bright red color were photographed under inverted phase contrast microscopy. For quantification of staining, 100 mM cetylpyridinium chloride solution was added for 1 h in each well to solubilise and to release calcium-bound alizarin red into solution. A 100 μl of the supernatant from each well were transferred in 96 well plate in triplicate and the absorbance was recorded at 570 nm by a microplate reader.

Cellular DNA content

Cell cycle phase distribution with cellular DNA content was analyzed using flow cytometry with some modification [24]. Osteoblasts were planted in 6-wells plate at a density 1×10^6 cells/well and treated with different concentrations (10–100 μg/ml) of extract for 48 h. E2 at the concentration of 10 nM was used as a positive control. Cultured cells were washed with cold PBS and fixed in 70% ethanol at −20°C for 2 h. Fixed cells were treated with RNase A (10 mg/ml) and stained with PI dye in the dark for 30 min at room temperature. The PI dye fluorescence of individual nuclei was measured by using a flow cytometer (BD FACS Calibur, Becton Dickinson, USA) and data were analyzed using Cell Quest Pro V 3.2.1 software (Becton Dickinson, USA).

Quantitative real-time PCR (qPCR)

The total RNA was isolated from cultured osteoblasts treated with PG extract using RNAiso Plus reagent. Aliquots of 2.0 μg of total RNA in a 10 μl reaction volume were subjected to PCR using a cDNA synthesis kit. Quantitative real-time PCR was performed in light cycler PCR system (LightCycler 480, Roche, USA) using SYBER green kit following manufacturer's instruction. Runx2 gene expression in calvarial osteoblasts was determined by qPCR using an optimized protocol [25]. Sequence of primer pairs of the genes used in the present study were; runx2- CCACAGAGCTATTAAAGTGACAGTG (F), AACAAACTAGGTTTAGAGTCATCAAGC (R) and GAPDH (housekeeping gene) - CAGCAAGGATACTGA GAGCAAGAG (F), GGATGGAATTGTGAGGGAGATG (R). All the data were normalized to GAPDH expression to study the relative expression of the targeted gene.

Statistics

All results were represented as the means ± SEM of results from all replicates and statistically significance was determined by one-way analysis of variance (ANOVA) followed by Dunnett's multiple comparison tests. Probability values of $p < 0.05$ were considered to be statistically significant. All analysis was conducted using the Graph Pad Prism (Ver. 5.1) software.

Results and discussion

Microscopic observation of osteoblastic cells

The morphological changes of untreated (control) and treated osteoblasts with different concentrations of PG extract at 48 h are shown in Figure 1A. The typical spindle shaped with fibroblastic appearance was observed in control under inverted phase contrast microscope. The concentrations 10 and 25 μg/ml of extract enhanced the cell proliferation, moreover, 50 and 100 μg/ml of PG showed the more dense appearance with increased number of cells as compared to control that attributed differentiation of osteoblastic cells. The results revealed that cells exposed to PG extract induce differentiation of osteoblasts as a function of dose due to their morphological alterations and number of cells increment [26].

Effect of PG on the cell proliferation of osteoblasts

The effect of different doses (10–100 μg/ml) of PG extract on osteoblastic cell proliferation was tested at 48 h (Figure 1B). As compared to control group (cells without extract treatment), PG significantly increased the cell proliferation to 13.03 ($p < 0.05$) and 24.28% ($p < 0.001$) at 10 and 25 μg/ml, respectively. Moreover, 50 and 100 μg/ml of PG extract induced cell proliferation to 39.64 and 62.59% ($p < 0.001$) respectively. The results revealed that PG extract induced the significant cell proliferation in a dose dependent manner. Exposure of cells to 1 nM of 17β-estradiol as a positive control, increased the cell proliferation to 41.72% ($p < 0.001$) as compared to control. The proliferative effects of PG extract might be due to their estrogenic nature of its contents, including quercetin, kaempferol, estrone and estradiol, which promote bone cell proliferation [11]. A study has shown that PG promoted osteoblast MC3T3-E1 cell proliferation up to approximately 2-fold at 250 μg/ml of plant extracts [7]. Both osteoblast and MCF-7 (human breast adenocarcinoma) cells are an estrogen receptor positive (ER^+) cells. A similar study has also revealed that MCF-7 cells exposed to legume extracts containing quercetin, daidzein, genistein and kaempferol glycosides at various concentrations (1–1000 μg/ml) showed a maximum cell proliferation at 100 μg/ml of the extracts [27].

Effect of PG on ALP activity of osteoblasts

Quantitative estimation of alkaline phosphatase activity is one of the biochemical methods, which described the early cell differentiation of osteoblastic cells [28]. Fast blue BB salt-ASMX-phosphate complex acted on ALP activity which appeared to be blue in color. The qualitative data showed that PG extract stimulated ALP stain by increasing the rate of osteoblast cell differentiation in a dose dependent manner (Figure 2A). As observed from numerical data (Figure 2B), concentrations 10 and 25 μg/ml of extract induced ALP level to 9.66% ($p < 0.05$) and 22.49% ($p < 0.01$) significantly as compared to control. Also, 50 and 100 μg/ml of extract induced the significant ALP level to 34.67 and 43.95% ($p < 0.01$) respectively as compared to control. Exposure of cells to 1 nM of E2 increased ALP activity to 36.66% ($p < 0.01$) as compared to control. Results of ALP assay were the consistent with

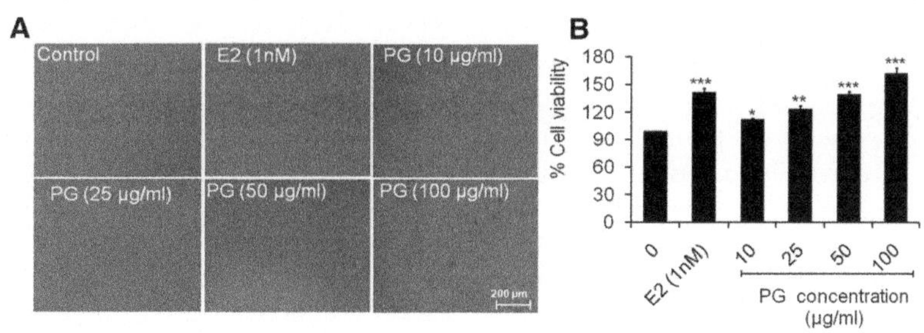

Figure 1 Percent cell proliferation of primary osteoblasts. (A) Morphology of osteoblasts under inverted phase contrast microscope treated with different concentrations of PG extract at 48 h **(B)** Percent cell proliferation of osteoblasts treated with 10–100 μg/ml of PG extract. Values were obtained from three independent experiments and expressed as mean ± SEM. $^*p < 0.05$, $^{**}p < 0.01$ and $^{***}p < 0.001$ as compared with control.

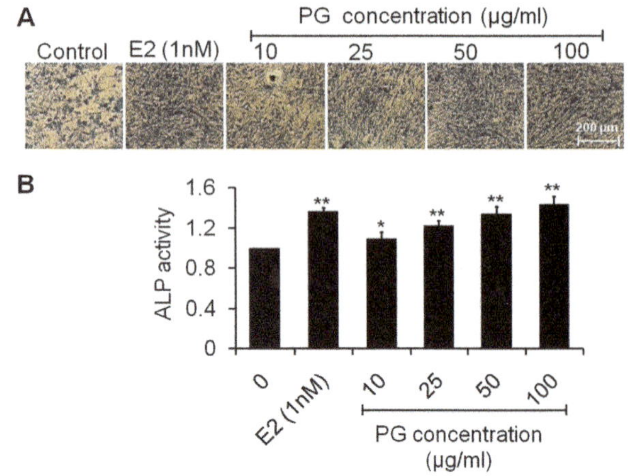

Figure 2 Measurement of ALP activity. (A) Photomicrographs stained with fast blue BB salt-ASMX-phosphate complex showing increased formation of ALP in osteoblasts treated with increasing concentrations (10–100 µg/ml) of PG extract at 48 h **(B)** Quantitative data of ALP level presented in the form of ALP activity relative to control. Values are obtained from three independent experiments and expressed as mean ± SEM. *p < 0.05 and **p < 0.01 as compared with control.

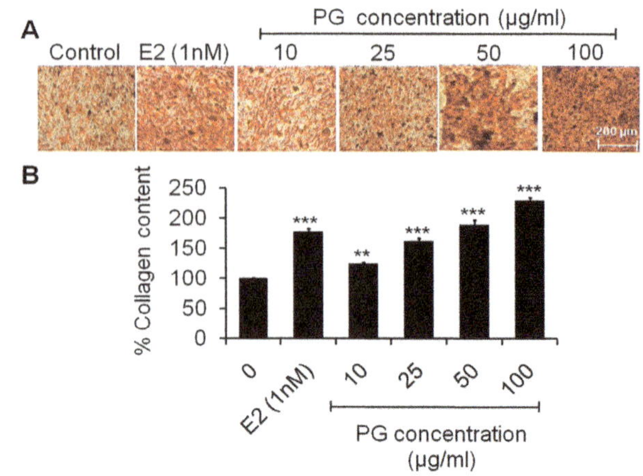

Figure 3 Collagen formation assay of osteoblasts. (A) Photomicrographs stained with Sirius Red dye showing increased formation of collagen matrix of osteoblasts treated with increasing concentrations (10–100 µg/ml) of PG extract at 48 h **(B)** Quantitative data of collagen content expressed in the form of percent collagen content respective to control. Data represented as mean ± SEM of three independent experiments. **p < 0.01 and ***p < 0.001 as compared with control.

MTT assay data which suggested that cell proliferation also correlate with cell differentiation. These results indicate that PG extract induces regeneration of osteoblasts as a function of dose might be due to the presence of estrogenic compounds. PG containing estrogenic compounds daidzein and genistein has been reported to possess stimulatory effects synthesizing alkaline phosphatase by osteoblasts *in vitro* [29].

Effect of PG on collagen deposition by osteoblasts

Sirius Red stain was used to assess the extent of collagen (predominantly collagen type I and III fibers) deposited by osteoblasts which developed dense and cross-linked collagen. Collagen comprises 85-90% of the total organic bone matrix [30]. Histological analysis showed that PG extract increases collagen content in osteoblasts in a dose dependent manner as compared to control. PG extract exposed on cells was able to enhance in the collagen density significantly as evident by dark red clusters of collagen evenly distributed throughout the stimulated region (Figure 3A). Further, quantitative measurement of the Sirius Red staining intensity in osteoblasts culture showed a significant increment of 24.96 ($p < 0.01$), 62.40, 89.37 and 129.84% ($p < 0.001$) of collagen secretion at 10, 25, 50 and 100 µg/ml of PG exposure, respectively as compared to control (Figure 3B). Exposure of osteoblasts to 1 nM of E2 increased the collagen content to only 77.95% ($p < 0.001$) as compared to control. Bone shows a variety of structural organizations which is related to the balance between the amount of collagen and mineral [31]. However, not only mineral matrix deposition is essential to ensure a healthy bone, giving strength and rigidity in the skeletal system, but also the adequate deposition of organic matrix (collagen) contributes to bone architecture. Therefore, experiments were conducted to determine whether PG extract exposure enhances the organic matrix deposition. PG treated osteoblasts progressively deposited more collagen (Figure 3A and B) suggesting the collagen deposition induced by PG is a function of dose. A study has reported that ascorbic acid stimulates the formation of collagen matrix at multiple levels, including gene expression, hydroxylation of proline and lysine in collagen during post-translational modification [32].

Effect of PG on osteoblast mineralization

Mineralized nodule formation describes the final stages of osteoblastic differentiation at 21 days. As observed from photomicrographs, osteoblastic cells in proliferation period exhibited a fibroblastic morphology monolayer in control cells. As the progress in mineralization, the cells continued growing slowly and formed a mosaic like multiple layers which was greater at 100 µg/ml of PG extract (Figure 4A). The percent calcification data of Alizarin stain showed that treatment of osteoblasts at 10, 25, 50 and 100 µg/ml of extract significantly increased mineralized nodule formation that signifying by 26.15 ($p < 0.01$), 44.55, 65.64 and 82.81% ($p < 0.001$), respectively as compared to control (Figure 4B). Exposure of

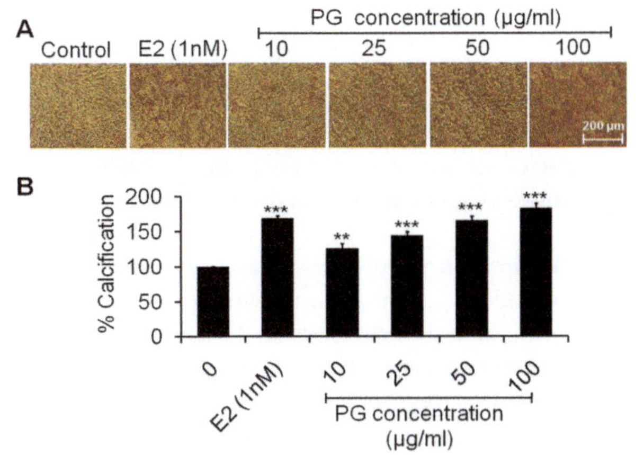

Figure 4 Mineralization assay of osteoblasts. (A) Photomicrographs stained with Alizarin Red S showing increased formation of mineralized nodules of osteoblasts treated with increasing concentrations (10–100 µg/ml) of PG extract at 21 days **(B)** Quantitative data of Alizarin Red-S extraction expressed in the form of percent calcification. Data represented as mean ± SEM of three independent experiments. **p < 0.01 and ***p < 0.001 as compared with control.

osteoblasts to 1 nM of E2 increased the mineralization content to 68.85% ($p < 0.001$) as compared to control. Increased mineralization is synonymous to increased calcium deposition. The ability to form an extracellular matrix that can undergo regulated mineralization is the ultimate phenotypic expression of an osteogenic tissue [33]. PG treatment increased the calcium content notably in the mineralized matrix at 21 days of osteoblasts when compared with untreated cells. In this context, the phytoestrogen genistein has been previously found to stimulate bone mineralization *in vitro* [34].

Effect of PG on cellular DNA content and cell cycle distribution of osteoblasts

The cellular DNA content and proportion of cells in different phases of the cell cycle was analyzed by using flow cytometry. Osteoblastic cells were treated with one lower (25 µg/ml) and one higher concentration (100 µg/ml) of the PG extract for 48 h and observed the different phases of the cell cycle. As evident from the results (Figure 5), a normal distribution of cell cycle was observed in the control group. At 25 µg/ml of PG extract, the accumulation of cells (DNA content) in S phase was sharply increased from 12.67 to 31.54% as compared to control. Moreover, 100 µg/ml concentration of the extract resulted to an incredible increment of DNA content in S phase by 78.72% as compared to control. Exposure of osteoblasts to 1 nM of E2 increased the DNA content in S phase by 44.08% greater at 25 µg/ml of PG treatment. These data indicate that the PG extract induce the cell proliferation by accumulating the DNA content in S phase of the cell cycle. A similar study has reported that estradiol induced the expression of estrogen receptor by promoting S phase of cell cycle in human osteosarcoma cell lines and pilose antler polypeptides promoted chondrocytes proliferation by accelerating cell cycle progression in S phase [35,24].

Effect of PG on osteogenic gene runx2 expression

To determine these results could be extended to another protein present in the organic bone matrix and effect of PG on the expression of Runx2 gene. Runx2 is a noncollagenous, highly conserved transcription factor involved in the regulation of mineralized matrix of bone. Increased expression of osteogenic gene was observed by qPCR in osteoblasts treated with PG extract at 48 h. As cleared from results (Figure 6), 10 µg/ml of PG extract significantly elevated the Runx2 expression as compared to

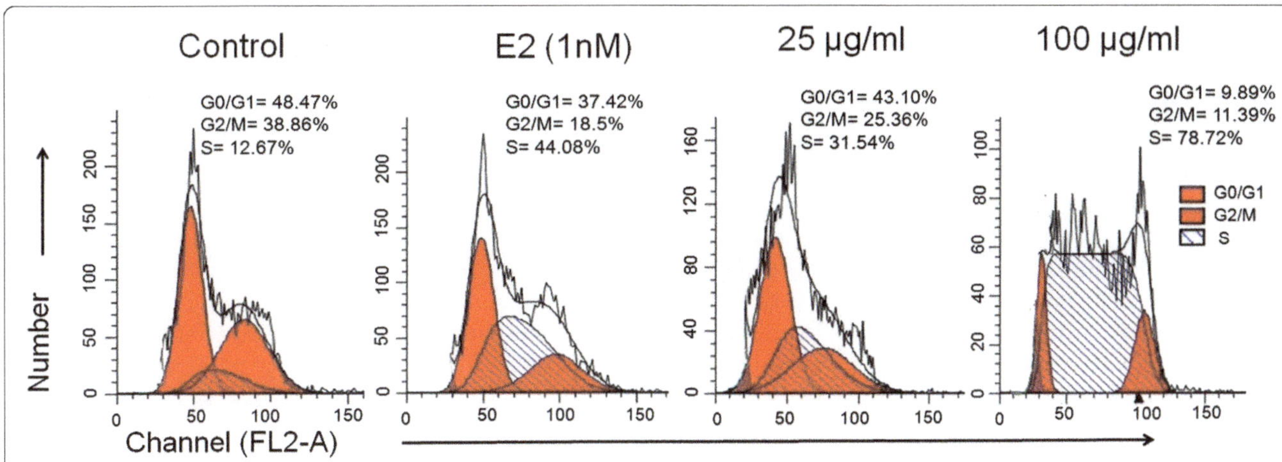

Figure 5 Analysis of DNA content by flow cytometry. Pictorial graph showing the proportion of osteoblastic cells in different phases of cell cycle stained with PI dye of treated with 1 nM of E2 as a positive control and 25 and 100 µg/ml of PG extract at 48 h.

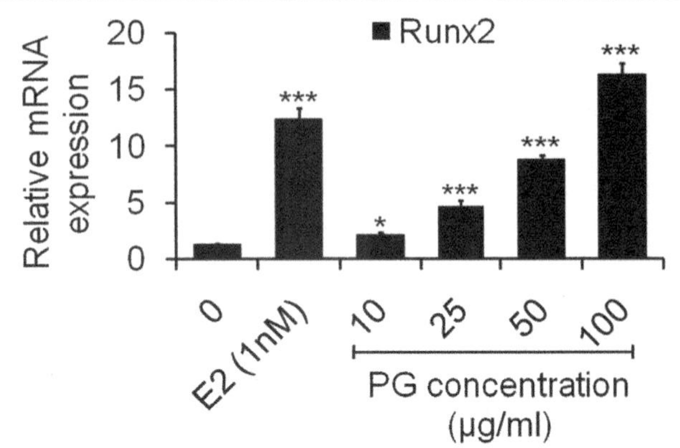

Figure 6 Analysis of mRNA levels of Runx2 gene by qPCR. Osteoblasts were treated with (10–100 μg/ml) of PG for 48 h. qPCR for Runx2 mRNAs was performed. At each concentration, PG increased the mRNA levels when compared to control. Fold changes in mRNA levels are indicated by the numbers derived after normalizing with GAPDH mRNA levels used as an internal control. Values are obtained from three independent experiments in triplicate and expressed as mean ± SEM; $^{*}p < 0.05$, $^{*}p < 0.01$ and $^{***}p < 0.001$ as compared with control.

control ($p < 0.05$). Moreover, concentrations 25, 50 and 100 μg/ml of PG increased the remarkable Runx2 level in a dose dependent manner ($p < 0.001$) as compared to control. It has been reported that Runx2 bonds to the osteoblast specific cis acting element which is found in the promoter region of all major osteoblast specific genes like osteocalcin, type-I collagen, BSP, OPN, ALP and control their expression [36]. Hence, it is reasonable to speculate that the estrogenic compounds such as β-sitosterol present in PG could have acted in a manner to induce mRNA expression of ALP, collagen and their protein levels and consequently increased Runx2 gene expression in osteoblastic cells. Furthermore, flavonoids have also been shown to increase the expression of Runx2 [37,38]. Thus, β-sitosterol and flavonoids present in PG might be responsible for the increased expression and transcriptional activity of Runx2.

Conclusion

The present study showed that osteogenic potential of PG extract in primary calvaria osteoblasts is based on two salient features. (1) Cytochemical studies including cell proliferation, ALP stain, collagenation, matrix mineralization and DNA content in the S phase of the cell cycle in osteoblasts are the key parameters, which favor the osteogenic potential of PG. (2) A molecular marker Runx2 is a highly conserved osteogenic transcription factor involved in the regulation of bone cells proliferation and differentiation, which is also favors the osteogenic nature of PG.

Even though E2 used as a positive control shows the slightly higher effect on the proliferation, differentiation, collagenation, mineralization, DNA content and Runx2 gene expression of osteoblasts than lower doses, however, the side effects of the long-term use of estrogen, such as a higher incidence of endometrial cancer, cardiovascular disease and breast carcinoma, could not be ignored.

Thus, the results from this study suggest that PG promotes the function of osteoblasts and plays an important role in remodeling of the bone, which indicated that it may be one of anti-osteoporotic herbal candidate free from side effects. Accordingly, PG might be useful for alternative pharmacological agent of osteoporosis and skeletal tissues may benefit from the consumption of PG.

Abbreviations

ALP: Alkaline phosphatase; α-MEM: Alpha modified minimum essential medium; E2: 17β-estradiol; BMPs: Bone morphogenetic proteins; Cbfα1: Core-binding factor alpha-1; DMSO: Dimethyl sulfoxide; ELISA: Enzyme linked immunosorbent assay; FBS: Fetal bovine serum; FDA: Food and drug administration; HRT: Hormone replacement therapy; MTT: (3-(4,5-dimethylthiazol-2-yl)-2,5-diphenyltetrazolium bromide); PBS: Phosphate buffered saline; PG: *Punica granatum*; pNPP: *p*-nitrophenyl phosphate; PTH: Parathyroid hormone; PI: Propidium iodide; qPCR: Quantitative real-time PCR; Runx2: Runt-related transcription factor 2; SEM: Standard error mean; SERMs: Selective estrogen receptor modulators; TGFβ: Transforming growth factors.

Competing interests

The authors declare that they have no competing interests.

Authors' contributions

SS and MA participated in the design of the study. SS performed the experimental work and data interpretation. SS and MA involved in review of the paper. Both authors read and approved the final version of the manuscript.

Authors' information

Sahabjada Siddiqui, M.Sc. in Biotechnology; Md Arshad, Ph.D. in Endocrinology, CDRI, Lucknow and Assistant Professor at University of Lucknow.

Acknowledgments

Authors are thankful to UGC Major Research Project File No. 37-436/2009 (SR), New Delhi, India for financial support. Author Sahabjada Siddiqui is thankful to ICMR, New Delhi, India for the award of Senior Research Fellowship (No. 45/26/2013/BMS/TRM). Authors are thankful to the Director, Azad Institute of Pharmacy and Research, Lucknow for providing research facilities for animal experiment.

References

1. Kaunitz AM, Mcclung MR, Feldman RG: **Post menopausal osteoporosis: fracture risk and prevention.** *J Fam Pract* 2009, **58:**S1–S6.
2. Maclaughlin EJ, Sleeper RB, McNatty D, Raehl CL: **Management of age-related osteoporosis and prevention of associated fractures.** *Ther Clin Risk Manag* 2006, **2:**281–295.
3. Rizzoli R, Reginster JY, Boonen S, Bréart G, Diez-Perez A, Felsenberg D, Kaufman JM, Kanis JA, Cooper C: **Adverse reactions and drug-drug interactions in the management of women with postmenopausal osteoporosis.** *Calcif Tissue Int* 2011, **89:**91–104.
4. Dixit P, Khan MP, Swarnkar G, Chattopadhyay N, Maurya R: **Osteogenic constituents from *pterospermum acerifolium* willd. Flowers.** *Bioorg Med Chem Lett* 2011, **21:**4617–4621.

5. John MR, Arai M, Rubin DA, Jonsson KB, Jüppner H: **Identification and characterization of the murine and human gene encoding the tuberoinfundibular peptide of 39 residues.** *Endocrinology* 2002, **143**:1047–1057.
6. Wang W, Olson D, Cheng B, Guo X, Wang K: **Sanguis Draconis resin stimulates osteoblast alkaline phosphatase activity and mineralization in MC3T3-E1 cells.** *J Ethnopharmacol* 2012, **142**:168–174.
7. Kim YH, Choi EM: **Stimulation of osteoblastic differentiation and inhibition of interleukin-6 and nitric oxide in MC3T3-E1 cells by pomegranate ethanol extract.** *Phytother Res* 2009, **23**:737–739.
8. van Elswijk DA, Schobel UP, Lansky EP, Irth H, van der Greef J: **Rapid dereplication of estrogenic compounds in pomegranate (*punica granatum*) using on-line biochemical detection coupled to mass spectrometry.** *Phytochemistry* 2004, **65**:233–241.
9. Trivedi R, Kumar A, Gupta V, Kumar S, Nagar GK, Romero JR, Dwivedi AK, Chattopadhyay N: **Effects of Egb 761 on bone mineral density, bone microstructure, and osteoblast function: Possible roles of quercetin and kaempferol.** *Mol Cell Endocrinol* 2009, **302**:86–91.
10. Heftmann E, Ko ST, Bennett RD: **Identification of estrone in pomegranate seeds.** *Phytochemistry* 1966, **5**:1337–1339.
11. Jurenka J: **Therapeutic applications of pomegranate (*punica granatum* L.): a review.** *Alterm Med Rev* 2008, **13**:128–144.
12. Pérez-Vicente A, Gil-Izquierdo A, García-Viguera C: ***In vitro* gastrointestinal digestion study of pomegranate juice phenolic compounds, anthocyanins, and vitamin C.** *J Agric Food Chem* 2002, **50**:2308–2312.
13. Konar N: **Non-isoflavone phytoestrogenic compound contents of various legumes.** *Eur Food Res Technol* 2013, **236**:523–530.
14. Spilmont M, Léotoing L, Davicco MJ, Lebecque P, Mercier S, Miot-Noirault E, Pilet P, Rios L, Wittrant Y, Coxam V: **Pomegranate seed oil prevents bone loss in a mice model of osteoporosis, through osteoblastic stimulation, osteoclastic inhibition and decreased inflammatory status.** *J Nutr Biochem* 2013, **24**:1840–1848.
15. Mori-Okamoto J, Otawara-Hamamoto Y, Yamato H, Yoshimura H: **Pomegranate extract improves a depressive state and bone properties in menopausal syndrome model ovariectomized mice.** *J Ethnopharmacol* 2004, **92**:93–101.
16. Jazayeri SB, Amanlou A, Ghanadian N, Pasalar P, Amanlou M: **A preliminary investigation of anticholinesterase activity of some Iranian medicinal plants commonly used in traditional medicine.** *Daru* 2014, **22**:17.
17. Yamaguchi A, Komori T, Suda T: **Regulation of osteoblast differentiation mediated by bone morphogenetic proteins, hedgehogs, and Cbfa1.** *Endocr Rev* 2000, **21**:393–411.
18. Komori T: **Regulation of osteoblast differentiation by Runx2.** *Adv Exp Med Biol* 2010, **658**:43–49.
19. Orriss IR, Taylor SE, Arnett TR: **Rat osteoblast cultures.** *Methods Mol Biol* 2012, **816**:31–41.
20. Ashfaq M, Singh S, Sharma A, Verma N: **Cytotoxic evaluation of the hierarchal web of carbon micro-nanofibers.** *Ind Eng Chem Res* 2013, **52**:4672–4682.
21. Moutahir-Belqasmi F, Balmain N, Lieberrher M, Borzeix S, Berland S, Barthelemy M, Peduzzi J, Milet C, Lopez E: **Effect of water soluble extract of nacre (pinctada maxima) on alkaline phosphatase activity and Bcl-2 expression in primary cultured osteoblasts from neonatal rat calvaria.** *J Mater Sci Mater Med* 2001, **12**:1–6.
22. Tullberg-Reinert H, Jundt G: ***In situ* measurement of collagen synthesis by human bone cells with a sirius red-based colorimetric microassay: effects of transforming growth factor beta2 and ascorbic acid 2-phosphate.** *Histochem Cell Biol* 1999, **112**:271–276.
23. Weivoda MM, Hohl RJ: **Effects of farnesyl pyrophosphate accumulation on calvarial osteoblast differentiation.** *Endocrinology* 2011, **152**:3113–3122.
24. Lin JH, Deng LX, Wu ZY, Chen L, Zhang L: **Pilose antler polypeptides promote chondrocyte proliferation via the tyrosine kinase signaling pathway.** *J Occup Med Toxicol* 2011, **6**:27.
25. Dixit P, Chand K, Khan MP, Siddiqui JA, Tewari D, Ngueguim FT, Chattopadhyay N, Maurya R: **Phytoceramides and acylated phytosterol glucosides from *pterospermum acerifolium* willd. Seed coat and their osteogenic activity.** *Phytochemistry* 2012, **81**:117–125.
26. Abiramasundari G, Sumalatha KR, Sreepriya M: **Effects of *tinospora cordifolia*** (menispermaceae) on the proliferation, osteogenic differentiation and mineralization of osteoblast model systems *in vitro*. *J Ethnopharmacol* 2012, **141**:474–480.
27. Zhao QW, Li B, Weber N, Lou YJ: **Estrogen-like effects of ethanol extracts from several Chinese legumes on MCF-7 cell.** *Eur Food Res Technol* 2005, **221**:828–833.
28. Bhargavan B, Gautam AK, Singh D, Kumar A, Chaurasia S, Tyagi AM, Yadav DK, Mishra JS, Singh AB, Sanyal S, Goel A, Maurya R, Chattopadhyay N: **Methoxylated isoflavones, cajanin and isoformononetin, have non-estrogenic bone forming effect via differential mitogen activated protein kinase (MAPK) signalling.** *J Cell Biochem* 2009, **108**:388–399.
29. Sugimoto E, Yamaguchi M: **Stimulatory effect of daidzein in osteoblastic MC3T3-E1 cells.** *Biochem Pharmacol* 2000, **259**:471–475.
30. Sasano Y, Li HC, Zhu JX, Imanaka-Yoshida K, Mizoguchi I, Kagayama M: **Immunohistochemical localization of type I collagen, fibronectin and tenascin C during embryonic osteogenesis in the dentary of mandibles and tibias in rats.** *Histochem J* 2000, **32**:591–598.
31. Landis WJ: **The strength of a calcified tissue depends in part on the molecular structure and organization of its constituent mineral crystals in their organic matrix.** *Bone* 1995, **16**:533–544.
32. Franceschi RT, Iyer BS, Cui Y: **Effects of ascorbic acid on collagen matrix formation and osteoblast differentiation in murine MC3T3-E1 cells.** *J Bone Miner Res* 1994, **9**:843–854.
33. Muthusami S, Senthilkumar K, Vignesh C, Ilangovan R, Stanley J, Selvamurugan N, Srinivasan N: **Effects of *cissus quadrangularis* on the proliferation, differentiation and matrix mineralization of human osteoblast like SaOS-2 cells.** *J Cell Bioch* 2011, **112**:1035–1045.
34. Morris C, Thorpe J, Ambrosio L, Santin M: **The soybean isoflavone genistein induces differentiation of MG63 human osteosarcoma osteoblasts.** *J Nutr* 2006, **136**:1166–1170.
35. Ikegami A, Inoue S, Hosoi T, Kaneki M, Mizuno Y, Akedo Y, Ouchi Y, Orimo H: **Cell cycle-dependent expression of estrogen receptor and effect of estrogen on proliferation of synchronized human osteoblast-like osteosarcoma cells.** *Endocrinology* 1994, **135**:782–789.
36. Ducy P, Starbuck M, Priemel M, Shen J, Pinero G, Geoffroy V, Amling M, Karsenty G: **A Cbfa1-dependent genetic pathway controls bone formation beyond embryonic development.** *Genes Dev* 1999, **13**:1025–1036.
37. Chen CH, Ho ML, Chang JK, Hung SH, Wang GJ: **Green tea catechin enhances osteogenesis in a bone marrow mesenchymal stem cell line.** *Osteoporos Int* 2005, **16**:2039–2045.
38. Qian G, Zhang X, Lu L, Wu X, Li S, Meng J: **Regulation of Cbfa1 expression by total flavonoids of Herba epimedii.** *Endocr J* 2006, **53**:87–94.

Raloxifene adjunctive therapy for postmenopausal women suffering from chronic schizophrenia: a randomized double-blind and placebo controlled trial

Gilda Kianimehr[1], Farzad Fatehi[2], Sara Hashempoor[3], Mohammad-Reza Khodaei-Ardakani[3], Farzin Rezaei[4], Ali Nazari[4], Ladan Kashani[5] and Shahin Akhondzadeh[6*]

Abstract

Background: Cumulative evidence from epidemiological, preclinical and clinical studies suggests estrogens may have psychoprotective effects in schizophrenic patients. Selective Estrogen Receptor Modulators could have therapeutic benefits in schizophrenia for both sexes without being hazardous to gynecological tissues or having feminizing effects. Few studies have been conducted regarding the effects of raloxifene on postmenopausal women suffering from schizophrenia. We conducted this placebo-controlled trial to compare the add-on effect of raloxifene to risperidone versus risperidone with placebo.

Methods: This was an 8-week, parallel-group, placebo-controlled trial undertaken at two universities affiliated psychiatric Hospitals in Iran. Forty-six postmenopausal women with the definite diagnosis of schizophrenia were enrolled in the study. Patients received risperidone (6 mg/day in 3 divided doses) combined with either placebo (N = 23) or 120 mg/day of raloxifene (N = 23) for 8 weeks. Patients were assessed by a psychiatrist at baseline and at 2 and 8 weeks after the start of medical therapy. Efficacy was defined as the change from baseline to endpoint in score on Positive and Negative Syndrome Scale (PANSS).

Results: For PANSS scores, the main effect comparing two types of intervention was not significant [$F(1, 48) = 1.77$, $p = 0.18$]. For positive subscale scores, there was marginal significant interaction between intervention type and time [$F(2, 47) = 2.93$, $p = 0.06$] and there was substantial main effect for time [$F(2, 47) = 24.39$, $p = 0.001$] within both groups showing reduction in positive subscale scores across the three time periods. In addition, the main effect comparing two types of intervention was significant [$F(1, 48) = 3.78$, $p = 0.02$]. On the other hand, for negative subscale scores, the main effect comparing two types of intervention was not significant [$F(1, 48) = 1.43$, $p = 0.23$]. For general subscale scores, the main effect comparing two types of intervention was not significant [$F(1, 48) = 0.03$, $p = 0.86$].

Conclusions: According to our findings, raloxifene as an adjunctive treatment to risperidone was only superior in improvement of positive symptoms and it was not effective in treating negative and general psychopathology symptoms.

Trial registration: The trial was registered at the Iranian registry of clinical trials: IRCT201205131556N42

Keywords: Schizophrenia, Menopause, Raloxifene, Selective estrogen receptor modulators

* Correspondence: S.akhond@neda.net
[6]Psychiatric Research Center, Roozbeh Psychiatric Hospital, Tehran University of Medical Sciences, South Kargar Street 13337, Tehran, Iran
Full list of author information is available at the end of the article

Background

Cumulative evidence from epidemiological, preclinical and clinical studies suggests estrogens may provoke psychoprotective effects in schizophrenic patients [1]. In addition, Selective Estrogen Receptor Modulators (SERMs) could have therapeutic benefits on both sexes with schizophrenia without any hazard to gynecological tissues or feminizing effects [1]. There are several lines of evidence that support the estrogen hypothesis of schizophrenia [2]. Most antipsychotics cause prolactin-inducing effects, and ensuing negative feedback on estrogen levels [2]. Sex differences in the incidence, onset and course of schizophrenia have led to the hypothesis that estrogens play a protective role in the pathophysiology of this disorder [3]. Estrogen treatment may boost the recovery of schizophrenia in women. However, adverse effects on uterine and breast tissue and other physical side effects may limit the long-term therapeutic use of estrogen [4-6]. Raloxifene hydrochloride is a selective estrogen receptor modulator that acts as an estrogen antagonist in breast tissue and may have agonistic actions in the brain, potentially offering mental health benefits with few estrogenic side effects [4].

Prognosis and severity of schizophrenia is different between males and females and as a result, it is suggested that estrogen may play a role in the pathogenesis of schizophrenia [1,3]. sex differences is a fascinating aspect of schizophrenia, which have been described for nearly all features of the illness, including the peak age of onset, symptoms and treatment response [7]. Estradiol and some SERMs are neuroprotective in a variety of experimental models of neurodegeneration; they could lessen the inflammatory response of glial cells, decrease anxiety and depression, and endorse cognition. Moreover, they are able to modulate synaptic plasticity in the hippocampus of rodents [8]; however, long term estrogen application may cause significant complications especially in menopausal women. Therefore, administration of Selective Estrogen Receptor Modulators (SERMs) may reduce such side effects. Raloxifene is a SERM that has similar dopaminergic and serotonergic effects as estrogen. Few studies have been conducted regarding the effects of raloxifene on postmenopausal women suffering from schizophrenia [9,10]. However, the sample size of these studies was relatively small [9.10]. We conducted this placebo-controlled trial to compare the add-on effect of raloxifene to risperidone in comparison with risperidone and placebo.

Methods

Trial organization

This was an 8-week, parallel-group, placebo-controlled trial undertaken at two universities affiliated psychiatric Hospitals in Iran (Roozbeh and Razi Hospital) from June 2012 to December 2013. The trial protocol was approved by the Institutional Review Board (IRB) of Tehran University of Medical Science (Grant No: 17215) and was conducted in agreement with the Declaration of Helsinki and its subsequent revisions. The trial was registered at the Iranian registry of clinical trials (www.irct.ir; registration number: (IRCT201205131556N42). Written informed consent was obtained from all eligible patients and/or their legally authorized representatives. Patients were informed that they are free to withdraw from the study at any time without any influence on their relationship with their health care provider.

Study population

Forty-six postmenopausal women with the definite diagnosis of schizophrenia were enrolled in the study. The diagnosis of schizophrenia was made according to DSM-IV TR. Diagnosis was made based on a Structured Clinical Interview for DSM-IV-TR Axis I Disorders (SCID) and was confirmed with chart review and senior physician interview. Inclusion criteria were postmenopausal (be in postmenopause is defined as period of one year spontaneous amenorrhea, a serum FSH level of >20 and clinical symptoms such as hot flashes,...) women who met the diagnostic criteria for schizophrenia according to DSM IV-TR consisting of Positive and Negative Syndrome Scale (PANSS) [11] score above 60 and disease onset over 2 years. Exclusion criteria were the concurrent presence of neurologic or organic disorders; IQ lower than 70; illicit drug use in past 6 months, consumption of antipsychotic drugs in the previous week or a long-acting antipsychotic drug in previous 2 months, receiving any antidepressant and mood stabilizer drugs during the trial, former hormone replace therapy, electroconvulsive therapy in past 2 weeks; endocrine abnormality; hepatic or renal dysfunction; and history of thromboemboli, abnormal uterine bleeding or breast and uterine cancer, and stroke.

Study design

Forty-six postmenopausal women with DSM-IV-TR diagnosed chronic schizophrenia received risperidone (6 mg/day in 3 divided doses) (Janssen Pharmaceuticals, Toronto, Canada; 2 mg tablet) combined with either placebo (N = 23) or 120 mg/day of raloxifene (Eli Lilly) (N = 23) for 8 weeks. Patients were assessed by a psychiatrist at baseline and at 2 and 8 weeks after the start of medical therapy. Efficacy was defined as the change from baseline to endpoint in score on PANSS.

Outcome measurement

PANSS is one of the most important rating tools for computing symptom severity in patients with schizophrenia. It comprises 3 subscales (positive scale, negative scale, and general psychotherapy scale) with 30 items in total ranging in score between 1 and 7 which leads to a minimum total score of 30. PANSS has been used in a number of trials in Iran [12-15]. The mean decline in PANSS scale as well as subscales from baseline was regarded as the main outcome measure of response in schizophrenia to treatment. The scale was measured at baseline, week 2 and week 8. Efficacy will be defined as change from baseline to endpoint in score on PANSS. Adverse events were evaluated using a 25 –item checklist and Extra-pyramidal Symptoms Rating Scale (ESRS) [16].

Statistical analysis

SPSS software, version 20.0 for Windows, was used to analyze the data. Continuous data are presented as mean ± standard deviation (SD). We used Kolmogorov-Smirnov Z test to determine the normal distribution of all continuous variables and due to normal distribution of PNSS score and subscales (positive, negative, general), we used parametrical tests to analyze data. A mixed between-within subjects analysis of variance was conducted to assess the impact of two different interventions (Risperidone + Raloxifene, Risperidone + placebo) on patient scores on PANSS score, positive subscale, negative subscale, and general psychotherapy subscale, across three time periods (the start of study, week 2, and week 8).

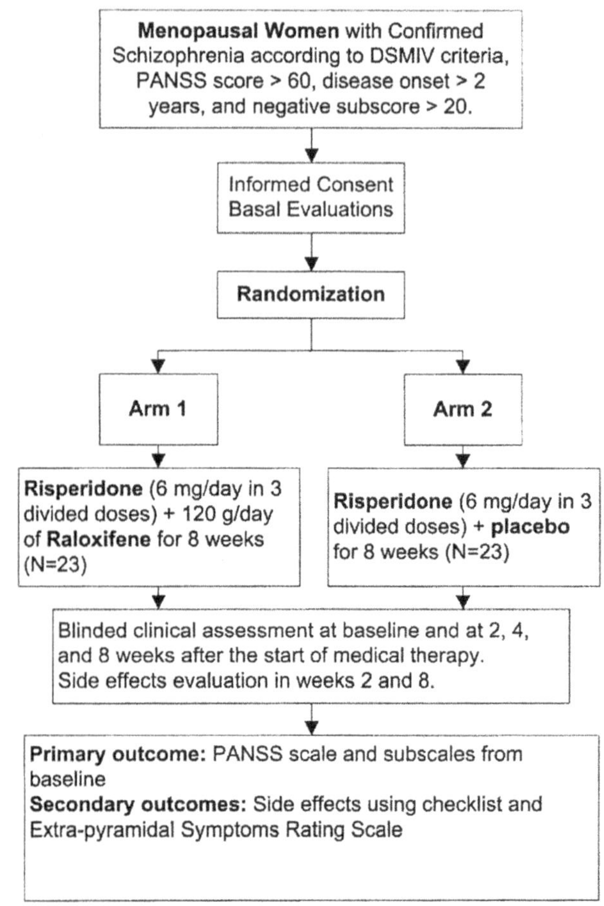

Figure 1 **Trial flow diagram of adjunctive Raloxifene versus placebo.**

Results

Figure 1 shows flow diagram of the patients. The mean age (±SD) of the raloxifene group was 61.96 ± 4.49 years versus 60.44 ± 5.28 years in the placebo group (non significant). Demographic data of the patients is presented in Table 1.

For PANSS scores, there was no significant interaction between intervention type and time [Wilks' Lambda = 0.89, F (2, 47) = 2.79, p = 0.07]. There was substantial main effect for time [Wilks' Lambda = 0.36, F (2, 47) = 42.56, p < 0.01] within both groups showing a reduction in PANSS scores across three time periods (Table 2, Figure 2). Furthermore, the main effect comparing two types of intervention was not significant [F (1, 48) = 1.77, p = 0.18].

For positive subscale scores, there was marginal significant interaction between intervention type and time [Wilks' Lambda = 0.89, F (2, 47) = 2.93, p = 0.06] and there was substantial main effect for time [Wilks' Lambda = 0.44, F (2, 47) = 24.39, p < 0.01] within both groups showing a reduction in positive subscale scores across the three time periods (Table 2, Figure 3). In addition, the main effect comparing two types of intervention was significant [F (1, 48) = 3.78, p = 0.02] suggesting superior effectiveness of Risperidone plus Raloxifene over Risperidone plus Placebo.

For negative subscale scores, there was no significant interaction between intervention type and time [Wilks' Lambda = 0.99, F (2, 47) = 0.12, p = 0.73]. There was substantial main effect for time [Wilks' Lambda = 0.46, F (2, 47) = 55.65, p < 0.01] within both groups showing a reduction in negative subscale scores across three time periods (Table 2, Figure 4). Additionally, the main effect comparing two types of intervention was not significant [F (1, 48) = 1.43, p = 0.23] suggesting no difference in effectiveness of the two therapies on negative subscale scores.

For general subscale scores, there was significant interaction between intervention type and time [Wilks' Lambda = 0.78, F (2, 47) = 6.78, p < 0.01]. There was substantial main effect for time [Wilks' Lambda = 0.34, F (2, 47) = 46.13, p < 0.01] within both groups showing a reduction in general subscale scores across the three time periods (Table 2, Figure 5). However, the main effect comparing two types of intervention was not significant [F (1, 48) = 0.03, p = 0.86] suggesting no difference in the effectiveness of the two therapies on general subscale scores.

Main adverse events included constipation (3 patients in Raloxifene group and 2 patients in placebo group), tremor (1 in each group), dry mouth (2 patients in raloxifene group), restless leg syndrome (1 patient in Raloxifene

Table 1 Demographic data of the raloxifene group versus the placebo group

		Risperidone + Raloxifene group (N = 25)	Risperidone + Placebo group (N = 25)	p-value
Age (±SD)		61.96 ± 4.49	60.44 ± 5.28	p > 0.05
Education	Illiterate	4 (36.36%)	7 (63.64%)	p > 0.05
	School	17 (51.52%)	16 (48.48%)	
	University	3 (50%)	3 (50%)	
Positive family history		13 (42%)	15 (60%)	p > 0.05
Age of onset		34.96 ± 11.69	29.40 ± 8.57	p > 0.05
Duration		17.24 ± 12.03	13.64 ± 12.41	p > 0.05
Previous treatment	Risperidone	7 (41.12%)	10 (58.88%)	p > 0.05
	Other atypical	3 (75.0%)	1 (25.0%)	
	Typical	11 (50.0%)	11 (50.0%)	
	Combination	4 (57.14%)	3 (42.86%)	
IQ	Normal	24 (52.17%)	22 (47.83%)	p > 0.05
	Borderline	1 (25.0%)	3 (75.0%)	

group), drowsiness (2 patients in placebo group), and loss of appetite (1 patient in placebo group). In addition, there was no ESRS difference between the two groups at weeks 2 and 8 [F (1, 48) = 1.04, p = 0.30].

Discussion

Adjunctive therapy and polypharmacy is used routinely for several chronic diseases. Medications with different mechanisms of action are used in polypharmacy. The use of adjunctive therapy in schizophrenia has been a major concern especially in recent years. The potential therapeutic efficacy of estrogens in schizophrenia is being identified and Selective Estrogen Receptor Modulators (SERMs) seem to be a better option in view of safety concerns. According to our findings, Raloxifene as an adjunctive treatment to risperidone was only superior for positive symptoms and it was not effective in treating negative and general psychopathology symptoms.

Recently, some studies have pointed to the adjunctive efficacy of raloxifene in improving schizophrenic symptoms [17]. In a 12-week, double-blind, randomized, placebo-controlled study [10], 33 postmenopausal women with schizophrenia were randomized to receive either adjuvant raloxifene (16 women) or adjuvant placebo (17 women) for three months. The addition of raloxifene produced significant differences in some aspects of memory and executive function in patients treated with raloxifene. In another 12-week, double-blind, randomized, placebo-controlled study, 33 postmenopausal women with schizophrenia and prominent negative symptoms were randomized to either adjunctive raloxifene or adjunctive placebo for 12 weeks [9]. The addition of raloxifene

Table 2 PANSS and subscale scores for the intervention type across three time periods

		Risperidone + Raloxifene (n = 25)	Risperidone + Placebo (n = 25)
	Time period	Mean ± SD	Mean ± SD
PANSS score	Week 0	105.52 ± 16.96	105.00 ± 11.68
	Week 2	89.08 ± 16.14	94.16 ± 19.78
	Week 8	68.32 ± 21.04	82.00 ± 26.14
Positive subscale	Week 0	25.76 ± 8.00	26.68 ± 7.04
	Week 2	20.92 ± 5.41	24.28 ± 6.33
	Week 8	14.32 ± 4.33	21.12 ± 7.07
Negative subscale	Week 0	28.04 ± 8.64	30.76 ± 9.09
	Week 2	24.88 ± 8.76	28.12 ± 10.88
	Week 8	19.60 ± 8.66	23.08 ± 12.08
General Psychopathology subscale	Week 0	50.44 ± 9.92	47.52 ± 6.46
	Week 2	43.56 ± 9.30	41.88 ± 9.76
	Week 8	34.56 ± 10.78	37.84 ± 11.89

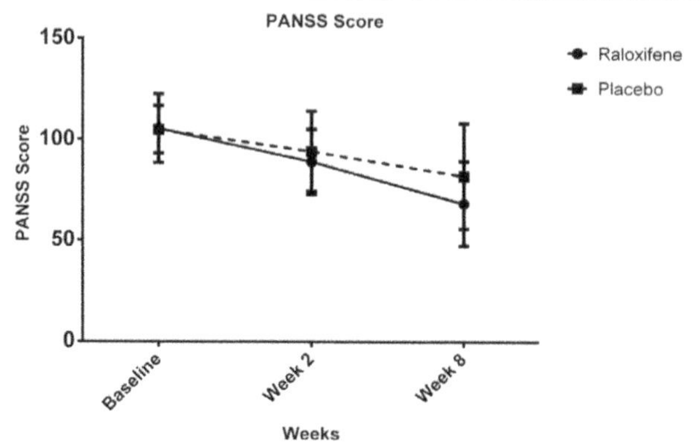

Figure 2 PANSS scores for the intervention type across three time periods (Raloxifene group: solid line, Placebo group: dashed line).

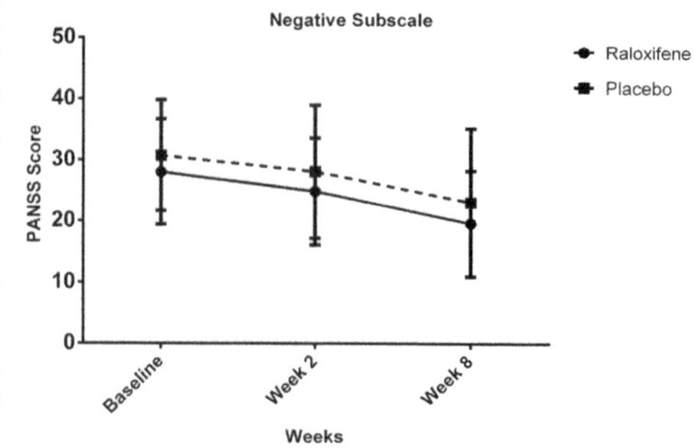

Figure 4 Negative subscale scores for the intervention type across three time periods (Raloxifene group: solid line, Placebo group: dashed line).

(60 mg/d) to regular antipsychotic treatment significantly reduced negative, positive, and general psychopathology symptoms compared to the placebo group.

In a randomized clinical trial [4], 35 postmenopausal women with schizophrenia received 120 mg/day adjunctive raloxifene compared to either adjunctive raloxifene HCl (60 mg/day) or placebo. A significantly greater recovery of total and general PANSS symptoms was noted in patients receiving 120 mg/day adjunctive raloxifene compared to either 60 mg/day adjunctive raloxifene HCl or placebo. In addition, adjunctive Raloxifene has been successfully used in single case reports for menstruating women suffering from resistant schizophrenia. A 29-year-old woman, with drug-resistant schizophrenia, experienced significant improvement in socio-occupational functioning, with reduction in symptom severity, over a 7-month follow-up period, [18].

It is significant that we encountered no adverse effects in the raloxifene group compared to the placebo group. The safer raloxifene profile compared with estrogenic compounds, makes it a preferred drug when adjunctive hormonal therapy of schizophrenia for post-menopausal women is considered. The lack of adverse effects on breast and uterine tissue is an imperative advantage of Raloxifene over estrogen [19].

The ovarian hormone 17β-estradiol acts in the central nervous system to regulate neuroendocrine events and reproduction. Estradiol controls gene expression, neuronal survival, neuronal and glial differentiation, and synaptic transmission and has anti-inflammatory, protective and reparative properties in the brain [20,21]. A number of studies seem to indicate that raloxifene acts on brain dopamine and serotonin systems in a way that is similar to that of conjugated estrogens [22].

It is proposed that conjugated estrogens may exercise their therapeutic potential either by modulating brain neurotransmission or through neuroprotective effects. On the other hand, the incidence of schizophrenia in men is consistently observed to be approximately 1.5 times higher than its in women [23] and there is a male predominance in incidence in the early twenties, but a

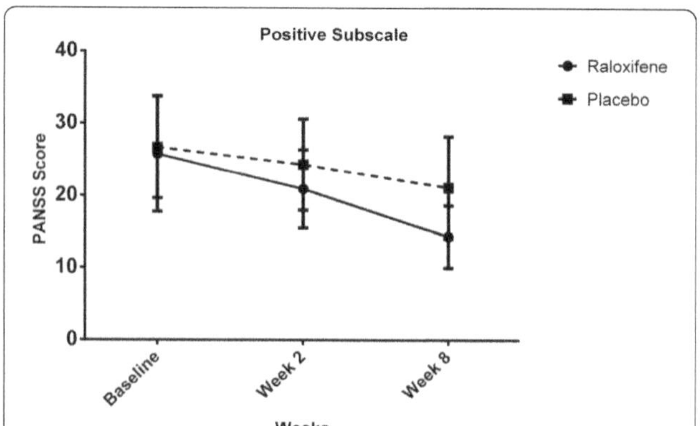

Figure 3 Positive subscale scores for the intervention type across three time periods (Raloxifene group: solid line, Placebo group: dashed line).

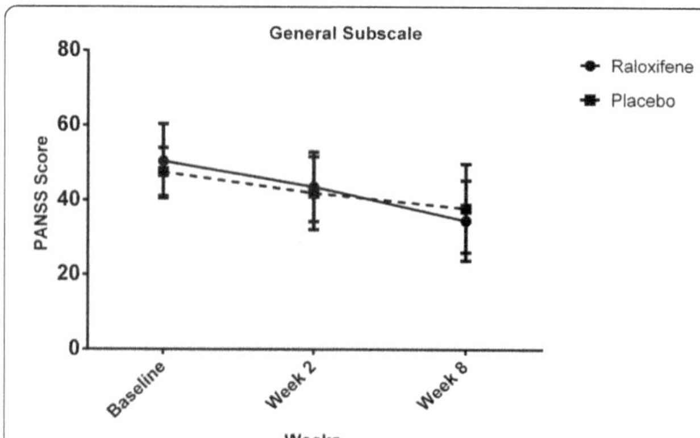

Figure 5 General Psychopathology subscale scores for the intervention type across three time periods (Raloxifene group: solid line, Placebo group: dashed line).

female predominance in older middle age [24]. Estrogen may have an impact on schizophrenia by several mechanisms. Short-term, it seems to have fast membrane effects by modifying functional activity in the dopaminergic synapse; for longer periods, it may appear to have genomic effects by altering synthesis at dopamine receptors. There is also evidence to suggest that estrogen alters serotonergic systems. Estrogen can also promote neuronal regeneration and block mechanisms of neuronal death [4]. In addition, numerous studies have described association between serotonin 1A receptor and major psychiatric disorders, such as schizophrenia and bipolar disorder [25]. Both serotonin and estrogen have been involved in modulation of mood and cognition. Even though substantial functional relations between estrogen and serotonin are recognized, the nature of their relationship has not been fully illuminated [26]. This study has some limitations which should be considered. The sample size was relatively small and the study course and follow-up period were relatively short. We did not measure the effect of raloxifene on menopausal symptoms as well. Furthermore, lack of cognitive assessments is another limitation of the present study.

Conclusions

In conclusion, it seems that according to our findings, raloxifene as an adjunctive treatment was shown to be superior to placebo in improving the positive symptoms in patients receiving risperidone. However, this drug did not show a benefit in treating the negative and general symptoms of schizophrenia when was added to risperidone therapy.

Abbreviations

SERMs: Selective estrogen receptor modulators; PNASS: Positive and negative syndrome scale.

Competing interests

No conflict of interest exists for any of the authors associated with the manuscript and there was no source of extra-institutional commercial funding. The funding organization had no role in the design and conduct of the study; in the collection, analysis, and interpretation of the data; or in the preparation, review, or approval of the manuscript and the decision to submit the paper for publication.

Authors' contributions

GK, SH and AN: Sample collection, FF: Statistical Analysis, Article writing, SA, LK, MK and FR: Designer and project manager, Article writing. All authors read and approved the final manuscript.

Acknowledgments

This study was supported by a grant from Tehran University of Medical Sciences to Prof. Shahin Akhondzadeh (Grant No: 17215). This study was Dr. Gilda Kianimehr's postgraduate thesis toward the Iranian Board of Psychiatry.

Author details

[1]Psychiatric Research Center, Roozbeh Hospital, Tehran University of Medical Sciences, Tehran 13337, Iran. [2]Shariati Hospital, Neurology Department, Tehran University of medical Sciences, Tehran, Iran. [3]Razi Psychiatric Hospital, University of Social Welfare and Rehabilitation, Tehran, Iran. [4]Qods Hospital, Kurdistan University of Medical Sciences, Sanandaj, Iran. [5]Infertility Ward, Arash Hospital, Tehran University of Medical Sciences, Tehran, Iran. [6]Psychiatric Research Center, Roozbeh Psychiatric Hospital, Tehran University of Medical Sciences, South Kargar Street 13337, Tehran, Iran.

References

1. Kulkarni J, Gavrilidis E, Worsley R, Hayes E: **Role of estrogen treatment in the management of schizophrenia.** *CNS Drugs* 2012, **26**(7):549–557.
2. Mortimer AM: **Relationship between estrogen and schizophrenia.** *Expert Rev Neurother* 2007, **7**(1):45–55.
3. Begemann MJ, Dekker CF, van Lunenburg M, Sommer IE: **Estrogen augmentation in schizophrenia: a quantitative review of current evidence.** *Schizophr Res* 2012, **141**(2-3):179–184.
4. Kulkarni J, Gurvich C, Lee SJ, Gilbert H, Gavrilidis E, de Castella A, Berk M, Dodd S, Fitzgerald PB, Davis SR: **Piloting the effective therapeutic dose of adjunctive selective estrogen receptor modulator treatment in postmenopausal women with schizophrenia.** *Psychoneuroendocrinology* 2010, **35**(8):1142–1147.
5. Akhondzadeh S, Nejatisafa AA, Amini H, Mohammadi MR, Larijani B, Kashani L, Raisi F, Kamalipour A: **Adjunctive estrogen treatment in women with chronic schizophrenia: a double-blind, randomized, and placebo-controlled trial.** *Prog Neuropsychopharmacol Biol Psychiatry* 2003, **27**(6):1007–1012.
6. Akhondzadeh S, Mokhberi K, Amini H, Larijani B, Kashani L, Hashemi L, Nejatisafa AA, Shafaei AR: **Is there a relationship between estrogen serum level and symptom severity throughout the menstrual cycle of patients with schizophrenia?** *Therapy* 2005, **2**(5):745–751.
7. Wu YC, Hill RA, Gogos A, van den Buuse M: **Sex differences and the role of estrogen in animal models of schizophrenia: interaction with BDNF.** *Neuroscience* 2013, **239**:67–83.
8. Velazquez-Zamora DA, Garcia-Segura LM, Gonzalez-Burgos I: **Effects of selective estrogen receptor modulators on allocentric working memory performance and on dendritic spines in medial prefrontal cortex pyramidal neurons of ovariectomized rats.** *Horm Behav* 2012, **61**(4):512–517.
9. Usall J, Huerta-Ramos E, Iniesta R, Cobo J, Araya S, Roca M, Serrano-Blanco A, Teba F, Ochoa S: **Raloxifene as an adjunctive treatment for postmenopausal women with schizophrenia: a double-blind, randomized, placebo-controlled trial.** *J Clin Psychiatry* 2011, **72**(11):1552–1557.
10. Huerta-Ramos E, Iniesta R, Ochoa S, Cobo J, Miquel E, Roca M, Serrano-Blanco A, Teba F, Ochoa S: **Effects of raloxifene on cognition in postmenopausal women with schizophrenia: A double-blind, randomized, placebo-controlled trial.** *Eur Neuropsychopharmacol* 2014, **24**(2):223–231.
11. Kay SR, Fiszbein A, Opler LA: **The positive and negative syndrome scale (PANSS) for schizophrenia.** *Schizophr Bull* 1987, **13**(2):261–276.
12. Farokhnia M, Azarkolah A, Adinehfar F, Khodaie-Ardakani MR, Hosseini SM, Yekehtaz H, Tabrizi M, Rezaei F, Salehi B, Sadeghi SM, Moghadam M, Gharibi F, Mirshafiee O, Akhondzadeh S: **N-acetylcysteine as an adjunct to risperidone for treatment of negative symptoms in patients with chronic schizophrenia: a randomized, double-blind, placebo-controlled study.** *Clin Neuropharmacol* 2013, **36**(6):185–192.
13. Farokhnia M, Sabzabadi M, Pourmahmoud H, Khodaie-Ardakani MR, Hosseini SM, Yekehtaz H, Tabrizi M, Rezaei F, Salehi B, Akhondzadeh S: **A double-blind, placebo controlled, randomized trial of riluzole as an adjunct to risperidone for treatment of negative symptoms in patients with chronic schizophrenia.** *Psychopharmacology (Berl)* 2014, **231**(3):533–542.
14. Khodaie-Ardakani MR, Mirshafiee O, Farokhnia M, Tajdini M, Hosseini SM, Modabbernia A, Rezaei F, Salehi B, Yekehtaz H, Ashrafi M, Tabrizi M, Akhondzadeh S: **Minocycline add-on to risperidone for treatment of negative symptoms in patients with stable schizophrenia: Randomized double-blind placebo-controlled study.** *Psychiatry Res* 2014, **215**(3):540–546.
15. Hosseini SM, Farokhnia M, Rezaei F, Gougol A, Yekehtaz H, Iranpour N, Salehi B, Tabrizi M, Tajdini M, Ghaleiha A, Akhondzadeh S: **Intranasal desmopressin as an adjunct to risperidone for negative symptoms of schizophrenia: A randomized, double-blind, placebo-controlled, clinical trial.** *Eur Neuropsychopharmacol* 2014, **24**(6):846–855.
16. Chouinard G, Margolese HC: **Manual for the Extrapyramidal Symptom Rating Scale (ESRS).** *Schizophr Res* 2005, **76**(2–3):247–265.
17. Kulkarni J, Gavrilidis E, Wang W, Worsley R, Fitzgerald PB, Gurvich C, Van Rheenen T, Berk M, Burger H: **Estradiol for treatment-resistant**

schizophrenia: a large-scale randomized-controlled trial in women of child-bearing age. *Mol Psychiatry* 2014, doi:10.1038/mp.2014.33.
18. Raveendranathan D, Shivakumar V, Jayaram N, Rao NP, Venkatasubramanian G: **Beneficial effects of add-on raloxifene in schizophrenia.** *Arch Womens Ment Health* 2012, **15**(2):147–148.
19. Chua WL, de Izquierdo SA, Kulkarni J, Mortimer A: **Estrogen for schizophrenia.** *Cochrane Database Syst Rev* 2005, **4:** CD004719.
20. Spencer JL, Waters EM, Romeo RD, Wood GE, Milner TA, McEwen BS: **Uncovering the mechanisms of estrogen effects on hippocampal function.** *Front Neuroendocrinol* 2008, **29**(2):219–237.
21. Vegeto E, Benedusi V, Maggi A: **Estrogen anti-inflammatory activity in brain: a therapeutic opportunity for menopause and neurodegenerative diseases.** *Front Neuroendocrinol* 2008, **29**(4):507–519.
22. Usall J, Coromina M, Araya S, Ochoa S: **Effect of raloxifene (a Selective Estrogen Receptor Modulator (SERM)) as coadjuvant to antidepressant treatment: a case report.** *Actas Esp Psiquiatr* 2011, **39**(5):334–336.
23. Welham J, Isohanni M, Jones P, McGrath J: **The antecedents of schizophrenia: a review of birth cohort studies.** *Schizophr Bull* 2009, **35**(3):603–623.
24. Abel KM, Drake R, Goldstein JM: **Sex differences in schizophrenia.** *Int Rev Psychiatry* 2010, **22**(5):417–428.
25. Kishi T, Okochi T, Tsunoka T, Okumura T, Kitajima T, Kawashima K, Yamanouchi Y, Kinoshita Y, Naitoh H, Inada T, Kunugi H, Kato T, Yoshikawa T, Ujike H, Ozaki N, Iwata N: **Serotonin 1A receptor gene, schizophrenia and bipolar disorder: an association study and meta-analysis.** *Psychiatry Res* 2011, **185**(1–2):20–26.
26. Amin Z, Canli T, Epperson CN: **Effect of estrogen-serotonin interactions on mood and cognition.** *Behav Cogn Neurosci Rev* 2005, **4**(1):43–58.

8

Evaluation of antitumor activity of a TGF-beta receptor I inhibitor (SD-208) on human colon adenocarcinoma

Abolfazl Akbari[1], Saeid Amanpour[2], Samad Muhammadnejad[2], Mohammad Hossein Ghahremani[1,3], Seyed Hamidollah Ghaffari[4], Ahmad Reza Dehpour[5], Gholam Reza Mobini[1], Fatemeh Shidfar[1], Mahdi Abastabar[6], Ahad Khoshzaban[7], Ebrahim Faghihloo[9], Abbas Karimi[10] and Mansour Heidari[7,8*]

Abstract

Background: Transforming growth factor-β (TGF-β) pathway is involved in primary tumor progression and in promoting metastasis in a considerable proportion of human cancers such as colorectal cancer (CRC). Therefore, blockage of TGF-β pathway signaling via an inhibitor could be a valuable tool in CRC treatment.

Methods: To evaluate the efficacy of systemic targeting of the TGF-β pathway for therapeutic effects on CRC, we investigated the effects of a TGβRI (TGF-β receptor 1) or TβRI kinase inhibitor, SD-208, on SW-48, colon adenocarcinoma cells. In this work, *in vitro* cell proliferation was studied by methyl thiazolyl tetrazolium (MTT) and bromo-2′-deoxyuridine (BrdU) assays. Also, the histopathological and immunohistochemical evaluations were conducted by hematoxylin and eosin, and Ki-67 and CD34 markers were stained, respectively.

Results: Our results showed no significant reduction in cell proliferation and vessel formation (170 ± 70 and 165 ± 70, $P > 0.05$) in treated SW-48 cells with SD-208 compared to controls.

Conclusion: Our data suggested that SD-208 could not significantly reduce tumor growth and angiogenesis in human colorectal cancer model at least using SW-48 cells.

Keywords: SD-208, Colorectal cancer, SW-48, Immunohistochemistry staining

Background

Colorectal cancer (CRC) is the second leading cause of cancer death among adults, making it as an excellent and desirable area for clinicians and researchers to study [1,2]. It has been also found that a large proportion of cancers such as CRC display inactivation of the growth factors specially transforming growth factor-β (TGF-β) pathway but they are characterized by increasing the factor production. In man, three isoforms of TGF-β including TGF-β1, TGF-β2 and TGF-β3 have been well characterized [3,4]. The homology searching has revealed that these proteins share up to 75% amino acid sequences. In spite of the fact that they have demonstrated comparable signaling activities, they are differentially expressed in cell lineages and tissues. It has been also frequently reported that TGF-β is the most effective growth inhibitor for normal epithelial, hematopoietic and immune cells. Studies showed that TGF-β acts as a double-edged sword in the biological processes [3-6]. In addition, it plays important roles in primary tumor progression and in promoting metastasis and has become an attractive target for therapy [5-7]. TGF-β exerts its effects by acting on two types of transmembrane receptors: type I (TGβRI) and type II (TGβRII). These receptors are involved in signal transduction, triggers through interaction of the TGF-β with TGβRII. Once TGF-β binds to TGβRII leads to the recruitment, phosphosphorylation, and activation of TGβRI. Activation of the TGβRI invokes several TGF-β signaling pathway targets and downstream genes [7,8]. Based on the literature, targeting of TGF-β signaling could be a valuable tool to treatment of human cancers such as CRC, glioblastoma and breast cancer [6-10]. Several studies

* Correspondence: mheidari@sina.tums.ac.ir
[7]Stem Cells Preparation Uinte, Farabi Eye Hospital, Tehran University of Medical Sciences, Tehran, Iran
[8]Department of Medical Genetics, School of Medicine, Tehran University of Medical Sciences, Tehran, Iran
Full list of author information is available at the end of the article

reported that a series of pyridopyrimidine-based TGβRI kinase inhibitors such as SD-208 could be a powerful approach for the treatment of various cancers. SD-208 is a small-molecule kinase inhibitor that bind to the ATP-binding site of the TGβRI kinase and maintains the enzyme in its inactive configuration [11-13]. Despite advances in our understanding of the molecular and genetic basis of CRC, effective treatment of the disease remains a clinical challenge. As pointed out, TGF-β promotes cell proliferation, development, invasion and metastasis in several types of tumors. It is thought that TGβRI inhibitor may have a therapeutic benefit in CRC; therefore, pharmacological blockade of the TGF-β signaling pathway has been proposed as a benefit strategy for CRC therapy. In the current study, SW-48, colon adenocarcinoma cell line was treated with different doses of SD-208, an anti-cancer agent. We evaluated the effects of SD-208 on cell proliferation and differentiation *in vitro* and *in vivo*.

Methods

Cell culture

Human colorectal adenocarcinoma cell line with pathologic differentiation grade of the original tumors IV, SW-48, was obtained from National Cell Bank of Iran (NCBI) affiliated to Pasteur Institute (Tehran, Iran). The cell line was grown in RPMI-1640 medium (Gibco; Germany) containing 25 mM D-glucose, 4 mM L-glutamine and 1 mM sodium pyruvate and supplemented with 5% (v/v) heat inactivated fetal bovine serum (FBS) (Gibco; Germany), 2 mM glutamax (Gibco; Germany), 100 units/ml penicillin, 100 μg/ml streptomycin and 250 ng/ml amphoterycin (Gibco; Germany) in culture flask 25 cm^2 (SPL Life Sciences; South Korea). The cells were kept at 37°C in a humidified 95% atmosphere, 5% CO_2 atmosphere incubator designated as culture at a steady-state condition. Cell viability was assessed using trypan blue exclusion test and routinely found to all flasks contain more than 95% viable cells.

Chemical description and biological activity TGβRI kinase inhibitor, SD-208

SD-208 (Sigma Aldrich; Belgium) is a selective and orally active pyridopyrimidine type TGβRI kinase inhibitor with an IC50 of approximately 35 nmol/L against TβRI kinase activity *in vitro*. The drug was dissolved in 100% dimethylsulfoxide (DMSO; Sigma Aldrich; Belgium) and prepared as stock solutions of 5 mM in DMSO and kept at −20°C until use.

MTT assay

The *in vitro* growth inhibitory effect of SD-208 was measured by the MTT assay (Roche Applied Science; Germany). This assay is dependent on the ability of viable cells to reduce a yellow tetrazolium salt (MTT) metabolically to a purple formazan product. This reaction takes place when the cell is viable and mitochondrial reductase enzymes are active. Briefly, monolayer cultures were trypsinized in exponential growth phase, and viable cell counts were assessed using trypan blue exclusion. Then, cells were seeded in 96-well flat-bottom microtitration plates (SPL Life Sciences; South Korea) at a density of 5×10^4 cells/well (200 μL media/well). After 24 h, once the cells reached ~85% confluence they were treated with different concentrations of SD-208 (0.5 μM, 1 μM and 2 μM). Following 24 h drug exposure, for the recovery period, the cells were washed two times with fresh and free-FBS medium and the culture continued (Figure 1). Subsequently, fresh medium containing FBS was replaced for removal of efflux and unbound drug. In all *in vitro* experiments, control cells were incubated with dimethylsulfoxide (DMSO) alone (with the final concentration 0.2%). Complete medium was replaced with 100 μl MTT after 48 h incubations. The cells were incubated for 3 h at 37°C then MTT was removed, and 300 μl DMSO were added to each well. Finally, the optical densitometry was measured at a wavelength of 490 nm with background subtraction at 630 nm using a spectrophotometric microplate reader (BioTek Elx 808). The growth inhibition rate was calculated using the following formula:

$$\text{Growth inhibition rate } (\%) = 1-\left(OD_{\text{drug exposure}}/OD_{\text{control}}\right) \times 100$$

BrdU assay

The BrdU assay was performed using BrdU ELISA kit according to the manufacturer's instructions (Roche Applied

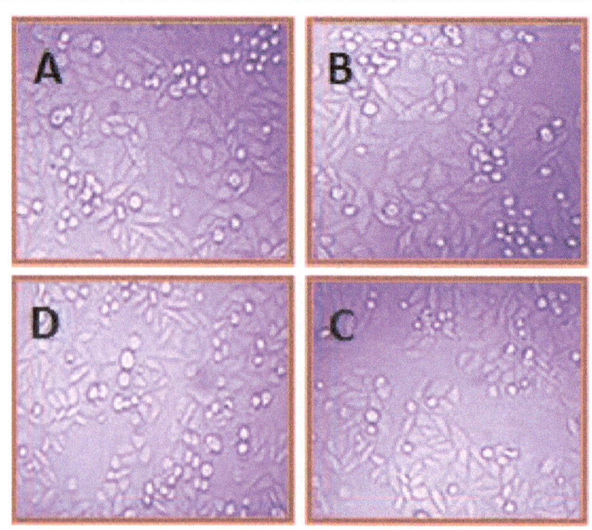

Figure 1 Continuous culture of SW-48 cells and treatment with SD-208. The cells were grown as monolayer epithelial-like morphology. SW-48 cells after treatment by DMSO alone as control **(A)**, SD-208 concentrations 0.5 μM **(B)**, 1 μM **(C)** and 2 μM **(D)**.

Science; Germany) for the quantification of cell proliferation base on the measurement of BrdU incorporation during DNA synthesis. Briefly, the SW-48 cells were seeded in 96-well flat-bottom microtitration plates at a density of 5 × 10^4 cells/well (100 μl media/well). After 24 h at 37°C, the cells were treated with different concentrations of SD-208 (0.5 μM, 1 μM and 2 μM). Every well, except for the background controls, received 10 μl marker solution (1:100 dilution with a sterile medium) and the cells were further incubated for 5 h at 37°C under 5% CO_2. Removal of the medium from the wells was followed by incubation of the cells in 200 μl FixDenat for 30 min. The FixDenat was removed, and the cells were further incubated for 75 min with the antibody solution. The cells were then washed three times with 200 μl washing buffer (1:10 dilution) and then incubated in 100 μl substrate solution (tetramethylbenzidine) for 15 min. Absorbance was measured at a wavelength of 490 nm using a spectrophotometric microplate reader (BioTek Elx 808). Cells from the same population and treatment that were not BrdU-labeled were used as the background controls. The cell proliferation was calculated using the following formula:

$$\text{Cell proliferation } (\%) = \left(OD_{\text{drug exposure}}/OD_{\text{control}}\right) \times 100$$

Animal model implanted with adenocarcinoma cell line (SW-48) and treatment protocol

6–week–old female athymic C56BL/6 nude mice (n = 8 per group) were obtained from Omid Institute for Advanced Biomodels (Tehran, Iran). Animals were kept under optimized hygienic conditions in an individually ventilated cage system. The mice were fed with autoclaved commercial diet and water ad libitum. All animal experiments were carried out according to the Tehran University of Medical Sciences, Ethical Committee Acts and were approved by the TUMS Ethical Committee. In order to establish the xenograft model of SW-48 cell line, the cells were cultured in RPMI 1640 containing 10 percent FBS in 75 cm^2 cell culture flasks. The cells were trypsinized and harvested. After washing, totally 5 × 10^6 cells were resuspended and inoculated subcutaneously at a 200 μl volume of serum–free medium into the flank of the animals. Tumor growth was measured twice a week. The volume of tumors was calculated by standard formula (Length × width^2 × 0.52) and growth curve was drawn (Tomayko, 1989). Xenograft tumors were allowed to reach a size of 100 mm^3. Then, the animals were randomly divided into two groups of 8 to receive either SD-208 (50 mg/kg/d) or vehicle orally for three weeks. Control animals were received daily drug-free and DMSO-containing deionized water (vehicle). At the end of the treatment period, mice were killed by CO_2 inhalation and obtained tumors after isolating from animal were fixed in 10% buffered formalin and were subjected to histopathological staining.

Histopathological diagnosis and immunohistochemistry

Hematoxylin and eosin (H&E) staining for SW-48 tumor confirmation and immunohistochemistry (IHC) staining for Ki-67 and CD34 markers were done. Then, five sections at routine thickness (5 μm) were prepared from the formalin-fixed paraffin-embedded tissue blocks and floated onto charged glass slides (Super-Frost Plus, Fisher Scientific). The slides then were dried overnight at 60°C. For the revision of the histopathological diagnosis and confirmation of developed the SW-48 cell-derived tumors, two hemotoxylin and eosin stained sections were obtained from tissue blocks. Immunohistochemistry carried out for the evaluation of SD-208 effects on proliferation and angiogenesis (Ki-67 and CD34 marker, respectively) in the tumor xenografts. For this, three sections were deparaffinized and hydrated using graded concentrations of ethanol to deionized water from each block. These sections were stained immunohistochemically using three steps-indirect streptavidin method for Monoclonal Mouse Anti-Human Ki-67 Antigen (MIB-1), clone M 7240 (Dako; Denmark) and Monoclonal Mouse Anti-Human CD34, clone QBEnd-10 (Dako; Denmark). Negative controls were obtained by omitting the primary antibody for aforementioned markers under identical test condition. Sections from a lymph node with follicular lymphoid hyperplasia known to be immunoreactive for Ki-67 and CD34 were used as a positive control (as recommended by the manufacturer).

Statistical analysis

Statistical analysis was performed, and statistical significance of differences between data was evaluated by independent sample Student's *t*-test for tumor markers (Ki-67 and CD34) and one-way analysis of variance (ANOVA) followed by Tukey's post tests for multiple comparisons of differences between treatment groups. Data were expressed as mean ± SEM (the standard error of the mean). P values less than 0.05 were considered to indicate statistically significant differences between data sets.

Results

In vitro effects of SD-208 on SW-48 cell line

In order to examine the growth inhibitory effect of SD-208 on CRC, the SW-48 cell line was cultured with different SD-208 concentrations (0.5 μM, 1 μM and 2 μM) for 48 h (Figure 1). As shown in Table 1, evaluation of *in vitro* growth inhibition by MTT (Figure 2A) and BrdU assays (Figure 2B) revealed no significant changes in treated versus untreated cells ($P > 0.05$).

Table 1 Effects of SD-208 on growth of SW-48 cell line

Inhibition rate (IR)%	P value	OD value (mean ± SEM)	Concentration of SD-208 (μM)
MTT assay			
		2.06 ± 0.085	Untreated
2.36	0.69	1.64 ± 0.098	Control (DMSO)
2.57	0.63	1.61 ± 0.093	0.5
3.4	0.6	1.54 ± 0.099	1
3.64	0.57	1.51 ± 0.098	2
BrdU assay			
		2.14 ± 0.079	Untreated
2.24	0.68	1.73 ± 0.081	Control (DMSO)
2.32	0.64	1.71 ± 0.087	0.5
2.6	0.63	1.69 ± 0.097	1
3.2	0.59	1.62 ± 0.098	2

Colon adenocarcinoma model

To determine the potential toxicity effects of SD-208, the appropriate numbers of SW-48 cells were injected into nude mice. Subsequently, animals were treated with or without SD-208 (as described in the Methods section). Following SD-208 treatment, we could not observe any changes in animal behavior, body weight and lifespan. These data suggest that SD-208 lacks toxic effects on mice bearing SW-48 tumor (data not shown).

Ten days after the subcutaneous inoculation, all 24 nude mice with an observed tumor growth survived with a balanced diet (Figure 3). Based on the standards of cancer-bearing models, 24 mice were selected for further experiments. The mice were sacrificed, and their tumor tissues were excised for pathological examinations.

The H&E staining demonstrates marked cellularity with profound hyperchromatism and pleomorphism (Figure 4). Pleomorphic malignant epithelial cells with the clearly nucleolus were visible. In tumor cells, the ratio of nucleus to the cytoplasm was 1/1. Also, high mitotic index and atypical areas were observed in both samples (treated versus controls). The pattern of adenocarcinoma was identical with the human origin in which the cancerous cells were poorly differentiated. Figure 4 indicates H&E staining of tumor tissues from studied animals. These results revealed no major differences in the sizes and the histology of the tumors (P > 0.05).

Immunohistochemistry

Immunohistochemical analysis was conducted using Ki-67 and CD34 antibodies. Immunoreactive SW-48 cells to anti- Ki-67 are brown nuclear with a diffuse pattern. It was scored by counting about 1000 cells in 10 different fields. Each brown stained nucleus was considered positive, regardless of intensity (Figure 5). Immunohistochemical staining of treated and untreated nude mice's

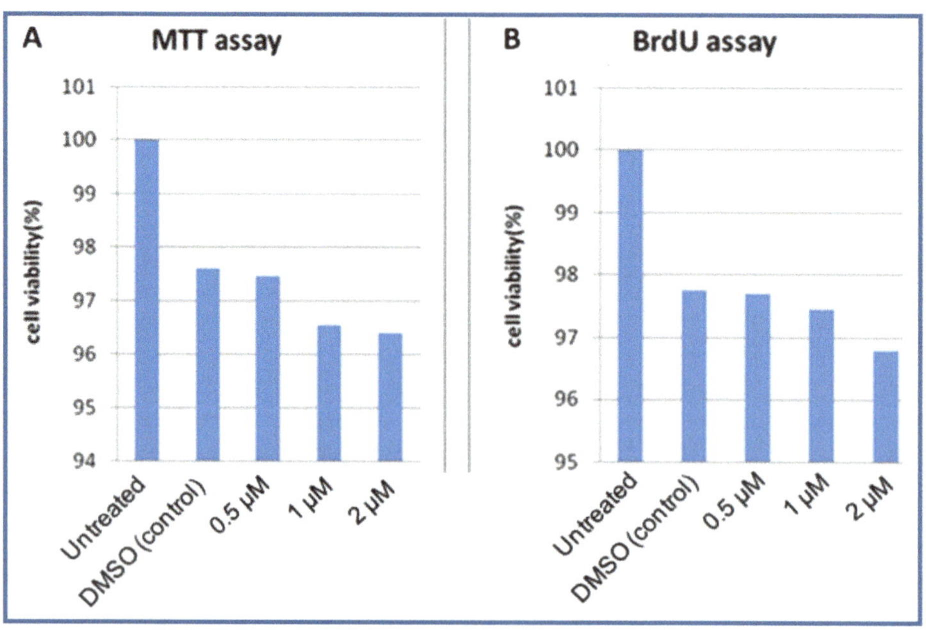

Figure 2 Effect of SD-208 on the cell growth and proliferation of the SW-48 cells. SW-48 cells were treated by 0.5, 1 and 2 μM for 48 h. Cell proliferation was examined by MTT and BrdU assays as described in methods. **A**: MTT assay of SW-48 cells after treatment with SD-208 in comparison with controls (untreated and treated with DMSO). **B**: BrdU assay of SW-48 cells after treatment with SD-208 comparison with controls (untreated and treated with DMSO). All data are reported as the percentage change in comparison with the controls, which were arbitrarily assigned 100% cell proliferation. Analysis of one-way ANOVA was used to compare the cell proliferation of SW-48 cells in different concentrations of SD-208 to control. P value < 0.05 was regarded as statistically significant. Results are expressed as the mean ± SEM from three independent experiments.

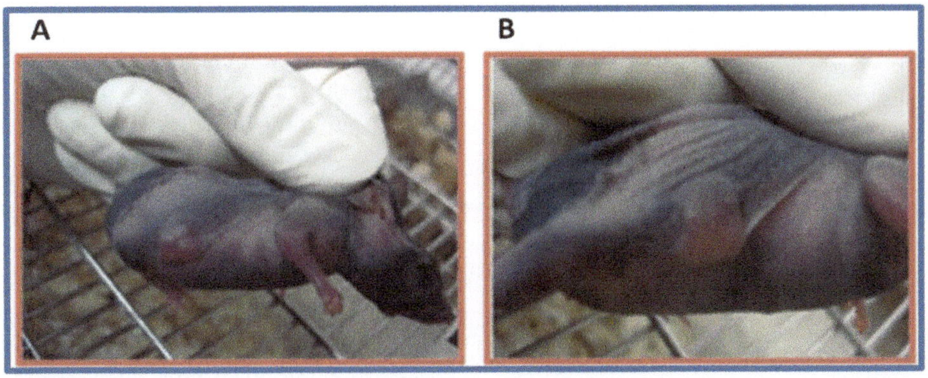

Figure 3 A representative of colorectal adenocarcinoma model. Tumor implantation; athymic nude mice implanted by SW-48 cell line, the cells were grown as tumor xenografts after 10 days. Cancer-bearing nude mice were treated with 50 mg/kg/day of SD-208 **(A)** or without SD-208 **(B)**.

tissues using anti-CD34 (as shown in the Figure 6) showed no significant changes among studied samples.

Ki-67 and CD34 expressions in the tumor xenografts

The results from the immunochemical assay indicated that Ki-67 was predominantly expressed in the nucleus. As already pointed out, the immunohistochemically stained tumors with anti-Ki-67 showed positively brown nuclear in the studied tissues (Figure 5). The Ki-67 expression levels between the test and control groups did not show significant changes ($P > 0.05$). Immunohistochemical staining using anti-CD34 antibody on tumor tissues from either treated or untreated nude mice with SD-208 showed cytoplasmic membrane of endothelial cells in brown color and marked microvessels proliferation (Figure 6).

Discussion

Despite aggressive surgery, radiotherapy and chemotherapy, treatment of malignant CRC remains formidable. Even though that TGF-β suppresses proliferation of certain carcinoma cells and is well-known to be a tumor suppressor, it promotes tumor development, progression and metastasis in human cancers including CRC, glioma, osteosarcoma, breast, lung and pancreatic cancers [14-16]. The insights into the role of the TGF-β signaling in carcinogenesis importantly have come due to experimental study on animal models. Understanding the mechanisms by which TGF-β signaling regulates tumor development and progression is critical for designing the beneficial therapeutic strategies for the cancers [14,16-18]. In the last few years, because of availability and easily drug delivery, the targeting of receptor kinases by small-molecule inhibitors has been a profound area of experimental cancer studies [16,17,19].

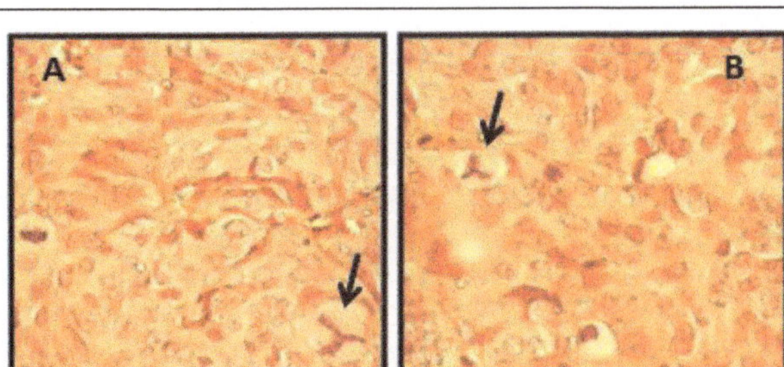

Figure 4 A representative results of pathological examinations of nude mice tumors with or without SD-208 treatment. A: tumors of nude mice treated with 50 mg/kg/day stained with H&E. **B**: H&E staining of tumor tissues of control. No significant difference histologically was observed ($P > 0.05$).

It is thought that pharmacological blockade of the TGF-β signaling pathway by TGβRI inhibitors may be as a potential strategy for cancer therapy [17-19]. For the first time, we evaluated the efficacy of systemic targeting of the TGF-β pathway by a TGβRI kinase inhibitor, SD-208, on a high-grade colon adenocarcinoma cell line, SW-48, *in vitro* and in developed heterotopic colon tumors in model that shares similarities with human colon cancer. Our findings using MTT and BrdU assays demonstrated that treatment of SW-48 cells with SD-208 using different doses had no significant inhibitory effects on cell growth and proliferation. Our *in vitro* results were consistent with one study revealing SD-208 can not reduce viability or proliferation of human malignant glioma cells [17]. However, this study showed that SD-208 regulates the growth of glioma in syngeneic mice without changes in proliferation, apoptosis or angiogenesis. Also, other investigators demonstrated that SD-208 failed to inhibit R3T tumor growth or metastasis in athymic nude mice [20]. On the other hand, some studies suggested that the various kinase inhibitors including SD-208, were able to inhibit TGF-β-evoked migration and invasion [20-22]. These results indicated that reduction of tumors was due to regulation of immune

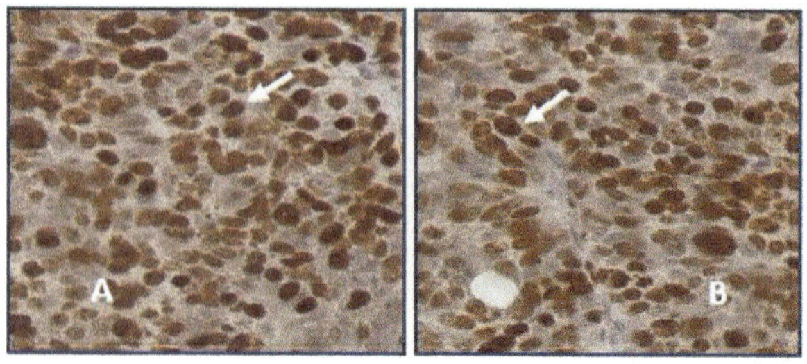

Figure 5 Colon adenocarcinoma (grade IV) stained immunohistochemically with anti-Ki-67. Positive immunoreactive showing brown nuclear expression of Ki-67 with a large number (~80%) of stained nuclei reflecting active cellular proliferation in the treated nude mice with SD-208 **(A)** and control **(B)**: Immunohischemical assay showed no significant difference between tests and controls in terms of cellular proliferation ($P > 0.05$).

surveillance and importantly correlated with tumor-reactive immune regulation and increased immune infiltration [21,22]. Thereby, it has been commented that SD-208 could be a promising agent for the treatment of human malignancy and other conditions associated with pathological TGF-β activity.

In addition, we revealed that when drinking water contains SD-208 daily, the drug could not inhibit the growth of established heterotopic SW-48 tumors and its progression in nude mice. Further histological analysis indicated that SD-208 had no significant effects on proliferation (Ki-67 positivity) or the number of blood vessels and angiogenesis (CD34 positivity). This is consistent with reports by others showing SD-208 had no effect on the growth of primary and metastatic R3T mammary tumors in athymic nude mice [18]. In the agreement with our results and previous studies, it has been shown that an inhibitor of TGF-β receptor 1 kinase, SM16, lost efficacy against the AB12 mesothelioma model in SCID mice [21].

Also, we found that SD-208 is not effective in limiting heterotopic tumor growth and not proper to treat established primary tumors settings at least in SW-48 colorectal cancer cells. The failure of SD-208 to inhibit SW-48 tumor growth in nude mice suggests that the suppression of angiogenesis and proliferation could be dependent on cell lineage and cell context [23]. Our results are not the first report suggesting the inability of SD-208 to inhibit angiogenesis and proliferation. Some researchers reported that SD-208 was unable to cause differences in microvessel density in gliomas [17]. Furthermore, a study of two TGF-βR1 inhibitors, SD-093 and SD-208, on two murine mammary carcinoma cell lines (R3T and 4 T1) revealed that SD-208 failed to inhibit R3T tumor growth or metastasis in athymic nude mice. However, SD-208 treatment led to a reduction in microvessel density in mammary tumors [20].

It is quite understandable that the efficacy of this kinase inhibitor is a controversial issue in cancer treatment [20]. In this regard, several scenarios could be proposed to elucidate the failure of SD-208 as an anti-tumor: (1) genetic alterations such as chromosomal abnormalities and (2) gene mutation in any TGF-β signaling pathway.

Conclusion

We have demonstrated that SD-208, a TGβRI kinase inhibitor, was not able to reduce tumor growth and angiogenesis in a heterotopic human colorectal cancer model. Our results also for the first time indicated that this anti-cancer agent could not potentially have a therapeutic benefit in at least proportion of CRC. To get more insight into the potential biological effects of SD-208 on CRC, different CRC cells with various differentiated status are required to treat with SD-208. Moreover, because of the complexity of TGF-β signaling role and crosstalk with other factors (such as immunochemotactic and angiogenic agents) in the derived

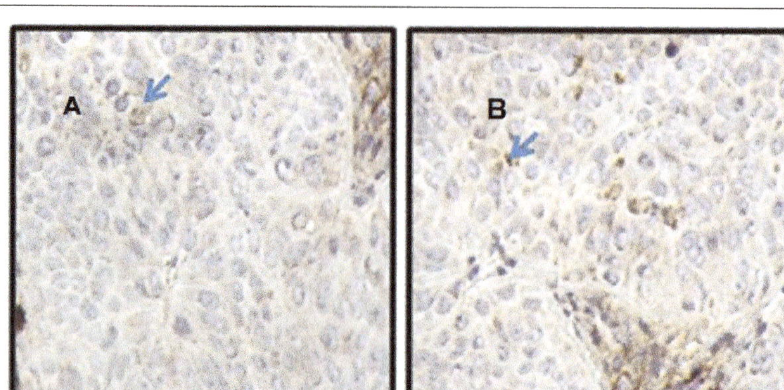

Figure 6 Colon adenocarcinoma (grade IV) stained immunohistochemically with anti-CD34. The paraffin embedded sections of tumor tissues were stained with anti-CD34 antibody and positive immunoreactive indicating brown cytoplasmic membrane of endothelial cells and marked microvessel's proliferation. Microvessel density (MVD) was ~40 microvessel/mm^2. SD-208-treated tumors **(A)** vs controls **(B)** revealed no significant immunohistologically differences ($P > 0.05$). Note the prominent vascularity. Arrows indicate CD34 staining of the cytoplasmic membrane.

tumor microenvironment, designing therapeutic intervention strategies for targeting tumors in this field, should be very carefully.

Abbreviations

TGF-β: Transforming growth factor-β; CRC: Colorectal cancer; TGβRI or TβRI: TGF-β receptor 1, TGβRII or TβRII, TGF-β receptor 2; SW-48: A colon adenocarcinoma cell line; SD-208: A TGF-β receptor I kinase inhibitor; MTT: Methyl thiazolyl tetrazolium; BrdU: Bromo-2′-deoxyuridine; H&E: Hematoxylin and Eosin; IHC: Immunohistochemistry.

Competing interests

The authors declare they have no competing interests.

Authors' contributions

MH and AA contributed to idea and study design; ARD contributed to the supervision of sections of the study. MHG, SHG, GRM and FS assisted with cell culture study and experimentation and provided scientific advice, MA assisted with analysis of the data. SM and SA assisted with IHC staining and data analysis. AA prepared the manuscript which SM, MH and AK significantly revised. All authors read and approved the final manuscript.

Acknowledgements

This study represents a part of a Ph.D. dissertation by Abolfazl Akbari. We wish to thank the School of Advanced Medical Technologies, the Tehran University of Medical Sciences (TUMS) for financially supporting this study.

Author details

[1]Department of Molecular Medicine, School of Advanced Medical Technologies, Tehran University of Medical Sciences, Tehran, Iran. [2]Cancer Research Center, Cancer Institute of Iran, Tehran University of Medical Sciences, Tehran, Iran. [3]Department of Pharmacology and Toxicology, Faculty of Pharmacy, Tehran University of Medical Sciences, Tehran, Iran. [4]Hematology, Oncology and Stem Cell Transplantation Research Center, Shariati Hospital, Tehran University of Medical Sciences, Tehran, Iran. [5]Department of Pharmacology, School of Medicine, Tehran University of Medical Sciences, Tehran, Iran. [6]Invasive Fungi Research Center, Department of Medical Mycology and Parasitology, School of Medicine, Mazandaran University of Medical Sciences, Sari, Iran. [7]Stem Cells Preparation Uinte, Farabi Eye Hospital, Tehran University of Medical Sciences, Tehran, Iran. [8]Department of Medical Genetics, School of Medicine, Tehran University of Medical Sciences, Tehran, Iran. [9]Department of Virology, School of Public Health, Tehran University of Medical Sciences, Tehran, Iran. [10]Department of Molecular Medicine, Faculty of Advanced Technologies in Medicine (FATiM), Iran University of Medical Sciences, Tehran, Iran.

References

1. Jemal A, Siegel R, Ward E, Hao Y, Xu J, Murray T, Thun MJ: **Cancer statistics.** *CA Cancer J Clin* 2008, **58:**71–96.
2. Kinzler KW, Vogelstein B: **The Genetic Basis of Human Cancer.** 2nd edition. New York: McGraw-Hill; 2002:583–612.
3. Luo K, Lodish HF: **Signaling by chimeric erythropoietin-TGF-β receptors: homodimerization of the cytoplasmic domain of the type I TGF-β receptor and heterodimerization with the type II receptor are both required for intracellular signal transduction.** *EMBO J* 1996, **15:**4485–4496.
4. Siegel PM, Massague J: **Cytostatic and apoptotic actions of TGF-β in homeostasis and cancer.** *Nature Rev Cancer* 2003, **3:**807–821.
5. Moustakas A, Heldin CH: **Non-Smad TGF-β signals.** *J Cell Sci* 2005, **118:**3573–3584.
6. Miriam Barrios R, Kevin R, Barish O, Rohit B, Zhong L, RS D, Fukiko SH, Yongmei L, Joanna D, Taylor IW, Valbona L, Mark R, Harukazu S, Yoshihide H, Igor J, Jeffrey LW: **High-throughput mapping of a dynamic signaling network in mammalian cells.** *Science* 2005, **307:**1621–1625.
7. Bierie B, Moses HL: **TGF-β and cancer.** *Cytokine Growth Factor Rev* 2006, **17:**29–40.
8. Levy L, Hill CS: **Alterations in components of the TGF-β superfamily signaling pathways in human cancer.** *Cytokine Growth Factor Rev* 2006, **17:**41–58.
9. Yingling JM, Blanchard KL, Sawyer JS: **Development of TGF-β signaling inhibitors for cancer therapy.** *Nature Rev Drug Discov* 2004, **3:**1011–1022.
10. Jean-Jacques L: **The dual role of TGF in human cancer: from tumor suppression to cancer metastasis.** *ISRN Molecular Biology* 2012, **7:**1–28.
11. Peng SB, Yan L, Xia X, Watkins SA, Brooks HB, Beight D, Herron DK, Jones ML, Lampe JW, McMillen WT, Mort N, Sawyer JS, Yingling JM: **Kinetic characterization of novel pyrazole TGF-β receptor I kinase inhibitors and their blockade of the epithelial-mesenchymal transition.** *Biochemistry* 2005, **44:**2293–2304.
12. Hill R, Song Y, Cardiff RD, Van Dyke T: **Selective evolution of stromal mesenchyme with p53 loss in response to epithelial tumorigenesis.** *Cell* 2005, **123:**1001–1011.
13. Inman GJ, Nicolás FJ, Callahan JF, Harling JD, Gaster LM, Reith AD, Laping NJ, Hill CS: **SB-431542 is a potent and specific inhibitor of transforming growth factor-β superfamily type I activin receptor-like kinase (ALK) receptors ALK4, ALK5, and ALK7.** *Mol Pharmacol* 2002, **62:**65–74.
14. Bruna A, Darken RS, Rojo F, Ocaña A, Peñuelas S, Arias A, Paris R, Tortosa A, Mora J, Baselga J, Seoane J: **High TGFbeta-Smad activity confers poor prognosis in glioma patients and promotes cell proliferation depending on the methylation of the PDGF-B gene.** *Cancer Res* 2003, **63:**7791–7798.
15. Qipeng F, Miao H, Tao S, Xiaoli Z, Mala S, Bruce L, Xingbo Z, Jing Wu X: **Requirement of TGF Signaling for SMO-mediated Carcinogenesis.** *J Biol Chem* 2010, **47:**36570–36576.
16. Bierie B, Harold LM: **TGFβ: the molecular Jekyll and Hyde of cancer.** *Nat Rev Cancer* 2006, **6:**506–520.
17. Uhl M, Steffen A, Jörg W, Markus W, Jing Ying M, Ramona A, Ruban M, Yu-Wang L, Michael P, Ulrich H, Alison M, Darren H, Wolfgang W, Higgins LS, Michael W: **SD-208, a novel transforming growth factor-β receptor I kinase inhibitor, inhibits growth and invasiveness and enhances immunogenicity of murine and human glioma cells *in vitro* and *in vivo*.** *Cancer Res* 2004, **64:**7954–7961.
18. Subramanian G, Schwarz RE, Linda H, Glenn M, Sarvajit C, Sundeep D, Michael R: **Targeting endogenous transforming growth factor-β receptor signaling in SMAD4-deficient human pancreatic carcinoma cells inhibits their invasive phenotype1.** *Cancer Res* 2004, **64:**5200–5211.
19. Leung SY, Niimi A, Noble A, Oates T, Williams AS, Medicherla S, Protter AA, Chung KF: **Effect of transforming growth factor-beta receptor I kinase inhibitor 2,4-disubstituted pteridine (SD-208) in chronic allergic airway inflammation and remodeling.** *J Pharmacol Exp Ther* 2006, **319:**586–594.
20. Ge R, Rajeev V, Ray P, Lattime E, Rittling S, Medicherla S, Protter A, Murphy A, Chakravarty J, Dugar S, Schreiner G, Barnard N, Reiss M: **Inhibition of growth and metastasis of mouse mammary carcinoma by selective inhibitor of transforming growth factor-beta type I receptor kinase *in vivo*.** *Clin Cancer Res* 2006, **12:**4315–4330.
21. Suzuki E, Kim S, Cheung HK, Corbley MJ, Zhang X, Sun L, Shan F, Singh J, Lee WC, Albelda SM, Ling LE: **A novel small-molecule inhibitor of transforming growth factor β type I receptor kinase (SM16) inhibits murine mesothelioma tumor growth *in vivo* and prevents tumor recurrence after surgical resection.** *Cancer Res* 2007, **67:**2351–2359.
22. Khalid SM, Delphine J, Pierrick GJ, Maria N, Ryan M, Xiang HP, Duong V, Lauren KD, Alain M, Theresa AG: **TGF-β-RI kinase inhibitor SD-208 reduces the development and progression of melanoma bone metastases.** *Cancer Res* 2011, **71:**175–184.
23. Medicherla S, Li L, Ma JY, Kapoun AM, Gaspar NJ, Liu YW, Mangadu R, O'Young G, Protter AA, Schreiner GF, Wong DH, Higgins LS: **Antitumor activity of TGF-β inhibitor is dependent on the microenvironment.** *Anticancer Res* 2007, **27:**4149–4158.

Non-addictive opium alkaloids selectively induce apoptosis in cancer cells compared to normal cells

Monireh Afzali[1], Padideh Ghaeli[2], Mahnaz Khanavi[3], Maliheh Parsa[1], Hamed Montazeri[1], Mohammad Hossein Ghahremani[1] and Seyed Nasser Ostad[1*]

Abstract

Background: Cytotoxic effects of some of the members of papaveraceae family have been reported in Iranian folk medicine. Recent reports has indicated that alkaloids fraction of opium may be responsible for its cytotoxic effect; however, the mechanism of this effect is not fully understood. This study has been designed to investigate the selective cytotoxic, genotoxic and also apoptosis induction effects of noscapine, papaverine and narceine, three non-addictable opium alkaloids, on HT29, T47D and HT1080 cancer cell lines. Mouse NIH3T3 cell line was chosen to present non-cancerous cells and Doxorubicin was selected as the positive control.

Methods: Cells were treated by different concentrations of Noscapine, Papaverine, Narceine and doxorubicin; viability was assessed by MTT assay. The genotoxicity and apoptosis induction were tested with comet assay and Annexin-V affinity when the concentration of each these drugs is less than its IC50. In addition, the DNA damage and caspase activity of the T47D cells were examined and the results were compared.

Results: This study noted the cytotoxicity and genotoxicity of noscapine and papaverine, specifically on cancerous cell lines. Furthermore, papaverine induces apoptosis in all studied cancer cell lines and noscapine showed this effect in T47D and HT29 cells but not in NIH-3 T3 cells as noncancerous cell line. narceine also showed genototoxicity in the studied cell lines at its IC50 concentration.

Conclusions: This experiment suggests that noscapine and papaverine may be of use in cancer treatment due to their specific cytotoxicity and genotoxicity. However, further in vivo studies are needed to confirm its usefulness in cancer treatment.

Keywords: Cancer cell, Cytotoxicity, Genotoxicity, Narceine, Noscapine, Papverine

Background

The agents which have the potential for induction of apoptosis may be considered as good candidates for cancer therapy due to their effect on the uncontrolled proliferation of malignant cells. In spite of excellent anti-tumor activities of common chemotherapy drugs, treatment will be restricted in some cases due to drug-resistance, low therapeutic index, severe side effects and different routes of administration [1]. Recently, in search for new treatments for cancer, there has been an emphasis on herbal and natural compounds. Cytotoxic effects of some members of Papaveraceae family have been considered in Iranian and Indian medicine [2]. *Papaverine somniferum L.* (opium poppy) has been traditionally used in Chinese and Indian herbal medicine to cure some disorders including chronic cough, dysentery, diarrhea, rectum prolapse and gastrointestinal problems [3]. The contents of opium alkaloids include morphine, codeine, tebaine, noscapine, papaverine, narceine as well as little percentage of some other compounds [4]. Many studies revealed a remarkable anti-tumor activity of the alkaloid noscapine, a naturally-occurring benzylisoquinoline alkaloid that constitutes about 2-10% of the alkaloid content of opium [5,6]. Furthermore, the anti-tumor activities of noscapine and its tubulin-binding property have been mentioned in many studies [7-12]. Noscapine inhibits the progression of melanoma, lymphoma, leukemia, breast cancer, colon cancer, ovarian carcinoma, glioblastoma, non-small cell lung

* Correspondence: ostadnas@tums.ac.ir
[1]Department Toxicology & Pharmacology, Faculty of Pharmacy, Toxicology & Poisoning Research Center, Tehran University of Medical Sciences, 14155/6451 Tehran, Iran
Full list of author information is available at the end of the article

cancer and prostate cancer while it has a little or no significant toxicity to the kidney, heart, liver, bone marrow, spleen and small intestine [8,12-16]. Papverine and narceine are two other benzylisoquinoline alkaloids constituting 0.5-3% and <0.5% of the alkaloid contents of opium, respectively. Papaverine has been used clinically as smooth muscle relaxant, anti-spasmodic for gastrointestinal disorders, cough suppressant and for treatment of erectile dysfunction (an unlabeled use). Although cytotoxic effect of papaverine and some of its derivatives has been observed in breast cancer, melanoma and prostate cancer [17-20], their mechanism of action has not been fully understood. Based on our knowledge, no previous study has examined the anti-cancer activities of narceine.

In this study three different human cancer cell lines have been chosen. HT29 colorectal carcinoma and T47D breast cancer cells as two of the most common types of human tumors and HT1080 fibrosarcoma cells as one of the most resistant cell lines to anti-cancer therapy. In addition, non-cancerous NIH-3 T3 cell line has been chosen to compare the effect of the agents between cancerous and non-cancerous cells and doxorubicin has been chosen as positive control. The purpose of this study is to show whether papaverine and narcein have selective cytotoxicity, genotoxicity and induction of apoptosis in cancerous cell lines as has been demonstrated in noscapine and was claimed in the traditional medicine.

Methods

Cell lines and chemicals

T47D (Breast, ductal-carcinoma, Human), HT-29 (Colon, epithelial-like carcinoma, Human), HT-1080 (connective tissue, fibro sarcoma, Human) and NIH-3 T3 (Swiss mouse embryo fibroblast) cell lines were all obtain from National Cell Bank (Pasture institute of Iran, Tehran). The cells were cultured in RPMI 1640 medium (Biosera, England) that was supplemented with 10% heat-inactivated fetal bovine serum (FBS; Biosera, England) as well as antibiotic vials containing 100 U/ml penicillin and 100 μg/ml streptomycin (Gibco, USA); then were incubated in a humidified atmosphere with 5% CO_2 at 37°C.

The materials used in the present study and the manufacturers provided them are as following: noscapine hydrochloride, agarose and low melting point agarose (LMP) from Sigma-Aldrich (USA), papaverine hydrochloride and ethanol from TEMAD Co. (Tehran, Iran), narceine trihydrate from Seqchem (UK), doxorubicin from Sobhan-daru (Tehran, Iran), MTT (3-[4,5-dimethylthiazol-2yl] -2,5-diphenyl tetrazolium bromide) powder and Caspase Assay fluorometric kit from Roche (Germany) and annexine V-PE apoptosis detection kit from Abcam (UK).

In vitro cytotoxicity assay

The cells in logarithmic phase of growth were seeded into 96-well plates at a density of 10^4 cells per well and allowed to incubate overnight at 37°C. Cells were treated with different concentrations of noscapine, papaverine, narceine and doxorubicin and were incubated for 48 hours and then cell viability was determined by MTT assay. Briefly, 25 μl of 5 mg/ml MTT solution in phosphate-buffered saline was added and incubated for four hours at 37°C. The medium was removed and 100 μl dimethylsulfoxide (DMSO) was added to each well. The formazan salts were quantified by reading the absorbance at a test wavelength of 570 nm and a reference wavelength of 690 nm [21-23]. The IC50 values were calculated from their cytotoxity dose–response curves.

Single cell gel electrophoresis (SCGE)/comet

The treated cells were diluted with RPMI 1640 + 10% FBS to final concentration of 175000 cells/ml. Cells were treated with 0.4% methanol in the CO_2 incubator for 3 hours. Each sample of 50 ul was harvested; then, immediately suspended in 450 μl of solution composed of 10 μl PBS and 75 μl 0.5% LMP agarose. The samples were then immediately coated on a uniform background of each rough microscope slide that had been previously prepared by 1% agarose. The agarose on the microscope slides was allowed to harden at 4°C for 10 minutes. After coating with supportive layer (LMP), slides were then placed in a chilled (4°C) lysis buffer (2.5 M sodium chloride, 100 mM EDTA, pH = 10, 10 mM Trise base, 1% sodium lauryl sarcosinate, 0.01% triton x-100) for 30 minutes to unwind the nuclear DNA at 4°C and drip dried. Slides were then immersed in the same buffer for 30 minutes at 24 V and 250 mA at room temperature. DNA damage was recognized by ethidium bromide and florescence microscope after neutralizing the gel with Tris buffer [24-26]. Pictures were captured electronically with an image analysis system and analyzed for fluorescence intensity. DNA damage was evaluated using the tail length and compared with the control group.

Examination of PS exposure

Surface exposure of phosphatidyl serine (PS) by apoptotic cells was examined according to manufacturer's protocol. Briefly, cells were seeded in 6-well plates (3 × 10^5 Cells/well) and treated with the agents for 24 hours. Cells were collected and resuspended in binding buffer (10 mM HEPES/NaOH, pH 7.4, 140 mM NaCl, 2.5 mM $CaCl_2$) then were incubated with Annexin V-FITC and PI for 15 minutes at room temperature and darkness. The fluorescent intensity of the cells was measured in FL1 (for FITC) and FL2 (for PI) using flow cytometry technique.

DNA fragmentation

Following drug treatments, 2 × 106 cells were collected and incubated in lysis buffer in ice for 20 minutes. The cells were centrifuged at 4°C at 12000 g for 30 minutes and then the supernatant was extracted after being centrifuged using 1:1 mixture of phenol: chloroform. Two equivalences of cold ethanol with one-tenth equivalence of sodium acetate were added; nucleic acid contaminant was decanted and exposed to water-RNase solution for 30 minutes at 37°C. The samples were electrophoresed through 1.5% agarose gel that contained ethidium bromide at 5 V for 5 minutes and then the voltage increased to 100 V for an hour [27].

Caspase activity assay

The caspase activity was investigated based on the Homogeneous Caspases Assay fluorimetric kit. According to the protocol, the cells were cultured in a "black microplate with clear bottom" and were treated. Caspase Substrate in lysis buffer was added and was then incubated at 37°C for 2 hours. The free substrate was determined fluorimetrically at 521 nm and the activity of caspases was quantified by a calibration curve.

Statistical analysis

The results were analyzed using one way ANOVA followed by Tukey-Kramer Posttest. The p-value less than 0.05 ($p < 0.05$) was considered significant.

Any experimental research that is reported in this manuscript have been approved by ethics committee of pharmaceutical sciences research center of Tehran University of Medical Sciences.

Results

Cytotoxicity of noscapine, papaverine, narceine and doxorubicin on breast cancer, colorectal carcinoma and connective tissue fibro sarcoma cell lines and non-cancerous cell line

The MTT curve showed that noscapine and papaverine had a dose-dependent cytotoxic effect on T47D, HT-29 and HT-1080 cell lines, with no cytotoxic effect on non-cancerous NIH-3 T3 cells. Narceine did not show any toxic effect on the studied cell lines and doxorubicin-induced cytotoxicity was demonstrated on both cancerous and noncancerous cells. The results are presented in Figure 1.

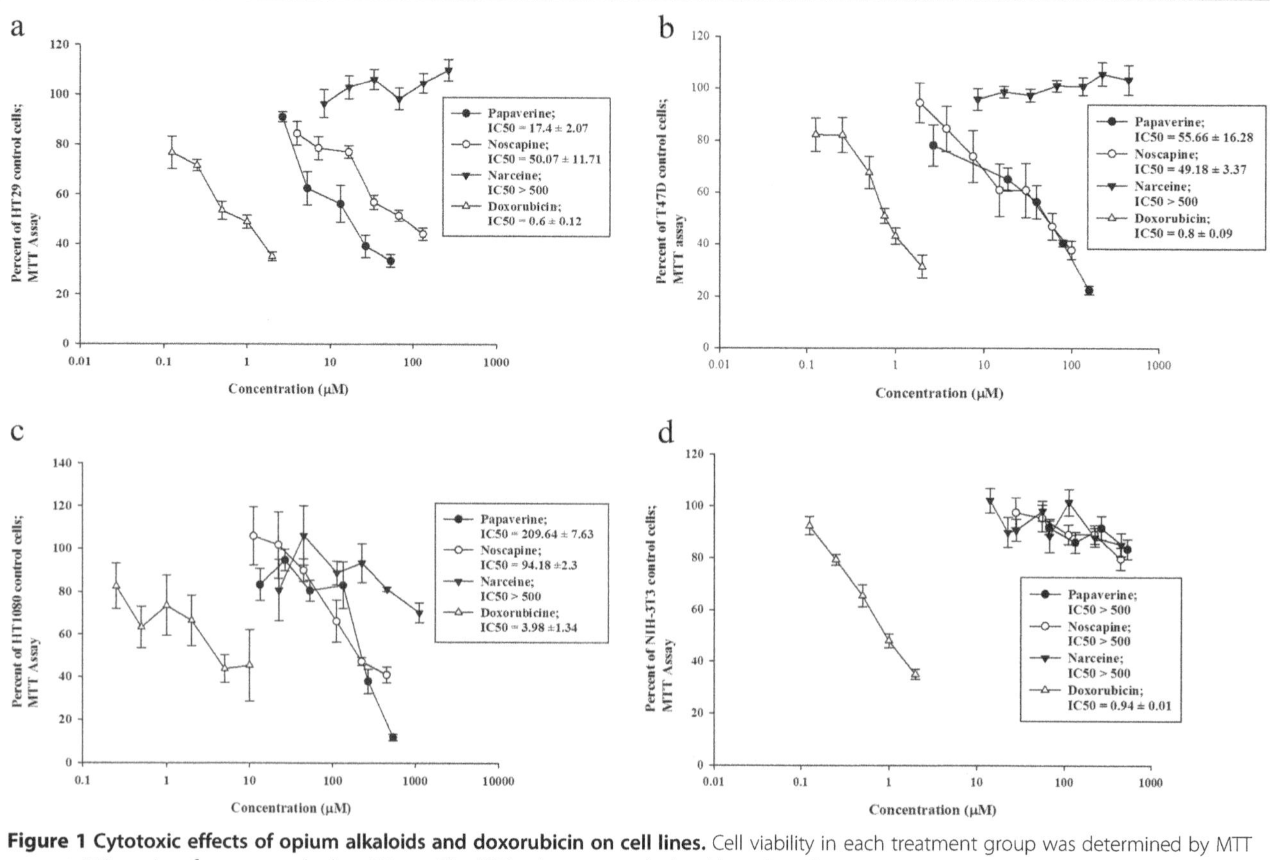

Figure 1 Cytotoxic effects of opium alkaloids and doxorubicin on cell lines. Cell viability in each treatment group was determined by MTT assay at 570 nm in reference standard at 690 nm. The IC50 values were calculated based on their cytotoxicity dose–response curve using Sigmaplot software and the results are expressed as Mean ± SD. **a**: HT29, **b**: T47D, **c**: HT1080 and **d**: NIH-3 T3.

Effect of noscapine, papaverine and narceine on DNA damage

The cells were evaluated with an image analysis system (CASP Comet assay Software Project) and the results are expressed in terms of L tail (length of tail) and are presented in Figure 2. Noscapine and papaverine selectively enhanced DNA damage on cancerous cells when compared with noncancerous cells ($p < 0.001$). On the other hand, DNA damage was observed on all the cell lines after administration of doxorubicin ($p < 0.001$). However, narceine induced DNA damage only on HT-1080 cells.

Effect of noscapine, papaverine, narceine on induction of apoptosis

Cell membrane asymmetry was investigated by translocation of phosphatidylserine to the cell surface in order to determine whether or not apoptosis was the major mechanism of cell death [28,29]. Based on this method, the apoptosis percentage has been reported and was compared with that in the control group (Figure 3). Results showed that doxorubicin has induced apoptosis in all the cell lines. However, noscapine and papaverine have induced apoptosis on HT-29 and T47D without any significant effect on NIH-3 T3 cell lines. However, the effects of narceine were different from the other two alkaloids. Narceine showed no apoptotic effect on the cell lines.

DNA fragmentation in T47D cells treated by noscapine, papaverine, narceine and compared to doxorubicin

To further determine if apoptosis was the major mechanism of the drug-induced cell death, DNA fragmentation was investigated in T47D cells. Figure 4 shows clear

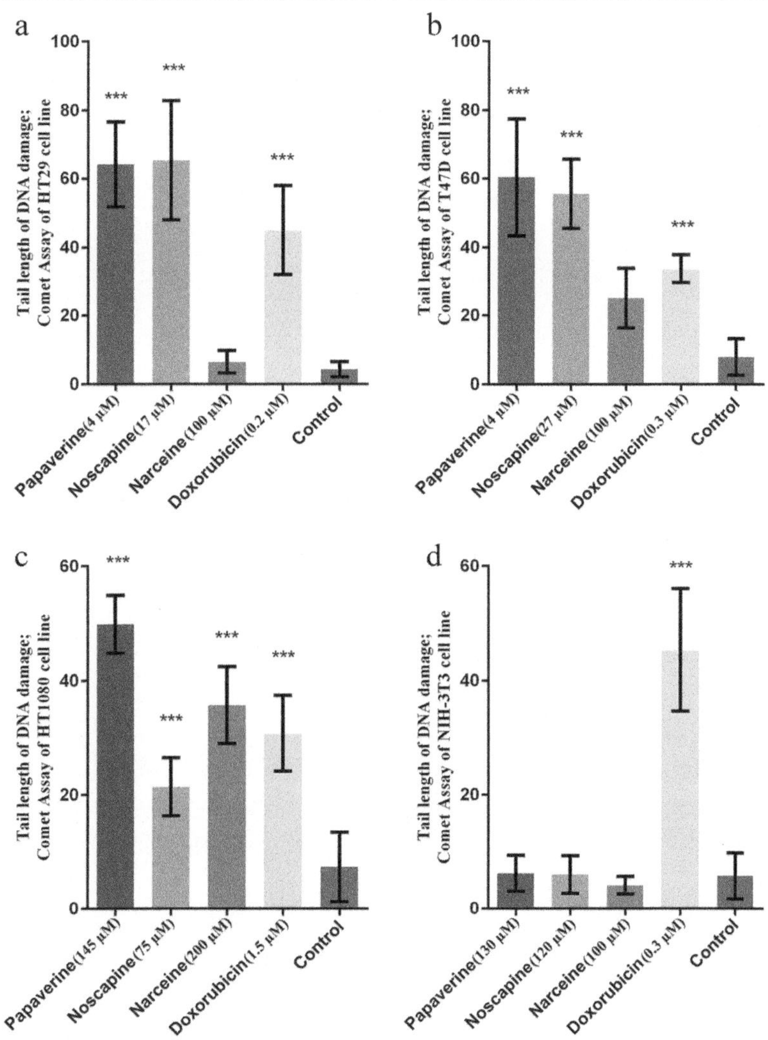

Figure 2 The DNA damage detected in treated cells compared to control group. The concentrations less than IC50 were used for treatment. The tail length of comet assay has been shown (Mean ± SD) and p-value has been reported. **a**: HT29, **b**: T47D, **c**: HT1080 and **d**: NIH-3 T3.

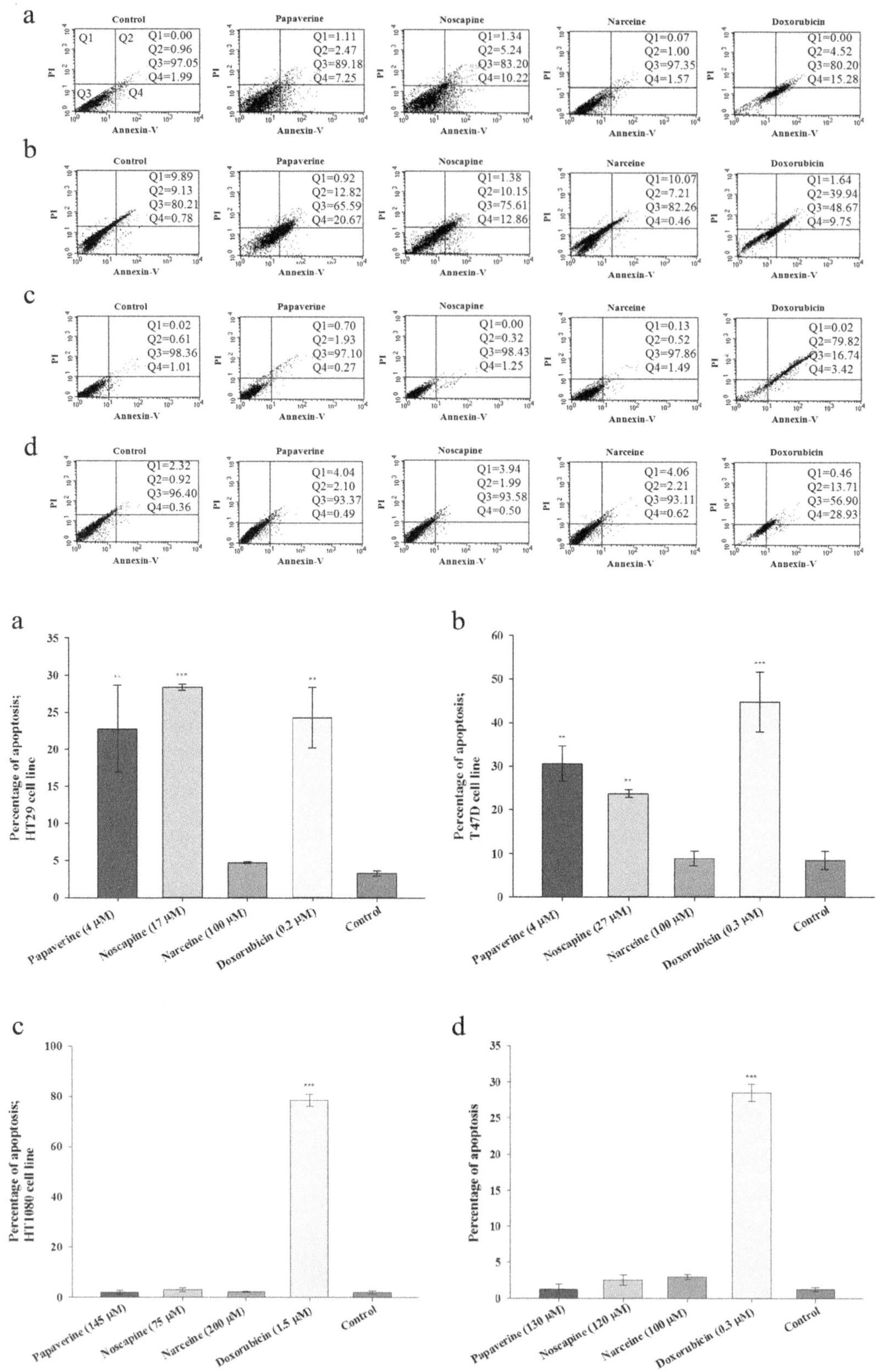

Figure 3 The membrane asymmetry comparison between treated cells compared to control group. The concentrations less than IC50 were used for treatment. The percentage of cell population of each quadrant has been shown and the quantitative average of percentage of apoptotic cells of repeated examinations (Mean ± SD) and p-value has been reported. **a**: HT29, **b**: T47D, **c**: HT1080 and **d**: NIH-3 T3.

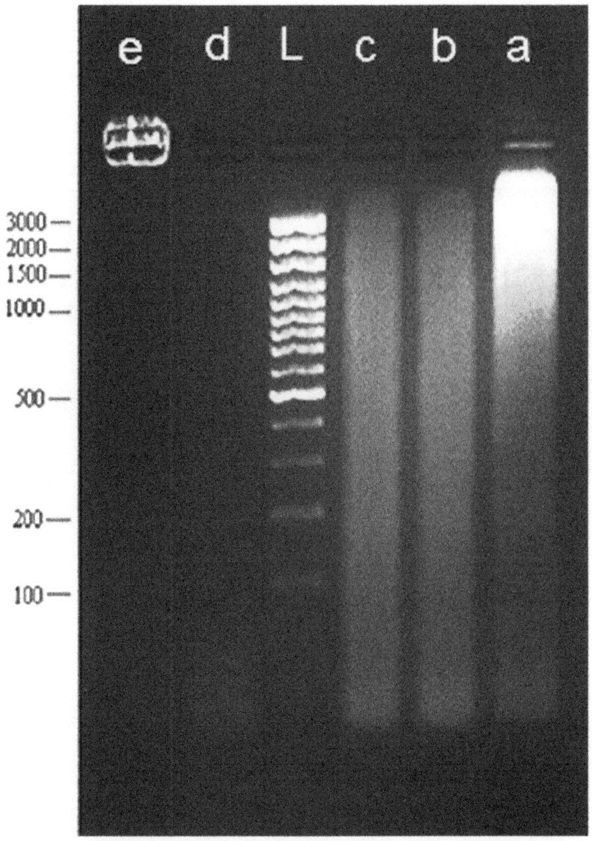

Figure 4 Internucleosomal fragmentation of T47D cells. The cells were treated with a: doxorubicin, b: noscapine, c: papaverine and d: narceine then DNA laddering was measured after 48 hours. e: negative control and L: Laddering marker are presented in figure as well.

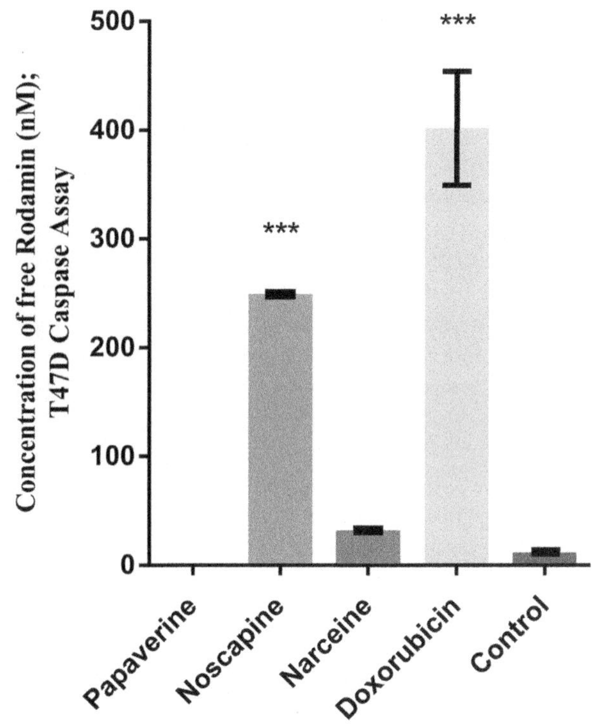

Figure 5 The activity of caspase-3 after 48 hours incubation of post-treatment T47D cells. Data are reported as mean ± SD. It is shown significant increase in caspase 3 activities after treatment by doxorubicin and noscapine ($p < 0.001$).

DNA fragmentation in cells treated by doxorubicin as positive control. Noscapine and papaverine induced DNA fragmentation in smaller sizes which were distinguishable from negative control group.

Caspase activity in T47D cells treated by noscapine, papaverine, narceine and compared to doxorubicin

Caspase-3 activity was measured by the cleavage of the substrate -Rodamin110- fluorimerically and was quantified by calibration curve (Figure 5). According to Figure 5 and in opposite to doxorubicin and noscapine, papaverine did not increase caspase activity.

Discussion

The present study noted that noscapine and papaverine had dose-dependent cytotoxic effects on cancer cell lines, without any cytotoxic effect on noncancerous NIH-3 T3 cells. Minor, non-significant increases are visible in cytotoxicity curves that maybe related to the non-specific toxicity caused by high concentrations of all three alkaloids used in this study. Therefore the selective toxicity observed in the present project as well as the unselective doxorubicin-induced toxicity could have affected both cancerous and noncancerous cells. To determine whether or not apoptosis was considered as the major cell death pathway, the cell lines were examined by using annexin -V affinity, Comet assay, DNA laddering and Caspase assay. The annexin V assay has been widely accepted as a marker of apoptosis. Annexin V, a calcium-dependent phospholipid-binding protein, binds to PS residues on the cell membrane that are translocated to the outside of the cell due to apoptosis [28,29]. DNA damage is a hallmark of cell death [30] and alkaline single cell gel electrophoresis (SCGE) or comet assay is a very sensitive assay for detection of some kinds of DNA damage including single strand DNA breakage, alkaline-labile sites and other damage that generates DNA breaks [25,30]. Based on the results of this study, noscapine and papaverine induced DNA damage followed by apoptosis on HT-29 and T47D cell lines without significant effect on NIH-3 T3 as a noncancerous cell line. Apoptotic effect of noscapine was confirmed by the results of DNA fragmentation and caspase assay. It should be mentioned that even though many other studies have previously noted apoptosis induced by noscapine on cancer cells, a limited number of research has focused on noncancerous cell lines [12,31]. Recently, noscapine has been recognized as a kinetic stabilizer compound. Interestingly, noscapine binds to different site of tubulin when compared to other known tubulin-binding agents. Additionally, even though noscapine's binding to tubulin site is not very strong, it is adequate enough to arrest the cell cycle [31]. Therefore, this feature might explain the selective cytotoxicity of noscapine. Based on the results of the present study and in contrast to noscapine and what was expected, papaverine did not increase caspase activity. Several studies have shown the apoptotic effect of papaverine [17,19,20,32]. However, a study on human promyelocytic leukemia HL60 cells declined cytotoxic and apoptotic effects of this alkaloid [33]. According to the results of DNA damage and apoptotic annexin-V assays, papaverine produced genotoxicity through induction of apoptosis in cancer cells. This lack of caspase activity has been also reported previously by Rubis et al. [20]. The results of the later study as well as our study may indicate that caspase-independent apoptosis pathways are involved in the programmed cell death related to papaverine. Further studies seem to be necessary to better clarify the exact mechanisms of papaverine-dependent apoptosis. Furthermore, in spite of DNA damage in HT-1080 after alkaloids treatment (Figure 2), apoptosis was not confirmed as a cell death pathway in this cell line. This contradiction might be related to intracellular repair system. However, the effects of narceine were different from those seen with the other two alkaloids on the cells in our study. Among the cells tested in this study, only HT-1080 cells were affected by DNA damage induced by narceine. However this damage did not result in apoptosis. It should be mentioned that all the findings about narceine were obtained despite the fact that no cytotoxicity was present when MTT assay was performed. Part of these findings may be related to other pathways of cell toxicity or death. However, more studies are needed to determine anti-tumor activity of narceine.

Conclusion

In the present study, we demonstrated that noscapine and papaverine inserted selective cytotoxicity effects on cancer cell lines in comparison to doxorubicin which showed unselective cytotoxic effects on both malignant and non-malignant cell lines. This effect may present a new approach for using non-addictive opium alkaloids in the treatment of cancer. Further investigations are needed to clarify and confirm the selective cytotoxic effects of these alkaloids on other noncancerous cell lines.

Competing interests

The authors declare that they have no competing interests.

Authors' contributions

MA carried out the practical activities, participated in the design of the study and drafted the manuscript. PG helped to draft and edited the manuscript. MK participated in the sequence alignment. MP participated in practical activities, data analysis and helped to draft the manuscript. HM participated in practical activities and data analysis. MHG participated in design of the study, data analysis and helped to draft the manuscript. SNO participated in study design, coordination and data analysis and helped to draft the manuscript. All authors read and approved the final manuscript.

Acknowledgment

This project was supported by of deputy of research at Tehran University of medical sciences (TUMS) (grant number 8960) and was a part of Dr. Afzali's thesis toward graduation to receive Pharm.D degree.

Author details

[1]Department Toxicology & Pharmacology, Faculty of Pharmacy, Toxicology & Poisoning Research Center, Tehran University of Medical Sciences, 14155/6451 Tehran, Iran. [2]Department Clinical Pharmacy, Faculty of Pharmacy & Rational Drug Use Research Center, Tehran University of Medical Sciences, 14155/6451 Tehran, Iran. [3]Department Pharmacognosy, Faculty of Pharmacy, Tehran University of Medical Sciences, 14155/6451 Tehran, Iran.

References

1. Goodman LS, Gilman A, Brunton LL, Parker KL, Blumenthal DK, Buxton ILO. Goodman & Gilman's manual of pharmacology and therapeutics. New Delhi: McGraw-Hill; 2008.
2. Aruna K, Sivaramakrishnan V. Anticarcinogenic effects of some Indian plant products. Food Chem Toxicol. 1992;30:953–6.
3. Healthcare T. PDR for Herbal Medicines. 4, illustrated edn. Montvale: Thomson Healthcare; 2007.
4. Evans WC. Trease and Evans. WB Saunders Harcourt Publishers Ltd. 2002;292:357–75.
5. Aneja R, Miyagi T, Karna P, Ezell T, Shukla D, Vij Gupta M, et al. A novel microtubule-modulating agent induces mitochondrially driven caspase-dependent apoptosis via mitotic checkpoint activation in human prostate cancer cells. Eur J Cancer. 2010;46:1668–78.
6. Ye K, Ke Y, Keshava N, Shanks J, Kapp JA, Tekmal RR, et al. Opium alkaloid noscapine is an antitumor agent that arrests metaphase and induces apoptosis in dividing cells. P Natl Acad Sci. 1998;95:1601.
7. Zhou J, Gupta K, Aggarwal S, Aneja R, Chandra R, Panda D, et al. Brominated derivatives of noscapine are potent microtubule-interfering agents that perturb mitosis and inhibit cell proliferation. Mol Pharmacol. 2003;63:799–807.
8. Aneja R, Lopus M, Zhou J, Vangapandu SN, Ghaleb A, Yao J, et al. Rational design of the microtubule-targeting anti-breast cancer drug EM015. Cancer Res. 2006;66:3782–91.
9. Aneja R, Vangapandu SN, Lopus M, Chandra R, Panda D, Joshi HC. Development of a novel nitro-derivative of noscapine for the potential treatment of drug-resistant ovarian cancer and T-cell lymphoma. Mol Pharmacol. 2006;69:1801–9.
10. Heidari N, Goliaei B, Moghaddam PR, Rahbar-Roshandel N, Mahmoudian M. Apoptotic pathway induced by noscapine in human myelogenous leukemic cells. Anticancer Drugs. 2007;18:1139–48.
11. Jaiswal AS, Aneja R, Connors SK, Joshi HC, Multani AS, Pathak S, et al. 9-bromonoscapine-induced mitotic arrest of cigarette smoke condensate transformed breast epithelial cells. J Cell Biochem. 2009;106:1146–56.
12. Mahmoudian M, Rahimi-Moghaddam P. The anti-cancer activity of noscapine: a review. Recent Pat Anticancer Drug Discov. 2009;4:92–7.
13. Aneja R, Ghaleb AM, Zhou J, Yang VW, Joshi HC. p53 and p21 determine the sensitivity of noscapine-induced apoptosis in colon cancer cells. Cancer Res. 2007;67:3862–70.
14. Jackson T, Chougule MB, Ichite N, Patlolla RR, Singh M. Antitumor activity of noscapine in human non-small cell lung cancer xenograft model. Cancer Chemother Pharmacol. 2008;63:117–26.
15. Chougule M, Patel AR, Sachdeva P, Jackson T, Singh M. Anticancer activity of Noscapine, an opioid alkaloid in combination with Cisplatin in human non-small cell lung cancer. Lung Cancer. 2011;71:271–82.

16. Chougule MB, Patel AR, Jackson T, Singh M. Antitumor activity of noscapine in combination with doxorubicin in triple negative breast cancer. PloS one. 2011;6:e17733.
17. Helson L, Lai K, Young CW. Papaverine-induced changes in cultured human melanoma cells. Biochem Pharmacol. 1974;23:2917–20.
18. Goto T, Matsushima H, Kasuya Y, Hosaka Y, Kitamura T, Kawabe K, et al. The effect of papaverine on morphologic differentiation, proliferation and invasive potential of human prostatic cancer LNCaP cells. Int J Urol. 1999;6:314–9.
19. Nohl H, Rohr-Udilova N, Gille L, Bieberschulte W, Jurek D, Marian B, et al. Ubiquinol and the papaverine derivative caroverine prevent the expression of tumour-promoting factors in adenoma and carcinoma colon cancer cells induced by dietary fat. Biofactors. 2005;25:87–95.
20. Rubis B, Kaczmarek M, Szymanowska N, Galezowska E, Czyrski A, Juskowiak B, et al. The biological activity of G-quadruplex DNA binding papaverine-derived ligand in breast cancer cells. Invest New Drugs. 2009;27:289–96.
21. Morgan DML. Tetrazolium (MTT) assay for cellular viability and activity. Methods Mol Biol. 1997;79:179–83.
22. Plumb JA. Cell sensitivity assays: the MTT assay. Methods mol med. 2004;88:165–70.
23. Burton JD. The MTT assay to evaluate chemosensitivity. Methods Mol Med. 2005;110:69–78.
24. Lah B, Gorjanc G, Nekrep FV, Marinsek-Logar R. Comet assay assessment of wastewater genotoxicity using yeast cells. Bull Environ Contam Toxicol. 2004;72:607–16.
25. Kopjar N, Milas I, Garaj-Vrhovac V, Gamulin M. Alkaline comet assay study with breast cancer patients: evaluation of baseline and chemotherapy-induced DNA damage in non-target cells. Clin Exp Med. 2006;6:177–90.
26. Dhawan A, Bajpayee M, Parmar D. Comet assay: a reliable tool for the assessment of DNA damage in different models. Cell Biol Toxicol. 2009;25:5–32.
27. DNA Fragmantation Assays for Apoptosis Protocol. [hedricklab.ucsd.edu/Protocol/DNAFRAG.html]
28. Miller E. Apoptosis Measurement by Annexin V Staining. In: Langdon SP, editor. Cancer cell culture: methods and protocols, vol. Volume 88. Totowa: Springer; 2004. p. 191–202.
29. Jones S, Howl J. Applications of cell-penetrating peptides as signal transduction modulators for the selective induction of apoptosis. In: Langel U, editor. Methods in molecular biology, vol. Volume 683. Clifton: springer; 2011. p. 291–303.
30. Roos WP, Kaina B. DNA damage-induced cell death by apoptosis. Trends Mol Med. 2006;12:440–50.
31. Dhiman N, Sood A, Sharma A. Noscapine: An Anti-Mitotic Agent. 2013.
32. Gao YJ, Stead S, Lee RMKW. Papaverine induces apoptosis in vascular endothelial and smooth muscle cells. Life Sciences. 2002;70:2675–85.
33. Rosenkranz V, Wink M. Induction of apoptosis by alkaloids, non-protein amino acids and cardiac glycosides in human promyelotic HL-60 cells. Zeitschrift fur Naturforschung C-Journal of Biosciences. 2007;62:458.

Alteration in brain-derived neurotrophic factor (BDNF) after treatment of mice with herbal mixture containing Euphoria longana, Houttuynia cordata and Dioscorea japonica

Songhee Jeon[1], Chia-Hung Lee[2], Quan Feng Liu[2], Geun Woo Kim[3], Byung-Soo Koo[4*] and Sok Cheon Pak[5]

Abstract

Background: Literature data indicate that brain-derived neurotrophic factor (BDNF), cyclic-AMP response element-binding protein (CREB) and phospho-CREB (pCREB) may have a place in depression. BDNF belongs to the neurotrophin family that plays an important role in proliferation, survival and differentiation of different cell populations in the mammalian nervous system. The herbal mixture used in the present study consists of *Euphoria longana*, *Houttuynia cordata* and *Dioscorea japonica*. The purpose of the present study was to determine the neuroprotective effect of herbal mixture. We also tested the hypothesis that administration of herbs reverses memory deficits and promotes the protein expression of BDNF in the mouse brain.

Methods: Mice were randomized into four different treatment groups (n = 10/group). Normal and stress groups received regular lab chow without stress and under stress conditions, respectively, for 3 weeks. The animals in the stress group were immobilized for 4 hours a day for 2 weeks. Different doses of herbal mixture (206 and 618 mg/kg) were administered for 3 weeks to those mice under stress conditions. Mice were analyzed by behavioral tests and immunoblotting examination in the hippocampus and cortex. An additional in vitro investigation was performed to examine whether herbs induce neurotoxicity in a human neuroblastoma cell line, SH-SY5Y cells.

Results: No significant toxicity of herbs on human neuroblastoma cells was observed. These herbs demonstrated an inductive effect on the expression of BDNF, pCREB and pAkt. For spatial working memory test, herbal mixture fed mice exhibited an increased level of spontaneous alternation ($p < 0.01$) compared to those in stress conditions. Moreover, herbal mixture produced highly significant ($p < 0.01$) reduction in the immobility time in the tail suspension test. Mice in the herbal mixture groups demonstrated lower serum corticosterone concentration than mice in the stress group ($p < 0.05$). Effects of the oral administration of herbal mixture on protein levels of BDNF in the hippocampi and cortices were significant.

Conclusions: Our study showed that herbal mixture administration has antidepressant effects in mice. It is proposed that adverse events such as stress and depression can modulate the expression of molecular players of cellular plasticity in the brain.

Keywords: Stress, Depression, BDNF, Memory, *Euphoria longana*, *Houttuynia cordata*, *Dioscorea japonica*

* Correspondence: koobs@dongguk.ac.kr
[4]Department of Korean Neuropsychiatry, Dongguk University Ilsan Oriental Hospital, Goyang, Republic of Korea
Full list of author information is available at the end of the article

Background

Specific data from the Global Burden of Disease 2010 study confirmed that mental and substance use disorders account for 7.4% of disease burden worldwide which is greater than HIV/AIDS and tuberculosis (5.3%), diabetes (2%) or transport injuries (3.3%) [1]. Depression in particular is projected to become the leading cause of disability and the second leading contributor to the global burden of disease in approximately 10 years [2]. As a heterogeneous disorder with unclear etiology, depression includes disturbance of neurogenesis, genetic predisposition, deficiency of monoamines, hypercortisolemia, reduction of neurotrophins, inflammation and oxidative stress [3].

It has been proposed that brain-derived neurotrophic factor (BDNF), as one of neurotrophins, may be a key player in depression since it is involved in regulation of neuronal differentiation, survival, function and plasticity [4]. This neurotrophic hypothesis of depression claims that decreased levels of BDNF contribute to the hippocampal atrophy seen in depressed patients [5]. Depressive symptoms are also associated with decreased serum level of BDNF [6]. These evidences have already led to clinical trials of antidepressant medications for treating major depression, although there are some gaps in the clinical outcomes depending on the classes of psychotropic drugs and uncertainty about whether drugs that specifically target depressive symptoms are feasible and safe. The transcription of BDNF is dependent on cyclic-AMP response element-binding protein (CREB).

CREB is a transcriptional factor implicated in the control of adaptive neuronal responses. It has been found that calcium ions in neurons bind to a calcium response element within the BDNF gene which triggers phosphorylation of CREB and subsequent activation of BDNF transcription [7]. Depression is accompanied by down-regulated and decreased phosphorylated CREB (pCREB). A growing number of clinical and experimental studies have demonstrated that structural and functional modifications of hippocampus from antidepressant treatments most likely require the transcription and protein expression of CREB, despite some inconsistencies in its mRNA and protein levels depending on the brain regions where such molecule is expressed [7]. CREB is regulated by several pathways including protein kinase B (PKB/Akt).

Antidepressant medications are effective at treating depression, but discontinuation rates are high because adverse effects are common [8]. For example, selective serotonin reuptake inhibitors (SSRIs) frequently cause gastrointestinal problems, insomnia, headache, anxiety and sexual dysfunction although they are the most commonly prescribed antidepressants [9]. Considering the side effects of synthetic antidepressants, natural plants can be alternative sources of new antidepressant drugs due to their more tolerable and less toxic properties. Therefore, the current study was performed as the progress toward finding reliable alternatives to depression.

Three different ingredients of traditional Korean medicine for depression were selected to observe the effects of them in cell culture and animal experiment. *Euphoria longana* Lam., especially a dried longan seed extract, contain high levels of antioxidant polyphenolic compounds [10]. Longan seed extracts are found to possess anticancer properties by inducing apoptosis [11]. *Houttuynia cordata* Thunb. is a single species of its genus and the whole plant of *H. cordata* is used for the treatment of diabetes [12]. Reported pharmacological activities of plant include anti-cancer [13], anti-inflammatory [13] and antioxidant [14]. The rhizome of *Dioscorea japonica* Thunb. has been used to strengthen stomach function, improve anorexia, eliminate diarrhea, dilute sputum, and moisturize skin in traditional Chinese medicine [15]. An ethanol extract of the rhizome of *D. japonica* showed considerable cytotoxic activity against some human tumor cell lines [16]. These three natural plants have been used as traditional herbal medicines in the treatment of neurological disorders in Korea. However, few studies have evaluated their anti-depressant effects. The effects of these three herbs on BDNF, pCREB and pAkt are currently unknown. In this experiment, one human neuroblastoma cell line was used to investigate the neuroprotective effect of herbs. We also tested the hypothesis that administration of herbs reverses memory deficits and promotes the protein expression of BDNF in the mouse brain. To test the hypothesis, three different settings of neuronal cell culture, behaviour study and their brains have been used in the present study.

Methods

Preparation of herbal extracts

All medicinal herbs used were purchased from DY Herb (Seoul, Korea). Each herb was boiled in 30% ethanol mixed filter-purified drinking water for 2 h at 100°C in a reflux condenser. For the cellular experiment, aqueous extract of each herb was freeze-dried and the dried extract was reconstructed with distilled water and filtered through 0.2 μm filter (Millipore, MA, USA). In addition, the resulting dry powder of each herb was mixed with the same ratio and added into the feed in the animal studies.

Cell culture

Human neuroblastoma SH-SY5Y cells were obtained from American Type Culture Collection (Rockville, MD, USA). Cells were maintained in Dulbecco's modified Eagle's minimum essential medium (DMEM, Invitrogen, Carlsbad, CA, USA) supplemented with 10% fetal bovine serum (FBS, Invitrogen, Carlsbad, CA, USA), 100 unit/ml penicillin and 100 μg/ml streptomycin (Gibco-BRL, Rockville, MD, USA) with further addition of trypsin-

EDTA (Gibco-BRL, Rockville, MD, USA) in condition of 95% air and 5% CO_2 at 37°C.

Cell viability assay

Cell viability was determined by 3-(4,5-dimethylthizaol-2-yl)-2,5-diphenyltetrazolium bromide (MTT, Abcam, Cambridge, MA, USA) assay. SH-SY5Y cells were seeded in 12-well plates (Corning Incorporated, USA) at a density of 5×10^3 cells/well, stabilized at 37°C for 16 h in DMEM medium supplemented with FBS and cultured with the indicated concentrations of herbs for 24 h. The medium was removed and the cells were incubated with 2 mg/ml of MTT solution. After incubation for 4 h at 37°C and 5% CO_2, the supernatants were removed and dimethyl sulfoxide (DMSO, Sigma, USA) was added. The reactants were measured in terms of optical density (OD) at 580 nm with a microplate reader (UV max, Molecular Devices, USA). The optical densities were converted into percentages using the following formula: Cell viability (%) = OD sample/OD negative control × 100. Negative control cells were treated with complete DMEM alone.

Quantification of BDNF/pCREB/pAkt expression by Western blot analysis

SH-SY5Y cells were maintained in serum-free medium with herbs at 30 μg/ml for 24 h. Cells were then washed twice with ice-cold PBS and lysed in lysis buffer containing 62.5 mmol/L Tris–HCl, pH 6.8, 2% SDS, 20% glycerol, 10% 2-mercaptoethanol and protease inhibitors. After incubation for 30 min on ice, cell lysates were centrifuged and protein concentrations were determined using bicinchoninic acid method (Pierce). Samples of cell lysate containing 50 μg of total protein were separated by 4-12% SDS-PAGE and transferred onto nitrocellulose membrane (Amersham Pharmacia Biotech, Buckinghamshire, UK) by electroblotting. After blocking with 5% skim milk in Tris-buffered saline (50 mmol/L Tris–HCl, pH 7.6, 150 mmul/L NaCl, 0.1% Tween-20) for more than 30 min, the membranes were incubated for 16 h at 4°C with primary antibodies (anti-BDNF, anti-phosphorylated-CREB, anti-phosphorylated-Akt, β-actin antibody) and further incubated with horseradish peroxidase-conjugated secondary antibodies for 1 h. The membranes were visualized by an enhanced chemiluminescence system (ECL kit; Pierce, Rockford, IL, USA). Densitometric analysis was performed by Quantity One (Bio-Rad, Hercules, CA) to scan the signals. Further assay was carried out to detect BDNF protein expression in the hippocampus and cortex. The treated hippocampal and cortical tissues removed and homogenized in lysis buffer containing 50 mM Tris-base (pH 7.5), 150 mM NaCl, 2 mM EDTA, 1% glycerol, 10 mM NaF, 10 mM Na-pyrophosphate, 1% NP-40 and protease inhibitors (0.1 mM phenylmethylsulfonylfluoride, 5 μg/ml aprotinin, and 5 μg/ml leupeptin). Thirty μg of tissue lysate were electrophoresed using SDS-polyacrylamide gels and transferred to nitrocellulose membranes, which were then incubated with anti-BDNF (Cell signaling technology, Beverly, MA, USA) for 16 h at 4°C. After washing with TBS-T (0.05%), the blots were incubated with horseradish peroxidase-conjugated anti-rabbit or anti-mouse IgG, and the bands were visualized using the ECL system (Thermo Fisher Scienctific, USA). Band images were obtained by using a Molecular Imager ChemiDoc XRS$^+$ (Bio-Rad, Hercules, CA, USA) and band intensity was analyzed using Image Lab™ software version 2.0.1 (Bio-Rad).

Experimental animals

Protocols for animal use were reviewed and approved by the Institutional Animal Care and Use Committee at the Dongguk University Ilsan Hospital and were in accordance with National Institute of Health guidelines. Healthy male ICR mice (20–26 g, 6 weeks old) were obtained from OrientBio (Seoul, Korea) and were allowed 1 week for quarantine and acclimatization. Animals were housed under the conditions of constant temperature (22 ± 1°C), relative humidity (55 ± 1%) and 12 h light/12 h dark cycle (light on at 7:00 am). They were housed in polycarbonate cages and given tap water and commercial rodent chow (Samyang Feed, Daejeon, Korea) ad libitum. Forty mice were blindly randomized into four different treatment groups (n = 10/group). Normal and stress groups received regular lab chow without stress and under stress conditions, respectively, for 3 weeks. The animals in the stress group were immobilized for 4 h a day for 2 weeks by being gently inserted into a flexible triangle shaped vinyl screen that was closed and secured with nonallergic adhesive tape. Different doses of herbal mixture (206 and 618 mg/kg which are equivalent to the recommended adult human dose of 1000 and 3000 mg/kg, respectively) were administered for 3 weeks to those mice under stress conditions. The herbal mixture of *E. longana*, *H. cordata* and *D. japonica* was in a ratio of 1:1:1 by weight. Lab chow with or without herbal mixture was prepared for a mouse to have 1 g/kg/day which is equivalent to 7 g/60 kg/day for human and was gamma-irradiated. In order to examine the nutritional status, body weight was evaluated in mice that were fed with normal or herb mixture diet. At the end of experiment period, all animals were immediately decapitated, and their hippocampus and cortex of brains were collected and frozen at −80°C for following analysis. Blood was collected from the heart by cardiac puncture prior to the excision of brain, then after centrifugation serum aliquots were stored at −70°C for further corticosterone determination. The concentration of serum corticosterone was measured with the Corticosterone EIA Kit (Enzo Life Sciences, Farmingdale, NY, USA) in accordance with the manufacturer's instructions.

Step-through passive avoidance test

The apparatus (AP model; O'Hara Co., Tokyo, Japan) for the step-through passive avoidance test consisted of two compartments, an illuminated compartment [100 mm · 120 mm · 100 mm; light at the top of compartment (27 W, 3000 lx)] and a dark compartment (100 mm · 170 mm · 100 mm). The compartments were separated by a guillotine door. During the training trial, a mouse was placed in the safe, illuminated compartment. As the compartment was lit, the mouse stepped through the opened guillotine door into the dark compartment. The time spent in the illuminated compartment was defined as the latency time. Three seconds after the mouse entered the dark compartment, a foot shock (0.3 mA, 50 V, 50 Hz ac for 3 seconds) was delivered to the floor grids in the dark compartment. The mouse could escape from the shock only by stepping back to the safe illuminated compartment. Mice remaining in the light chamber for more than 120 seconds during the learning stage were excluded from the following retention trial. The retention trials were carried out at 24 h after the training trial to evaluate the retention of avoidance memory. The latency time was measured for up to 300 seconds without delivering a foot shock. It was judged that the mouse retained the avoidance memory when it stayed in the illuminated safe compartment for 300 seconds.

Y-maze test

This behavioral test was performed at 48 h after the passive avoidance test. The maze was made of black painted wood; each arm was 40 cm long, 12 cm high, 3 cm wide at the bottom and 10 cm wide at the top. The arms converged at an equilateral triangular central area that was 4 cm at its longest axis. Each mouse was placed at the centre of the apparatus and allowed to move freely through the maze for 8 min. The series of arm entries was recorded visually. Alternation was defined as successive entry into the three arms on overlapping triplet sets. Alternation behavior (%) was calculated as the ratio of actual alternations to possible alternations (defined as the number of arm entries minus two) multiplied by 100.

Forced swimming test

Mice were placed in a Plexiglas cylinder 25 cm in height with a 15 cm internal diameter containing water at a temperature of 25 ± 1°C and a depth of 10 cm so they could not escape and could not touch the bottom. Water was changed between each swim session to prevent possible effects of an alarm substance released by mice during the swim session. There were two swim sessions. The first was 15 min pre-test swim for 3 days in a row and a second 5 min swim test. The pre-test facilitates the development of immobility during the test session and increases the sensitivity for detecting antidepressant behavioral effects. The 5 min swim test was used for analysis of behavior such as swimming, climbing and immobility.

Tail suspension test

Mice both acoustically and visually isolated were suspended individually by their tails 40 cm above the tabletop with the use of an adhesive tape placed approximately 1 cm from the tip of the tail. After a few minutes of vigorous activity, the mice hung passively and completely motionless. The total immobility period in number of seconds was scored throughout the 6 min test. Mice were considered immobile with the absence of any limb or body movements, except for those caused by respiration. A

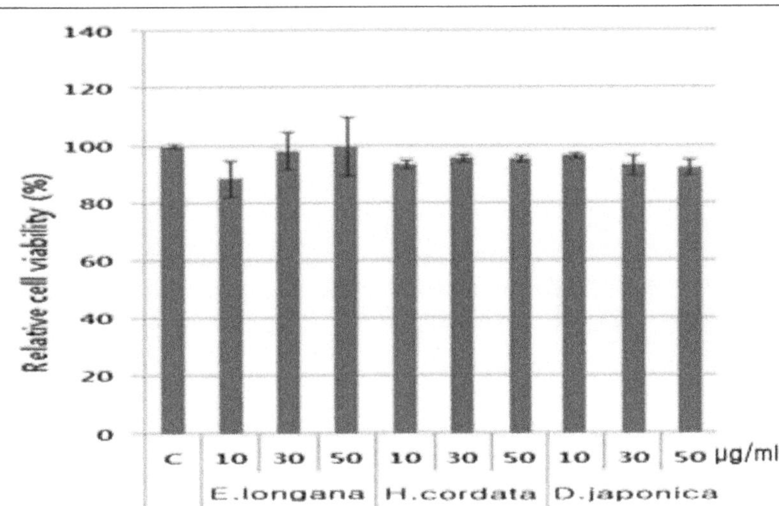

Figure 1 Effect of herbs on the cell viability measured by MTT assay. The human neuroblastoma SH-SY5Y cells were incubated at concentrations of 10, 30 and 50 µg/ml of each herb for 24 h. Values are presented as means ± SEM of six determinations.

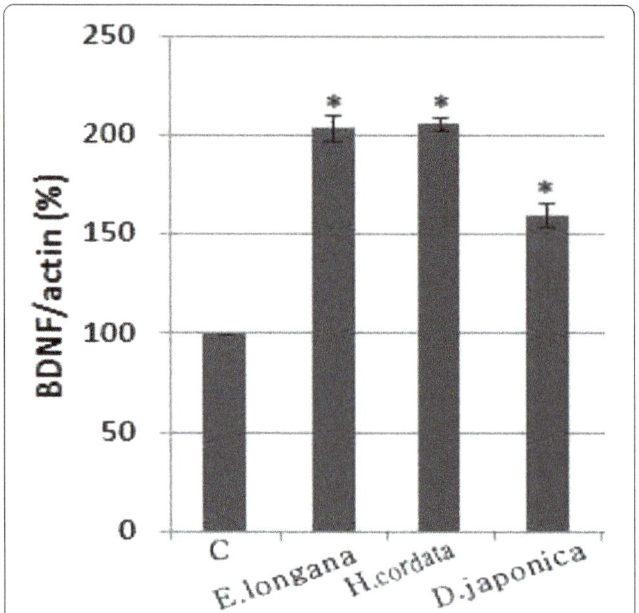

Figure 2 Measurement of BDNF level in neuroblastoma SH-SY5Y cells. To evaluate the protein level of BDNF expression, cells were incubated with 30 μg/ml herb. For the control, nonincubated cells were analyzed. The BDNF level in cell lysates was measured by immunoblotting. Data are presented as means ± SEM of three determinations. *$P < 0.05$ vs. control.

decrease in the duration of immobility is indicative of an antidepressant-like effect [17].

Data analysis

All statistical analyses were conducted with SPSS (ver. 19, Somers, NY, USA). Values are expressed as means ± SEM. All data were analyzed using Student's t-test. Statistical significance was accepted at a p value less than 0.05.

Results

Effect of herbs on cell viability

In order to measure the cytotoxicity of herbs on SH-SY5Y neuroblastoma cells, a cell viability using MTT assay was utilized. Cells were treated with herbs at concentrations of 10, 30 and 50 μg/ml for 24 h (Figure 1). The percentages of viable cells were as follows: *E. longana* 10 μg/ml, 88.53 ± 6.3%; 30 μg/ml, 98.25 ± 6.4%; 50 μg/ml, 99.73 ± 10.1%; *H. cordata* 10 μg/ml, 93.76 ± 1.6%; 30 μg/ml, 95.83 ± 1.2%; 50 μg/ml, 95.61 ± 1.0%; and *D. japonica* 10 μg/ml, 96.58 ± 0.9%; 30 μg/ml, 93.22 ± 3.4%; 50 μg/ml, 92.38 ± 2.8%. No significant toxicity of herbs on SH-SY5Y was observed at the indicated concentrations.

Effect of herbs on BDNF/pCREB/pAkt expression

We looked at the inductive effects of herbs on the expression of BDNF, pCREB and pAkt in cell extracts. For the control, nonincubated SH-SY5Y cells were analyzed. The BDNF expression in the SH-SY5Y cell extracts treated with herbs was significantly higher than that in the control

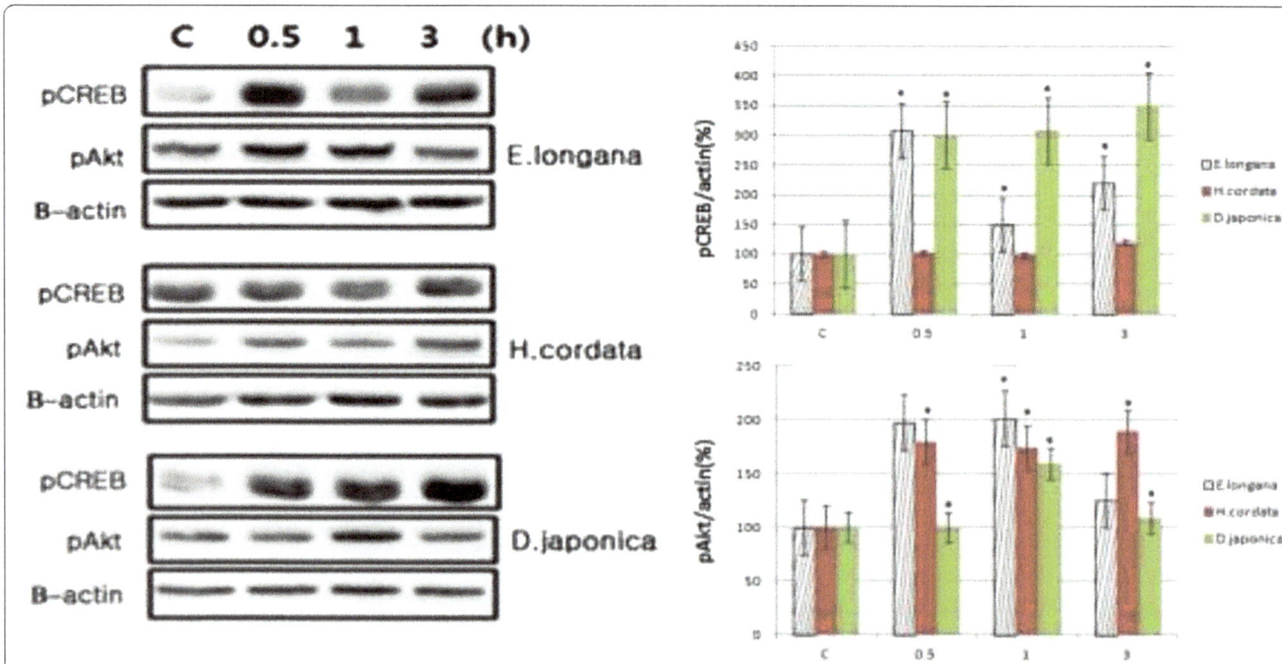

Figure 3 Time course of expression of pCREB and pAkt in neuroblastoma SH-SY5Y cells. To evaluate the protein level of pCREB and pAkt expression, cells were incubated with 30 μg/ml herb. For the control, nonincubated cells were analyzed. The level of pCREB and pAkt in cell lysates was measured by immunoblotting. Data are presented as means ± SEM of three determinations. *$P < 0.05$ vs. control.

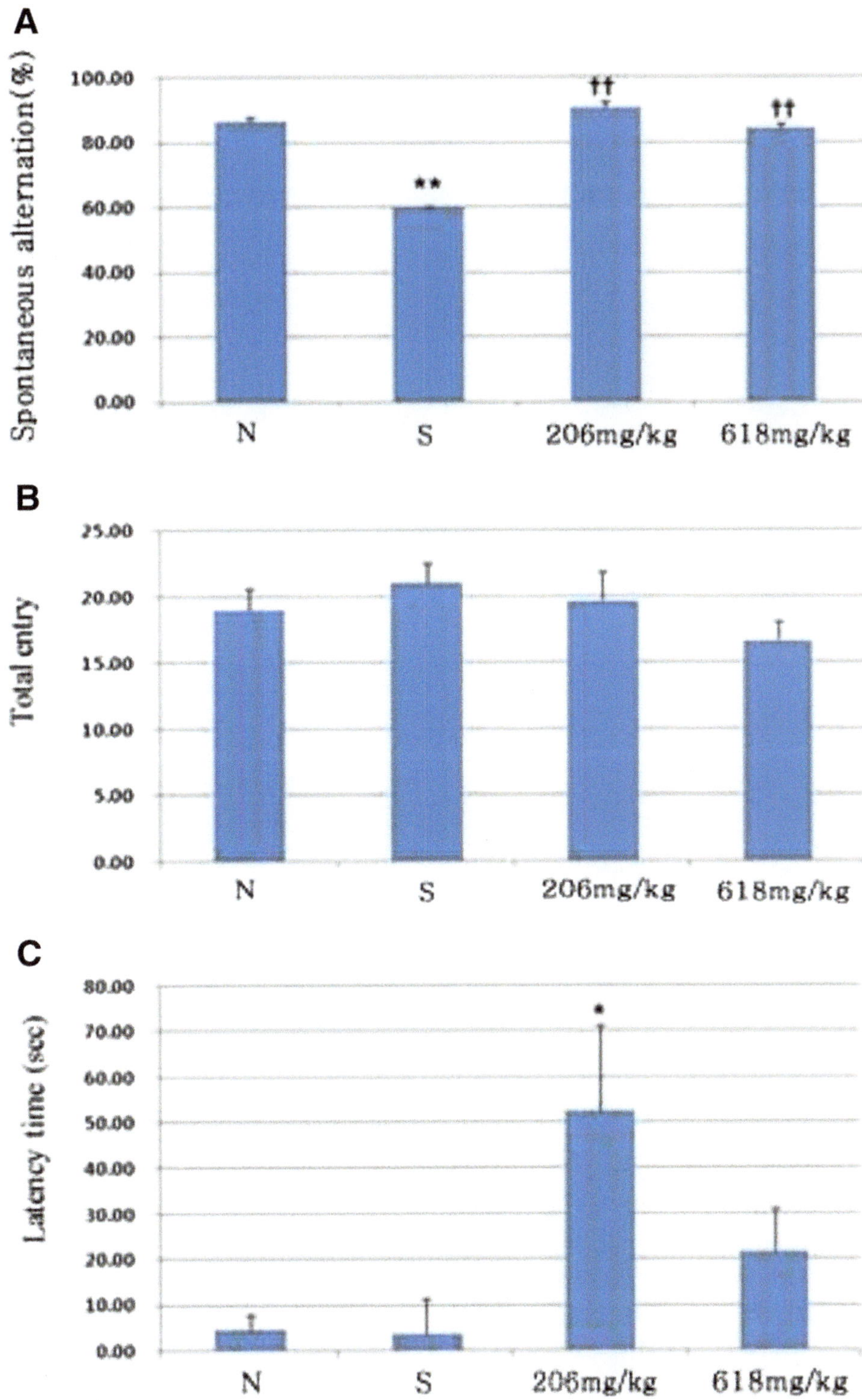

Figure 4 Attenuated effect of herb mixture on stress induced impairment of the Y-maze task and passive avoidance task in mice. Spontaneous alternation in behavior **(A)** and the number of arm entries **(B)** were measured. **(C)** Mice were subjected to the training trial and the step-through latency time was measured. Data are presented as means ± SEM of three determinations. $^{*}P < 0.05$ vs. stress, $^{**}P < 0.01$ vs. normal, $^{††}P < 0.01$ vs. normal.

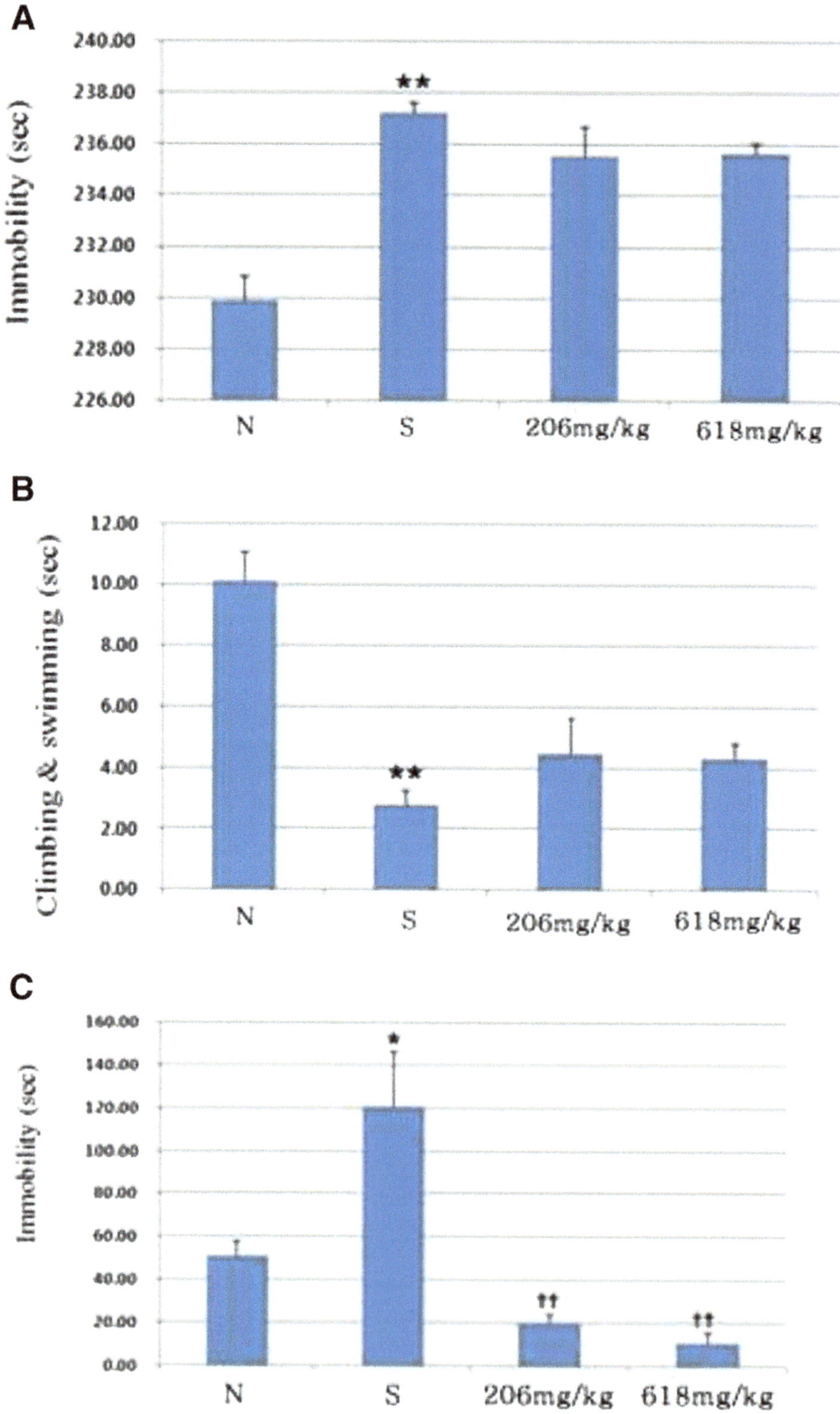

Figure 5 Effect of herbal mixture on duration of immobility (A), swimming and climbing (B) behaviors in mice when sampled during the 5 min swim test. (C) Effect of herbal mixture on the amount of immobility in mice during the tail suspension test. Behavior was observed during the 6 min test period and scored as mobile or immobile. Data are presented as means ± SEM of three determinations. $^{*}P < 0.05$ vs. normal, $^{**}P < .01$ vs. normal, $^{††}P < 0.01$ vs. stress.

cells (Figure 2). Immunoblotting analysis confirmed these results (figure not shown). To determine the expression of pCREB and pAkt, the cultures were harvested at 30 min, 1 h and 3 h and immunoblotting was performed on the cell extracts (Figure 3). Compared to the control, the expression of pCREB treated with 30 μg/ml of *E. longana* was 308 ± 8%, 150 ± 11% and 220 ± 10% at 30 min, 1 h and 3 h, respectively. For *H. cordata*, it was 102 ± 11%, 98 ± 15% and 120 ± 12% at 30 min, 1 h and 3 h, respectively. In the case of *D. japonica*, it was 302 ± 11%, 308 ± 15% and 350 ± 14% at 30 min, 1 h and 3 h, respectively. The pAkt expression in the cell extracts that were incubated with 30 μg/ml of *E. longana* was 198 ± 11%, 202 ± 15% and 126 ± 16% at 30 min, 1 h and 3 h, respectively. For *H. cordata*, it was 180 ± 11%, 175 ± 10% and 190 ± 9% at 30 min, 1 h and 3 h, respectively. In the case of *D. japonica*, it was 100 ± 10%, 160 ± 12% and 109 ± 17% at 30 min, 1 h and 3 h, respectively. Overall each herb was able to induce the expression of pCREB and pAkt regardless of time course.

Antidepressant effect of herbal mixture

We examined whether herbal mixture attenuated depression in mice under stress conditions. We first performed the Y-maze test for spatial working memory. Only the stress mice displayed a reduced level of spontaneous alternation in the Y-maze test compared to that of the normal control group ($p < 0.01$, Figure 4A). However, mice in the experimental group, which were fed herbal mixture for 3 weeks, exhibited an increased level of spontaneous alternation ($p < 0.01$, Figure 4A). In addition, the total number of maze arm entries was not different among the groups (Figure 4B). We then examined the effects of herbal mixture on learning and memory using a passive avoidance test. Administration of low dose herbal mixture attenuated the learning memory impairment induced by stress ($p < 0.05$, Figure 4C). This finding indicates that herbal mixture improved the stress induced memory impairment under stress conditions. We further examined the effect of herbal mixture on the forced swim test. In 5 min swim test, normal mice were immobile for 229.91 ± 1.0 sec and stress mice were immobile for 237.20 ± 0.4 sec ($p < 0.01$, Figure 5A). The immobility was the sum of the durations of floating, twitching and kicking behaviors. We observed that herbal mixture administration did not induce any significant change in immobility when compared to the stress group. But it trended in favor of herbal mixture. When climbing and swimming behaviors were combined, stress mice were less active with 2.80 ± 0.4 sec than those in normal group with 10.09 ± 1.0 ($p < 0.01$, Figure 5B). Herbal mixture caused improvement of activity compared with stress group but as a non-significant trend. The effects on immobility and swimming observed after the administration of high dose of herbal mixture were similar to those observed after the administration of low dose of herbal mixture. On the other hand, herbal mixture produced highly significant reduction in the immobility time in the tail suspension test ($p < 0.01$, Figure 5C). Figure 6 illustrates the serum corticosterone concentration among groups. Mice in the herbal mixture groups demonstrated lower serum corticosterone concentration than those in the stress group ($p < 0.05$). As expected, mice exposed to the chronic stress paradigm had elevated corticosterone level compared to those in the normal group ($p < 0.05$). Effects of the oral administration of herbal mixture on protein levels of BDNF in the hippocampi and cortices are shown in Figure 7. Statistical analysis indicated a significant effect of administration with herbal mixture. There were 54.55% ($p < 0.01$) and 52.15% ($p < 0.01$) increase in the levels of BDNF in the hippocampal tissues after administration with 206 and 618 mg/kg herbal mixture as compared with stress group,

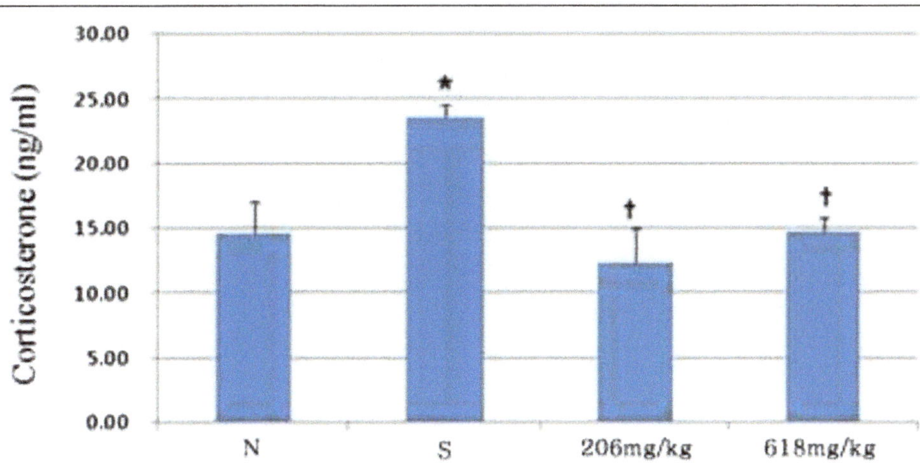

Figure 6 Effects of exposure to chronic stress and herbal mixture on corticosterone levels. Data are presented as means ± SEM of ten mice per group. *$P < 0.05$ vs. normal, †$P < 0.05$ vs. stress.

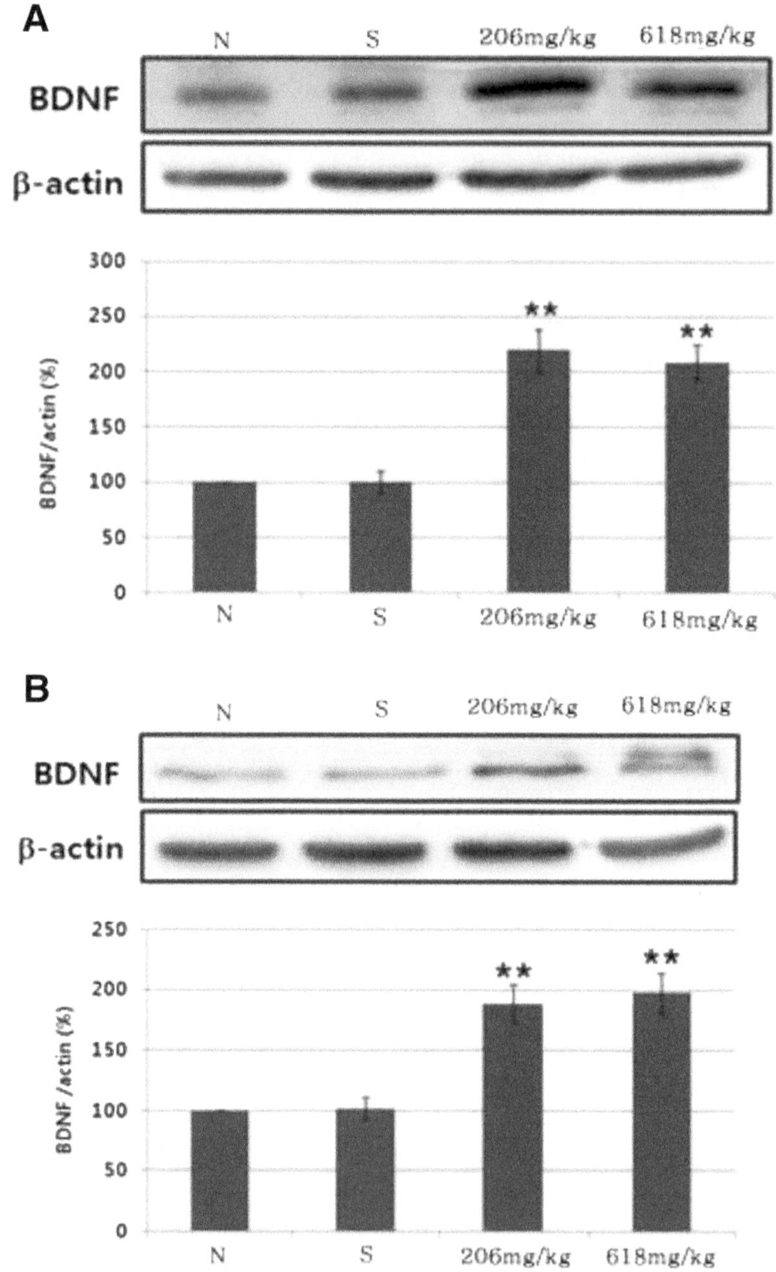

Figure 7 Effects of the oral administration of herbal mixture on protein levels of BDNF in the hippocampi (A) and cortices (B). Data are presented as means ± SEM of three determinations. $^{**}P < 0.01$ vs. stress.

respectively. In the cortical tissues, 206 mg/kg herbal mixture significantly increased the BDNF level (46.03%, $p < 0.01$ vs. stress) similar to that of 618 mg/kg herbal mixture (48.49%, $p < 0.01$ vs. stress).

Discussion

Numerous medicinal herbs have been employed as a form of mixture or decoction since their effects can be manifested after total and final reaction by their constituent compounds when administered to humans. The herbal mixture used in the present study consists of *E. longana*, *H. cordata* and *D. japonica* which demonstrated an inductive effect on the expression of BDNF, pCREB and pAkt. These herbs have been used as a therapeutic agent for cerebral disease especially in Korea in conjunction with Sasang Constitutional Medicine which takes a typological constitution approach to holistic medicine by balancing an individual's psychological, social and physical aspects to achieve wellness and increased longevity.

The present study demonstrated that oral administration of herbal mixture in both doses (206 and 618 mg/kg) alleviated stress induced learning and memory deficits for mice by remaining in the well-lit side of a two compartment apparatus and not entering the dark where it received the electrical stimulus. Since mouse innately gravitates to darkness, the animal has to suppress this instinct through pairing the aversive stimulus (electrical stimulus) with the desired compartment (dark chamber). Animals that do not remember the aversive stimulus will cross over earlier than animals that remember. In addition, it was clear that the level of exploratory activities was not affected by the spatial working memory of mice. Herbal mixture treatment also decreased the immobility time in the tail suspension test. In order to understand the molecular mechanism of herbal mixture induced antidepressant effects in the brain, the present study investigated BDNF protein levels in hippocampus and cortex of mice under stress and compared values with herbal mixture fed mice under stress. Treatment with herbal mixture showed a significant increase in BDNF translation level.

Chronic stress may lead to psychotic symptoms including depression and suicide [18]. Studies have shown that the hippocampus is affected by stress. Depression invoked by stress has been associated with neuronal atrophy and decreased volume of hippocampus [19-21]. Several clinical reports have shown depression-induced deregulation of serum BDNF concentration. Depressed patients were characterized by low serum BDNF levels [6,22,23], implying an inverse relationship between serum BDNF levels and the severity of depression. Support for this comes from a number of studies demonstrating that treatment with antidepressants has been shown to increase BDNF levels in serum [6,23,24] and plasma [25]. It is speculated that lower BDNF levels may be caused by dysregulation of BDNF expression. This was evidenced with decreased BDNF mRNA and protein levels in postmortem hippocampus and frontal cortex of suicide victims [26]. Recent reports further support the speculation that antidepressant treatment increased BDNF protein levels in serum [27] and in both prefrontal cortex and hippocampus [28]. In the current study, herbal mixture administration with low and high dose increased the BDNF protein levels in hippocampus and cortex compared to the stress group. Herbal mixture might have significantly increased the BDNF transcript levels as well although they were not evaluated in our study.

Several types of stressors have been known to disrupt BDNF expression. For example, single (one day) or repeated (7 days) immobilization for 2 hours per day markedly reduced BDNF mRNA levels in the dentate gyrus and hippocampus [29]. This was later confirmed by other investigators who used the same stress paradigm [30]. Other types of stressors such as footshock [31], early maternal deprivation [32], social defeat [33] and chronic unpredictable stress before pregnancy [34] were correlated with decreased BDNF expression. In our study using immobilization as a stressor, no significant changes in BDNF protein level were observed in hippocampus and cortex. It can be proposed that stress induced changes in BDNF protein level may be involved in other brain regions. The other hypothesis is that immobilization stress duration was too long enough to neutralize the downregulation of BDNF expression. Interestingly, brief immobilization stress can induce BDNF expression as part of a compensatory response to preserve hippocampal homeostasis to cope with new stress [35].

Our study provides further data that herbal mixture is able to modulate serum corticosterone level in mice under stress conditions. This effect could be either of peripheral origin through a direct action of herbal mixture on adrenal glands, or of central origin via the hypothalamic-pituitary-adrenal axis. The inverse relationship between memory performance and corticosterone level in stress conditions from our study confirms the past report that chronic stress in rodents has mostly impairing effects on memory [36]. Moreover, a long term immobilization stress has been shown to affect spatial memory [37] which is in accordance with our data of short term immobilization paradigm.

Conclusions

In conclusion, our study showed that herbal mixture administration has antidepressant effects in mice. Each herb induced the expression of BDNF, pCREB and pAkt. The administration of herbal mixture significantly increased BDNF protein expression in mouse hippocampus and cortex.

Competing interests

The authors declare that they have no competing interests.

Authors' contributions

SJ and CL designed the study. QFL and GWK carried out the experiment. BK and SCP drafted the manuscript. All authors read and approved the final manuscript.

Author details

[1]Dongguk University Research Institute of Biotechnology, Seoul 100-715, Republic of Korea. [2]Department of Neuropsychiatry, Graduate School of Oriental Medicine, Dongguk University, Gyeongju, Republic of Korea. [3]Department of Korean Neuropsychiatry, Dongguk University Bundang Oriental Hospital, Sungnam, Republic of Korea. [4]Department of Korean Neuropsychiatry, Dongguk University Ilsan Oriental Hospital, Goyang, Republic of Korea. [5]School of Biomedical Sciences, Charles Sturt University, Bathurst, NSW 2795, Australia.

References

1. Baxter AJ, Ferrari AJ, Erskine HE, Charlson FJ, Degenhardt L, Whiteford HA: **The global burden of mental and substance use disorders: changes in estimating burden between GBD1990 and GBD2010.** *Epidemiol Psychiatr Sci* 2014, **23**:1–11.

2. Bryant K, Wicks MN, Willis N: **Recruitment of older African American males for depression research: lessons learned.** *Arch Psychiatr Nurs* 2014, **28**:17–20.
3. Hung CJ, Wu CC, Chen WY, Chang CY, Kuan YH, Pan HC, Liao SL, Chen CJ: **Depression-like effect of prenatal buprenorphine exposure in rats.** *PLoS One* 2013, **8**:e82262.
4. Davies AM: **The role of neurotrophins in the developing nervous system.** *Neurobiol* 1994, **25**:1334–1348.
5. Duman RS, Monteggia LM: **A neurotrophic model for stress-related mood disorders.** *Biol Psychiatry* 2006, **59**:1116–1127.
6. Shimizu E, Hashimoto K, Okamura N, Koike K, Komatsu N, Kumakiri C, Nakazato M, Watanabe H, Shinoda N, Okada S, Iyo M: **Alterations of serum levels of brain-derived neurotrophic factor (BDNF) in depressed patients with or without antidepressants.** *Biol Psychiatry* 2003, **54**:70–75.
7. Tao X, Finkbeiner S, Arnold DB, Shaywitz AJ, Greenberg ME: **Ca2+ influx regulates BDNF transcription by a CREB family transcription factor-dependent mechanism.** *Neuron* 1998, **20**:709–726.
8. Crawford AA, Lewis S, Nutt D, Peters TJ, Cowen P, O'Donovan MC, Wiles N, Lewis G: **Adverse effects from antidepressant treatment: randomised controlled trial of 601 depressed individuals.** *Psychopharmacol (Berl)* 2014, **231**:2921–2931.
9. Ferguson JM: **SSRI antidepressant medications: adverse effects and tolerability.** *Prim Care Companion J Clin Psychiatry* 2001, **3**:22–27.
10. Rangkadilok N, Worasuttayangkurn L, Bennett RN, Satayavivad J: **Identification and quantification of polyphenolic compounds in Longan (Euphoria longana Lam.) fruit.** *J Agric Food Chem* 2005, **53**:1387–1392.
11. Panyathep A, Chewonarin T, Taneyhill K, Vinitketkumnuen U, Surh YJ: **Inhibitory effects of dried longan (Euphoria longana Lam.) seed extract on invasion and matrix metalloproteinases of colon cancer cells.** *J Agric Food Chem* 2013, **61**:3631–3641.
12. Kumar M, Prasad SK, Krishnamurthy S, Hemalatha S: **Antihyperglycemic activity of Houttuynia cordata Thunb. in streptozotocin-induced diabetic rats.** *Adv Pharmacol Sci* 2014, **2014**:809438.
13. Kim SK, Ryu SY, No J, Choi SU, Kim YS: **Cytotoxic alkaloids from Houttuynia cordata.** *Arch Pharm Res* 2001, **24**:518–521.
14. Cho EJ, Yokozawa T, Rhyu DY, Kim SC, Shibahara N, Park JC: **Study on the inhibitory effects of Korean medicinal plants and their main compounds on the 1,1-diphenyl-2-picrylhydrazyl radical.** *Phytomedicine* 2003, **10**:544–551.
15. Wu JN: *Chinese Materia Medica.* New York: Oxford University Press; 2005:264.
16. Kim KH, Choi SU, Choi SZ, Son MW, Lee KR: **Withanolides from the rhizomes of Dioscorea japonica and their cytotoxicity.** *J Agric Food Chem* 2011, **59**:6980–6984.
17. Saleem AM, Taufik Hidayat M, Mat Jais AM, Fakurazi S, Moklas M, Sulaiman MR, Amom Z: **Antidepressant-like effect of aqueous extract of Channa striatus fillet in mice models of depression.** *Eur Rev Med Pharmacol Sci* 2011, **15**:795–802.
18. Dwivedi Y: **Brain-derived neurotrophic factor: role in depression and suicide.** *Neuropsychiatr Dis Treat* 2009, **5**:433–449.
19. Sala M, Perez J, Soloff P, Ucelli di Nemi S, Caverzasi E, Soares JC, Brambilla P: **Stress and hippocampal abnormalities in psychiatric disorders.** *Eur Neuropsychopharmacol* 2004, **14**:393–405.
20. Campbell S, Marriott M, Nahmias C, MacQueen GM: **Lower hippocampal volume in patients suffering from depression: a meta-analysis.** *Am J Psychiatry* 2004, **161**:598–607.
21. Frodl T, Schaub A, Banac S, Charypar M, Jäger M, Kümmler P, Bottlender R, Zetzsche T, Born C, Leinsinger G, Reiser M, Möller HJ, Meisenzahl EM: **Reduced hippocampal volume correlates with executive dysfunctioning in major depression.** *J Psychiatry Neurosci* 2006, **31**:316–323.
22. Karege F, Perret G, Bondolfi G, Schwald M, Bertschy G, Aubry JM: **Decreased serum brain-derived neurotrophic factor levels in major depressed patients.** *Psychiatry Res* 2002, **109**:143–148.
23. Gonul AS, Akdeniz F, Taneli F, Donat O, Eker C, Vahip S: **Effect of treatment on serum brain-derived neurotrophic factor levels in depressed patients.** *Eur Arch Psychiatry Clin Neurosci* 2005, **255**:381–386.
24. Yoshimura R, Mitoma M, Sugita A, Hori H, Okamoto T, Umene W, Ueda N, Nakamura J: **Effects of paroxetine or milnacipran on serum brain-derived neurotrophic factor in depressed patients.** *Prog Neuropsychopharmacol Biol Psychiatry* 2007, **31**:1034–1037.
25. Lee HY, Kim YK: **Plasma brain-derived neurotrophic factor as a peripheral marker for the action mechanism of antidepressants.** *Neuropsychobiology* 2008, **57**:194–199.
26. Dwivedi Y, Rizavi HS, Conley RR, Roberts RC, Tamminga CA, Pandey GN: **Altered gene expression of brain-derived neurotrophic factor and receptor tyrosine kinase B in postmortem brain of suicide subjects.** *Arch Gen Psychiatry* 2003, **60**:804–815.
27. Huang TL, Lee CT, Liu YL: **Serum brain-derived neurotrophic factor levels in patients with major depression: effects of antidepressants.** *J Psychiatr Res* 2008, **42**:521–525.
28. Réus GZ, Stringari RB, Ribeiro KF, Ferraro AK, Vitto MF, Cesconetto P, Souza CT, Quevedo J: **Ketamine plus imipramine treatment induces antidepressant-like behavior and increases CREB and BDNF protein levels and PKA and PKC phosphorylation in rat brain.** *Behav Brain Res* 2011, **221**:166–171.
29. Smith MA, Makino S, Kvetnansky R, Post RM: **Stress and glucocorticoids affect the expression of brain-derived neurotrophic factor and neurotrophin-3 mRNAs in the hippocampus.** *J Neurosci* 1995, **15**:1768–1777.
30. Ueyama T, Kawai Y, Nemoto K, Sekimoto M, Toné S, Senba E: **Immobilization stress reduced the expression of neurotrophins and their receptors in the rat brain.** *Neurosci Res* 1997, **28**:103–110.
31. Rasmusson AM, Shi L, Duman R: **Downregulation of BDNF mRNA in the hippocampal dentate gyrus after re-exposure to cues previously associated with footshock.** *Neuropsychopharmacology* 2002, **27**:133–142.
32. Roceri M, Hendriks W, Racagni G, Ellenbroek BA, Riva MA: **Early maternal deprivation reduces the expression of BDNF and NMDA receptor subunits in rat hippocampus.** *Mol Psychiatry* 2002, **7**:609–616.
33. Pizarro JM, Lumley LA, Medina W, Robison CL, Chang WE, Alagappan A, Bah MJ, Dawood MY, Shah JD, Mark B, Kendall N, Smith MA, Saviolakis GA, Meyerhoff JL: **Acute social defeat reduces neurotrophin expression in brain cortical and subcortical areas in mice.** *Brain Res* 2004, **1025**:10–20.
34. Huang Y, Shi X, Xu H, Yang H, Chen T, Chen S, Chen X: **Chronic unpredictable stress before pregnancy reduce the expression of brain-derived neurotrophic factor and N-methyl-D-aspartate receptor in hippocampus of offspring rats associated with impairment of memory.** *Neurochem Res* 2010, **35**:1038–1049.
35. Marmigère F, Givalois L, Rage F, Arancibia S, Tapia-Arancibia L: **Rapid induction of BDNF expression in the hippocampus during immobilization stress challenge in adult rats.** *Hippocampus* 2003, **13**:646–655.
36. Wolf OT: **HPA axis and memory.** *Best Pract Res Clin Endocrinol Metab* 2003, **17**:287–299.
37. Kitraki E, Kremmyda O, Youlatos D, Alexis M, Kittas C: **Spatial performance and corticosteroid receptor status in the 21-day restraint stress paradigm.** *Ann N Y Acad Sci* 2004, **1018**:323–327.

11

Adenosine deaminase activity modulation by some street drug: molecular docking simulation and experimental investigation

Massoud Amanlou[1*], Ali-akbar Saboury[2], Roya Bazl[2], Mohammad Reza Ganjali[2] and Shokoofeh Sheibani[3]

Abstract

Background: Adenosine deaminase (ADA) is an enzyme that plays important roles in proliferation, maturation, function and development of the immune system. ADA activity may be altered by variety of substances including synthetic or natural products. Morphine, cocaine and their analogs exert immune suppressive activities by decreasing immune system function. The purpose of this study is to confirm that this possible effect may be modulated by interaction of these substances with ADA activity by experimental and computational method.

Methods: The structural changes in ADA have been studied in presence of cocaine, ethylmorphine, homatropine, morphine and thebaine by determination of ADA hydrolytic activity, circular dichroism and fluorescence spectroscopy in different concentrations. Docking study was performed to evaluate interaction method of test compound with ADA active site using AutoDock4 software.

Results: According to in-vitro studies all compounds inhibited ADA with different potencies, however thebaine activated it at concentration below 50 μM, ethylmorphine inhibited ADA at 35 μM. Moreover, fluorescence spectra patterns were differed from compounds based on structural resemblance which were very considerable for cocaine and homatropine.

Conclusion: The results of this study confirms that opioids and some other stimulant drugs such as cocaine can alter immune function in illegal drug abusers. These findings may lead other investigators to develop a new class of ADA activators or inhibitors in the near future.

Keywords: Adenosine deaminase, Opioid, Cocaine, Immune system, Docking

Introduction

Adenosine deaminase (ADA) is an enzyme that irreversibly converts adenosine to inosine [1]. This enzyme exists in all human tissues, but the highest levels and activity are found in the lymphoid system such as lymph nodes, spleen, and thymus [2]. It is also essential for the proliferation, maturation and function of T lymphocyte cells. It is assumed that ADA plays a crucial role in development of the immune system, while its innate deficiency causes severe combined immunodeficiency (SCID) [3]. Moreover, ADA activity changes in a variety of other diseases including acquired immunodeficiency syndrome (AIDS), anemia, various lymphomas, tuberculosis, and leukemia [4,5]. On the other hand, ADA regulates the levels of endogenous adenosine which results in immune system suppression by inhibiting lymphoid or myeloid cells [6,7], including neutrophils [8], macrophages [9], lymphocytes [10,11] and platelets [12].

Two distinct isoenzymes of ADA, known as ADA_1 and ADA_2, are found in mammalian [13-15]; former has highest levels of activity in spleen, and thymus whereas latter is found in other parts of body [15]. As the most abundant type of white blood cells that responds to infection and attacks of foreign invaders, neutrophils might possess more than one type of adenosine receptor [16], and adenosine regulates neutrophil function in an opposing manner through the ligation of ADA_1 (immunostimulatory) and ADA_2 (immunosuppressive) receptors [17].

* Correspondence: amanlou@tums.ac.ir
[1]Department of Medicinal Chemistry, Faculty of Pharmacy, Pharmaceutical Sciences Research Center, Tehran University of Medical Sciences, Tehran, Iran
Full list of author information is available at the end of the article

A number of ADA inhibitors with various degrees of potency have been reported [18]. In one study, immunosuppressive and anti-inflammatory effects of FR234938, as a non-nucleoside inhibitor of ADA, were investigated [19]. Moreover, deoxycoformycin, another ADA inhibitor, has been investigated in treatment of colon carcinoma cells [20,21] and hematological neoplasms [22]. By contrast, ibuprofen [23] and medazepam [24] effects on immune deficiency have been reported. This revealed that purine compound may act as ADA activator; but still more experiments are needed to confirm this finding.

Opioids have variety of clinical applications. Naltrexone in low dosage can suppress human ovarian cancer and provides novel non-toxic therapies for the treatment of this lethal neoplasia [25]. The idea that opioids suppress the immune system and reduce resistance to infections is not new [26]. Several studies on animals and humans have illustrated that opioids can exert immunosuppressive effects by interfering B and T cell function [27-29]. In this regard, Sacerdote et al. have reported that immune function is affected by morphine and tramadol [30]. In other investigations, chronic treatment with morphine has been shown to affect the function of T cells and reduce immunity by directly interacting with cells of the immune system [28,30-34]. On the other hand, studies about heroin abusers showed that patients were suffering from a disease that diminishes their immunity, by affecting T-lymphocyte function and therefore cause (HIV) infection [33,34]. In addition, long term usage of cocaine and homatropine leads to a heart attack, tremors, and apnea, cardiac arrest respectively. The possible involvement of adenosine in opioid antinociception has been supported by Ho et al. [34]. Interaction between an opioid and an adenosine receptor has been proposed. Yet, binding efficiency of ADA1 is reduced in the presence of morphine [35,36]. Also, transferring of opioids to the pontine reticular formation (PRF) and substantia innominata (SI) causes adenosine to decrease in the PRF and SI [37].

Although the knowledge about effects of opioids on immune responses has been improved, there is relatively little information about these immunosuppressive effects. Therefore, the present investigation was conducted to find the effects of this group of opiates and two other alkaloid compounds on ADA activity; by means of computational and experimental methods to found new compounds for modulation of adenosine deaminase activity.

Material and methods

Materials

Adenosine deaminase (EC 3.5.4.4) extracted from bovine spleen was purchased from sigma, and all other used materials were of analytical grade and acquired from Merck. PBS that is used in assay was adjusted at 7.4, at which, enzyme has optimal activity in [38,39]. All solutions were prepared in MilliQ (Millipore, USA) water.

Biological assays

Released ammonia resulted by enzyme activity was determined by specific Berthelot colorimetric method which was used for micro determination of ADA activity in serum [40]. Briefly, this method is based on the reaction of liberated ammonia with hypochlorite (OCl^-) to form a monochloramine and subsequent reaction of this intermediate with phenol to produce blue-colored indophenols that absorbance is measured at 625 nm. In this process sodium nitroprusside is used as the catalyst. The reaction was initiated by addition of adenosine as a substrate at 37°C to preincubated enzyme with different concentrations of tested compounds at different concentrations (5–300 μM). Finally, the enzymatic reaction was stopped at the end of 30 minutes of incubation by adding phenol nitroprusside solution. The mixture kept again for 30 minutes at 37°C before absorbance determination.

Obtained absorbance was normalized through blank sample, and IC_{50} values were calculated by Prism software (Ver. 5, GraphPad Software Inc., San Diego CA,).

Circular dichroism spectroscopy

CD spectra were measured in the far-UV (200–260 nm) region with JASCO J-715 spectropolarimeter (Japan). JASCO J-715 software not only gave us the possibility of data smoothing, but also used to predict the secondary structure changes of the protein according to the statistical method [41]. Each scan was recorded in 1 nm increments at 37°C, repeated three times, and averaged. The protein was in 0.1 M PBS buffer, pH = 7.4, and its concentration was adjusted to 2 mg/ml in 1 cm path length cuvette. The results were expressed in molar ellipticity [θ] (deg $cm^2.dmol^{-1}$).

Fluorescence spectroscopy

Fluorescence spectroscopy was performed on a Hitachi fluorescence spectrophotometer model MPF-4 with 1 cm path length fluorescence cuvette and final volume of 400 μL. The excitation wavelength was adjusted in 290 nm, and the emission was scanned every 1 nm in the range of 300 to 400 nm. The final concentration of enzyme was 6 μM and different concentrations of tested compounds were changed from 1.7 to 73.4 μM.

Docking simulation

To have a better understanding about the inhibitory mechanism of the test compounds and clarification of type of interactions, docking were performed using the AutoDock 4.2 package [42]. The ability of software in next predictions was determined with re-docking of co-crystallized inhibitor of protein x-ray structure pdb ID:

1ADD and compared to inhibitor orientation in crystal structure. This crystal structure has been used since its > 80% similarity in structure with bovine spleen and active site amino acids conservation. The structure of all compound have sketched by Marvin sketch applet (Marvin package, Chemaxon Company). AutoDockTools (ADT) 1.5.6 was used for preparing input files using Autodock 4.2 atom types and calculating all needed charges [42]. Adding polar hydrogens and rotatable bonds were done with ADT; docking with a maximum number of 25×10^6 energy evaluations using the Lamarckian Genetic Algorithm (LGA) were performed. All other parameters were set to default values. The docked conformations of each ligand were ranked into clusters based on the binding energy. After clustering analysis, conformation with the most favourable binding energy was selected.

Table 1 IC_{50} values and binding energies of test compounds in presence of 2 mg/ml adenosine deaminase enzyme

No.	Name	Structure	IC_{50} (μM)	ΔG° binding (kcal/mol)
1	Thebaine	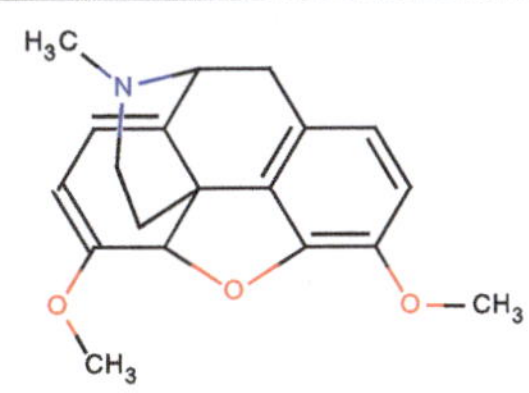	50*/163	−7.2
2	Morphine	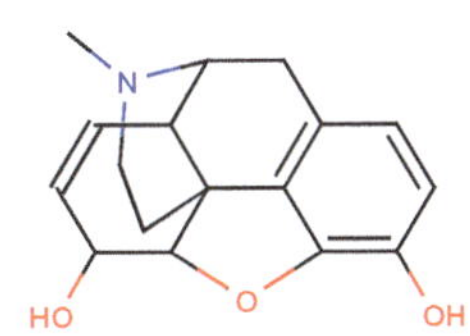	43.7	−8.1
3	Ethylmorphine	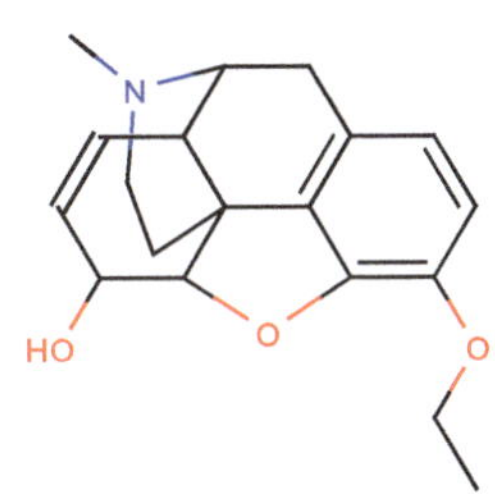	35	−8.0
4	Cocaine	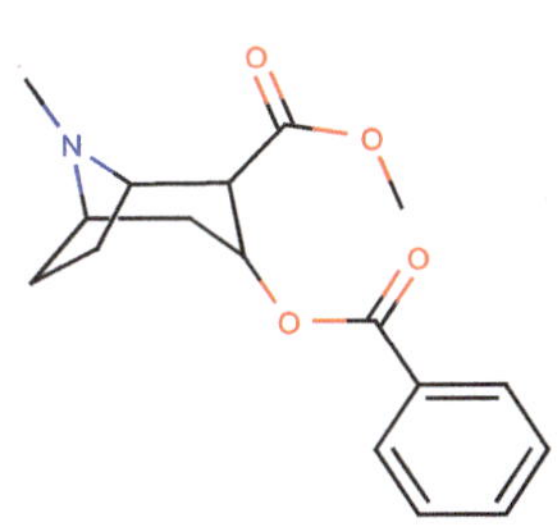	180	−6.8
5	Homatropine	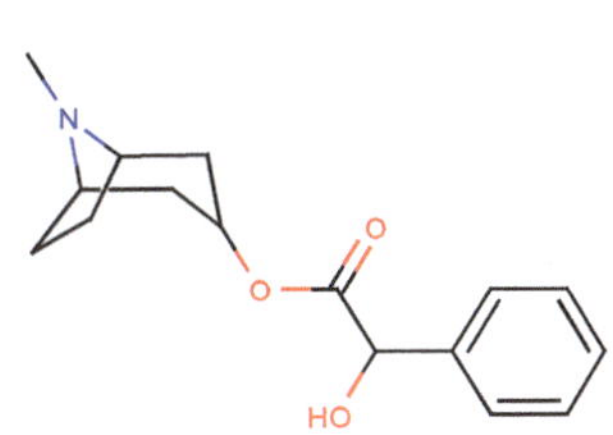	96	−7.2

*Thebaine was activated ADA till this concentration.

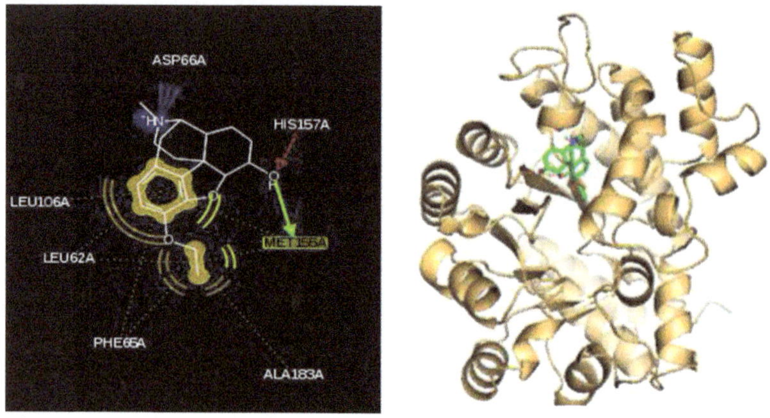

a) b)

Figure 1 Ethylmorphine binding site of adenosine deaminase 2D (a) and 3D (b) demonstration.

Results and discussion

Determination of ADA activity

The target compounds were evaluated against ADA enzymatic activity in vitro and obtained IC_{50} values are summarized in Table 1. As shown in Table 1 all tested compounds inhibit ADA activity in micromolar range. In general, compounds in group1 (consisted of ethylmorphine, morphine and thebaine) showed better inhibitory activities than compounds in the other structurally related group (group 2: cocaine and homatropine). As shown, despite of partially closed binding energies, each compound inhibits the enzyme in variety of concentrations. Enhance in inhibition potency may be due to a decrease in conformational flexibility and better stabilization in inhibition site. In first group the order of inhibitory activities showed the potency of ethylmorphine > morphine > thebaine. This tendency is due to the presence of different substitute on A and C rings of perhydrophenanthrene structure. Ethylmorphine with ethoxy group on A ring shows better potency (IC_{50}: 35 μM) than those with hydroxyl and methoxy substitutes. Upon further modification on C-ring in thebaine, the activity further decreased. This drop in inhibition activity may be due to inappropriate stabilization of compound to bind to target amino acids or inappropriate interactions which was confirmed by the molecular docking study. The binding energy of thebaine was calculated −7.2 kcal/mol compare to ethylmorphine (ΔG°: −8 kcal/mol). Interestingly in this series, thebaine activated enzyme hydrolytic activity till 50 μM and up to this level showed inhibition effect with IC_{50}: 163 μM (Table 1). However, thebaine, cocaine and homatropine shows IC_{50} higher than other inhibitors (ethylmorphine and morphine), it can imply some immunity problem in the opioid consumers may result by ADA inhibition.

In another group hydroxyl substitution may be responsible for the homatropine inhibition efficiency which might build H-bond with adjacent residues at active site of ADA. In addition, cocaine showed weaker inhibitory activity which indicated the influence of position and size of the substitute on tropan ring on the inhibitory activity. For more insight to obtained IC_{50} values and interaction site recognition the docking study has been performed.

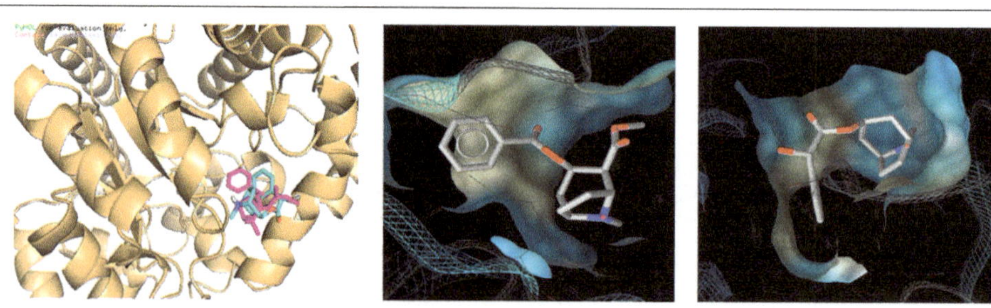

a) b) c)

Figure 2 Docking pose of cocaine and homatropine in the adenosine deaminase binding pocket at their lowest energy of binding conformation: a) Overlay of cocaine and homatropine. b) Cocaine and c) Homatropine.

Docking experiments

Docking studies are used at different stages of drug discovery such as in the prediction of ligand-receptor interaction and also to rank the compounds based on the binding energies. Docking of co-crystallized inhibitor with ADA was performed to evaluate the efficacy of docking software and the reasonable RMSD of 0.39 Å was obtained. Docking of tested compounds with the ADA enzyme was performed, and corresponded binding energies were determined as shown in Table 1. The interacting energies followed the order of the in vitro IC_{50} values with rational correlation (R^2: 0.84). All compounds posed in ADA active site entrance or partially penetrated in active site.

For the most potent inhibitor, ethylmorphine, the hydroxyl group of C-ring formed a hydrogen bond with Met155 and His157. Moreover, presence of ethoxy group in ring A resulted in hydrophobic interactions with Leu62,

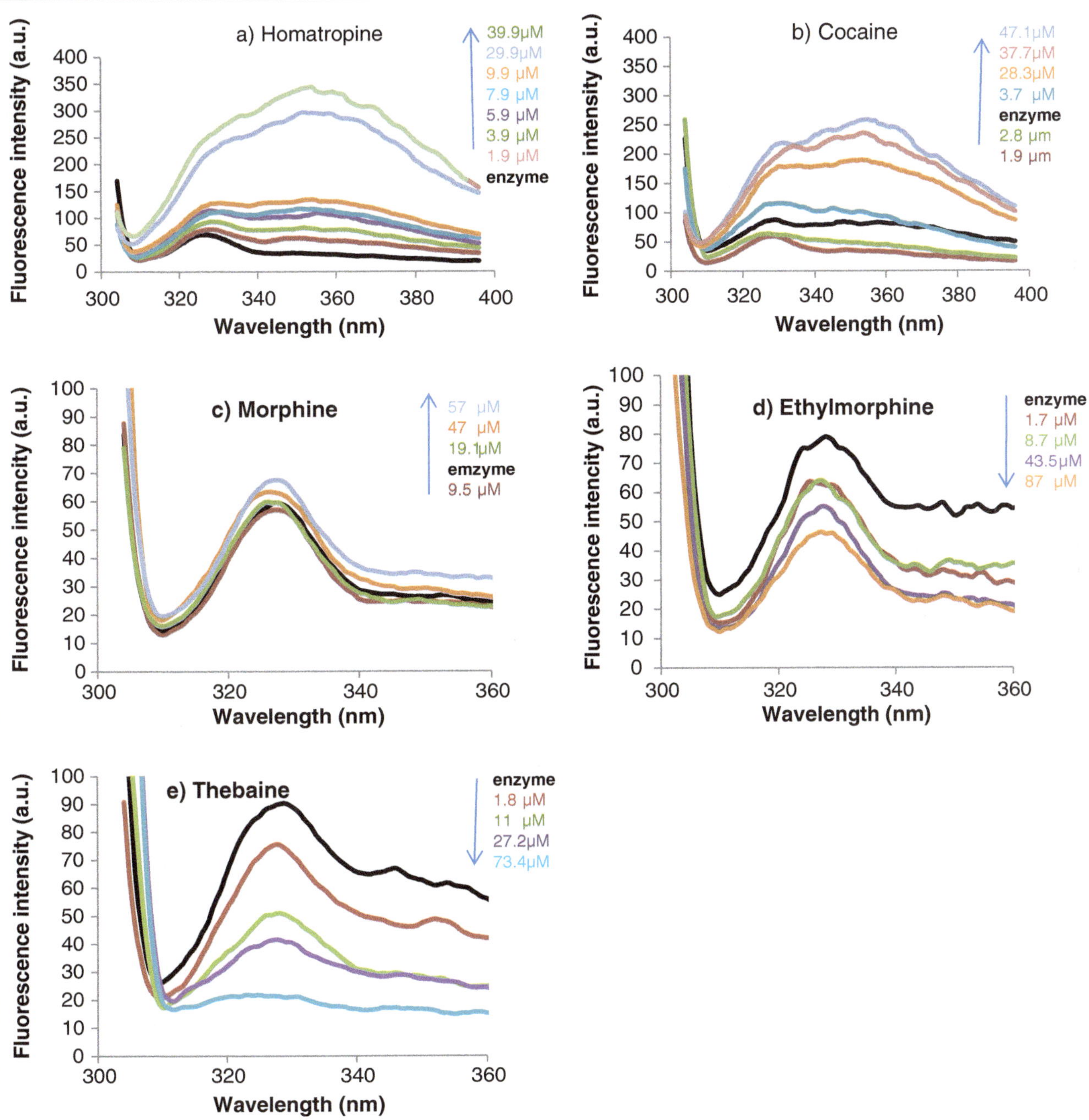

Figure 3 Change in fluorescence spectra of adenosine deaminase in presence of different concentration of a), Homatropine, b) Cocaine, c) Morphine, d) Ethylmorphine, and e) Thebaine in pH: 7.4.

Phe65, Leu106, Met155 and Ala183 as well as electrostatic interaction of nitrogen atom made it much more stabilized in binding site (Figure 1). Thebaine exhibited binding energy of "-7" kcal/mol which correlated with the experimentally observed activity due to flat T-shape structure which resulted in less penetration into active site. On the other hand, in comparison to morphine replacing of hydroxy with methoxy group on C-ring caused

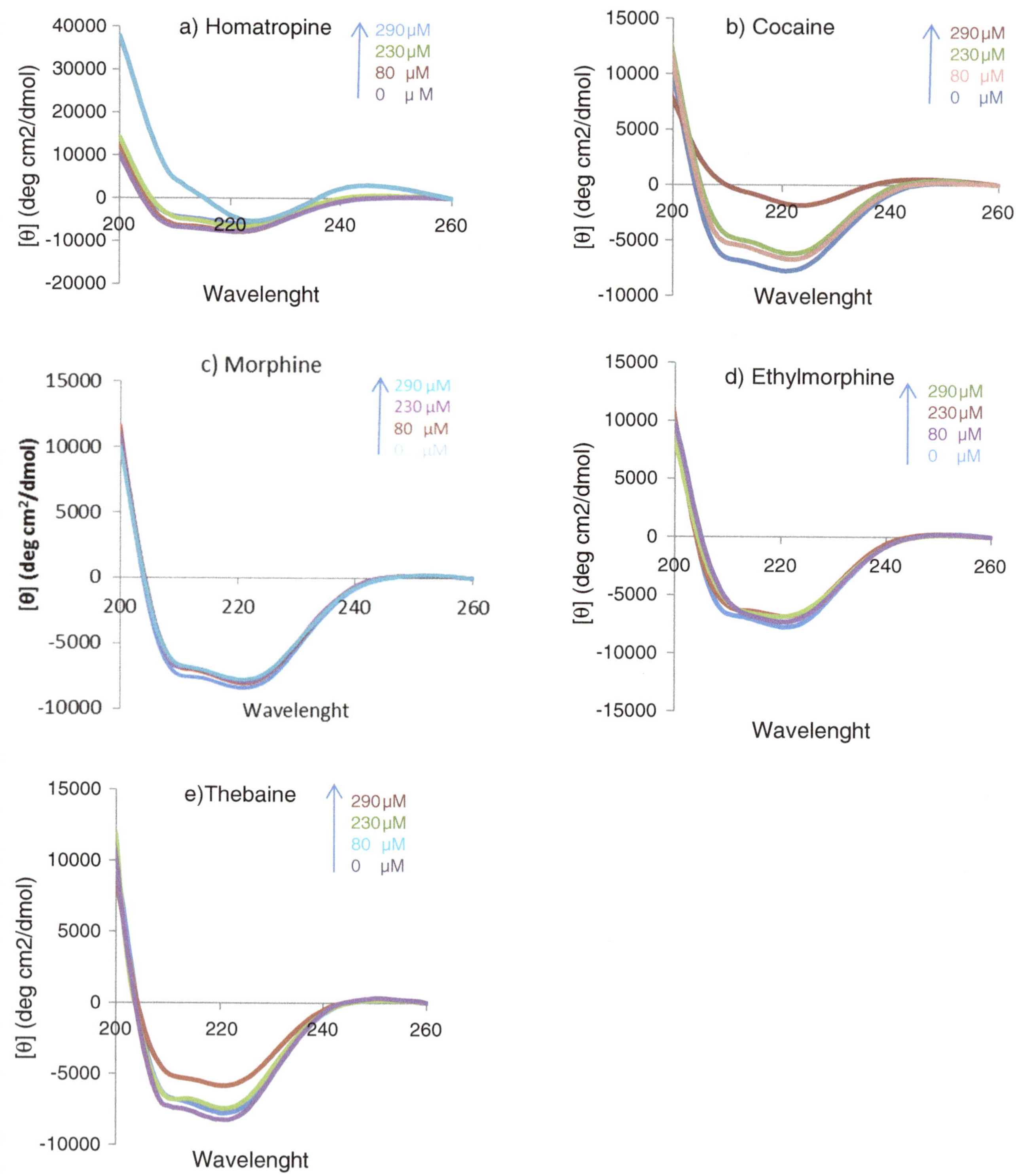

Figure 4 CD spectra of adenosine deaminase in presence of different concentration (0–300 µM) of a) Homatropine, b) Cocaine, c) Morphine, d) Ethylmorphine, e) Thebaine in pH: 7.4.

removing of H-bond with His157, consequently resulted in lower efficiency. This effect was illustrated in ethylmorphine which in existing H-bond made it more stabilized in binding site. In the other group, homatropine binds to ADA with lower binding energy than cocaine with IC_{50} 96 and 180 μM respectively. As it shown in Figure 2 cocaine doesn't diffuse into active site because of bulkier substitute, and just poses on enzyme active site entrance. In contrast, homatropine enters from phenyl part and OH group makes H-bond with Leu62.

Fluorescence spectroscopy

Interaction of tested compounds with Trp residues can be studied by change in emission spectra of ADA in 320-340 nm. In other words, any environmental alteration as well as three-dimensional structure changes in Trp amino acid and enzyme respectively, can change the innate spectrum of Trp residues in enzyme. As shown in Figure 3, there are two totally different patterns in interaction with Trp residues. In the first group, homatropine and cocaine in high concentrations, demonstrate bathochromic shift. This change may be probably due to severe change of three dimensional structure of the enzyme. In the other series: morphine, ethylmorphine and thebaine do not show noticeable change and shift in fluorescence spectra; indeed compounds with bulkier structure don't penetrate efficiently in binding pocket, and place in longer distance with Trp residues. Thebaine and ethylmorphine in this group decrease Trp emission as their concentration increase. This could be an indication that these compounds have bonded with the active sites or other sites of the ADA enzyme and therefore the Trp amino acid is out of access. According to the Berthelot test results, thebaine till 50 μM stimulates enzyme to break down faster, but above this concentration the activity of thebaine slows down and the concentration of 163 μM, results in 50% of inhibition.

Circular dichroism spectroscopy

CD spectra of ADA in the presence of different concentration of compounds have been illustrated in Figure 4. ADA showed two transitions in 210 and 222 nm which are attribute to $n \rightarrow \pi^*$ and $\pi \rightarrow \pi^*$ respectively. According to percent of different patterns of 2D structure of enzyme, among α-helix structure has been undergone sever changes, and mostly convert to random coil. This effect can be explained by compounds intercalation between helix residues and broken of H-bonds. According to the Figure 3 in high concentrations of cocaine, bathochromic shift in the fluorescence spectra was observed. On the other hand as it shown in Figure 4, in cocaine concentration around 180 μM drastic changes in CD spectra were observed. Also, based on in-vitro studies 50% of enzyme's activity has been diminished in 180 μM, so it can infer from this point despite of strong alteration in overall ADA structure or active site remains much more intact.

Conclusion

Regarding to immunosuppressive effects of opioids, evaluation of enzyme activity studies was performed parallel to structural changes caused by different concentrations of test compounds. Thebaine activated ADA in certain low concentrations; while in higher concentrations it inhibited the enzyme. On the contrary, all other compounds inhibited the enzyme in studied range (0-300 μM). The interaction site as well as existing interactions in stabilization of each compound was obtained by docking studies. Finally, changes in two and three dimensional structures of ADA (based on Circular dichroism and fluorescence spectroscopy Figure 3 and 4) revealed that only cocaine and homatropine, had major effects on the enzyme (made drastic changes in the enzyme); while these changes were not significant for morphine, etylmorphine and thebaine in studied concentrations.

Regarding that the adenosine deaminase enzyme has a very important role in the immune system activity, so the inhibition of this enzyme's natural function in the human body can lead to debilitation of the immune system. Therefore, the results of this experiment support the idea that persons with addiction and regular drug abuse have a weaker immune system than others. This study can also help other researchers to develop a new class of ADA activators or inhibitors in the near future to manage malfunction of the immune system.

Competing interest

There are no other conflicts of interest related to this publication.

Authors' contributions

All authors contributed to the concept and design, making and analysis of data, drafting, revising and final approval. MA is responsible for the study registration, financial and administrative support. RB & SHSH are responsible for biological assays. RB & MA were involved for docking studies. AAS & MRG were responsible for experimental analysis. All authors were participated in data assembly and analysis, interpretation and manuscript writing. They read and approved the final manuscript.

Acknowledgments

This study was supported by a grant from the Research Council of Tehran University of Medical Sciences.

Author details

[1]Department of Medicinal Chemistry, Faculty of Pharmacy, Pharmaceutical Sciences Research Center, Tehran University of Medical Sciences, Tehran, Iran. [2]Institute of Biochemistry and Biophysics, University of Tehran, Tehran, Iran. [3]Center of Excellence in Electrochemistry, Faculty of Chemistry, University of Tehran, Tehran, Iran.

References

1. Brady T: **Adenosine deaminase.** *Biochem J* 1942, **36**:478–484.

2. Gorrell MD, Gysbers V, McCaughan GW: **CD26: a multifunctional integral membrane and secreted protein of activated lymphocytes.** *Scand J Immunol* 2001, **54**:249–264.
3. Resta R, Thompson LF: **SCID: the role of adenosine deaminase deficiency.** *Immunol Today* 1997, **18**:371–374.
4. Gakis C, Calia C, Naitana A, Pirino D, Semi G: **Serum adenosine deaminase activity in HIV positive subjects: a by pothesis on the significance of ADA-2.** *Panminerva Med* 1989, **31**:107–113.
5. Glader BE, Backer K, Diamond LK: **Elevated erythrocyte adenosine deaminase activity in congenital hypoplastic anemia.** *Eng J Med* 1983, **309**:1486–1490.
6. Ohta A, Sitkovsky M: **Role of G-protein-coupled adenosine receptors in down regulation of inflammation and protection from tissue damage.** *Nature* 2001, **414**:916–920.
7. Sitkovsky MV, Lukashev D, Apasov S, Kojima H, Koshiba M, Cald-well C, Ohta A, Thiel M: **Physiological control of immune response and inflammatory tissue damage by hypoxia-inducible factors and adenosine A2A receptors.** *Annu Rev Immunol* 2004, **22**:657–682.
8. Fredholm BB: **Purines and neutrophil leukocytes.** *Gen Pharmacol* 1997, **28**:345–350.
9. Murphree LJ, Sullivan GW, Marshall MA, Linden J: **Lipopolysac-charide rapidly modifies adenosine receptor transcripts in murine and human macrophages: role of NF-kappa B in A2A, adenosine receptor induction.** *Biochem J* 2005, **391**:575–580.
10. Lappas CM, Rieger JM, Linden J: **A2A adenosine receptor induction inhibits IFN-gamma production in murine CD^{4+} T cells.** *J Immunol* 2005, **174**:1073–1080.
11. Koshiba M, Rosin DL, Hayashi N, Linden J, Sitkovsky MV: **Patterns of A2A extracellular adenosine receptor expression in different functional subsets of human peripheral T cells. Flow cytometry studies with anti-A2A receptor monoclonal antibodies.** *Mol Pharmacol* 1999, **55**:614–624.
12. Varani K, Gessi S, Dalpiaz A, Borea PA: **Pharmacological and biochemical characterization of purified A2a adenosine receptors in human platelet membranes by 3[H]-CGS 21680 binding.** *Br J Pharmacol* 1996, **117**:1693–1701.
13. Van Der Weyden MB, Kelly WN: **Human adenosine deaminase. Distribution and properties.** *J Biol Chem* 1976, **251**:5448–5456.
14. Hirschhorn R, Ratech H: **Isozymes of adenosine deaminase.** In *Current Topics in Biological and Medical Research*, Volume 1. Edited by Ratazzi MC, Scandalia JG, Whitt GS. New York: Alan R Liss; 1980:132–157.
15. Kurata N: **Adenosine deaminase.** *Nihon Rinsho* 1995, **53**:122–127.
16. Rose FR, Hirschhorn R, Weissmann G, Cronstein BN: **Adenosine promotes neutrophil chemotaxis.** *J Exp Med* 1988, **167**:1186–1194.
17. Haskó G, Cronstein BN: **Adenosine: an endogenous regulator of innate immunity.** *Trends Immunol* 2004, **25**:33–39.
18. Cristalli G, Costanzi S, Lambertucci C, Lupidi G, Vittori S, Volpini R, Camaioni E: **Adenosine deaminase: functional implication and different classes of inhibitors.** *Med Res Rev* 2001, **21**:105–128.
19. Kuno M, Seki N, Tsujimoto S, Nakanishi I, Kinoshita T, Nakamura K, Terasaka T, Nishio N, Sato A, Fujii T: **Anti-inflammatory activity of FR234938.** *Eur J Pharmacol* 2006, **534**:241–249.
20. Bemi V, Tazzini N, Banditelli S, Giorgelli F, Pesi R, Turchi G, Mattana A, Sgarrela F, Tozzi MG, Camici M: **Deoxyadenosine metabolism in a human colon-carcinoma cell line LoVo, in relation to its cytotoxic effect in combination with deoxycoformycin.** *Int J Cancer* 1998, **75**:713–720.
21. Camici M, Turriani M, Tozzi MG, Turchi G, Cos J, Alemany C, Miralles A, Noe V, Ciudad CJ: **Purine enzyme profile in human colon carcinoma cell lines and differential sensitivity to deoxycoformycin and 2'-deoxyadenosine in combination.** *Int J Cancer* 1995, **17**:176–183.
22. Pettitt AR: **Mechanism of action of purine analogues in chronic lymphocytic leukaemia.** *Br J Haematol* 2003, **121**:692–702.
23. Kalantari S, Rezaei-Tavirani M, Khodakarim S: **Effects of different therapeutical doses of ibuprofen on the adenosine deaminase activity at physiologic and pathologic temperatures.** *Koomesh* 2011, **13**:50–56.
24. Centelles JJ, Franco R, Bozal J: **Purification and partial characterization of brain adenosine deaminase: Inhibition by purine compounds and by drugs.** *J Neurosci Res* 1988, **19**:258–267.
25. Donahue RN, McLaughlin PJ, Zagon IS: **The opioid growth factor OGF, and low dose naltrexone LDN, suppress human ovarian cancer progression in mice.** *Gynecol Oncol* 2011, **122**:382–388.
26. Vallejo R, de Leon-Casasola O, Benyamin R: **Opioid therapy and immunosuppression.** *Am J Ther* 2004, **11**:354–365.
27. Peterson PK, Molitor TW, Chunc CC: **Mechanism of morphine induced immunomodulation.** *Biochem Pharmacol* 1993, **46**:343–348.
28. Sacerdote P, Manfredi B, Mantegazza P, Panerai AE: **Antinociceptive and immunosuppressive effects of opiate drugs: a structure-related activity study.** *Br J Pharmacol* 1997, **121**:834–840.
29. Eisenstein TK, Hilburger ME: **Opioid modulation of immune responses: effects on phagocyte and lymphoid cell populations.** *J Neuroimmunol* 1998, **83**:36–44.
30. Sacerdote P, Bianchi M, Gaspani L, Manfredi B, Maucione A, Terno G, Ammatuna M, Panerai AE: **The Effects of Tramadol and Morphine on Immune Responses and Pain After Surgery in Cancer Patients.** *Anesth Analg* 2000, **90**:1411–1414.
31. Zhang EY, Xiong J, Parker BL, Chen AY, Fields PE, Ma X: **Depletion and recovery of lymphoid subsets following morphine administration.** *Br J Pharmacol* 2011, **164**:1829–1844.
32. Ho IK, Loh HH, Way EL: **Cyclic adenosine monophosphate antagonism of morphine analgesia.** *J Pharmacol Exp Ther* 1973, **185**:336–346.
33. Risdahl JM, Khanna KV, Peterson PK, Molitor TW: **Opiates and infections.** *J Neuroimmunol* 1998, **83**:4–18.
34. Donahoe RM, Vlahov D: **Opiates as potential cofactors in progression of HIV-1 infections to AIDS.** *J Neuroimmunol* 1998, **83**:77–87.
35. Matthes HW, Maldonado R, Simonin F, Valverde O, Slowe S, Kitchen I, Befort K, Dierich A, Le Meur M, Dollé P, Tzavara E, Hanoune J, Roques BP, Kieffer BL: **Loss of morphine-induced analgesia, reward effect and withdrawal symptoms in mice lacking the mu-opioid-receptor gene.** *Nature* 1996, **383**:819–823.
36. Bailey A, Matthes H, Kieffer B, Slowe S, Hourani SM, Kitchen I: **Quantitative autoradiography of adenosine receptors and NBTI-sensitive adenosine transporters in the brains and spinal cords of mice deficient in the mu-opioid receptor gene.** *Brain Res* 2002, **943**:68–79.
37. Nelson AM, Battersby AS, Baghdoyan HA, Lydic R: **Opioid induced decreases in rat brain adenosine levels are reversed by inhibiting adenosine deaminase.** *Anesthesiology* 2009, **111**:1327–1333.
38. Brady TG, O'Connell W: **A purification of adenosine deaminase from the superficial mucosa of calf intestine.** *Biochim Biophys Acta* 1962, **62**:216–229.
39. Saboury AA, Divsalar A, Ataie G, Amanlou M, Moosavi-Movahedi AA, Hakimelahi GH: **Inhibition study of adenosine deaminase by caffeine using spectroscopy and isothermal titration calorimetry.** *Acta Biochim Pol* 2003, **50**:849–855.
40. Martinek RG: **Micromethod for estimation of serum adenosine deaminase.** *Clin Chem* 1963, **102**:620–625.
41. Yang JT, Wu CS, Martinez HM: **Calculation of protein conformation from circular dichroism.** *Meth Enzymol* 1986, **130**:208–269.
42. Morris GM, Huey R, Lindstrom W, Sanner MF, Belew RK, Goodsell DS, Olson AJ: **AutoDock4 and AutoDockTools4: Automated docking with selective receptor flexibility.** *J Comput Chem* 2009, **16**:2785–2791.

12

Nanoparticles as potential new generation broad spectrum antimicrobial agents

Clarence S. Yah[1,2*] and Geoffrey S. Simate[3]

Abstract

The rapid emergence of antimicrobial resistant strains to conventional antimicrobial agents has complicated and prolonged infection treatment and increased mortality risk globally. Furthermore, some of the conventional antimicrobial agents are unable to cross certain cell membranes thus, restricting treatment of intracellular pathogens. Therefore, the disease-causing-organisms tend to persist in these cells. However, the emergence of nanoparticle (NP) technology has come with the promising broad spectrum NP-antimicrobial agents due to their vast physiochemical and functionalization properties. In fact, NP-antimicrobial agents are able to unlock the restrictions experienced by conventional antimicrobial agents. This review discusses the status quo of NP-antimicrobial agents as potent broad spectrum antimicrobial agents, sterilization and wound healing agents, and sustained inhibitors of intracellular pathogens. Indeed, the perspective of developing potent NP-antimicrobial agents that carry multiple-functionality will revolutionize clinical medicine and play a significant role in alleviating disease burden.

Introduction

In recent past, microbial infections have become a global health burden due to emerging and resistant strains of viruses [1], bacteria [2], pathogenic fungi [3] and protozoa [4] defying clinical treatment. Consequently, this has culminated into prolonged treatment, higher health expenditure, mortality risk, and low life expectancy [2]. In view of ineffective antimicrobial agents, there is need to seek new alternative and safer antimicrobial agents against these "super bugs" of viruses, bacteria, fungi and protozoa. With the development of biomedical nanomaterials, new antimicrobial agents have begun to emerge either as novel and/or augmenting the activities of the current conventional antimicrobials. This is motivated by the vast physiochemical and functionalization (ligand attachment) properties of nanoparticles (NPs) [5–7]. The NPs physiochemical properties are highly diverse in nature and are highly applicable in biomedical field including antimicrobial and drug delivery [6, 8, 9]. Some examples of these biomedical NPs include silver nanoparticles (AgNPs) [10], carbon nanotubes (CNTs) [11], gold NPs (AuNPs) [12], zinc oxide NPs (ZnO-NPs) [13], and iron oxide NPs (FeO-NPs) [14].

The antimicrobial actions of NPs include cidal destruction of cell membranes, blockage of enzyme pathways, alterations of microbial cell wall, and nucleic materials pathway [1]. However, the antimicrobial mechanisms of the actions are yet to be fully elucidated since some of the NPs drugs are still at their infancy. The high potency of NPs antiviral, antibacterial, antifungal and antiprotozoal activities may revolutionize and bring another turning point in pharmacological therapy. In that regard, this review looks at the status quo of nanomaterials as alternative antimicrobial agents in terms of their broad spectrum ability, the crossing of difficult membrane barriers, delivery and sustained inhibition of intracellular pathogens and sterilization abilities as shown in Fig. 1. This perspective status quo of NP antimicrobial agents with multiple functions will play a significant impact on the treatment of diseases.

Broad spectrum nanoparticle-antimicrobial agents

The global emergence of multidrug-resistant microorganisms (viruses, bacteria, fungi and protozoa) has made conventional treatment of infectious diseases difficult. Therefore, the discovery of alternative new classes of antiviral [15], antibiotics [16], antifungal [17], and

* Correspondence: cyah@nmmu.ac.za
[1]Department of Biochemistry and Microbiology, Nelson Mandela Metropolitan University, Port Elizabeth, South Africa
[2]Department of Epidemiology, Johns Hopkins Bloomberg School of Public Health, E7146, 615 N. Wolfe Street, Baltimore 21205, MD, USA
Full list of author information is available at the end of the article

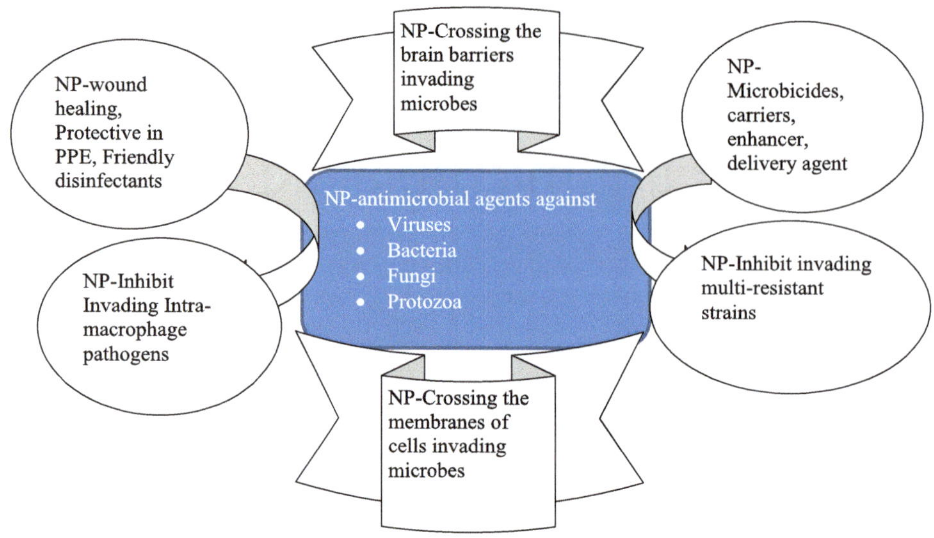

Fig. 1 Multiple functionality and broad spectrum activities of nanoparticles antimicrobial agents. The diverse vast antimicrobial uses of nanoparticle bioconjugates. Used for wound healing, use as anticancers, anti multi-resistant pathogens, aid drugs to cross the blood brain barriers, help in the inhibition of microbes that hide in macrophages. NP = acronyms for Nanoparticles. PPE = Personal Protective equipment incorporated with nanoparticles capable of destroying microbes

antiprotozoal [18] agents that can treat resistant strains is paramount. Research has shown that these emerging broad-spectrum antimicrobial nanomaterial can knock-out diverse pathogenic organisms of different phyla, across diverse and/or within species of viruses, bacteria and fungi [19–22]. For example, Fig. 2 shows the broad spectrum NP-antimicrobial effect of AgNPs. The AgNP antimicrobial agent has multi-functionality of antibacterial [22], antifungal [22], antiviral [23], anti-parasitic [4], and anti-inflammatory properties [14, 24].

One of the mechanisms of NP-antimicrobial actions is cell wall lysis. For example, a study by Addae et al. [12] in an attempt to produce a transducer agent for photothermal therapy (PTT) found the destruction of *Bacillus*

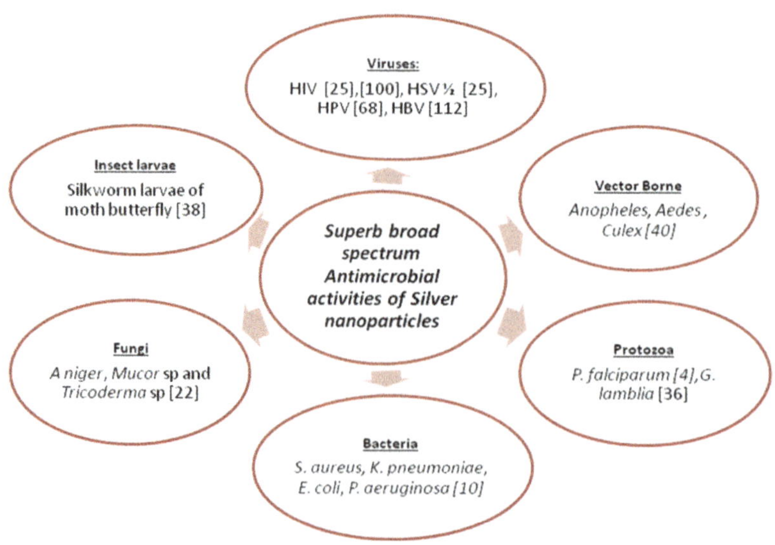

Fig. 2 Broad spectrum NP-antimicrobial activities of silver nanoparticles. The Figure describes the antimicrobial spectrum of silver bio-conjugate nanoparticles against diverse genera of microorganisms. HIV = Human immunodeficiency virus, HSV = Herpes Simplex Virus 1, HPV = Human papillomavirus, HBV = Hepatitis B virus, *P. falciparum* = *Plasmodium falciparum*, *G. lamblia* = *Gardia lamblia*, *S. aureus* = *Staphylococcus aureus*, *E. coli* = *Escherichia coli*, *P. aeruginosa* = *Pseudomonas aeruginosa*, sp = species

species cell membranes when treated with Au/CuS NPs. The destruction of *Bacillus* species in this study proved that Au/CuS NPs are potent NP-antimicrobial agents.

The NPs are potential broad spectrum antibiotics because they can inhibit wide range of multidrug-resistant strains of bacteria that have defied most antibiotic treatment. For example, in the study by Adeli et al. [10] it was found that AgNPs were able to inhibit pan-multidrug resistant strains of *S. aureus, K. pneumoniae, E. coli,* and *P. aeruginosa* that were resistant to all the antibiotic drugs including imipenem. Another similar study by Kathiravan et al. [22] showed that AgNPs can inhibit both bacteria (*S. aureus, E coli, B subtilis*) and fungi species (*A niger, Mucor* sp and *Tricoderma* sp). In addition, earlier findings by Fayaz et al. [25] showed that the AgNPs-coated condom have antiviral (against HIV-1 and HSV-1/2), antibacterial (against *E. coli, S. aureus, M. luteus, K. pneumonia*) and anti-fungi (against *Candida* spp.) properties. This suggests that AgNPs can be used to treat all multi-drug resistant pathogens from diverse phyla from all clinical sources.

The broad spectrum antimicrobial activities have also been demonstrated by CNTs. For example, a study by Tank et al. [26] showed that silica coated silicon nanotubes (SCSNTs) exhibit enhanced antimicrobial activities when compared to other non-silica coated silicon nano-particles. Other studies also found that CNTs containing lysine such as multiwalled CNT (MWCNT)-epilsonpolylysine [27], and SWCNT-poly(L-lysine) (PLL), and poly(L-glutamic acid) [28] exhibit very strong broad antimicrobial activities against a wide range of bacteria. A study by Amiri et al. [29] showed MWCNT-lysine exhibiting very strong broad antimicrobial activity against *S. aureus, S. agalactiae, S. dysgalactiae, E.coli, K. pneumonia* and *Salmonella typhimurium.*

In addition to antimicrobial activities, hybrids of nanomaterials such as cholesterol-containing liposomes phytonanosilver and CNTs have been found to exhibit high antioxidant activity as well as antimicrobial activities against *E. coli, Staphylococcus aureus* and *Enterococcus faecalis* [30]. This shows that when two or more NPs are combined, they tend to enhance the broad spectrum activity of the nano-antimicrobial agents. The hydrid behaviour was equally found when CNTs and AgNP-based nanomaterials were combined and the resulting hybrid biocomposite was found to exhibit stronger and excellent antimicrobial properties [27]. Similarly, chitosan-CNT hybrid showed excellent antimicrobial activities against bacteria and fungi [9]. Other CNTs antimicrobial hybrids include ZnO coated MWCNTs (ZnO/MWCNTs) [13], Triad CNT-NPs/Polymer nanocomposites [11], functionalized MWCNTs-CdS and functionalized-MWCNTs-Ag2S [31], and CdTe QDs/single-walled aluminosilicate nanotubes [32]. Furthermore, Cefalexin-immobilized multi-walled CNTs have been found to broadly enhance the antimicrobial activities against a wide range of pathogens including *E. coli, P. aeruginosa, S. aureus* and *Bacillus subtilis* [8] as shown in Table 1. The combination of AgNPs and CNTs including MWCNT-AgNPs [33] on fiber membrane has also been found to enhance the filtration and antimicrobial potentials against all types of bacteria. In addition, Poly(N-vinylcarbazole) (PVK)-SWCNT nanocomposite coated membrane for water purification were found to destroy all bacterial species including spore forming organisms such as *Bacillus subtilis* [34]. Apart from filtration and demonstration of antimicrobial activities the MWCNT-AgNPs hybrid composite membrane has been found to significantly reduce biofilm formation which can easily be extended to other types of support membranes [33]. Table 1 summaries the types of NPs and their susceptibility to various organisms.

Nanoparticle anti-parasitic effect

Despite the efforts made in the treatment of parasitic infections, infections by parasites particularly those of giardiasis, schistosomiasis, trypanosomiasis, malaria, leishmaniasis, dengue fevers, Japanese encephalitis, and filariasis continue to increase particularly in tropical and low income countries [24, 35, 36]. The problems associated with parasitic infections include drug toxicity, ineffectiveness, and developments of resistance to conventional anti-parasitic drugs. Furthermore, treatment costs are high, thus limiting supply of drugs in low income countries [37]. As a results of the limitation in anti-parasitic drugs, newer approaches such as nano-biotechnology have shown significant improvement in the treatment of parasitic infections [24]. This is based on the unique properties of NPs including those of AgNPs, AuNPs, chitosan, selenium oxide, and other metallic oxide based NPs that have shown excellent inhibitory effects against parasitic infections including insect larvae [24, 35–38].

Parasites such as *Leishmania* can reside and survive inside macrophages without being exposed to cell damage by reactive oxygen species (ROS) and anti-parasitic drugs [37]. However, AgNPs, because of their trans-membrane mechanisms and sustained anti-parasitic delivery, can inhibit intracellular *Leishmania* and enhance their destruction via ROS [37].

Other NPs including the combination of silver, chitosan, and curcumin nanoparticles have been used in the treatment of *Giardia lamblia* as demonstrated in experimental animals [36]. The findings also showed that *Giardia lamblia* can be successfully eradicated from stool and intestine [36]. The potential of NPs if fully optimized may lead to the development of newer synergic antimicrobials where two or more nano-antimicrobials are combined to generate an effective efficacy in the

Table 1 Summary of the types of nanoparticles susceptibility to organisms

Type of NP	Method of NPs characterization	Size of NP	Types organisms inhibited	Outcome	Toxicity	Author
Fe-Oxide NP & AgNP	UV–vis spectroscopy, Fourier Transform Infrared Spectroscopy (FTIR), Transmission Electron Microscopy (TEM)	Fe-oxide NP 20–40 nm, AgNP 10–20 nm	*Bacillus, E. coli* and *Staphylococcus* species	Fe-Oxide NPs were sensitive against *Bacillus, E. coli* and *Staphylococcus* species.	The very smaller size AgNP were toxic against the pathogens	[14]
Ag NPs.	TEM, Field Emission Transmission Electron Microscopy (FESEM), FTIR, UV–Vis spectra, Raman spectroscopy, X-ray Difraction (XRD)	Average 18–20 nm	*Escherichia coli, Pseudomonas* spp. *Bacillus* species, *Staphylococcus* species, *Aspergillus niger, Aspergillus flavus, Penicillium*	Inhibited the growth and multiplication of *E. coli, Pseudomonas* species, *Bacillus* spp. and *Staphylococcus* species, *A. niger, A. flavus, Penicillium* spp	ND	[98]
Silver, chitosan, and curcumin nanoparticles	NA	-	*Giardia lamblia*	The highest effect was achieved by combining the three nanoforms. The parasite was found to be eradicated from stool and intestine.	None of the nanoparticle exhibited toxic effect	[36]
AgNPs	UV spectra, TEM	2–30 nm; averagely 20 nm	*S. aureus, Klebsiella pneumoniae, Escherichia coli,* and *Pseudomonas aeruginosa*	The AgNPs produced had strong antibacterial effect against all the pathogenic bacteria	ND	[10]
polyvinylpyrrolidone (PVP)-coated silver nanoparticles	-	1–10 nm	HIV-1	PVP-coated AgNP exhibit potent cyto-protective and post-infected anti-HIV-1 activities toward Hut/CCR5 cells.	ND	[99]
PVP-coated silver nanoparticles	-	30–50 nm	HIV-1	PVP-coated AgNPs Inhibited cell-associated HIV-1 and cell-free HIV-1 transmission.	PVP-coated AgNPs were non toxic to cells explant	[100]
mercaptoethane sulfonate (MES)-coated silver and gold nanoparticles	-	4 nm	Herpes simplex virus type 1 (HSV-1)	The MES-coated silver and gold nanoparticles inhibited HSV-1 infec tion in cell culture	The MES-coated silver and gold were non toxic to host cells	[101]
PVP-coated silver nanoparticles	-	69 nm +/− 3 nm	Respiratory syncytial virus (RSV)	Inhibited RSV infection	showed low toxicity to cells	[102]
AgNP and polysaccharide-coated AgNP	-	10–80 nm	Monkey pox virus (MPV)	The AgNPs of approximately 10 nm inhibit MPV infection in vitro, as an anti-viral	Non of te GgNPs were cytotoxic (Vero cell monolayer sloughing)	[103]
AgNPs	-	10–50 nm	Hepatitis B virus (HBV)	AgNPs inhibited in vitro HBV RNA and extracellular virions	ND	[104]
AgNPs and polysaccharide-coated AgNP	-	10 nm	Tacaribe virus (TCRV)	AgNPs inhibited the TCRV infection in vitro	ND	[105]
Ag-NPs-coated PUC	High resolution Scanning Electron Microscopy (HrSEM), UV Spectra	30–60 nm	*E. coli, S. aureus, M. luteus, K. pneumoniae,* and *Candida tropicalis, Candida krusei, Candida glabrata,* and *Candida albicans and* HIV-1	Ag-NPs-coated PUC with HIV-1 and HSV-1/2 was able to inactivate their infectiousness as well as bacterial and fungal species	ND	[25]

Table 1 Summary of the types of nanoparticles susceptibility to organisms *(Continued)*

Mycosynthesized silver nanoparticles	UV spectra, TEM, Nanosight-LM 20;	4–46 nm	HSV 1 and 2 and with human parainfluenza virus type 3.	Smaller-sized AgNPs were able to inhibit the infectivity of the viruses	ND	[23]
AgNPs	UV–vis spectroscopy, SEM, TEM, FTIR and XRD.	18 to 45 nm with an average size of 32 nm	*Anopheles stephensi, Aedes aegypti*, and *Culex quinquefasciatus*	AgNPs showed biolarvicidal effect to *A. stephensi, A. aegypti*, and *C. quinquefasciatus.*	ND	[39]
AgNPs	UV–vis spectroscopy, SEM, FTIR and XRD.	41–60 nm.	*Anopheles stephensi, Aedes aegypti*, and *Culex quinquefasciatus*	The AgNPs were effective in destroying the vectors of mosquito vector blood born parasites	ND	[40]
AgNPs	Atomic force microscopy (AFM), UV–vis spectroscopy, FTIR	60–95 nm	3 instar larvae of Culex quinquefasciatus	AgNPs exhibited high mortality against larvae of *Culex quinquefasciatus*	ND	[78]
AgNPs	UV–vis spectroscopy, SEM, energy-dispersive X-ray (EDX) spectroscopy.	43.52 to 142.97 nm	Aedes aegypti	The Bt-AgNPs showed larvicide ef fect against mosquito larva A. aegypti	ND	[106]
Polyvinyl-N-carbazole (PVK) and single-walled carbon nanotubes (SWNTs) (PVK:SWNT)	UV vis spectra, FTIR, SEM	NA	*E. coli* MG 1655 and *B. subtilis*-102	The nano-composite showed anti microbial activity against both Gram-positive and negative bacterial isolates.	The PVK-SWNT were non toxic to fibroblast cells	[34]
MWCNT-lysine functionalized	FTIR, Thermal gravimetric analysis (TGA), Raman spectra and TEM	N/A	*S. aureus, Streptococcus agalactiae, S. dysgalactiae, E. coli, K. pneumonia, S. typhimurium*	The functionalized MWCNT with lysine expressed high antimicrobial effect against all bacterial cells	ND	[29]
MWCNT-AgNPs	Inductively coupled plasma atomic emission spectroscopy (ICP-AES), XRD, FTIR	3 to 30 nm	*Escherichia coli*	MWCNT-AgNPs exhibited strong antimicrobial activities and reduce biofilm formation.	ND	[33]
Silicon nanotubes (SNTs), silicon nanoparticles (SNPs)	SEM–EDX, TEM, Brunauer-Emmett-Teller (BET), STM, Raman spectroscopy.	average diameter of 14	Multidrug-resistant *Staphylococcus aureus*	SCSNTs were effective in limiting the growth of multidrug-resistant *S aureus*	ND	[26]
Ag–Fe/SWCNTs	TEM, SEM, XRD, Raman spectra	1–10 nm Ag-Fe NP dispersed and tightly attached to the outer surfaces of SWCNTs	*Escherichia coli.*	Purified Ag–Fe/SWCNT hybrid nanoparticles were effective against *E. coli.*	ND	[104]
SWCNTs combine with H_2O_2 or NaOCl	TEM, SEM-EDX	SWCNTs 1–1.5 nm	*Bacillus anthracis* Spores	The combined effect of SWCNTs and H_2O_2 or NaOCl exhibited sporicidal effect on *B. anthracis* spores	ND	[87]
SWNT/PLL/PGA	Uv spectra, TEM, SEM, Quartz crystal microgravimetry	SWNT is 0.8–1.2 nm	*E. coli* and *S. epidermidis*	SWNT/PLL/PGA highly inactivated *E. coli* and *S. epidermidis*	ND	[28]
Zirconia (ZrO2) nanoparticles	SEM, EDX, AFM, U vis spectra, FTIR	50e100 nm, average size 50 nm	*Staphylococcus aureus, Escherichia coli, Candida albicans, Aspergillus niger*	Zirconia (ZrO2) nanoparticles exhibited antifungal and antibacterial against the test organisms.	ND	[111]

Table 1 Summary of the types of nanoparticles susceptibility to organisms *(Continued)*

Au/CuS core/shell nanoparticles (NPs)	HRTEM, SEM, energy dispersive X-ray spectroscopy (EDS)	2–5 nm.	*B. anthracis* spores and cells	The Au/CuS NPs were highly efficient in inactivating *B. anthracis* cells, but not effective to the spores.	ND	[12]
Sialic-acid functionalized gold nanoparticles	TEM	2 nm and 14 nm	Influenza virus	The NPs inhibition influenza virus infection	The functionalized AuNPs were nontoxic to the cells	[107]
Titanium dioxide nanoparticles (TiO2 NPs)	XRD, FTIR, SEM, EDX, AFM.	Average size of 70 nm.	Pediculus humanus capitis De Geer (Phthiraptera: Pediculidae); larvae of cattle tick Hyalomma anatolicum (a.) anatolicum Koch (Acari: Ixodidae), and fourth instar larvae of malaria vector Anopheles subpictus Grassi (Diptera: Culicidae).	The TiO_2 NPs showed significant mortality against the vectors borne organisms	ND	
Chrysosporium tropicum mediated silver and gold nanoparticles	Microscan reader, XRD, TEM, SEM	AuNPs: 2–15 nm and AgNP: 20–50 nm	*Aedes aegypti* larvae.	The AuNPs used as an efficacy enhancer shown mortality 3 times higher *Aedes aegypti* larvae.	ND	[41]
Zinc oxide nanoparticles (ZnO NPs)	UV–visible spectroscopy, XRD, FTIR, SEM	60–120 nm.	larvae of cattle tick Rhipicephalus (Boophilus) microplus, Canestrini (Acari: Ixodidae); head louse Pediculus humanus capitis, De Geer (Phthiraptera: Pediculidae); larvae of malaria vector, Anopheles subpictus, Grassi; and filariasis vector, Culex quinquefasciatus, Say (Diptera: Culicidae). R. microplus larvae	The ZnO NPs had significant inhibitory effect on the parasites	ND	[110]
Cobalt nanoparticles (CoNPs)	XRD, FTIR FESEM with energy dispersive X-ray spectroscopy, and TEM	average size of 84.81 nm.	malaria vector Anopheles subpictus and dengue vector *Aedes aegypti (Diptera: Culicidae).*	The larvicidal effect was observed in the cobalt acetate solution and against the *A. subpictus* and *A. aegypti*	ND	[108]
Copper(II) nanohybrid solids, $LCu(CH_3COO)_2$ and $LCuCl_2$	TEM, dynamic light scattering, and IR spectroscopy	5–10 and 60–70 nm of $LCu(CH_3COO)_2$ and $LCuCl_2$	*Plasmodium falciparum* (MRC 2).	The two compounds showed significant antimalarial activities against the parasites	The copper(II) nanohybrid solids were nontoxic to human hepatocellular carcinoma cells	[109]

eradication and probably the elimination of parasitic infections. Some studies have shown that modified *Plasmodium berghei* sporozoite (Tg-Pb/PfCSP) and self-assembling protein NP (SAPN) vaccine presenting *Plasmodium falciparum* circumsporozoite protein epitopes (PfCSP-SAPN) can stimulate humoral and cellular responses against *Plasmodium falciparum* using the complement classical pathway cascade [4]. The results indicates the potential application of the circumsporozoite protein epitopes (PfCSP-SAPN) in the development of protective effector memory CD8+ T-cells [4] capable of generating strong long-lived IgG.

Nanoparticle anti-vector borne diseases

As a result of the increase in the prevalence of vector borne diseases, the production of environmentally friendly and safe NP insecticides synthesized from plants are currently available. These include those of AgNPs synthesized from the leaf extracts of *Heliotropium indicum* [39], and *Azadirachta indica* [40]. These insecticides have shown maximum efficacy against blood feeding mosquitoes of *Anopheles stephensi, Aedes aegypti,* and *Culex quinquefasciatus* [39, 40]. This shows that eco-friendly NPs have the potential of controlling vector transmitted infections that have significantly contributed to disease burden, social debility, poverty and death in mostly low income countries [39, 40]. However, due to NPs non-specific actions to environmental organisms, this may deter their usefulness as vector control agents [40–42].

Wound healing and nanoparticles

Wound dressing and wound healing are very important components of reducing morbidity and mortality of wound related burden. A wound is a debilitated tissue that results from a breakdown in the skin giving rise to a physiological condition for microbial manifestation including opportunistic pathogens [43, 44] affecting wound healing [45]. Depending on the degree of wound, whether acute or chronic, wound care is necessary to reduce infection or abnormal bacterial presence that may cause stress and other health consequences [44, 46]. Over the years, wound dressing and healing have been problematic to clinicians [46]. Because there is no single appropriate wound dressing material that can act as a potent sterile antimicrobial agent capable of absorbing excess exudate, preserving the wound from external sources of infection, preventing excess heat at the wound, impermeable to gases, and a dressing that is easy to remove without further trauma to the wound [47] has complicated wound healing. Wound dressing materials such as gauze are associated with painful removal and may cause trauma and associated stress [48].

Nevertheless, the research on NPs in wound dressing materials has come at an opportune time. The NP wound dressing materials provide biocompatible antimicrobial agents that are inexpensive, soft, and flexible, and conform to the contours of the body [49, 50]. For example, AgNPs wound dressing antimicrobial nanomaterials have been introduced to supplement traditional wound dressing because the slow release of the AgNPs allow the dressing to be changed less frequently, but is highly effective and efficient in wound healing with less antimicrobial resistance [49]. Furthermore, a study by Guidelli et al. [51] showed that natural latex rubber blended with AgNPs gradually released the AgNPs, but was useful in promoting and facilitating wound healing as well as the reduction in scar formation [49]. The AgNPs may also mediate wound healing via reduced mitochondria activity that does not affect the host cell viability with rapid re-establishment of the body integrity [52]. According to a study by Tian et al. [53] AgNPs exert positive broad spectrum antimicrobial properties by reducing wound inflammation, and modulation of fibrogenic cytokines.

Similarly, other findings by John and Moro [54] showed that NPs hydrogel wound dressing consist of methacrylate backbone and terminal hydroxyl group capable of providing versatile and excellent wound healing. This is because the NPs hydrogel dressing powders have thermal insulators capable of absorbing some of the blood or wound exudate, thus providing an impermeable potent antimicrobial environment to wound pathogens as well as protecting the wound from external contamination [50, 54]. The NPs hydrogel are cost effective, user friendly, easy to apply, do not adhere to the wound and have minimal need for secondary dressing [54].

Apart from AgNPs, other NPs equally used in wound healings include those of gold [55], curcumin-encapsulated NPs [56], chitin/nanosilver composite with good blood clotting ability [57], conjugated iron oxide NPs [58], and nitric oxide releasing NPs [59]. However, the significant acceleration of wound healing by nanomaterials still remains a mystery and the mechanisms of action are still to be fully elucidated and unfold.

Nanoparticles microbicides activities

With the increase in sexually transmitted infections (STI) fuelling the HIV burden and other health problems, microbicides may be considered as alternative preventive methods of STI and HIV [60, 61]. Microbicides are antimicrobial agents that are self-applied on the vagina or rectum to protect against STIs [19, 62, 63]. Hence they act as chemical, biological and/or physical barriers that prevent transmission of pathogens during sexual intercourse [62, 64, 65]. They may be in gel, creams, rings, or films form and can be used with condoms, thus offering additional protection or used alone especially by those who do not appreciate the use of condoms [19]. The microbicides may be used by both HIV positive and heathy individuals to prevent transmission of the virus. Studies have shown that microbicides may provide prevention against HIV and STI infections for those practicing receptive anal and/or vaginal intercourse [63]. In addition, microbicides can provide individuals with protection especially those who are unaware of their partner HIV status including those on antiretroviral therapies (ART) and undetectable HIV viral load [63].

Research studies have shown that NPs-microbicides including those of dendrimer-nanoscale-microbicides hold potential safety efficacy against viruses [19, 66–68]. For example, the VivaGel™ (SPL7013Gel) dendrimer is carefully formulated against HIV and HSV and does not interfere with vaginal or rectal physiological pH [19, 69]. The dendrimer VivaGel™ microbicide is meant to disrupt and block viral attachment and/or prevent the viral adsorption from targeting cells of the rectum or vagina. In the case of HIV the gp120 of the virus are blocked from attaching to the CD4 receptors of human white blood cells [19]. In a study by Chonco et al. [60], it was found that carbosilane dendrimer microbicide are capable of exhibiting HIV thus blocking potential in epithelial monolayer in vitro model cells. Other dendrimers such as heparan sulfate-binding peptide were found to inhibit human papillomaviruses [68] thus, acting as promising antiviral microbicides.

Nanoparticles inhibition of intra-macrophage pathogens

Pathogenic organisms that traverse cell membranes or reside in nerve cells cause persistence infections and, thus are difficult to treat [70]. Bacteria such as *Brucella, Mycobacterium, Listeria* species and viruses including HIV, and herpes simplex are intracellular pathogens that invade treatment and persistently exhibit latent infections [70–72]. Therefore, some drugs find it difficult to reach such cells, thus complicating the elimination and eradication of such microbial pathogens [73]. Some of the pathogens may invade cells and exist as intra-macrophage pathogens and central nervous infections escaping drugs action as well as immunological responses [71, 73]. Health care workers (HCWs) find it very difficult and frustrating when providing treatment to such intravascular disease causing pathogens due to failure of conventional antimicrobial drugs to destroy such organisms. Drugs for treating such diseases including HIV, encephalopathy and cerebrovascular infections may not lack potency, but due to shortcomings of poor or inefficient intracellular penetration and sustained drugs concentration, may limit treatment efficiency and efficacy [73]. The problems associated with such drugs may include lack of solubility and bio-distribution to reach target areas, thus do not have sufficient drug delivery profile.

Nano-drugs such as polymeric NPs, dendrimers, polymer micelles, and solid lipid NPs have been shown to exhibit excellent antimicrobial profiles and have potent ligand conjugates that improve the pharmacological and therapeutic profile of such drugs to cross such cell membranes, internalize and render efficient antimicrobial potentials [70, 71, 73]. The delivery process provide NP-drugs with multiple functions of carrier, delivery, and antimicrobial capabilities [71, 73, 74]. These attributes are due to the small size (1–100 nm), vast NPs-functionalization ability, and the robust physiochemical properties, even if biodegradability and the toxicological challenges may be hindering beneficial health outcomes [75, 76].

As mentioned earlier, organisms such *Brucella* species, *Mycobacterium tuberculosis* exist as intra-macrophage pathogen rendering standard treatment very difficult [71, 72]. For example, *Brucella* species usually invade, reside and survive within phagocytic, dendritic and trophoblast cells, thus making treatment potential very difficult to clinicians [71]. Similarly, *Mycobacterium tuberculosis* bacteria responsible for tuberculosis reside inside macrophage resulting into persistent tuberculosis [77]. The same effect has been demonstrated by herpes simplex virus that hides and resides in nerve cells causing latent herpes zosters infections [78]. The use of NPs could be beneficial for such treatments because of the NPs antimicrobials potentials, ease membrane crossing ability and delivery potentials of materials into such cells. They play the role of carrier, delivery and sustain antimicrobials effect in such cells. For example, AgNPs have huge biocidal effect and have been shown to cross the macrophage cell wall and inhibit intra-macrophage *Bacillus abortus*; a maternal bacterium that tend to resist treatment and causes perinatal morbidity during pregnancy [79].

Furthermore, some pathogens are highly resistant to extreme temperatures and difficult to be eliminated by antibiotics or other chemicals. Nanomaterials and other emerging materials have been reported to be potent antimicrobial agents capable of destroying such pathogens that are tolerant to extreme temperatures and resistant to treat with conventional antibiotics [80]. For example, SWCNTs coupled within 20 minutes near infrared (NIR) treatment significantly increases the potential effect of antimicrobials against *Bacillus anthracis* spores when compared to non NIR treated SWCNTs [67]. In addition, a study by Martínez-Gutierrez et al. [81] found that 24 nm AgNPs were not only potent antibacterial agents against resistant strains of bacteria, but also had anti-coagulation activities as well as inflammatory response in macrophages. This indicates that nanomaterials can easily be modified as efficient intravascular agent for the destruction of intravascular pathogens as well as delivery agents since they are capable of crossing membrane cell walls without any cell damage or harm [82]. However, the mechanisms of cell membrane or pathways used by the NPs antimicrobial agents in crossing/cell uptake are still to be fully explained [82].

Nanoparticles penetration of the brain barriers and difficult to reach tissues or cells

Infections of the brain are often very difficult to treat because of the difficulty of most antimicrobial agents to cross the blood brain barrier and inhibit microbial agents [84]. This is due to the fact that the brain is made up of complex cell networks that filter foreign materials, protect and prevent the brain from injuries and diseases [83]. However, some small microbes such as viruses as well as some bacteria are still capable of bypassing and crossing the blood brain barrier [83, 84]. Substances entering the brain are mediated through a tight regulated systematic process of membrane transporters [82–84]. This tight regulatory system prevents most pharmacological antimicrobial agents from crossing the blood brain barrier and exercising their pharmacological activities [82–84]. In this regard nanotechnological antimicrobial agents could bring a novel dimensional approach that is capable of overcoming and bypassing the complex brain cell network, and inhibiting the brain pathogens, thus reducing the burden of microbial brain infections [85]. The NPs can potentially carry and potentially deliver antimicrobial across the blood brain barrier. In fact, it is known that NPs have very small nanosizes that exhibit vast physiochemical multifunctional properties that play a significant role of crossing the blood brain barrier with ease. These features of being able to transiting difficult biological system with ease without disrupting or damaging the cell membranes and sustaining the antimicrobials have made NPs and/or nanomaterials (nano-functionalized-ligands) very attractive for biomedical applications [5, 86]. For example, a single oral administration of polylactide-co-glycolide NP-encapsulated antituberculosis drugs consisting of rifampicin + isoniazid + pyrazinamide + ethambutol conjugate in murine mice was found to cross the blood brain barrier and sustained for 9 days in the brain [86]. Furthermore, based on colony forming unit enumerations and pathological examinations, the study showed that 5 oral doses administered every 10th day improved the pharmacologic activities of the polymer NP-antituberculosis drugs resulting in an undetectable level of *Mycobacterium tuberculosis* in the mice meninges [86].

The mechanisms of action of how the polymer- antituberculosis nanomaterials bypassed the complex cell network of blood brain barriers are yet to be uncovered. It is envisaged that the development of emerging novel NP-antimicrobial agents will soon revolutionize clinical medicine [86]. It is anticipated that the crossing of the blood brain barrier by NP-antimicrobial agents including other classes of drugs would reduce the burden of infections including meningitis caused by vast majority of pathogens.

Nanoparticles enhancement of antimicrobial activities of other agents

The NPs play a significant role in enhancing the activities of other agents leading to effective and efficient treatment action. For example, the combination of SWCNTs and hydrogen peroxide (H_2O_2) or NaOCl increases the sporicidal effect on the spores of organisms such as *Bacillus* species when compared to treatment with H_2O_2 or NaOCl alone at the same concentrations [87]. In such treatments, synergistic mechanisms of efficacy are established due to contribution of multiple antimicrobial effects. Further analysis shows that SWCNTs do not only play the role of antimicrobial effect, but also increases permeability/susceptibility of the *Bacillus* species pathogen to H_2O_2 or NaOCl, thus significantly developing high effective sporicidal effect [87]. Furthermore, findings by Gilbertson et al. [6] found that oxygen functional groups when functionalized on MWCNTs, enhances several MWCNT properties such as redox activity, electrochemical and antimicrobial activities. The redox activities include the ability to enhance the oxidation of glutathione, and the reduction of surface carboxyl groups that promote the functional performance of MWCNTs antimicrobial activities for biomedical application [6]. This synergetic effect has equally been shown by AgNPs which enhanced the angiogenic properties of natural latex rubber for cell growth and wound healing [51].

Nanoparticles disinfectants

The inventive approach of nanomaterials as disinfectant relate to their stability, homogeneity, high efficiency and efficacy of broad biocide spectrum of virucidal, bactericidal, fungicidal, antiparasitic and sporicidal as well as mycobactericidal and mycoplasmicidal potentials [88–90]. These excellent disinfectant properties as well as the additional ability of NPs surface functionalization and the dispersion on the NPs surfaces have been exhibited by a wide range of NPs [5–7]. Such functional groups provide very potent additional antimicrobial properties and include ligands such as hydroxyl, carboxyl, amine, and other chemical radicals [5]. The NPs including those of silver, copper and gold [91] have excellent cleaning and disinfecting properties. Some of these NPs are now being used as cleaning disinfectants in hospitals. In such instances, the surfaces may be coated with potent nanomaterials against nosocomial pathogens including the stubborn multi-drug resistant pathogens of Methicillin-resistant *Staphylococcus aureus*

(MRSA) that are responsible for most nosocomial infections [88, 92]. For example, silicone polymers of AuNPs have shown to actively reduce the microbial load on clinical surfaces, particularly, when the surfaces are activated with white light [93].

To minimize the risk of microbial and other contamination of hospital HCW during various clinical procedures and examination procedures, hospital protective equipment are re-enforced with nanomaterials-antimicrobial agents that have been developed. Some of the HCW antimicrobial protective materials include surgical mask, gloves and many other latex personal protective equipment (PPE). For example, mixtures of silver nitrate and titanium dioxide NP coated on hospital facemask used during very delicate clinical procedures have shown to have significant protection against infectious agents [91, 93, 94]. The use of NPs-antiseptics has also led to an increase in surface area to volume ratio, thus improving the lethal action of NPs-antiseptics against pathogens [91, 93].

As a result of the biocidal action and non-toxic nature of some NPs such as AgNPs, they are widely coated on medical devices to reduce infections [95]. In addition, nanomaterials of silver are being used in pet-animal shampoos as disinfection, cleaning and softening agents [96]. The AgNPs can also be coated on filters used for the purification of water. In some studies, PVK and SWNTs were found to destroy bacterial cell membranes [34].

Furthermore, NPs are currently being used as preservatives in packages to prevent food spoilage. For example, allyl isothiocyanate (AIT) and CNTs can be incorporated into packaging materials so as to prevent the contamination of food by *Salmonella choleraesuis* [97]. The allyl isothiocyanate (AIT) and CNTs work by providing an antimicrobial film that reduces the microbial contamination, control oxidation and reduces the colour changes for up to 40 days [97].

Nanoparticles antimicrobial mechanisms of action

Traditionally, most antimicrobial agents inhibit microbial growth through several mechanisms such as cell wall inhibition and lysis, inhibition of protein synthesis, alteration of cell membranes, inhibition of nucleic acid (NA) synthesis and antimetabolite activity [113]. The NP-antimicrobials, on the other hand, may encompass and differ slightly due to their vast physiochemical properties with respect to size, shape, surface area, surface energy, charge, crystallinity, agglomeration, aggregation and chemical composition [114–116]. Although most NP-antimicrobial mechanisms of action are still unknown and are currently under investigations [117], studies show that NPs can mediate bacterial cell membranes degradation [118–120]. For example, Li et al. [120] found the degradation of *S. aureus* by Catechin-Cu NPs. The Catechin-Cu NPs was also found to exert different mechanisms of action during *E. coli* cell wall degradation, which is an indication of different impacts on the Gram negative and Gram positive bacteria [120]. The multiple effects have also been observed in CuNP-antimicrobial actions which include the generation of reactive oxygen species and lipid peroxidation [118]. Other CuNP-antibacterial actions include protein oxidation and DNA degradation in *E. coli* cells [118]. Another study by Xie et al. [121] showed that zinc oxide (ZnO) NPs exerted bactericidal effect by disruption of the cell membrane and oxidative stress in *Campylobacter jejuni*. The NP-antimicrobials such as AgNP have also been shown to bind to lippopolysaccharides, surface proteins or porin, collapsing the microbial cell wall and limiting the membrane potential [122]. Similarly, AgNP have been found to induce efflux of phosphate, reduction of cellular ATP level, interacting with sulphahydryl (or thiol) group and altering cytoplasmic components as well as inhibiting the respiratory enzymes and blocking of DNA replication in both Gram negative and Gram positive bacterial pathogens [122]. These studies show that different NPs have very different physiochemical properties and thus exhibit different antimicrobial mechanisms of action.

Nanoparticles toxicity

The NPs antimicrobial agents have excellent potent and low tendency of inducing resistance when compared to non-NPs-antimicrobial agents [123]. However, the NP-antimicrobial agents' pharmacological properties may be hampered by potential toxicity [123, 124]. As stated in previous sections of this review paper, NPs facilitate the penetration and delivery of antimicrobial agents into biological membranes including microbial cells, thereby enhancing and increasing biological activities [76, 113]. This means that the toxicity of different NP-antimicrobial polymers needs a time-dependent understanding and characterization [125]. Generally, antimicrobial agents' biocompatibility inhibition cannot occur without producing some undesirable health effects, either local or systemic. In fact, the most deterring effect of most drugs is their potential toxicity to organisms of which NPs-antimicrobials agents are not an exception. Therefore, effective NP-antimicrobial agents' dose-related response is an important factor in relation to human exposure and other organisms. Few studies have described the toxicity of NP-antimicrobials (Table 1) with controversies. For example, a study by Cooper and Spitzer [126] shows that AgNPs antimicrobials at sub-lethal dose disrupt cytoskeleton and neurite dynamics when cultured in adult neural stem cells. For example, at sub-lethal dose of 1.0 µg/mL, AgNP cultured in neural stem cells induced the formation of f-actin inclusions, indicating a disruption of actin function [126]. Similar findings were reported by

Baram-Pinto [101] that AgNPs capped with Mercaptoethane Sulfonate showed some serious effects in mammalian cells. Some results showed that PVK-SWCNT-antimicrobial agents were nontoxic to fibroblast cells as opposed to pure SWCNTs [34]. Multivalent Sialic acid functionalized AuNPs-antimicrobials agents have also been shown to demonstrate no toxic effect on Madin-Darby canine kidney cells [107]. Similarly, copper (II) nanohybrid solids-antimicrobial have shown no toxic effect on human hepatocellular carcinoma cells [109]. In another study, no cytotoxicity was reported when rats were treated with antibacterial AgNP-loaded titanium nanotube [127]. The rat cells expressed no toxicity thus demonstrating the competence of NPs-antimicrobials as future antimicrobial agents. However, despite several studies, the current available information is insufficient to ascertain the adverse effects of NP-antimicrobials on human health. Therefore, it is imperative that further research is carried out to mitigate any toxicological problems that may arise.

Summary and future perspectives

Research has shown that the functionalization-immobilization and/or hybridization of NPs can enhance and improve the antimicrobial activities of the nanomaterials against a wide range of multi-resistant strains of pathogenic microorganisms. For example, a single type of NP-antimicrobial agent could show multiple antimicrobial properties against many pathogens. However, these characteristics may also alter the microbial flora of the body since their antimicrobial action is non-specific. Most of the studies reviewed showed that AgNPs were the widely used and have several antibacterial, antiviral, antifungal, anti-parasite, anti-insect and anti-vector borne properties. Generally, most NP-antimicrobial drugs were able to target and transit difficult membrane barriers, deliver and sustain the NP-antimicrobial doses resulting in disease clearance which is a difficult phenomenon for conventional antimicrobials. However, more information on the toxicological effects of NP-antimicrobial agents is needed so as to enhance and broaden their biomedical application [76]. In some instances, depending on the size of the NP, the particle tended to be toxic rather than demonstrating antimicrobial effect of inhibiting pathogens. For example, very small AgNPs were found to cover the pathogen, inhibiting oxygen supply to the pathogen thus reducing respiration and toxically killing the pathogen rather than inhibiting the microbial growth [14]. However, very small NPs may also be toxic to human pathogens. For example, AgNPs ranging from 10–20 nm were found to be toxic to *Bacillus* species, *E. coli* and *Staphylococcus* species. [14]. Therefore, it is imperative that further research is carried out to mitigate such problems.

Competing interest

The authors declare that they have no competing interests.

Authors' contributions

CSY conceived, CSY and GSS collected and CSY drafted the manuscript. CSY and GSS analysed the data and additional information. Both authors have read and approved the final manuscript.

Acknowledgements

We acknowledge the Social Aspects for HIV/AIDS Research Alliance (SAHARA) unit of the HIV/AIDS, STIs and TB (HAST) at the Human Sciences Research Council (HSRC) of South Africa for providing conducive infrastructural environment during the course of the sourcing and writing of the manuscript.

Disclaimer

The contents of this paper reflect authors views who are responsible for the accuracy of the information presented herein. This paper does not constitute a standard, specification, nor is it intended for design, construction, bidding, or permit purposes.

Author details

[1]Department of Biochemistry and Microbiology, Nelson Mandela Metropolitan University, Port Elizabeth, South Africa. [2]Department of Epidemiology, Johns Hopkins Bloomberg School of Public Health, E7146, 615 N. Wolfe Street, Baltimore 21205, MD, USA. [3]School of Chemical and Metallurgical Engineering, University of the Witwatersrand, P/Bag 3, Wits 2050, Johannesburg, South Africa.

References

1. Galdiero S, Falanga A, Vitiello M, Cantisani M, Marra V, Galdiero M. Silver nanoparticles as potential antiviral agents. Molecules. 2011;16:8894–918.
2. Tanwar J, Das S, Fatima Z, Hameed S. Multidrug resistance: an emerging crisis. Interdiscip Perspect Infect Dis. 2014;2014:541340. 7 pages.
3. Sharma RK, Ghose R. Synthesis of zinc oxide nanoparticles by homogeneous precipitation method and its application in antifungal activity against *Candida albicans*. Ceram Int. 2015;l41:967–75.
4. McCoy ME, Golden HE, Doll TA, Yang Y, Kaba SA, Zou X, et al. Mechanisms of protective immune responses induced by the *Plasmodium falciparum* circumsporozoite protein-based, self-assembling protein nanoparticle vaccine. Malar J. 2013;22:2–136.
5. Ngoy JM, Iyuke SE, Neuse WE, Yah CS. Covalent functionalization for multi-walled carbon nanotube (*f-MWCNT*) -folic acid bound bioconjugate. J Appl Sci. 2011;11(15):2700–11.
6. Gilbertson LM, Goodwin DG, Taylor AD, Pfefferle L, Zimmerman JB. Toward tailored functional design of Multi-Walled Carbon Nanotubes (MWNTs): electrochemical and antimicrobial activity enhancement via oxidation and selective reduction. Environ Sci Technol. 2014;48:5938–45.
7. Parise A, Thakor H, Zhang X. Activity inhibition on municipal activated sludge by single-walled carbon nanotubes. J Nanoparticle Res. 2014;16:2159.
8. Qi X, Gunawan P, Xu R, Chang MW. Cefalexin-immobilized multi-walled carbon nanotubes show strong antimicrobial and anti-adhesion properties. Chem Eng Sci. 2015;84:552–6.
9. Venkatesan J, Jayakumar R, Mohandas A, Bhatnagar I, Kim SK. Antimicrobial activity of chitosan-carbon nanotube hydrogels. Materials. 2014;7:3946–55.
10. Adeli M, Hosainzadegan H, Pakzad I, Zabihi F, Alizadeh M, Karimi F. Preparation of the silver nanoparticle containing starch foods and evaluation of antimicrobial activity. Jundishapur J Microbiol. 2013;6(4):e5075.
11. Subbiah R, Veerapandian M, Sadhasivam S, Yun K. Triad CNT-NPs/Polymer nanocomposites: fabrication, characterization, and preliminary antimicrobial study. Synth React Inorg Met-Org Nano-Met Chem. 2011;41:345–55.
12. Addae E, Dong X, McCoy E, Yang C, Chen W, Yang L. Investigation of antimicrobial activity of photothermal therapeutic gold/copper sulphide core/shell nanoparticles to bacterial spores and cells. J Biol Eng. 2014;8:11.
13. Sui M, Zhang L, Sheng L, Huang S, She L. Synthesis of ZnO coated multi-walled carbon nanotubes and their antibacterial activities. Sci Total Environ. 2013;452–453:148–54.

14. Sunitha A, Rimal IRS, Sweetly G, Sornalekshmi S, Arsula R, Praseetha PK. Evaluation of antimicrobial activity of biosynthesized iron and silver Nanoparticles using the fungi *Fusarium oxysporum* and *Actinomycetes sp.* on human pathogens. Nano Biomed Eng. 2013;5(1):39–45.
15. Hoffmann H-H, Kunz A, Simon VA, Palese P, Shawa ML. Broad-spectrum antiviral that interferes with de novo pyrimidine biosynthesis. Proc Natl Acad Sci U S A. 2011;108(14):5777–82.
16. Kollef MH. Broad-spectrum antimicrobials and the treatment of serious bacterial infections: Getting It Right Up Front. Clin Infect Dis. 2008;47(Supplement 1):S3–13.
17. Kwon DS, Mylonakis E. Posaconazole: a new broad-spectrum antifungal agent. Expert Opin Pharmacother. 2007;8(8):1167–78.
18. Navarrete-Vazquez G, Chávez-Silva F, Argotte-Ramos R, Rodríguez-Gutiérrez Mdel C, Chan-Bacab MJ, Cedillo-Rivera R, et al. Synthesis of benzologues of Nitazoxanide and Tizoxanide: a comparative study of their in vitro broad-spectrum antiprotozoal activity. Bioorg Med Chem Lett. 2011;21(10):3168–71.
19. Rupp R, Rosenthal SL, Stanberry LR. VivaGel™ (SPL7013 Gel): A candidate dendrimer –microbicide for the prevention of HIV and HSV infection. Int J Nanomedicine. 2007;2(4):561–6.
20. Marambio-Jones C, Hoek EMV. A review of the antibacterial effects of silver nanomaterials and potential implications for human health and the environment. J Nanoparticle Res. 2010;12:1531–51.
21. San CY, Don MM. Biosynthesis of silver nanoparticles from *Schizophyllum Commune*and *in-vitro* antibacterial and antifungal activity studies. J Phys Sci. 2013;24(2):83–96.
22. Kathiravan V, Ravi S, Ashokkumar S, Velmurugan S, Elumalai K, Khatiwada CP. Green synthesis of silver nanoparticles using Croton sparsiflorus morong leaf extract and their antibacterial and antifungal activities. Spectrochim Acta A Mol Biomol Spectrosc. 2015;139:200–5.
23. Gaikwad S, Ingle A, Gade N, Rai M, Falanga A, Incoronato N, et al. Antiviral activity of mycosynthesized silver nanoparticles against herpes simplex virus and human parainfluenza virus type 3. Int J Nanomedicine. 2013;8:4303–14.
24. Elmi T, Gholami S, Fakhar M, Azizi F. A review on the use of nanoparticles in the treatment of parasitic infections. J Mazand Uni Med Sci. 2013;23:127–34.
25. Fayaz AM, Ao Z, Girilal M, Chen L, Xiao X, Kalaichelvan P, et al. Inactivation of microbial infectiousness by silver nanoparticles-coated condom: a new approach to inhibit HIV- and HSV-transmitted infection. Int J Nanomedicine. 2012;7:5007–18.
26. Tank C, Raman S, Karan S, Gosavi S, Lalla NP, Sathe V, et al. Antimicrobial activity of silica coated silicon nano-tubes (SCSNT) and silica coated silicon nano-particles (SCSNP) synthesized by gas phase condensation. J Mater Sci Mater Med. 2013;24(6):1483–90.
27. Zhou J, Qi X. Multi-walled carbon nanotubes/epilson-polylysine nanocomposite with enhanced antibacterial activity. Lett Appl Microbiol. 2010;52:76–83.
28. Aslan S, Deneufchatel M, Hashmi S, Li N, Pfefferle LD, Elimelech M, et al. Carbon nanotube-based antimicrobial biomaterials formed via layer-by-layer assembly with polypeptides. J Colloid Interface Sci. 2012;388(1):268–73.
29. Amiri A, Zardini HZ, Shanbedi M, Maghrebi M, Baniadam M, Tolueinia BB. Efficient method for functionalization of carbon nanotubes by lysine and improved antimicrobial activity and water-dispersion. Mater Lett. 2012;72:153–6.
30. Barbinta-Patrascu ME, Ungureanu C, Iordache SM, Iordache AM, Bunghez IR, Ghiurea M, et al. Eco-designed biohybrids based on liposomes, mint-nanosilver and carbon nanotubes for antioxidant and antimicrobial coating. Mater Sci Eng C Mater Biol Appl. 2014;39:177–85.
31. Neelgund GM, Oki A, Luo Z. Antimicrobial activity of CdS and Ag2S quantum dots immobilized on poly(amidoamine) grafted carbon nanotubes. Colloids Surf B Biointerfaces. 2012;100:215–21.
32. Geraldo DA, Arancibia-Miranda N, Villagra NA, Mora GC, Arratia-Perez R. Synthesis of CdTe QDs/single-walled aluminosilicate nanotubes hybrid compound and their antimicrobial activity on bacteria. J Nanoparticle Res. 2012;14:1286.
33. Booshehri AY, Wang R, Xu R. The effect of re-generable silver nanoparticles/ multi-walled carbon nanotubes coating on the antibacterial performance of hollow fibermembrane. Chem Eng J. 2013;230:251–9.
34. Ahmed F, Santos CM, Mangadlao J, Advincula R, Rodrigues DF. Antimicrobial PVK:SWNT nanocomposite coated membrane for water purification: Performance and toxicity testing. Water Res. 2013;47:3966–75.
35. Santos-Magalhães NS, Mosqueira VC. Nanotechnology applied to the treatment of malaria. Adv Drug Deliv Rev. 2010;62(4–5):560–75.
36. Said DE, ElSamad LM, Gohar YM. Validity of silver, chitosan, and curcumin nanoparticles as anti-Giardia agents. Parasitol Res. 2012;111(2):545–54.
37. Allahverdiyev AM, Abamor ES, Bagirova M, Ustundag CB, Kaya C, Kaya F, et al. Antileishmanial effect of silver nanoparticles and their enhanced antiparasitic activity under ultraviolet light. Int J Nanomedicine. 2011;6:2705–14.
38. Das S, Bhattacharya A, Debnath N, Datta A, Goswami A. Nanoparticle-induced morphological transition of Bombyx mori nucleopolyhedrovirus: a novel method to treat silkworm grasserie disease. Appl Microbiol Biotechnol. 2013;97(13):6019–30.
39. Veerakumar K, Govindarajan M, Hoti SL. Evaluation of plant-mediated synthesized silver nanoparticles against vector mosquitoes. Parasitol Res. 2014;113:4567–77.
40. Poopathi S, De Britto LJ, Praba VL, Mani C, Praveen M. Synthesis of silver nanoparticles from Azadirachta indica—a most effective method for mosquito control. Environ Sci Pollut Res. 2015;22:2956–63.
41. Soni N, Prakash S. Efficacy of fungus mediated silver and gold nanoparticles against Aedes aegypti larvae. Parasitol Res. 2012;110:175–84.
42. Kramer MF, Cook WJ, Roth FP, Zhu J, Holman H, Knipe DM, et al. Latent herpes simplex virus infection of sensory neurons alters neuronal gene expression. J Virol. 2003;77(17):9533–41.
43. Sharman D. Moist wound healing: a review of evidence, application and outcome – Review. Diabet Foot J. 2003;6(3):112–20.
44. Yah SC, Enabulelel O, Eghafona NO, Udemezue OO. Prevalence of *Pseudomonas* in burn wounds at the University of Benin teaching Hospital. Benin City, Nigeria. J Exp Clin Anat (JECA). 2004;3(1):12–5.
45. Hiro ME, Pierpont YN, Ko F, Wright TE, Robson MC, Payne WG. Comparative evaluation of silver containing antimicrobial dressing on the In-vitro and In vivo processing of wound healing. ePlasty. 2012;12:409–19.
46. Yah SC, Yusuf EO, Haruna T. Patterns of antibiotics susceptibility of isolates and plasmid analysis of *Staphylococcus aureus* from Postoperative Wound Infections. Int J Biol Chem Sci. 2009;3(4):810–8.
47. Jones V, Grey JE, Harding KG. Wound dressings. BMJ. 2006;332:777–80.
48. Stashak TS, Farstvedt E, Othica A. Update on wound dressings: Indications and best use. Clin Tech Equine Pract. 2004;3:148–63.
49. Kwan KH, Liu X, Yeung KW. Silver nanoparticles improve wound healing. Nanomedicine. 2011;6(4):595–6.
50. Caló E, Khutoryanskiy VV. Biomedical applications of hydrogels: a review of patents and commercial products. Eur Polym J. 2015;65:252–67.
51. Guidelli EJ, Kinoshita A, Ramos AP, Baffa O. Silver nanoparticles delivery system based on natural rubber latex membranes. J Nanoparticle Res. 2013;15:1536.
52. Rigo C, Ferroni L, Tocco L, Roman M, Munivrana I, Gardin C, et al. Carlo Barbante 4 and Barbara ZavanActive silver nanoparticles for wound healing. Int J Mol Sci. 2013;14:4817–40.
53. Tian J, Wong KK, Ho CM, Lok CN, Yu WY, Che CM, et al. Topical delivery of silver nanoparticles promotes wound healing. Chem Med Chem. 2007;2:129–36.
54. John JS, Moro DG. Hydrogel wound dressing and biomaterials formed in situ and their uses. Patent US7910135 B2. 2011.
55. Leu JG, Chen SA, Chen HM, Wu WM, Hung CF, Yao YD, et al. The effects of gold nanoparticles in wound healing with antioxidant epigallocatechin gallate and α-lipoic acid. Nanomedicine. 2012;8(5):767–75.
56. Krausz AE, Adler BL, Cabral V, Navati M, Doerner J, Charafeddine RA, et al. Curcumin-encapsulated nanoparticles as innovative antimicrobial and wound healing agent. Nanomedicine. 2015;11(1):195–206.
57. Madhumathi K, Kumar PTS, Abhilash S, Sreeja V, Tamura H, Manzoor K, et al. Development of novel chitin/nanosilver composite scaffolds for wound dressing applications. J Mater Sci Mater Med. 2010;21920:807–13.
58. Ziv-Polat O, Topaz M, Brosh T, Margel S. Enhancement of incisional wound healing by thrombin conjugated iron oxide nanoparticles. Biomaterials. 2010;31(4):741–7.
59. Mihu MR, Sandkovsky U, Han G, Friedman JM, Nosanchuk JD, Martinez LR. The use of nitric oxide releasing nanoparticles as a treatment against *Acinetobacter baumannii* in wound infections. Virulence. 2010;1(2):62–7.
60. Chonco L, Pion M, Vacas E, Rasines B, Maly M, Serramía MJ, et al. Carbosilane dendrimer nanotechnology outlines of the broad HIV blocker profile. J Control Release. 2012;161(3):949–58.
61. Fields S, Song B, Rasoul B, Fong J, Works MG, Shew K, et al. New candidate biomarkers in the female genital tract to evaluate microbicide toxicity. PLoS ONE. 2014;9(10):e110980.

62. Gary AB, Nuttall J, Romano J. The future of HIV microbicides: challenges and opportunities. Antivir Chem Chemother. 2009;19:143–50.
63. Galea JT. Preparing for rectal microbicides: sociocultural factors affecting product uptake among potential South American users. Am J Public Health. 2014;104(6):e113–20.
64. Morris GC, Wiggins RC, Woodhall SC, Bland JM, Taylor CR , Jespers V, et al. MABGEL 1: first phase 1 trial of the anti-HIV-1 monoclonal antibodies 2F5, 4E10 and 2G12 as a vaginal microbicide. PLoS ONE. 2014;9(12):e116153.
65. Harper CC, Holt K, Nhemachena T, Chipato T, Ramjee G, Stratton L, et al. Willingness of clinicians to integrate microbicides into HIV prevention practices in southern Africa. AIDS Behav. 2012;16(7):1821–9.
66. McCarthy TD, Karellas P, Henderson SA, Giannis M, O'Keefe D F, Heery G, et al. Dendrimers as drugs: discovery and preclinical and clinical development of dendrimer-based microbicides for HIV and STI prevention. Mol Pharm. 2005;2:312–8.
67. Gong E, Matthews B, McCarthy T, Chu J, Holan G, Raff J, et al. Evaluation of dendrimer SPL7013, a lead microbicide candidate against herpes simplex viruses. Antivir Res. 2005;68:139–46.
68. Donalisio M, Rusnati M, Cagno V, Civra A, Bugatti A, Giuliani A, et al. Inhibition of human respiratory syncytial virus infectivity by a dendrimeric heparan sulfate-binding peptide. Antimicrob Agents Chemother. 2012;56(10):5278–88.
69. Price CF, Tyssen D, Sonza S, Davie A, Evans S, Lewis G R, et al. SPL7013 Gel (VivaGel®) retains potent HIV-1 and HSV-2 inhibitory activity following vaginal administration in humans. PLoS ONE. 2011;6(9):e24095.
70. Imbuluzqueta E, Gamazo C, Ariza I, Blanco-Prieto MJ. Drug delivery systems for potential treatment of intracellular bacterial infections. Front Biosci (Landmark Ed). 2010;15:397–417.
71. Alizadeh H, Salouti M, Shapouri M. Bactericidal effect of silver nanoparticles on intramacrophage brucella abortus 544. Jundishapur J Microbiol. 2014;7:e9039.
72. Xie S, Tao Y, Pan Y, Qu W, Cheng G, Huang L, et al. Biodegradable nanoparticles for intracellular delivery of antimicrobial agents. J Control Release. 2014;187:101–17.
73. Upadhyay RK. Drug delivery systems, CNS protection, and the blood brain barrier. Biomed Res Int. 2014;2014:869269. 37 pages.
74. Zhang L, Pornpattananangkul D, Hu CMJ, Huang CM. Development of nanoparticles for antimicrobial drug delivery. Curr Med Chem. 2010;17:585–94.
75. Yah CS, Iyuke SE, Simate GS. Nanoparticles toxicity and their routes of exposures. Pak J Pham Sci. 2012;25(2):477–91.
76. Simate GS, Yah CS. The use of carbon nanotubes in medical applications - is it a success story? Occup Med Health Aff. 2014;2(1):147.
77. Welin A. Survival strategies of Mycobacterium tuberculosis inside the human macrophage. Linköping University Medical Dissertations. Sweden Linköping University: Division of Medical Microbiology Department of Clinical and Experimental Medicine , Faculty of Health Sciences Linköping University SE-58185 Linköping; 2011.
78. Kumar KR, Nattuthurai N, Gopinath P, Mariappan T. Synthesis of eco-friendly silver nanoparticles from Morinda tinctoria leaf extract and its larvicidal activity against Culex quinquefasciatus. Parasitol Res. 2015;114:411–7.
79. Malone FD, Athanassiou A, Nores LA, Dalton ME. Poor perinatal outcome associated with maternal Brucella abortus infection. Obstet Gynecol. 1997;90(4 Pt 2):674–6.
80. Dong X, Tang Y, Wu M, Vlahovic B, Yang L. Dual effects of single-walled carbon nanotubes coupled with near-infrared radiation on *Bacillus anthracis* spores: inactivates spores and stimulates the germination of surviving spores. J Biol Eng. 2013;7:19.
81. Martinez-Gutierrez F, Thi EP, Silverman JM, de Oliveira CC, Svensson SL, Vanden Hoek A, et al. Antibacterial activity, inflammatory response, coagulation and cytotoxicity effects of silver nanoparticles. Nanomedicine. 2012;8(3):328–36.
82. Briones E, Colino CI, Lanao IM. Delivery systems to increase the selectivity of antibiotics in phagocytic cells. J Control Release. 2008;125:210–27.
83. Masserini M. Nanoparticles for brain drug delivery. ISRN Biochemistry. 2013;2013:238428. 18 pages.
84. Gandhi M, Bohra H, Daniel V, Gupta A. Nanotechnology in blood brain barrier. Int J Pharm Biol Arch. 2010;1(1):37–43.
85. Haque S, Md S, Alam MI, Sahni JK, AliN J, Baboota S. Nanostructure-based drug delivery systems for brain targeting. Drug Dev Ind Pharm. 2012;38(4):387–411.
86. Khuller GK, Pandey R. Oral nanoparticle-based antituberculosis drug delivery to the brain in an experimental model. J Antimicrob Chem. 2006;57:1146–52.
87. Lilly M, Dong X, McCoy E, Yang L. Inactivation of Bacillus anthracis spores by single-walled carbon nanotubes coupled with oxidizing antimicrobial chemicals. Environ Sci Technol. 2012;46(24):13417–24.
88. McDonnell G, Russell AD. Antiseptics and disinfectants: activity, action, and resistance. Clin Microbiol Rev. 1999;12(1):147–79.
89. Gutiérrez LG. Nanoparticulate titanium dioxide nanomaterial modified with functional groups and with citric extracts adsorbed on the surface, for the removal of a wide range of microorganisms. Patent. WO/2014/204290. 2010.
90. Vetten MV, Yah CS, Singh T, Gullumian M. Challenges facing sterilization and depyrogenation of nanoparticles: effects on structural stability and biomedical applications. Nanomedicine. 2014;10(7):1391–9.
91. Bouchard M, Bouchard J-M. Disinfectant cleaner. Patent no. US20110195131A1. 2011.
92. Turos E, Shim JY, Wang Y, Greenhalgh K, Reddy GS, Dickey S, et al. Antibiotic-conjugated polyacrylate nanoparticles: new opportunities for development of anti-MRSA agents. Bioorg Med Chem Lett. 2007;17(1):53–6.
93. Ismail S, Perni S, Pratten J, Parkin I, Wilson M. Efficacy of a novel light-activated antimicrobial coating for disinfecting hospital surfaces. Infect Control Hosp Epidemiol. 2011;32(11):1130–2.
94. Li Y, Leungb P, Yaoa L, Songa QW, Newtona E. Antimicrobial effect of surgical masks coated with nanoparticles. J Hosp Infect. 2006;62(1):58–63.
95. Reiche T, Lisby G, Jorgensen S, Christensen A B, Nordling J. A prospective, controlled, randomized study of the effect of a slow-release silver device on the frequency of urinary tract infection in newly catheterized patients. BJU Int. 2000;85:54–9.
96. Troncarelli MZ, Brandão HM, Gern JC, Guimarães AS, Langoni H. Nanotechnology and antimicrobials in veterinary medicine. Badajoz, Spain: FORMATEX; 2013.
97. Dias MV, Soares Nde F, Borges SV, de Sousa MM, Nunes CA, de Oliveira IR, et al. Use of allyl isothiocyanate and carbon nanotubes in an antimicrobial film to package shredded, cooked chicken meat. Food Chem. 2013;141(3):3160–6.
98. Ajitha B, Reddy YAK, Reddy PS. Biosynthesis of silver nanoparticles using Plectranthus amboinicus leaf extract and its antimicrobial activity. Spectrochim Acta A Mol Biomol Spectrosc. 2014;128:257–62.
99. Sun RW, Chen R, Chung NP, Ho CM, Lin CL, Che CM. Silver nanoparticles fabricated in Hepes buffer exhibit cytoprotective activities toward HIV-1 infected cells. Chem Commun (Camb). 2005;40:5059–61.
100. Lara HH, Nilda V, Ayala-Nuñez NV, Ixtepan-Turrent L, Rodriguez-Padilla C. Mode of antiviral action of silver nanoparticles against HIV-1. J Nanobiotechnol. 2010;8:1.
101. Baram-Pinto D, Shukla S, Perkas N, Gedanken A, Sarid R. Inhibition of herpes simplex virus type 1 infection by silver nanoparticles capped with mercaptoethane sulfonate. Bioconjug Chem. 2009;20:1497–502.
102. Sun L, Singh AK, Vig K, Pillai S, Shreekumar R, Singh SR. Silver nanoparticles inhibit replication of respiratory sincitial virus. J Biomed Biotechnol. 2008;4:149–58.
103. Rogers JV, Parkinson CV, Choi YW, Speshock JL, Hussain SM. A preliminary assessment of silver nanoparticles inhibition of monkeypox virus plaque formation. Nanoscale Res Lett. 2008;3:129–33.
104. Liu X, Yu L, Liu F, Sheng L, An K, Chen H, et al. Preparation of Ag–Fe-decorated single-walled carbon nanotubes by arc discharge and their antibacterial effect. J Mater Sci. 2012;47:6086–94.
105. Speshock JL, Murdock RC, Braydich-Stolle LK, Schrand AM, Hussain SM. Interaction of silver nanoparticles with Tacaribe virus. J Nanobiotechnol. 2010;8:19–27.
106. Banu AN, Balasubramanian C, Vinayaga MP. Biosynthesis of silver nanoparticles using Bacillus thuringiensis against dengue vector, Aedes aegypti (Diptera: Culicidae). Parasitol Res. 2014;113:311–6.
107. Papp I, Sieben C, Ludwig K, Roskamp M, Böttcher C, Schlecht S, et al. Inhibition of influenza virus infection by multivalent sialic-acid-functionalized gold nanoparticles. Small. 2010;6:2900–6.
108. Marimuthu S, Rahuman AA, Kirthi AV, Santhoshkumar T, Jayaseelan C, Rajakumar G. Eco-friendly microbial route to synthesize cobalt nanoparticles using Bacillus thuringiensis against malaria and dengue vectors. Parasitol Res. 2013;112(12):4105–12.
109. Mohapatra SC, Tiwari HK, Singla M, Rathi B, Sharma A, Mahiya K, et al. Antimalarial evaluation of copper(II) nanohybrid solids: inhibition of plasmepsin II, a hemoglobin-degrading malarial aspartic protease from Plasmodium falciparum. J Biol Inorg Chem. 2010;15(3):373–85.
110. Kirthi AV, Rahuman A, Rajakumar G, Marimuthu S, Santhoshkumar T, Jayaseelan C, et al. Acaricidal, pediculocidal and larvicidal activity of

synthesized ZnO nanoparticles using wet chemical route against blood feeding parasites. Parasitol Res. 2011;109:461–72.
111. Gowri S, Gandhi RR, Sundrarajan M. Structural, optical, antibacterial and antifungal properties of zirconia nanoparticles by biobased protocol. J Mater Sci Technol. 2014;30(8):782e790.
112. Lu L, Sun RW, Chen R, Hui CK, Ho CM, Luk JM, et al. Silver nanoparticles inhibit hepatitis B virus replication. Antivir Ther. 2008;13:253–62.
113. Pelczar M, Reid R, Chan ECS. Microbiologia. São Paulo: McGraw-Hill; 1980. p. 2008.
114. Senior K, Müller S, Schacht VJ, Bunge M. Antimicrobial precious-metal nanoparticles and their use in novel materials. Recent Pat Food Nutr Agric. 2012;4(3):200–9.
115. Yah CS. The toxicity of gold nanoparticles in relation to their physiochemical properties. Biomed Res. 2013;24(3):400–13.
116. Gatoo MA, Naseem S, Arfat MY, Dar AM, Qasim K, Zubair S. Physicochemical properties of nanomaterials: implication in associated toxic manifestations. Biomed Res Int. 2014;2014:498420.
117. Dorotkiewicz-Jach A, Augustyniak D, Olszak T, Drulis-Kawa Z. Modern therapeutic approaches against pseudomonas aeruginosa infections. Curr Med Chem. 2015;22(14):1642–64.
118. Chatterjee AK, Chakraborty R, Basu T. Mechanism of antibacterial activity of copper nanoparticles. Nanotechnology. 2014;25(13):135101.
119. Dong Q, Dong A, Morigen. Evaluation of novel antibacterial N-halamine nanoparticles prodrugs towards susceptibility of escherichia coli induced by DksA protein. Molecules. 2015;20(4):7292–308.
120. Li H, Chen Q, Zhao J, Urmila K. Enhancing the antimicrobial activity of natural extraction using the synthetic ultrasmall metal nanoparticles. Sci Rep. 2015;5:11033.
121. Xie Y, He Y, Irwin PL, Jin T, Shi X. Antibacterial activity and mechanism of action of zinc oxide nanoparticles against Campylobacter jejuni. Appl Environ Microbiol. 2011;77(7):2325–31.
122. Bawskar M, Deshmukh S, Bansod S, Gade A, Rai M. Comparative analysis of biosynthesised and chemosynthesised silver nanoparticles with special reference to their antibacterial activity against pathogens. IET Nanobiotechnol. 2015;9(3):107–13.
123. Piras AM, Maisetta G, Sandreschi S, Gazzarri M, Bartoli C, Grassi L, et al. Chitosan nanoparticles loaded with the antimicrobial peptide temporin B exert a long-term antibacterial activity in vitro against clinical isolates of Staphylococcus epidermidis. Front Microbiol. 2015;6:372.
124. Mogharabi M, Abdolahi M, Faramarzi MM. Toxicity of nanomaterials. Daru. 2014;22:9.
125. Nuñez-Anita RE, Acosta-Torres LS, Vilar-Pineda J, Martínez-Espinosa JC, de la Fuente-Hernández J, Castaño VM. Toxicology of antimicrobial nanoparticles for prosthetic devices. Int J Nanomedicine. 2014;9:3999–4006.
126. Cooper RJ, Spitzer N. Silver nanoparticles at sublethal concentrations disrupt cytoskeleton and neurite dynamics in cultured adult neural stem cells. Neurotoxicology. 2015;48:231–8.
127. Uhm SH, Lee SB, Song DH, Kwon JS, Han JG, Kim KN. Fabrication of bioactive, antibacterial TiO2 nanotube surfaces, coated with magnetron sputtered Ag nanostructures for dental applications. J Nanosci Nanotechnol. 2014;14(10):7847–54.

13

Thallium exists in opioid poisoned patients

Amir Ghaderi[1], Naser Vahdati-Mashhadian[2], Zohreh Oghabian[3], Valiallah Moradi[2], Reza Afshari[4,5*] and Omid Mehrpour[6]

Abstract

Background: Thallium (Tl) is a toxic heavy metal that exists in nature. Tl poisoning (thallotoxicosis) may occur in opioid addicts. This study was designed to evaluate the frequency and level of urinary Tl in opioid abusers. In addition, clinical findings were evaluated.

Methods: A total of 150 subjects were examined. Cases with a history of at least 3 years of abuse were admitted in the Imam Reza Hospital as the case group; 50 non-opioid abusers from the target population were included as the control group. Twenty-four hour urinary qualitative and quantitative Tl analyses were performed on both groups.

Results: Out of the 150 subjects, 128 (85 %) were negative for qualitative urinary Tl, followed by 5 % (trace), 7 % (1+), 2 % (2+), and 1 % (3+). Mean (standard error (SE), Min–Max) quantitative urinary Tl level was 14 μg/L (3.5 μg/L, 0–346 μg/L). Mean urinary Tl level in the case group was 21 μg/L (5 μg/L, 0–346 μg/L) and that in the controls was 1 μg/L (0.14 μg/L, 0–26 μg/L), which were significantly different ($P = 0.001$). The most frequent clinical findings were ataxia (86 %), sweating (81 %), and constipation (54 %). In all cases ($n = 150$), the mean (SE) value for cases with positive qualitative urinary Tl was 26.8 μg/L (0.9 μg/L) and that in the negative cases was 2.3 μg/L (0.2 μg/L), which were significantly different ($P = 0.002$).

Conclusions: This study showed that long-term opioid abuse may lead to Tl exposure. In opioid abusers with the clinical manifestation of thallotoxicosis, urinary Tl should be determined.

Keywords: Thallium, Opioid, Poisoning

Background

Thallium (Tl) is a highly toxic heavy metal with atomic number 81 and a molecular weight of 204.37 discovered by Sir William Crookes in 1861 [1]. It is a soft, bluish-white or gray water-insoluble metal but the salt forms are colorless, tasteless, and odorless. Tl is readily absorbed via ingestion, inhalation, and dermal contact [1–3]. Tl does not have any biological function in the body and the fatal dose is more than 10–15 mg/kg of body weight [4]. In the past, Tl was used as a hair remover and rodenticide because of its toxicity, but presently Tl administration is restricted to industrial usage such as optic lenses, and the radioisotope forms are used for medical purposes such as diagnosis of malignancies (such as melanoma) and tissue scintigraphy (such as cardiac scanning) [5]. Any amount of Tl in the body is abnormal [1]. In humans, Tl toxicity may occur occupationally (industrial exposure), accidentally (contact with Tl-containing material), or in cases of homicide; oral ingestion is the main route of Tl entrance in the body [1]. The clinical manifestation of thallotoxicosis has a wide spectrum but painful ascending peripheral neuropathy (both motor and sensory), gastrointestinal, and dermatologic manifestations (particularly alopecia) are major characteristics in Tl toxicity [5]. The exact mechanism of toxicity is still unclear, but because Tl ions are similar to potassium (K) ions, Tl may alter the number of K-dependent systems and enzymes in the body such as sulfhydryl groups, essential enzymes in the Krebs cycle, succinate dehydrogenase, and interactions with sodium-potassium ATPase and riboflavin [3, 6, 7]. Treatment includes early gastrointestinal decontamination, Prussian blue therapy (potassium ferric hexacyanoferrate), activated charcoal, laxatives, and enhanced elimination via forced diuresis and hemodialysis [3, 6, 8]. In Tl poisoning, early diagnosis and treatment is necessary for complete recovery; any

* Correspondence: AfshariR@mums.ac.ir
[4]Addiction Research Centre, Mashhad University of Medical Sciences, Imam Reza Hospital, Ibn-e-Sina Street, Mashhad 91735-348, Iran
[5]British Columbia Center for Disease Control, Vancouver, Canada
Full list of author information is available at the end of the article

delay may lead to permanent neurological disorders [6, 9]. Illicit opium may be adulterated with various substances such as sugars, quinine, caffeine, lactose, strychnine, paracetamol, and heavy metals such as lead [10, 11]. In fact, salesmen and smugglers may add any kind of heavy metals to opium to increase its weight for more profit. Recently, there have been reports of Tl toxicity in illicit opium users [12, 13]. We decided to evaluate Tl as an adulterant in opioid-like compounds from opium users, for the early diagnosis and treatment of thallotoxicosis.

Methods

Study design

This is a case–control study. One-hundred opioid-like abusers, raw opium, opium residue, crystal heroin, or mixed abusers for more than 3 years, aged 18–65 years, were recruited following admission to Imam Reza Hospital because of poisoning or rehabilitation as the case group. Controls were 50 non-abuser subjects with no history of drug use in the previous year. Urinary morphine tests using immunoassay tests were used to determine positive cases. Controls were verified to be opioid naïve via verbal conversation. All ethical approvals were considered and the aim of the study was explained to all subjects in both groups. Twenty-four hour urinary samples were taken on admission for qualitative and quantitative Tl analyses, and other data including demographic, neurological, dermal, and gastrointestinal clinical findings were entered into a predesigned checklist. Diphenoxylate, acetaminophen codeine, and tramadol users were excluded from the study.

Laboratory assessment

In acute poisoning, high concentrations of Tl appear in the kidney; thus, urine is the fluid of choice for Tl detection [14]. The normal concentration is <5 µg/L (<24.5 nmol/L) in a 24-h urine sample. The urine samples were placed in 100 mL urine collection containers (polyethylene) and stored at −20 °C until analysis [15]. The first 24-h urinary samples in the two groups were examined for Tl using a qualitative (semi-quantitative) survey. Reagents included: 1) cyanide reagent: 1.6 g of sodium hydroxide, 1.2 g of sodium-potassium tartrate, and 1.36 g of potassium cyanide dissolved in 10 mL of water. 2) Dithizone solution (250 mg/L) in chloroform prepared fresh: 12 mL urine sample and 1 mL cyanide reagent to dithizone solution (dithizone + chloroform) were combined, shaken for 2 min, and left for 3–5 min. Two-phase formation occurred, consisting of an upper urine phase and a lower chloroform phase. A pink-red color in the lower chloroform phase indicates the presence of Tl and indicates a positive result. According to semi-quantitative Tl-screening tests, <50 µg/L is considered negative, trace (50–100 µg/L), 1+ (100–200 µg/L), 2+ (200–300 µg/L), 3+ (300–400 µg/L), and 4+ (>400 µg/L) [16]. In the second step, quantitative analysis via graphite furnace atomic absorption spectrometry (Perkin Elmer, Model 3030 with HGA 400 Programmer), which is a highly sensitive spectroscopic technique that provides excellent detection limits for measuring concentrations of Tl in urine, was performed on all samples [17]. In this test, we applied a Tl standard solution, traceable to standard reference materials from National Institute of Standards and Technology thallium(I) nitrate in nitric acid 0.5 mol/L (1000 mg/L) TlCertipur®, provided from Merck. To measure TL in urine, after extraction with nitric acid, sulfuric acid, and Triton X- 100, the liquid phases were separated from the sediment. Next, 2 % ammonium monovanadate in 1 % sodium hydroxide was then added to neutralize acidity to prevent graphite tube damage. The solution was centrifuged at high speed for 5 min, and 25 µL from the upper layer was injected into the graphite. A thermal program was selected for drying; 130 °C, 300 °C for organic solvents, and 800 °C for inorganic solvents and ash removal, and 1700 °C for atomization. Absorbance was measured at 276.8 nm [18, 19]. Detection limits were 0.2 µg/L, precision 3.65 %, and accuracy 97.4 % of analyses were determined by repeated analyses of biological reference material (SERONORM urine trace element level 2, lot 1011645) [20]. We evaluated both qualitative and quantitative urinary Tl because they complement each other.

Statistical analysis

Data were analyzed with SPSS software (version 16). Student's *t* test and Spearman's coefficient test were used to analyze the data. *P* value was considered to be less than 0.05 throughout the study.

Results

Demographic findings

In total, 150 subjects, including 100 cases and 50 controls, were recruited. Among them, 134 (89 %) were male. Mean (standard error (SE), Min–Max) age was 41 (1.2, 19–85) years. Mean (SE) age in cases was 41 years (1.6) and in controls was 41 years (0.3), which were similar. Among cases, raw opium or opium residues were used by 66 % cases, followed by mixed (28 %), and crystal heroin (6 %). Cases only smoking were 49 %, those smoking and ingesting were 45 %, those only injecting were 3 %, and those using a mixture of methods were 3 %.

Clinical findings

Neurological

Frequency of ataxia in cases ($n = 100$) was 86 %, followed by tremor (85 %), insomnia (83 %), depression (82 %), blurred vision (79 %), memory deficits (78 %), weakness (77 %), fatigue (77 %), aggressiveness (77 %), jerking movements (76 %), vertigo (73 %), emotional liability

Table 1 Qualitative urinary thallium results ($n = 150$)

Qualitative Urinary Thallium Results	Cases n (%)	Controls n (%)	Total n (%)
Negative	80 (80)	48 (96)	128 (85)
Trace	6 (6)	1 (2)	7 (5)
1+	10 (10)	1 (2)	11 (7)
2+	3 (3)	0 (0)	3 (2)
3+	1 (1)	0 (0)	1 (1)
Total	100 (100)	50 (100)	150 (100)

(65 %), headache (59 %), paresthesia (40 %), tinnitus (38 %), seizure (36 %), delirium-psychosis-coma (30 %), and choreoathetosis (0 %).

Dermal: Frequency of sweating in cases ($n = 100$) was 81 %, followed by scalp hair loss (45 %), dry skin (36 %), acne (8 %), rashes (6 %), body hair loss (5 %), Mees' lines (0 %), and palmar erythema (0 %).

Gastrointestinal: Frequency of constipation in cases ($n = 100$) was 54 %, followed by nausea (20 %), vomiting (20 %), abdominal pain (16 %), and diarrhea (14 %).

Qualitative urinary Tl results

For all subjects, 128 (85 %) were negative for qualitative urinary Tl, followed by 5 % (trace), 7 % (1+), 2 % (2+), and 1 % (3+). The distribution of qualitative results is shown in Table 1. The two groups were significantly different ($P = 0.01$).

Quantitative urinary Tl level

The mean (SE, Min–Max) quantitative urinary Tl level was 14 μg/L (3.5 μg/L, 0–346 μg/L). Mean urinary Tl levels in the case group were 21 μg/L (5 μg/L, 0–346 μg/L) and in controls were 1 μg/L (0.14 μg/L, 0–26 μg/L), which were significantly different ($P = 0.001$).

Comparison of qualitative and quantitative results

In all cases ($n = 150$), the mean (SE) value for cases with positive qualitative urinary Tl levels was 26.8 μg/L (1 μg/L) and in negative cases was 2.3 μg/L (0.4 μg/L), which were significantly different ($P = 0.002$).

Duration of abuse was not associated with Tl levels ($r = 0.329$, $P = 0.099$). Positive Tl results were significantly higher for raw opium abusers in comparison with heroin abusers ($P < 0.001$). Table 2 summarizes these differences. Positive Tl results were significantly higher for smoke and ingestion compared with ingestion alone ($P = 0.001$). Table 2 summarizes these differences.

Discussion

Our results indicate that contaminated opiates could be a source of Tl poisoning. Substance abuse is one of the most preventable health hazards worldwide. Iran appears to have both traditional and modern drug use and abuse problems, and it appears to play an important transit role in the transfer of opium and other drugs from Afghanistan to western countries [21, 22]. Adding heavy metals such as lead adulterant to the drugs is already described [23, 24]. Opium is still a most frequently abused drug. Informal, and often illegal, laboratories refine opium into a sticky, brown paste, which is pressed into bricks and sun dried. This material can then be ingested or smoked. This process results in introduction of impurities such as lead into the product [25]. Salesmen and smugglers may add any number of heavy metals to opium to increase the weight for more profit. Although the amount of Tl in opium is usually small, when taken in large amounts, opium adulterated with Tl can produce clinical toxicity. However, very few reports describe unusual and exotic causes of chronic Tl poisoning as an adulterant to illicit drugs [12–14]. Afshari *et al.* reported three cases of suspected Tl poisoning after heroin abuse. Urine qualitative tests resulted in a range from negative to 4+ Tl, and three months after substitution of heroin, signs and symptoms of thallotoxicos returned; they concluded that contaminated heroin was responsible [13]. Questel *et al.* also reported two cases of Tl poisoning in heroin users [12].

In our study, the most frequent symptoms were ataxia, tremor, insomnia, neuropathy (both sensory and motor), sweating, scalp hair loss, dry skin, constipation, nausea, and vomiting, which were slightly different from previous studies that emphasized on polyneuropathy, paresis, abdominal pain, and alopecia [4, 6, 9, 21]. This dissimilarity may be because of the amount of Tl used or less severity of toxicity. There were significant differences in urinary Tl tests between case and control groups in addition to clinical findings. Surprisingly, nearly one-third of our patients had a history of seizure, possibly

Table 2 Comparison of qualitative urinary thallium results in different type of abused drugs ($n = 100$)

type of abused drugs	Qualitative test						Total
	Negative	Trace	1+	2+	3+	Positive	
(Crystal) Heroin	5(83 %)	0(0 %)	1(16 %)	0(0 %)	0(0 %)	1(16 %)	6(100 %)
Opium	51(77 %)	5(7 %)	7(10 %)	2(3 %)	1(1 %)	15(21 %)	66(100 %)
Mixed user	24(85 %)	1(3 %)	2(7 %)	1(3 %)	0(0 %)	4(13 %)	28(100 %)
Total	80(80 %)	6(6 %)	10(10 %)	3(3 %)	1(1 %)	20(20 %)	100(100 %)

because of abuse of tramadol or other unknown abuse of illicit drugs. In Iran, opium addicts have a great affinity for tramadol because of the euphoria experience or because of replacement of opiates [26–27]. Our study showed the most frequent illicit substance was raw opium and opium residue (66 %), and positive Tl results were significantly higher in this group in comparison with other abusers. In addition, ingestion and smoking was the most frequent route of consumption in the positive Tl group. Comparison between qualitative and quantitative results indicated that for exact diagnosis, it is better to incorporate both qualitative and quantitative analyses. Tl poisoning has a wide spectrum of clinical manifestation and any amount of Tl in the human body is abnormal. Moreover, it acts as a silent disease and diagnosis is sometimes difficult without suspicion. Our study showed that opium is a source of Tl in Iran and maybe in other parts of the world, so physicians should be aware of Tl exposure in opioid abusers, and they should be notified of its clinical symptoms. Although our findings suggested chronic Tl poisoning as an adulterant to illicit drugs, it should be noted that the findings may also result from cultivating opium poppies in Tl-contaminated soils or water.

Conclusion

As Tl is an accumulative poison [9], any illicit abuser subject with neuropathy, gastrointestinal complaints, and alopecia should be suspected of thallotoxicosis, and both urinary qualitative and quantitative Tl analyses would be helpful for exact diagnosis.

Limitations

This study is subjected to certain limitations because of the incontinency of opioid concentration and dose in the street drug abusers.

Competing interests

The authors declare that they have no competing interests.

Authors' contributions

AG clinical work and data collection. ZO drafting the manuscript NV and VM: Data collection RA: Research design, data interpretation, revising the manuscript. OM darafting the manuscript and revising the manuscript. All authors read and approved the final manuscript.

Acknowledgement

This research was supported by Addiction Research Center, Mashhad University of Medical Science (MUMS/2013-920441).

Author details

[1]Department of Addiction studies, School of Medical Kashan University of Medical Sciences, Kashan, Iran. [2]Departments of Pharmacodynamics and Toxicology, School of Pharmacy, Mashhad University of Medical Sciences, Mashhad, Iran. [3]Department of Clinical Toxicology, Kerman University of Medical Sciences, Kerman, Iran. [4]Addiction Research Centre, Mashhad University of Medical Sciences, Imam Reza Hospital, Ibn-e-Sina Street, Mashhad 91735-348, Iran. [5]British Columbia Center for Disease Control, Vancouver, Canada. [6]Atherosclerosis and Coronary Artery Research Center, Birjand University of Medical Science, Birjand, Iran.

References

1. Galván-Arzate S, Santamaría A. Thallium toxicity. Toxicol Lett. 1998;99(1):1–13.
2. Cvjetko P, Cvjetko I, Pavlica M. Thallium toxicity in humans. Arh Hig Rada Toksikol. 2010;61(1):111–9.
3. Mulkey JP, Oehme FW. A review of thallium toxicity. Vet Hum Toxicol. 1993;35(5):445–53.
4. Lech T, Sadlik JK. Thallium intoxication in humans. Toxicol Lett. 2007;172:S85.
5. Ibrahim D, Froberg B, Wolf A, Rusyniak DE. Heavy metal poisoning: clinical presentations and pathophysiology. Clin Lab Med. 2006;26(1):67–97. viii.
6. Misra UK, Kalita J, Yadav RK, Ranjan P. Thallium poisoning: emphasis on early diagnosis and response to haemodialysis. Postgrad Med J. 2003;79(928):103–5.
7. Hasan M, Chandra SV, Dua PR, Raghubir R, Ali SF. Biochemical and electrophysiologic effects of thallium poisoning on the rat corpus striatum. Toxicol Appl Pharmacol. 1977;41(2):353–9.
8. Ghannoum M, Nolin TD, Goldfarb DS, Roberts DM, Mactier R, Mowry JB, et al. Extracorporeal treatment for thallium poisoning: recommendations from the EXTRIP Workgroup. Clin J Am Soc Nephrol. 2012;7(10):1682–90.
9. Jha S, Kumar R, Kumar R. Thallium poisoning presenting as paresthesias, paresis, psychosis and pain in abdomen. J Assoc Physicians India. 2006;54:53–5.
10. Afshari R, Emadzadeh A. Short communication: case report on adulterated opium-induced severe lead toxicity. Drug Chem Toxicol. 2010;33(1):48–9.
11. Aghaee-Afshar M, Khazaeli P, Behnam B, Rezazadehkermani M, Ashraf-Ganjooei N. Presence of lead in opium. Arch Iran Med. 2008;11(5):553–4.
12. Questel F, Dugarin J, Dally S. Thallium-contaminated heroin. Ann Intern Med. 1996;124(6):616.
13. Afshari R, Mégarbane B, Zavar A. Thallium poisoning: one additional and unexpected risk of heroin abuse. Clin Toxicol. 2012;50(8):791–2.
14. Thallium health monitoring guidelines,PN10474 Version 2. Last updated June 2012.accessed 2014 April www.deir.qld.gov.au/workplace/…/ddp-thalliumguide.pdf.
15. Ćurković M, Sipos L, Puntarić D, Dodig-Ćurković K, Pivac N, Kralik K. Detection of thallium and uranium in well water and biological specimens of an eastern Croatian population. Arch Ind Hyg Toxicol. 2013;64(3):385–94.
16. Flanagan RJ, Braithwaite RA, Brown SS, Widdop B, Wolff FA. Basic Analytical Toxicology. 1st ed. Geneva: World Health Organization; 1995.
17. Ediger R. Atomic absorption analysis with the graphite furnace using matrix modification. Atomic Absorption Newsletter. 1975;14(5):127–30.
18. Christian G, Purdy W. Coulometric determination of thallium in blood and urine. Am J Clin Pathol. 1966;46(2):185.
19. Savory J, Roszel N, Mushak P, Sunderman F. Measurements of thallium in biologic materials by atomic absorption spectrometry. Am J Clin Pathol. 1968;50(4):505.
20. Fuller C. The effect of acids on the determination of thallium by atomic absorption spectrometry with a graphite furnace. Anal Chim Acta. 1976;81(1):199–202.
21. Karrari P, Mehrpour O, Afshari R, Keyler D. Pattern of illicit drug use in patients referredto addiction treatment centres in Birjand, Eastern Iran. J Pak Med Assoc. 2013;63(6):711–6.
22. Mehrpour O, Karrari P, Sheikhazadi A. Survey of factors related to criminal behavior in a sample of Iranian substance abusers. J Forensic Leg Med. 2013;20(8):1078–81.
23. Mehrpour O, Karrari P, Abdollahi M. Chronic lead poisoning in Iran; a silent disease. Daru. 2012;20(1):8.
24. Karrari P, Mehrpour O, Abdollahi M. A systematic review on status of lead pollution and toxicity in Iran: Guidance for preventive measures. Daru. 2012;20(1):2.
25. Jalili M, Azizkhani R. Lead toxicity resulting from chronic ingestion of opium. West J Emerg Med. 2009;10(4):244–146.
26. Mehrpour O. Addiction and seizure ability oftramadol in high-risk patients. Indian J Anaesth. 2013;57(1):86–7.
27. Taghaddosinejad F, Mehrpour O, Afshari R, Seghatoleslami A, Abdollahi M, Dart RC. Factors related to seizure in tramadol poisoning and its blood concentration. J Med Toxicol. 2011;7(3):183–8.

14

Curcumin as a double-edged sword for stem cells: dose, time and cell type-specific responses to curcumin

Fatemeh Attari[1,3], Maryam Zahmatkesh[1], Hadi Aligholi[1,3], Shahram Ejtemaei Mehr[4], Mohammad Sharifzadeh[5], Ali Gorji[3,7], Tahmineh Mokhtari[2], Mojtaba Khaksarian[6] and Gholamreza Hassanzadeh[1,2*]

Abstract

Background: The beneficial effects of curcumin which includes its antioxidant, anti-inflammatory and cancer chemo-preventive properties have been identified. Little information is available regarding the optimal dose and treatment periods of curcumin on the proliferation rate of different sources of stem cells.

Methods: In this study, the effect of various concentrations of curcumin on the survival and proliferation of two types of outstanding stem cells which includes bone marrow stem cells (BMSCs) and adult rat neural stem/progenitor cells (NS/PCs) at different time points was investigated. BMSCs were isolated from bilateral femora and tibias of adult Wistar rats. NS/PCs were obtained from subventricular zone of adult Wistar rat brain. The curcumin (0.1, 0.5, 1, 5 and 10 μM/L) was added into a culture medium for 48 or 72 h. Fluorescent density of 5-bromo-2′-deoxyuridine (Brdu)-positive cells was considered as proliferation index. In addition, cell viability was assessed by MTT assay.

Results: Treatment of BMSCs with curcumin after 48 h, increased cell survival and proliferation in a dose-dependent manner. However, it had no effect on NSCs proliferation except a toxic effect in the concentration of 10 μM of curcumin. After a 72 h treatment period, BMSCs and NS/PCs survived and proliferated with low doses of curcumin. However, high doses of curcumin administered for 72 h showed toxic effects on both stem cells.

Conclusions: These findings suggest that curcumin survival and proliferative effects depend on its concentration, treatment period and the type of stem cells. Appropriate application of these results may be helpful in the outcome of combination therapy of stem cells and curcumin.

Keywords: Curcumin, Bone marrow mesenchymal stem cells, Neural stem cells, Cell proliferation, Cell survival

Background

Curcumin (diferuloylmethane) is one of the active components of dietary spice turmeric (Curcuma longa Linn) which was first chemically characterized in 1910 [1, 2]. To date, a great number of studies have focused on the multifarious biological effects of curcumin including its antioxidant, anti-inflammatory and cancer chemo-preventive properties [3, 4]. In addition, some papers have reported that curcumin can decrease oxidative damage and improve cognitive deficiencies related to aging. Moreover, curcumin can also be useful for the treatment of neurodegenerative diseases such as Alzheimer's disease and brain ischemia [5, 6]. Furthermore, there are some reports on the synergistic effect of curcumin in conjunction with stem cell therapy vis-à-vis recovery from spinal cord injury [7]. In this regard, curcumin may enhance proliferation of stem cells for swift regeneration [7, 8]. Previous investigations have reported that curcumin has biphasic effects on the proliferation of some stem cells including spinal cord neural progenitor cells [9], embryonic neural progenitor cells [8] and 3 T3-L1 preadipocytes [10]. To find the optimal curcumin concentration as well as the administration time for treatment of different types of stem cells with curcumin, more studies are needed.

Among different sources of stem cells, bone marrow mesenchymal stem cells (BMSCs) are known to have

* Correspondence: hassanzadeh@tums.ac.ir
[1]Department of Neuroscience, School of Advanced Technologies in medicine, Tehran University of Medical Sciences, Tehran, Iran
[2]Department of Anatomy, School of Medicine, Tehran University of Medical Sciences, Tehran, Iran
Full list of author information is available at the end of the article

capacity for proliferation and differentiation into mesenchymal and non-mesenchymal lineages. In many previous study, these types of stem cells were used for cell and gene therapy due to their capacity for self-renewal in a number of non-hematopoietic tissues as well as their multi-potentiality for differentiation [11].

On the other hand, adult neural stem/progenitor cells (NS/PCs) are self-renewal and multi-potent cells located specially in the subventricular zone of the lateral wall of the lateral ventricle of an adult mammalian brain. These cells can be isolated and cultured in-vitro to produce true neural and glial cells and finally transplanted for the treatment of neurodegenerative diseases [12, 13]. Little is known about the effective dose and treatment periods of curcumin when it is utilized as a supportive element for BMSCs and NS/PCs. Hence, in this study, the effects of various concentrations of curcumin on survival and proliferation of BMSCs and NS/PCs at different time points were investigated.

Methods

BMSCs culture

BMSCs were extracted from the bone marrow of bilateral femora and tibias of 4 weeks old male Wistar rats. The cell suspension was centrifuged and plated on T-25 plastic flasks in Dulbecco's Modified Eagle Medium (DMEM/F12) (Invitrogen, USA), supplemented with 10 % fetal bovine serum (FBS, Invitrogen, USA), 100U/ml penicillin and 100 mg/ml streptomycin (Invitrogen, USA) and incubated at 37 °C with 5 % CO_2. When primary cultures became almost confluent, the cells were passaged by trypsinization and cultured in the above compound. All of the experiments were performed using cells at passages 10-18 [14].

NS/PCs culture

SVZ specimens were harvested from the brain of young adult male Wistar rats (150-200 g) and transported in 10 % penicillin-streptomycin solution (prepared with 0.1 M cold PBS, PH 7.2-7.4). Next, 500 μl of 0.05 % trypsin/ EDTA solution (Invitrogen, USA, 5 min at 37 °C) was used for tissue dissection. The reaction was brought to a halt by the addition of 500 μl of Soybean trypsin inhibitor (Sigma, USA) to the dissociated tissue. After centrifugation, the cells were placed on T-25 plastic flasks in 5 mL of DMEM/F12 containing 1 % N2 supplement (Invitrogen, USA), 3 % B27 supplement (Invitrogen, USA), 2 μg/mL heparin (Sigma, USA), 1 % glutamax (Invitrogen, USA), 1 % penicillin/streptomycin (Invitrogen, USA), 10 ng/ml basic fibroblast growth factor (bFGF; Millipore, Germany), 20 ng/ml epidermal growth factor (EGF; Miltenybiotech, Germany), at 37 °C in a humidified atmosphere with 5 % CO_2. Neurospheres were passaged by trypsinization and mechanically separated after 15 days [12, 15]. The NS/PCs obtained from the third passage were used for all experiments.

Cell viability assay

Cell viability was assessed by MTT (3-(4,5-dimethylthiazolyl-2) -2,5-diphenyltetrazolium bromide) assay. NS/PCs and BMSCs were seeded at a density of 1×10^4 cells in 96-well plates. Curcumin (Sigma, USA) was dissolved in Dimethyl Sulphoxide (DMSO) (Sigma, USA) and added in different concentrations of 0.1, 0.5, 1, 5 and 10 μM/L into the culture medium. In the control group, cells were treated with the DMSO. Forty-eight and seventy two hours after the treatment, the medium containing curcumin was replaced with fresh medium containing 1 mg/ml MTT solution in 0.01 M PBS. The plates were incubated at a temperature of 37 °C for 4 h. The mitochondrial dehydrogenase of viable cells broke down MTT and produced purple formazan. The cells were disrupted in DMSO. The purple formazan dye was then measured with ELISA reader at 595 nm absorbance [16]. Each experiment was repeated three times.

Immunofluorescent assay

The cells were fixed with 4 % paraformaldehyde in PBS for 1 h then rinsed with PBS three times for 5 min and incubated with blocker solution (5 % normal goat serum and 1 % bovine serum albumin in PBS) for 60 min. Mouse anti-Nestin (1:100; Abcam, USA) [12], rabbit anti-CD73 (1:200; Abcam, USA) or rabbit anti-CD105 (1:100; Abcam, USA) [17] were used at 4 °C over night. After washing with PBS, goat anti-Mouse IgG (alexa flour 647, 1:600; invitrogen, USA) or goat anti-Rabbit IgG (FITC; 1:700; Abcam, USA) were added to the cells for 60 min at room temperature and the nuclei were stained with 4,6-diamidino-2-phenylindole (DAPI, 1 g/ml, Santa Cruz, Germany) or Propidium Iodide (PI; invitrogen, USA). Immunolabeled cells were assessed by a fluorescent microscope (Olympus, japan). In control samples, the primary antibodies were eliminated in a reaction in which no immunoreactivity was detected.

Bromodeoxyuridine (BrdU) Immunocytochemistry

Cells were plated onto polyornithine (50 μg/ml) coated 96-well plates at a density of 1×10^4 cells. Cells were treated with either DMSO or curcumin at two time points (48 and 72 h). Adherent cells and neurospheres were then fixed in 4 % paraformaldehyde for 30 min. The cells were washed with 0.2 % Triton-X 100 in 0.1 M PBS (pH 7.4) three times for 5 min. DNA was denatured by exposing the cells to acid (2 M HCl, 30 min at 37 °C). After that, borate buffer (0.1 M) was added to the cells for 12 min at room temperature. Then, 5 % normal goat serum in 0.1 M PBS (pH 7.4) was added to block endogenous peroxidases. Next, the cells were incubated overnight with mouse anti-BrdU antibody (1:1000, Sigma, Germany) and thereafter exposed to FITC conjugate anti-mouse IgG (1:1000, Sigma, Germany) for BMSCs or Alexa-Fluor 647-conjugated anti-mouse IgG (1:500, Abcam USA) for NS/PCs for 2 h at room temperature. Each experiment was repeated three times.

Proliferating cells and neurospheres were incubated by 10 μM/l BrdU for 48 h and analyzed by immuno-staining [18]. Fluorescent density of Brdu positive cells were measured using image J software [19, 20]. The study had the endorsement of the ethical committee of Tehran University of Medical Sciences.

Statistical analysis

The statistical significance was determined using the *t*-test and One-Way Analysis of Variance (ANOVA) and a Tukey post-hoc test. The results are expressed as mean ± SEM. The null hypothesis was rejected at the 0.05 level of significance.

Results

Isolation of BMSCs and NS/PCs

After primary culture, BMSCs were obtained as monolayer cells which expressed mesenchymal stem cell markers CD105 and CD73. Cultivation of SVZ specimen resulted in the production of neurospheres which expressed nestin as a marker of NS/PCs (Fig. 1).

Effect of curcumin on proliferation of BMSCs

As indicated in Fig. 2, in the aftermath of 48 h administration, curcumin enhanced the BrdU positive BMSCs in a dose dependent manner, suchthat the doses of 5 and 10 μM of curcumin enhancement was statistically significant compared to the DMSO group ($P < 0.01$).

After 72 h treatment with different doses of curcumin, the above pattern was not seen, only the concentration of 0.5 μM of curcumin could considerably increase the BrdU positive BMSCs compared to the DMSO group ($P < 0.001$).

Effect of curcumin on proliferation of NS/PCs

There were no significant differences among the groups after 48 h treatment of NS/PCs with various doses of curcumin except for the 10 μM curcumin group in which the fluorescent density of BrdU was significantly decreased compared to the DMSO group ($P < 0.05$, Fig. 3).

After 72 h administration of curcumin, there was an increase in BrdU positive NS/PCs in doses of 0.1, 0.5 ($P < 0.01$) and 1 μM ($P < 0.001$) of curcumin compared to the DMSO group. The proliferation rate of NS/PCs significantly decreased following the administration of 5 or 10 μM of curcumin when compared with that of the DMSO group ($P < 0.05$, Fig. 3).

Effect of curcumin on survival of BMSCs

The results of MTT assay showed that all concentrations of curcumin including 0.1, 0.5, 1 ($P < 0.05$), 5 and 10 μM ($P < 0.01$) could enhance the viability of BMSCs after 48 h compared to the DMSO group (Fig. 4). Following 72 h treatment, the survival of BMSCs significantly increased with 0.5 μM of curcumin ($P < 0.001$), but this index considerably decreased with 5 and 10 μM of curcumin ($P < 0.05$) compared to the DMSO group.

Effect of curcumin on survival of NS/PCs

According to the results of MTT assay, curcumin with concentrations of 5 and 10 μM significantly reduced viability of NS/PCs compared to the DMSO group after 48 h (Fig. 5, $P < 0.05$). Moreover, following 72 h of NS/PCs encounter with curcumin, the highest cell viability was seen by using 1 μM of curcumin ($P < 0.001$ compared to the DMSO group). However, high doses of curcumin (5 and 10 μM) considerably decreased the viability of NS/PCs in comparison with the DMSO group ($P < 0.05$).

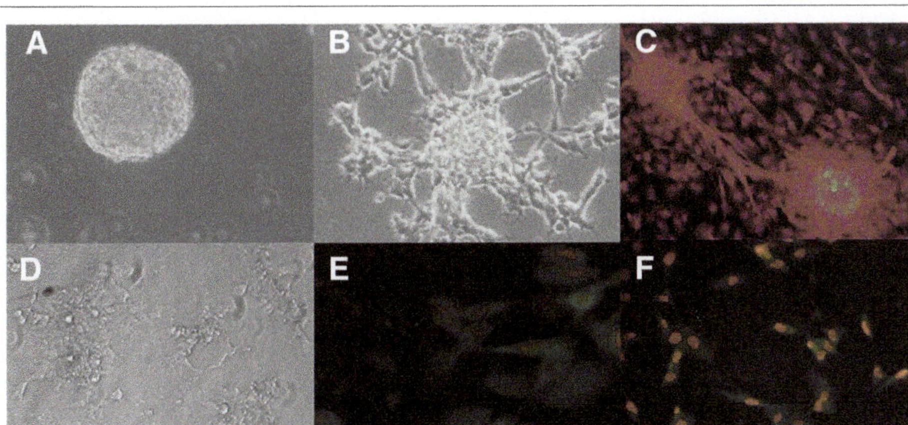

Fig. 1 Primary culture of NS/PCs and BMSCs. NS/PCs were cultured as flouting neurospheres (**a**) or slightly adherent cells (**b**) which expressed neural stem cell marker nestin (**c**). BMSCs were cultured as adherent cells (**d**) which expressed mesenchymal stem cell markers CD105 (**e**) and CD73 (**f**)

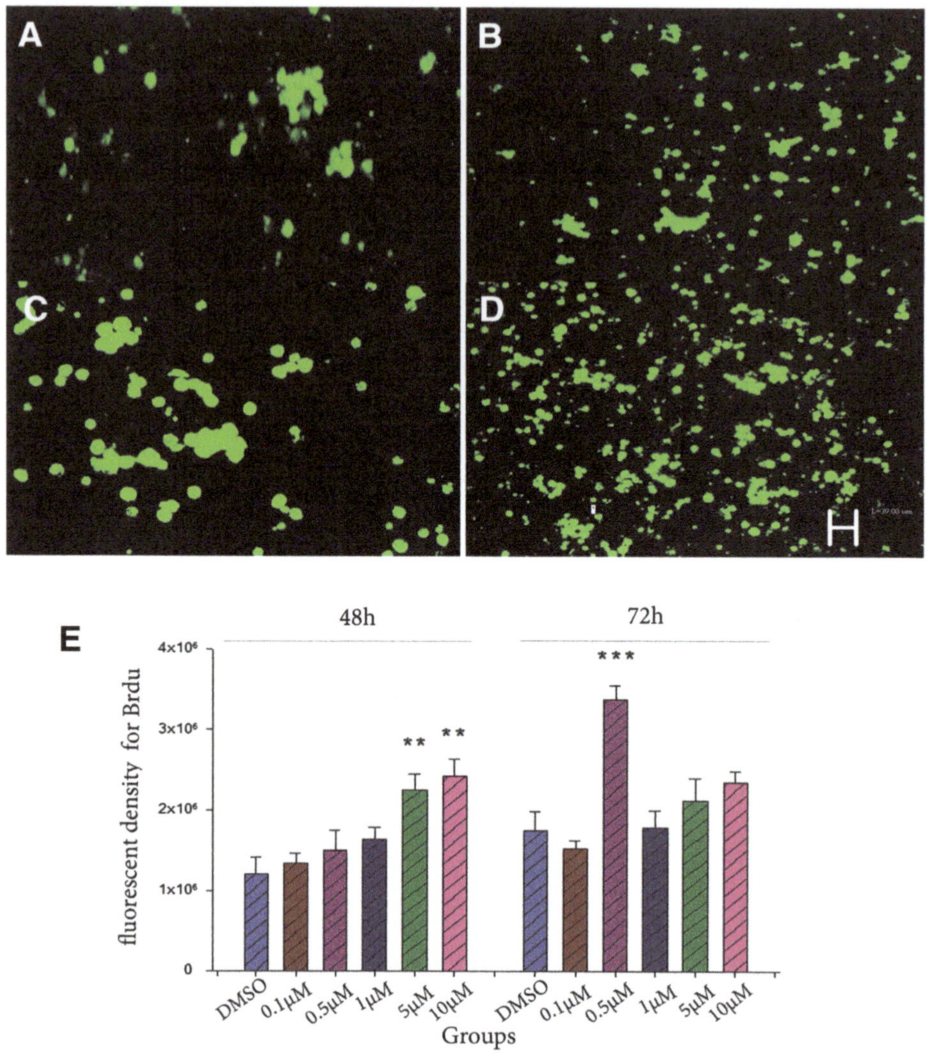

Fig. 2 The effect of various concentrations of curcumin on proliferation of BMSCs after 48 and 72 h. Different doses of curcumin (0.1, 0.5, 1, 5 and 10 μM) added 48 or 72 h into culture medium have various proliferative effects on BMSCs . The above pictures indicate the BrdU positive cells (green) in the DMSO 48 h group (**a**), 10 μM curcumin 48 h group (**b**), DMSO 72 h group (**c**) and 0.5 μM curcumin 72 h group (**d**). Scale bare:40 μm. **e**, fluorcent density for BrdU positive cells in different doses of curcumin after 48 or 72h, **: $P < 0.01$ or ***: $P < 0.001$ vs the DMSO group

Discussion

In the present study we observed multifarious effects of curcumin in terms of cell viability and stem cell proliferation. After administration of different doses of curcumin (0.1, 0.5, 1, 5 and 10 μM/L) to BMSCs, the high doses of curcumin enhanced the proliferation of BMSCs after 48 h However, when these cells were exposed to curcumin for 72 h, the increase in cell proliferation was seen only in doses of 0.5 μM of curcumin. On the other hand, the high doses of curcumin had adverse effects on the proliferation of NS/PCs while the doses of 0.1, 0.5 and 1 μM/L of curcumin administered for 72 h had beneficial effects on proliferation. The effect of curcumin on viability of BMSCs and NS/PCs was almost similar to its effect on proliferation of the cells.

Previous studies evaluated some of the effects of curcumin on the proliferation and viability of the cells. Kim et al. [8] revealed that after a 24 h treatment period, low concentration (0.5 μM) of curcumin was the most effective dose for increasing Brdu positive cells and cell viability of NS/PCs in cell culture. They opined that the stimulatory mechanism of low doses of curcumin on neural stem cells was facilitated by ERK and p38 MAP kinases [8]. In addition, Kim et al.[10] reported an increase in cell proliferation of preadipocytes with low concentrations of curcumin during a 24 h treatment period [10]. Moreover, Ormand et al. [7] reported that after 24 h, low doses of (0.5 μM) curcumin was the most effective concentration for increasing the neurosphere diameter of NS/PCs isolated from the adult rat SVZ, as

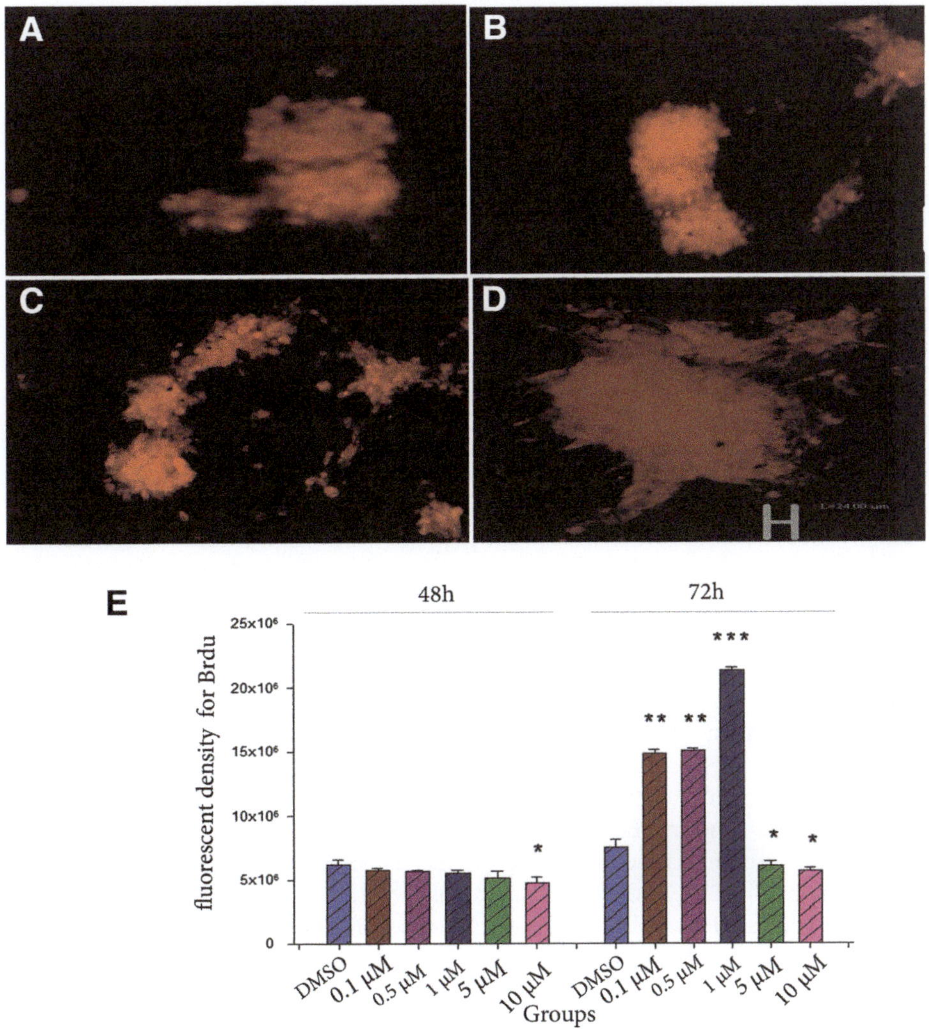

Fig. 3 The effect of various concentrations of curcumin on proliferation of NS/PCs after 48 and 72 h. Proliferation of NSCs was evaluated using fluorescent density for Brdu-positive cells. This index was different in the groups following 48 or 72 h treatment of NS/PCs with curcumin. The above photographs show the BrdU positive cells (red) in the DMSO 48 h group (**a**), 10 μM curcumin 48 h group (**b**), DMSO 72 h group (**c**) and 1 μM curcumin 72 h group (**d**). Scale bare:24 μm. **e**, fluorcent density for BrdU positive cells in different doses of curcumin after 48 or 72h, *: $P < 0.05$, **: $P < 0.01$ or ***: $P < 0.001$ vs the DMSO group

a proliferation index [7]. Previous studies have shown that curcumin can be utilized at low doses to induce heme oxygenase 1 at pharmacological levels, and its induction is accompanied by generation of non-lethal levels of reactive oxygen species [3]. On the other hand, Kim et al. [8] reported a cytotoxic effect with concentrations more than 10 μM of curcumin [8]. Ormand et al. [7] also demonstrated that curcumin at higher doses caused apoptosis [7]. Another report showed that the concentrations of 1-50 μM of curcumin increased cell viability while doses higher than 80 μM decreased it [16]. The discrepancies observed among the studies may be attributed in part to the different species, duration of curcumin exposure and the dose of curcumin. In the present study, the different doses of curcumin and treatment duration were chosen based on a pilot study as well as previous reports [10, 8]. It is important to point out that according to the results of the present study; it seems that the toxic effects of curcumin on NS/PCs were more sensitive than that on BMSCs.

Indeed, in the light of latest investigations and results, curcumin acts as a double-edged sword. In other words, it can be toxic to cells and can also be helpful. It depends on the dose and type of cells. Based on this fact, curcumin should be used cautiously in future treatment strategies. Recent studies have shown that curcumin could reduce oxidative damage related to aging and was beneficial in the treatment of neurodegenerative diseases such as Alzheimer diseases, Parkinson disease, and stroke in animal models [21–25]. Xu et al. [26] showed that curcumin could reverse

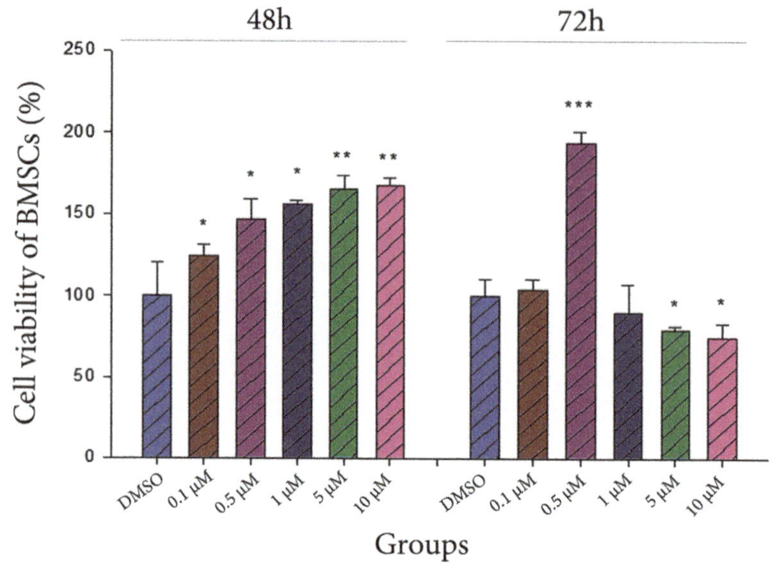

Fig. 4 The effect of various concentrations of curcumin on viability of BMSCs after 48 and 72 h. Cell viability of BMSCs was assessed using MTT assay method. The results indicated that dose and exposure time of curcumin were the factors infuence the cell viability. *: $P < 0.05$, **: $P < 0.01$ or ***: $P < 0.001$ vs the DMSO group

impaired hippocampal neurogenesis in rat model affected by chronic stress. Their results suggested that curcumin could increase the cell proliferation and neuronal populations in stress-induced behavioral abnormalities and hippocampal neuronal damage. Moreover, curcumin effects were induced by up-regulation of 5-HT_{1A} receptors and BDNF [26]. Fadhel et al. [24] indicated that administration of 200 mg/kg of curcumin by intraperitoneal method immediately, 3 h and 24 h after transient forebrain, ischemia model significantly reduced neuronal damage. This protective effect did not differ among these three different times. Fusheng et al. [21] reported that five months administration of 500 ppm curcumin in aged APP transgenic mice suppressed amyloid accumulation. Kim et al. showed that when curcumin was administered intraperitoneally at a dose of 500 nmol/kg body weight of adult mice once daily for 4 days, the Numbers of Newly Generated Cells in the Hippocampus increased [8]. However, the translation

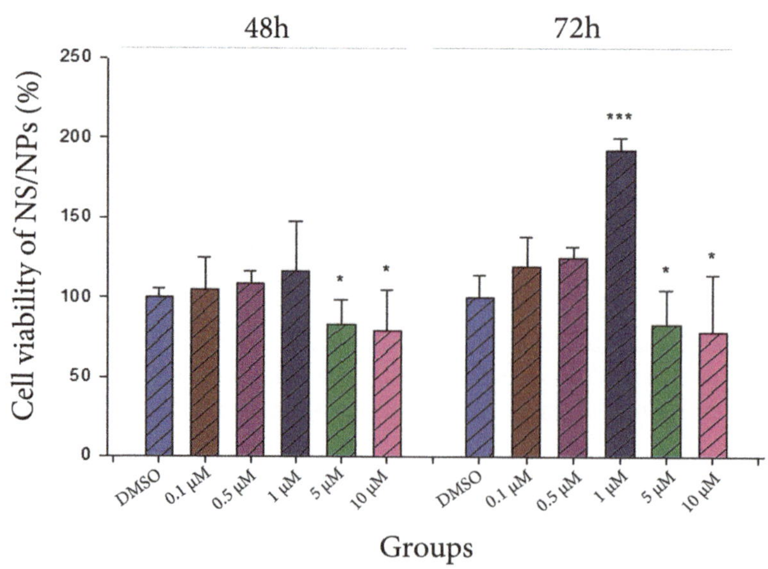

Fig. 5 The effect of various concentrations of curcumin on viability of NS/PCs after 48 and 72 h. Curcumin in different doses had various effects on survival of NS/PCs. In addition, the cell viabilty was affected by period of treatment. *: $P < 0.05$ or ***: $P < 0.001$ vs the DMSO group

of the results of animal studies to the clinic is not an easy job. The results of phase I clinical trials indicated that curcumin is safe even at high doses (12 g/day). Humans however exhibit poor bioavailability [27]. Considering the fact that curcumin in the face of stem cells exhibits a biphasic effect, further investigation is needed to determine specific effects of curcumin on different types of stem cells.

Conclusion

These findings suggest that curcumin proliferation effects depend on treatment period, its concentration, and the type of stem cells. These factors should be considered in stem cell therapy of degenerative and neurological disorders. Further studies are required to evaluate the synergistic effect of combination therapy of curcumin and stem cells.

Abbreviations

BMSCs: Bone marrow mesenchymal stem cells; NS/PCs: Neural stem/progenitor cells; DMEM/F12: Dulbecco's Modified Eagle Medium; DMSO: 3-(4, 5-dimethylthiazolyl-2)-2, Dimethyl Sulphoxide; MTT: 5-diphenyltetrazolium bromide; BrdU: Bromodeoxyuridine; ANOVA: One-Way Analysis of Variance.

Competing interests

The authors declare that they have no competing interests.

Authors' contributions

GH and FA carried out study concept and design, GH and AG carried out providing laboratory equipment, FA and GH carried out analysis and interpretation of data, FA carried out drafting of the manuscript, GH, MZ, HA, SE and MS carried out critical revision of the manuscript for important intellectual content, FA, TM and MK carried out statistical analysis. All authors read and approved the final manuscript.

Acknowledgments

This study was supported by a grant (90-3-87-14565) from Tehran University of Medical Sciences.

Author details

[1]Department of Neuroscience, School of Advanced Technologies in medicine, Tehran University of Medical Sciences, Tehran, Iran. [2]Department of Anatomy, School of Medicine, Tehran University of Medical Sciences, Tehran, Iran. [3]Shefa Neuroscience Research Center, Khatamolanbia Hospital, Tehran, Iran. [4]Department of Pharmacology, School of Medicine, Tehran University of Medical Sciences, Tehran, Iran. [5]Faculty of Pharmacy, and Pharmaceutical Sciences Research Center, Tehran University of Medical Sciences, Tehran, Iran. [6]Department of Physiology, Medical College, Lorestan University of Medical Sciences, Khorramabad, Iran. [7]Epilepsy Research Center, WestfälischeWilhelms-UniversitätMünster, Münster, Germany.

References

1. Milobedzka J, Kostanecki V, Lampe V. Structure. Chem Ber. 1910;43:2163.
2. Sharma R, Gescher A, Steward W. Curcumin: the story so far. Eur J Cancer. 2005;41(13):1955–68.
3. McNally SJ, Harrison EM, Ross JA, Garden OJ, Wigmore SJ. Curcumin induces heme oxygenase 1 through generation of reactive oxygen species, p38 activation and phosphatase inhibition. Int J Mol Med. 2007;19(1):165–72.
4. Goel A, Kunnumakkara AB, Aggarwal BB. Curcumin as "Curecumin": from kitchen to clinic. Biochem Pharmacol. 2008;75(4):787–809.
5. Ray B, Bisht S, Maitra A, Maitra A, Lahiri DK. Neuroprotective and neurorescue effects of a novel polymeric nanoparticle formulation of curcumin (NanoCurc™) in the neuronal cell culture and animal model: implications for Alzheimer's disease. J Alzheimers Dis. 2011;23(1):61–77.
6. Hatcher H, Planalp R, Cho J, Torti F, Torti S. Curcumin: from ancient medicine to current clinical trials. Cell Mol Life Sci. 2008;65(11):1631–52.
7. Ormond DR, Shannon C, Oppenheim J, Zeman R, Das K, Murali R, et al. Stem cell therapy and curcumin synergistically enhance recovery from spinal cord injury. PLoS One. 2014;9(2):e88916.
8. Kim SJ, Son TG, Park HR, Park M, Kim M-S, Kim HS, et al. Curcumin stimulates proliferation of embryonic neural progenitor cells and neurogenesis in the adult hippocampus. J Biol Chem. 2008;283(21):14497–505.
9. Son S, Kim K-T, Cho D-C, Kim H-J, Sung J-K, Bae J-S. Curcumin Stimulates Proliferation of Spinal Cord Neural Progenitor Cells via a Mitogen-Activated Protein Kinase Signaling Pathway. J Korean Neurosurg Soc. 2014;56(1):1–4.
10. Kim J-H, Park S-H, Nam S-W, Kwon H-J, Kim B-W, Kim W-J, et al. Curcumin stimulates proliferation, stemness acting signals and migration of 3T3-L1 preadipocytes. Int J Mol Med. 2011;28(3):429–35.
11. Chen J, Li Y, Wang L, Zhang Z, Lu D, Lu M, et al. Therapeutic benefit of intravenous administration of bone marrow stromal cells after cerebral ischemia in rats. Stroke. 2001;32(4):1005–11.
12. Aligholi H, Hassanzadeh G, Azari H, Rezayat SM, Mehr SE, Akbari M, et al. A new and safe method for stereotactically harvesting neural stem/progenitor cells from the adult rat subventricular zone. J Neurosci Methods. 2014;225:81–9.
13. Azari H, Rahman M, Sharififar S, Reynolds BA. Isolation and expansion of the adult mouse neural stem cells using the neurosphere assay. J Vis Exp. 2010;45:1–4.
14. Dahl J-A, Duggal S, Coulston N, Millar D, Melki J, Shandadfar A, et al. Genetic and epigenetic instability of human bone marrow mesenchymal stem cells expanded in autologous serum or fetal bovine serum. Int J Dev Biol. 2008;52(8):1033.
15. Azari H, Sharififar S, Rahman M, Ansari S, Reynolds BA. Establishing embryonic mouse neural stem cell culture using the neurosphere assay. J Vis Exp. 2011;47:1–4.
16. Ye J, Zhang Y. Curcumin protects against intracellular amyloid toxicity in rat primary neurons. Int J Clin Exp Med. 2012;5(1):44.
17. Dominici M, Le Blanc K, Mueller I, Slaper-Cortenbach I, Marini F, Krause D, et al. Minimal criteria for defining multipotent mesenchymal stromal cells. The International Society for Cellular Therapy position statement. Cytotherapy. 2006;8(4):315–7.
18. Zhang M, Jia G, Cheng J, Yang P, Lu Y, Wu X. In vitro analysis and in vivo tracing of BrdU-labeled rat bone marrow mesenchymal stem cells. Sichuan Da Xue Xue Bao Yi Xue Ban. 2012;43(2):266–70.
19. Jensen EC. Quantitative analysis of histological staining and fluorescence using image. J Anat R. 2013;296(3):378–81.
20. Wei W-L, Sun H-S, Olah ME, Sun X, Czerwinska E, Czerwinski W, et al. TRPM7 channels in hippocampal neurons detect levels of extracellular divalent cations. Proc Natl Acad Sci Proc Natl Acad Sci U S A. 2007;104(41):16323–8.
21. Yang F, Lim GP, Begum AN, Ubeda OJ, Simmons MR, Ambegaokar SS, et al. Curcumin inhibits formation of amyloid β oligomers and fibrils, binds plaques, and reduces amyloid in vivo. J Biol Chem. 2005;280(7):5892–901.
22. Calabrese V, Butterfield D, Stella A. Nutritional antioxidants and the heme oxygenase pathway of stress tolerance: novel targets for neuroprotection in Alzheimer's disease. Ital J Biochem. 2003;52(4):177–81.
23. Chen H, Zhang Z, Zhang Y, Zhou D. Curcumin inhibits cell proliferation by interfering with the cell cycle and inducing apoptosis in colon carcinoma cells. Anticancer Res. 1998;19(5A):3675–80.
24. Al-Omar FA, Nagi MN, Abdulgadir MM, Al Joni KS, Al-Majed AA. Immediate and delayed treatments with curcumin prevents forebrain ischemia-induced neuronal damage and oxidative insult in the rat hippocampus. Neurochem Res. 2006;31(5):611–8.
25. Zbarsky V, Datla KP, Parkar S, Rai DK, Aruoma OI, Dexter DT. Neuroprotective properties of the natural phenolic antioxidants curcumin and naringenin but not quercetin and fisetin in a 6-OHDA model of Parkinson's disease. Free Radic Res. 2005;39(10):1119–25.
26. Xu Y, Ku B, Cui L, Li X, Barish PA, Foster TC, et al. Curcumin reverses impaired hippocampal neurogenesis and increases serotonin receptor 1A mRNA and brain-derived neurotrophic factor expression in chronically stressed rats. Brain Res. 2007;1162:9–18.
27. Anand P, Kunnumakkara AB, Newman RA, Aggarwal BB. Bioavailability of curcumin: problems and promises. Mol Pharm. 2007;4(6):807–18.

15

Ionic liquid phase microextraction combined with fluorescence spectrometry for preconcentration and quantitation of carvedilol in pharmaceutical preparations and biological media

Mohsen Zeeb* and Behrooz Mirza

Abstract

Background: Carvedilol belongs to a group of medicines termed non-selective beta-adrenergic blocking agents. In the presented approach, a practical and environmentally friendly microextraction method based on the application of ionic liquids (ILs) was followed by fluorescence spectrometry for trace determination of carvedilol in pharmaceutical and biological media.

Methods: A rapid and simple ionic liquid phase microextraction was utilized for preconcentration and extraction of carvedilol. A hydrophobic ionic liquid (IL) was applied as a microextraction solvent. In order to disperse the IL through the aqueous media and extract the analyte of interest, IL was injected into the sample solution and a proper temperature was applied and then for aggregating the IL-phase, the sample was cooled in an ice water-bath. The aqueous media was centrifuged and IL-phase collected at the bottom of the test tube was introduced to the micro-cell of spectrofluorimeter, in order to determine the concentration of the enriched analyte.

Results: Main parameters affecting the accuracy and precision of the proposed approach were investigated and optimized values were obtained. A linear response range of 10–250 μg l^{-1} and a limit of detection (LOD) of 1.7 μg l^{-1} were obtained.

Conclusion: Finally, the presented method was utilized for trace determination of carvedilol in commercial pharmaceutical preparations and biological media.

Keywords: Carvedilol, Hydrophobic ionic liquid, Spectrofluorimetry, Real samples

Background

Carvedilol belongs to a group of medicines termed non-selective beta-adrenergic blocking agents (Figure 1). This drug is useful in treatment of congestive heart failure. In addition, carvedilol is applied to treat high blood pressure (hypertension) and for prevention of heart attacks [1,2].

In order to assay the presence of carvedilol in pharmaceutical and biological samples, some analytical approaches including chromatography [3-6], spectrophotometery [7], electrochemistry [8,9] and fluorimetry [10] have been developed. These methods suffer form some limitations including poor sensitivity, high cost of analysis, unsuitable selectivity and high time of analysis. One of the best choices for overcoming the mentioned problems is the combination of a practical sample enrichment method with analytical instruments.

In recent years, analytical chemists have developed some practical liquid phase microextraction methods and among these sample pretreatment methods, dispersive liquid-liquid microextraction (DLLME) has received much attention [11,12]. Unfortunately, one of the most important disadvantages of these microextraction methods is the usage of toxic solvents as the extraction solvent such as $CHCl_3$, CCl_4 and etc. In order to remove these toxic materials from microextraction procedures, ionic liquids (ILs) are the best choice. ILs offer many

* Correspondence: Zeeb.mohsen@gmail.com
Department of Applied Chemistry, Faculty of science, Islamic Azad University, South Tehran Branch, Tehran, Iran

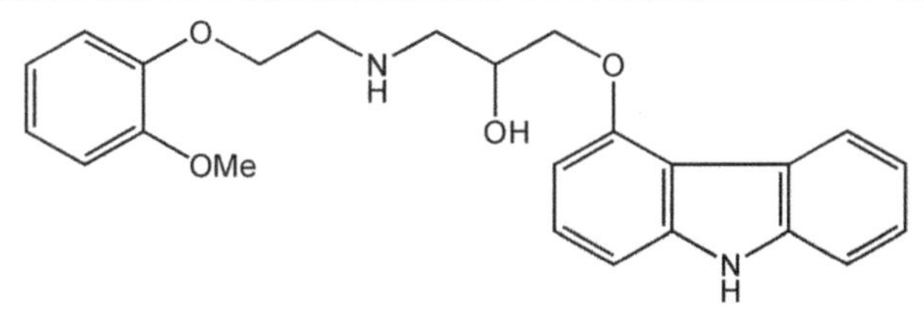

Figure 1 Structure of carvedilol.

advantages such as low vapor pressure, tunable solubility, desire thermal stability and etc. [13].

In recent years, some microextraction methods based on the application of ILs such as ionic liquid-based dispersive liquid-liquid microextraction (IL-DLLME) [14-16], ionic liquid cold-induced aggregation dispersive liquid-liquid microextraction (IL-CIA-DLLME) [17-19], ionic Liquid-based ultrasound-assisted in situ solvent formation microextraction [20], temperature-controlled ionic liquid dispersive liquid phase microextraction (TCIL-DLPME) [21], etc. have been introduced.

Solubility of ILs depends on the aqueous media temperature; hence it is possible to control the solubility of ILs by changing the temperature. In the presented ionic liquid phase microextraction, in order to disperse the IL-phase into the sample solution and increase the extraction recovery, a high temperature was applied. For collecting the IL-phase, sample solution was cooled and centrifuged.

Our previous studies revealed that the solubility of ILs depends on ionic strength of aqueous media, which has a negative influence on reproducibility and accuracy [18,19]. For solving this problem, a common ion of IL was introduced to the aqueous media. As a result, the solubility of IL phase was not affected by variations of ionic strength, and reproducible volume of enriched phase was obtained.

Some analytical instrument such as spectrofluorimetry offer many advantages such as proper sensitivity, selectivity, cost of analysis, speed of quantitative measurements and etc. In addition, by coupling a microextraction method with fluorescence spectrometry and due to the proper selectivity of this analytical technique, it is avoided the need of employing a high performance separation instrumental for pretreatment of biological samples prior to measurement.

As a part of our continuing efforts for quantitation of drugs using combination of new and benign sample enrichment methods with inexpensive, selective and sensitive analytical instrument [18,21], herein, for the first time a practical and environmentally friendly microextraction method based on the application of ILs was followed with spectrofluorimetry for trace determination of carvedilol in real samples. All variable were evaluated in details and optimized values were obtained.

Material and methods

Instrumentation

Detection of fluorescence signals were performed using a Perkin-Elmer LS 50 spectrofluorimeter. This instrument was equipped with xenon discharge lamp, and quartz micro-cell with a volume of 100 μl. Excitation and emission slits were fixed at 15 nm. In order to perform microextraction and optimization steps, a centrifuge from Hettich (Tuttlingen, Germany), a pH-meter, an adjustable sampler (10–100 μL) and a 1 ml syringe was prepared.

Reagents and materials

Analytical-reagent grade of 1-Hexyl-3-methylimidazolium hexafluorophosphate [Hmim][PF_6], acetone, acetonitrile, methanol, ethanol, HCl, NaOH and sodium hexafluorophosphate ($NaPF_6$) were obtained from Merck (Darmstadt, Germany). A working solution of $NaPF_6$ (250 mg ml^{-1}) was prepared. For preparing stock solution of carvedilol (1000 mg l^{-1}) (Fluka, Switzerland), proper amount of this drug was dissolved in methanol and diluted with ultra pure water. Standard solutions were prepared by dilution of the stock solution with ultra pure water. Tablets containing 12.5 mg and 25 mg carvedilol were purchased from a local pharmacy.

Sample pretreatment procedure

In this sample pretreatment method, ten milliliters of sample solution (10–250 μg l^{-1} of carvedilol) was transferred to a centrifuge tube. The pH of the solution was adjusted at 9. Afterwards, 60 mg of 1-Hexyl-3-methylimidazolium hexafluorophosphate [Hmim][PF_6] ionic liquid and 0.7 ml of hexafluorophosphate ($NaPF_6$) (250 mg ml^{-1}) was injected into the aqueous sample solution. After mixing the extractor with sample solution, the resultant solution was transferred into a hot water batch equipped with a thermostat. The temperature of the water batch was fixed at 50°C for 4 min. Under driving the temperature, IL-phase was dissolved and dispersed through the aqueous media. In order to aggregate the IL-phase, the sample was cooled at 0°C for 7 min. In order to collect the enriched phase, sample solution was centrifuged (6 min, 4000 r.p.m). After removing the aqueous media, the enriched phase was diluted with ethanol to 200 μl and transferred into the micro-cell of the spectrofluorimeter. Finally, quantitation of carvedilol was performed. Schematic diagram of the designed method is shown in Figure 2.

Preparation of pharmaceutical preparations, human urine and human plasma

To obtain pharmaceutical solutions for quantification, eight carvedilol tablets containing 12.5 or 25 mg drug were powdered, mixed and weighted. Required amount of the resultant material containing 10 mg carvedilol

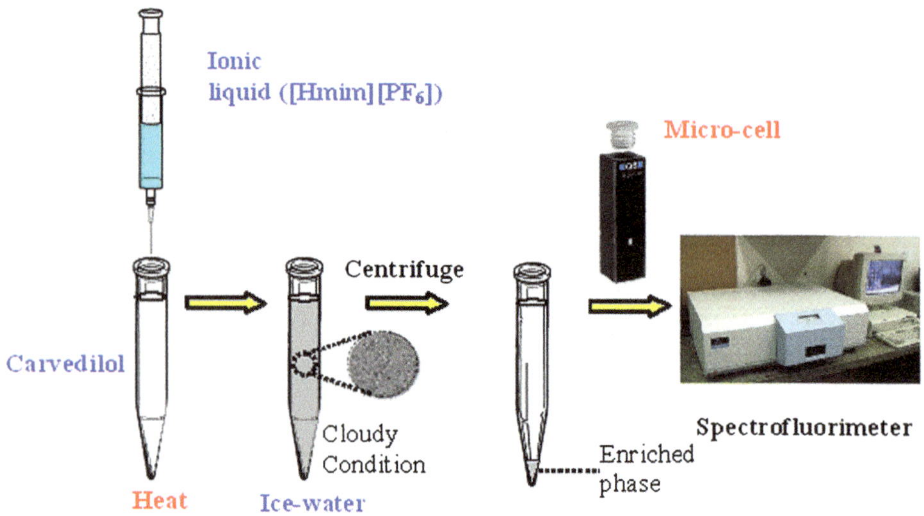

Figure 2 Schematic diagram of the proposed method.

was dissolved in methanol with signification. After filtration, the solution was transferred into a 100 ml volumetric vessel and diluted with ultra pure water. In order to set the concentration of carvedilol within the linear response range, further dilution was performed.

For preparing human plasma samples, different concentrations of carvedilol were added to one milliliter of human plasma. After this step, the real sample was deproteinized using 5 ml of acetonitrile. After centrifugation (12 min, 4000 r.p.m), 2.0 ml of the upper phase (clear condition) was diluted with ultra pure water and 10.0 ml of the obtained sample was utilized for quantitation.

In order to prepare human urine samples, ten milliliters of urine were centrifuged (5 min, 4000 r.p.m). Then, 2.0 ml of the upper clear phase was placed in centrifuge test tube and different amount of carvedilol was added to this and diluted to 10.0 ml. Finally, the defined quantitation procedure was performed.

Results and discussion

In recent work, a simple and benign sample pretreatment method based on the application of ILs was combined with fluorescence spectrometry for enrichment and determination carvedilol in real samples. Main parameters affecting the accuracy and precision of the proposed approach were investigated and optimized values were obtained.

Fluorescence spectra properties and linear dynamic range

Native Fluorescence intensities of molecules with π-electron and cyclic structure are relatively high. As a result, measurement of fluorescence intensity provides a

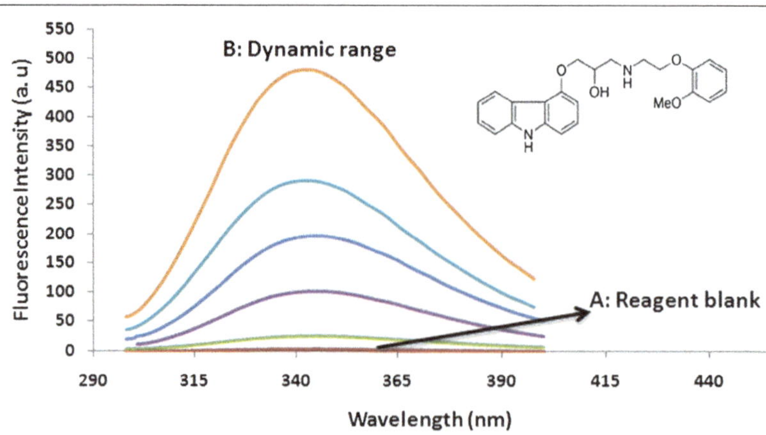

Figure 3 Fluorescence spectra of reagent blank and carvedilol. (A) Fluorescence spectrum of reagent blank after applying microextraction procedure. (B) Fluorescence spectra of carvedilol within linear dynamic range (10, 50, 100, 150, 250 μg l^{-1}) after applying microextraction procedure. Applied parameters: sample volume 10 ml; IL 60 mg; $NaPF_6$ 175 mg; pH 9; temperature 50°C; λ_{ex} 285 ± 5 nm; λ_{em} 345 ± 5 nm.

practical tool for sensitive quantitative analysis. After applying the designed microextraction procedure, fluorescence spectra of carvedilol (100 μg l^{-1}) was recorded (Figure 3). In this study, emission peaks were recorded at 345 ± 5 nm (excitation wave length was fixed at 285 ± 5 nm).

In order to evaluate the spectra properties of reagent blank, sample pretreatment method was performed without analyte of interest and the fluorescence spectra were recorded at 345 ± 5 nm. No main measurable influence of reagent blank on the quantitative analysis of carvedilol was observed. As a result, these excitation and emission wavelengths were selected for further quantitation of carvedilol.

Kind of ionic liquid

Based on the results obtained in our previous studies [18,19], three factors must be considered, in order to select a proper IL: (a) the density of IL as the extraction solvent must be higher than aqueous media, (b) IL must illustrate a desire hydrophobicity, (c) IL must be liquid and (d) these ionic material must be inexpensive. ILs with imidazolium scaffold which contain Cl^-, BF_4^- and $CF_3SO_3^-$ show hydrophilic properties and those contain PF_6^- and $(CF_3SO_2)_2N^-$ show hydrophobic properties.

According to these factors, [Hmim][PF_6] was used as an optimum microextraction solvent in all tests.

Optimization of diluting solvent

The viscosity of ionic liquids is relatively high; hence their direct transfer into the micro-cell of spectrofluorimeter for analyzing carvedilol is difficult. As a result, enriched-phase was conditioned and diluted. For this goal, some conditioner solvents such as methanol, ethanol, acetonitrile and acetone were evaluated as the diluting solvent. The obtained data showed that reproducible and sensitive signals were obtained in using ethanol as a conditioner agent. Due to the better data stability and ethanol environmental safety (less toxicity), this organic solvent was preferred and used in all experiments.

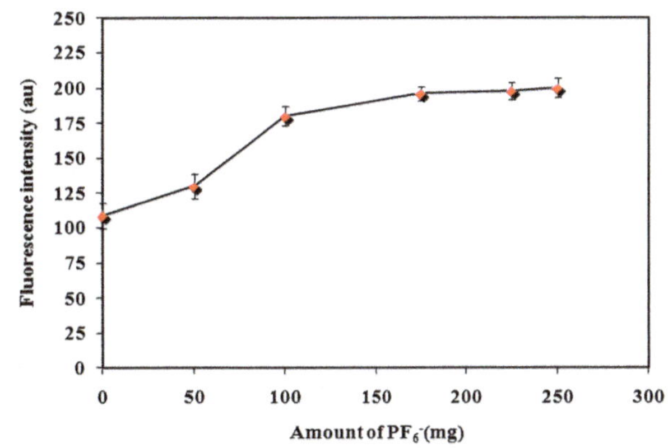

Figure 5 Effect of PF_6^- Applied parameters: Carvedilol concentration 100 μg l^{-1}; Sample volume 10 ml; IL 60 mg; pH 9; temperature 50°C; λ_{ex} 285 ± 5 nm; λ_{em} 345 ± 5 nm. Indicated analytical signals are the average of three independent measurements and error bars correspond to their standard deviations.

Optimization of IL amount

As it was mentioned, in this microextraction procedure, IL was applied as the microextraction phase. In this kind of sample pretreatment method, one of the major parameters affecting the performance is the amount of IL. This parameter has a significant effect on the reproducibility and sensitivity. In order to optimize the amount of extraction solvent, this parameter was tested within the range of 10–100 mg (Figure 4). Stable and sensitive fluorescence signals were obtained at 60 mg and this value was used for the rest of the work.

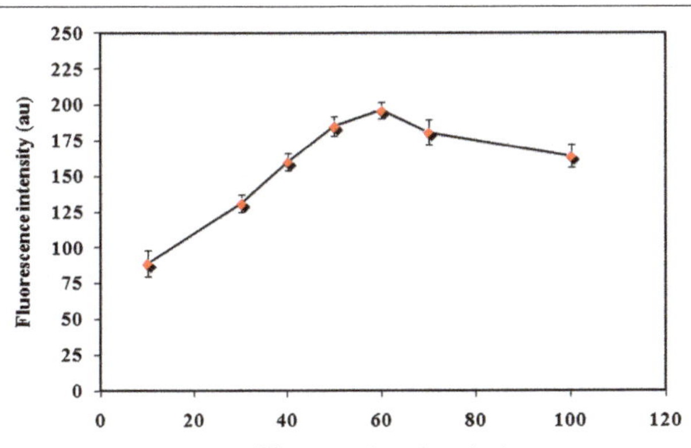

Figure 4 Effect of IL as the microextraction phase. Applied parameters: Carvedilol concentration 100 μg l^{-1}; sample volume 10 ml; $NaPF_6$ 175 mg; pH 9; temperature 50°C; λ_{ex} 285 ± 5 nm; λ_{em} 345 ± 5 nm. Indicated analytical signals are the average of three independent measurements and error bars correspond to their standard deviations.

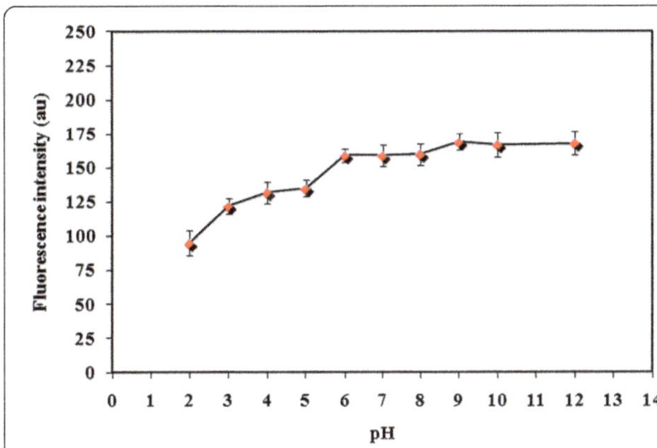

Figure 6 Effect of pH. Applied parameters: Carvedilol concentration 100 μg l^{-1}; sample volume 10 ml; IL 60 mg; $NaPF_6$ 175 mg; temperature 50°C; λ_{ex} 285 ± 5 nm; λ_{em} 345 ± 5 nm. Indicated analytical signals are the average of three independent measurements and error bars correspond to their standard deviations.

Table 1 Analytical characteristics of the presented work

Analytical factor	Values
Linear analytical response range (μg l^{-1})	10-250
Correlation coefficient (R^2)	0.9980
LOD[a] (μg l^{-1})	1.7
RSD[b] (%) (n = 4) ($C_{carvedilol}$ = 100 μg l^{-1})	3.8
PF[c]	50
Sample volume (mL)	10

[a]Limit of detection.
[b]Relative standard deviation.
[c]The ratio of diluted settled phase volume to aqueous volume gives the preconcentration factor (PF).

Optimization of PF_6^- amount and ionic strength

As it was demonstrated in our previous works [18,19], dissolving a common ion of IL like PF_6^-, significantly reduce the solubility of IL. This act improves the extraction performance of carvedilol and provides better analytical sensitivity. Effect of this parameter was examined in the range of 0–250 mg (see Figure 5). A value of 175 mg was selected as an optimum value, in order to obtain proper signal stability and reproducibility.

One of the most important parameters which affects on the extraction performance is ionic strength of the aqueous media. An increase in ionic strength causes a considerable increase in solubility of IL. As a result, the volume of the settled phase depends on the salt content of the sample solution. This phenomenon has a negative influence on the stability of analytical data. Fortunately, presence of PF_6^- (as a common ion) solves this problem and fixes the volume of the enrich phase. The effect of ionic strength was studied within the range of 0–40% (w/v) using $NaNO_3$ as an electrolyte. In the studied range, no significant influence on fluorescence signal was observed.

Table 2 Comparison of the proposed methodology with reported methods

Method	Sample	LOD (μg l^{-1})	LR (μg l^{-1})	Reference
DLLME-HPLC[a]	Human Urine, Human Plasma	4, 14	50-750, 20-1000	[6]
SPE-CE[b]	Human Urine	50	50-500	[23]
Synchronous fluorimetry	Pharmaceutical preparations	1	5-100	[24]
LLE-HPLC[c]	Human serum	2.5	5-500	[25]
Ionic liquid phase microextraction-spectrofluorimetry	Human Urine, Human Plasma, Pharmaceutical preparations	1.7	10-250	This work

[a]Dispersive liquid-liquid microextraction.
[b]Solid phase extraction-capillary electrophoresis.
[c]Liquid-liquid extraction.

Table 3 Results of recoveries of spiked biological samples

Sample	Carvedilol added (μg l^{-1})	Carvedilol found (μg l^{-1})[a]	RSD (%)	Recovery (%)
Urine	50	53.2	6.1	106.4
	100	98.3	5.9	98.3
	150	146.1	3.8	97.4
Plasma	50	44.6	5.6	89.2
	100	107.3	7.1	107.3
	150	154.8	4.2	103.2

[a]Average of four independent measurements.

Optimization of pH

In the case of microextraction of molecules like carvedilol, which have ionizable property, pH of the aqueous media reveals a significant role. In order to obtain the highest extraction efficiency, the uncharged condition of carvedilol must be prevalent (pK_a value of carvedilol is 7.97) [22]. The effect of sample pH on the analytical sensitivity and reproducibility was tested within the range of 2–12 (Figure 6). In the recent experiments, HCl and NaOH were used for adjusting the pH. Based on the results obtained in this study, in order to obtain a compromise between sensitivity and reproducibility, pH 9 was selected for further experiments.

Influence of temperature

In this microextraction procedure, IL-phase is dispersed into the aqueous media under increasing the temperature. The effect of this parameter was evaluated in the range of 25–80°C. Finally, a temperature of 50°C was used as an optimum value. In order to collect the IL-phase after extraction, the sample solution must be cooled. For the recent goal, the aqueous media was placed in ice-water bath and kept at 0°C for 7 min.

Interference study

For studying the possible interferences coming form other compounds, which exist in real samples, some ions and compounds were subjected to the recent combined methodology. In this investigation, the effect of 100-fold of K^+, Na^+, Mg^+, F^-, Cl^-, NO_3^-, SO_4^{2-}, glucose, urea, lactic acid, sucrose, ascorbic acid and fructose as the interfering or quenching agents on the determination of

Table 4 Analysis of carvedilol tablets by the present work and the reported method (5)

Claimed (mg/tablet)	Proposed method (mg)[a]	Reported method (mg)[a]	Error (%)[b]	Error (%)[c]
12.5	12.3 (±0.5)	12.6 (±0.4)	−1.6	−2.9
25	25.5 (±1.0)	25.7 (±1.1)	+2.0	−0.7

[a]Values in parenthesis give the standard deviation based on four determinations.
[b]Error against the tablet value.
[c]Error against the reported method.

carvedilol (100 μg L^{-1}) was evaluated. No change in signals over than 4.5% was observed.

Analytical figures of merits

Linear analytical response range was defined by analyzing standard solutions of carvedilol. The obtained results revealed that analytical responses are linear from 10 to 250 μg l^{-1}. Other analytical figures of merits obtained by the ionic liquid phase microextraction-spectrofluorimetry are shown in Table 1. Limit of detection (LOD) was determined using a conventional equation, LOD = ks_{bl}/m. This equation is resulted from the equation showed below:

$$S_m = S_{bl} + ks_{bl}$$
$$S_m = mc_m + S_{bl}$$
$$c_m = \frac{S_m - S_{bl}}{m} = \frac{ks_{bl}}{m}$$

S_m, S_{bl}, s_{bl}, K, m and C_m show the minimum distinguishable analytical signal, average of blank analytical signal, blank standard deviation, constant value equal with 3 (confidence level of 95%), calibration graph slope and detection limit, respectively. Using this way, a value of 1.7 μg l^{-1} carvedilol was achieved. In order to determine the relative standard deviation (RSD), four 100 μg l^{-1} of carvedilol was subjected to the designed methodology and finally a value of 3.8% was obtained.

Comparison with reported methods

In order to show the analytical advantages of the proposed method for the quantitation of carvedilol, some details were compared with reported methods in literature, and these results are shown in Table 2. As it can be seen, considerable LOD and relatively wide dynamic range were obtained. In addition, in most of the reported methods, tedious sample pretreatment procedures, toxic solvents and expensive analytical instrument have been used for quantification. In contrast, in the proposed method, a rapid, benign and simple ionic liquid phase microextraction was utilized for preconcentration and extraction of carvedilol. No hazardous material was used in this sample pre-treatment method. In addition, an inexpensive and sensitive analytical instrument was applied for quantitation.

Analysis of carvedilol in real samples

In order to demonstrate the analytical application of the presented technique, real samples including human urine and human plasma were spiked with different amounts of carvedilol and analyzed. Results of this investigation are shown in Table 3. At it can be seen, the averages of recoveries are placed in the range of 97.4-106.2% (urine) and 89.2-107.3% (plasma). It can be concluded that in the case of accuracy and reproducibility, satisfactory results were obtained. In the next step, some commercial pharmaceutical formulations involving carvedilol capsules and tablets were subjected to the designed method, in order to determine concentration of carvedilol (Table 4). The results obtained with the present work were compared with a reported method [5]. These data reveal the practical analytical application of the proposed method for analyzing the analyte of interest in pharmaceutical preparations.

Conclusion

A rapid, benign and simple ionic liquid phase microextraction was utilized for preconcentration and extraction of carvedilol. The enriched-phase was introduced to spectrofluorimeter for quantitation of carvedilol. No toxic and hazardous material was used in this sample pre-treatment method. In addition, an inexpensive and sensitive analytical instrument was applied for quantitative measurements. Finally, the combined methodology was successfully applied for quantitation of carvedilol in real samples.

Competing interests

The authors declare that they have no competing interests.

Authors' contributions

All authors contributed equally. Both authors read and approved the final manuscript.

Acknowledgment

Support of this investigation by the Islamic Azad University Tehran south branch through grant is gratefully acknowledged.

References

1. Packer M, Colicci WS, Sacker-Bernstein JD. Placebo-controlled study of the effects of carvedilol in patients with moderate to severe heart failure, the PRECISE trial. Circulation. 1996;94:2793–9.
2. Bristow MR, Gilbert EM, Abraham WT, Adams KF, Fowler MB, Hershberger RE, et al. Carvedilol produces dose related improvements in left ventricular function and survival in subjects with chronic heart failure. Circulation. 1996;94:2807–16.
3. Hokama N, Hobara N, Kameya H, Ohshiro S, Sakanashi M. Rapid and simple micro-determination of carvedilol in rat plasma by high performance liquid chromatography. J Chromatogr, B. 1999;732:233–8.
4. Machida M, Watanabe M, Takechi S, Kakinoki S, Nomura A. Measurement of carvedilol in plasma by high-performance liquid chromatography with electrochemical detection. J Chromatogr, B. 2003;798:187–91.
5. Zarghi A, Foroutan SM, Shafaati A, Khoddam A. Quantification of carvedilol in human plasma by liquid chromatography using fluorescence detection: application in pharmacokinetic studies. J Pharm Biomed Anal. 2007;44:250–3.
6. Zamani-Kalajahi M, Fazeli-Bakhtiyari R, Amiri M, Golmohammadi A, Afrasiabi A, Khoubnasabjafari M, et al. Analysis of losartan and carvedilol in urine and plasma samples using a dispersive liquid–liquid microextraction isocratic HPLC–UV method. Bioanalysis. 2012;4:2805–21.
7. Cardoso SG, Ieqqli CV, Pomblum SC. Spectrophotometric determination of carvedilol in pharmaceutical formulations through charge-transfer and ion-pair complexation reactions. Pharmazie. 2007;62:34–7.
8. Radi A, Elmogy T. Differential pulse voltammetric determination of carvedilol in tablets dosage form using glassy carbon electrode. Il Farmaco. 2005;60:43–6.

9. Soleymanpour A, Ghasemian M. Chemically modified carbon paste sensor for the potentiometric determination of carvedilol in pharmaceutical and biological media. Measurement. 2015;59:14–20.
10. Silva RA, Wang CC, Fernandez LP, Masi AN. Flow injection spectrofluorimetric determination of carvedilol mediated by micelles. Talanta. 2008;76:166–71.
11. Zeeb M, Ganjali MR, Norouzi P. Dispersive liquid-liquid microextraction followed by spectrofluorimetry as a simple and accurate technique for determination of thiamine (vitamin B_1). Michrochim Acta. 2010;168:317–24.
12. Bidari A, Jahromi EZ, Assadi Y, Hosseini MRM. Monitoring of selenium in water samples using dispersive liquid-liquid microextraction followed by iridium-modified tube graphite furnace atomic absorption spectrometry. Microchem J. 2007;87:6–12.
13. Zeeb M, Ganjali MR, Norouzi P, Kalaei MR. Separation and preconcentration system based on microextraction with ionic liquid for determination of copper in water and food samples by stopped-flow injection spectrofluorimetry. Food Chem Toxicol. 2011;49:1086–91.
14. Yao C, Anderson JL. Dispersive liquid-liquid microextraction using an in situ metathesis reaction to form an ionic liquid extraction phase for the preconcentration of aromatic compounds from water. Anal Bioanal Chem. 2009;395:1491–502.
15. Yao C, Li T, Wu P, Pitner WR, Anderson JL. Selective extraction of emerging contaminants from water samples by dispersive liquid-liquid microextraction using functionalized ionic liquids. J Chromatogr A. 2011;1218:1556–66.
16. Gharehbaghi M, Shemirani F, Baghdadi M. Dispersive liquid-liquid microextraction based on ionic liquid and spectrophotometric determination of mercury in water samples. Int J Environ Anal Chem. 2009;89:21–33.
17. Zeeb M, Sadeghi M. Modified ionic liquid cold-induced aggregation dispersive liquid-liquid microextraction followed by atomic absorption spectrometry for trace determination of zinc in water and food samples. Microchim Acta. 2011;175:159–65.
18. Zeeb M, Ganjali MR, Norouzi P. Modified ionic liquid cold-induced aggregation dispersive liquid-liquid microextraction combined with spectrofluorimetry for trace determination of ofloxacin in pharmaceutical and biological samples. Daru. 2011;19:446–54.
19. Zeeb M, Ganjali MR, Norouzi P. Preconcentration and Trace Determination of Chromium Using Modified Ionic Liquid Cold-Induced Aggregation Dispersive Liquid-Liquid Microextraction: Application to Different Water and Food Samples. Food Anal Method. 2013;6:1398–406.
20. Zeeb M, Mirza B, Zare-Dorabei R, Farahani H. Ionic Liquid-based Ultrasound-Assisted In Situ Solvent Formation Microextraction Combined with Electrothermal Atomic Absorption Spectrometry as a Practical Method for Preconcentration and Trace Determination of Vanadium in Water and Food Samples. Food Anal Method. 2014;7:1783–90.
21. Zeeb M, Tayebi-Jamil P, Berenjian A, Ganjali MR, Talei BOMR. Quantitative analysis of piroxicam using temperature controlled ionic liquid dispersive liquid phase microextraction followed by stopped-flow injection spectrofluorimetry. Daru. 2013;6:1398–406.
22. Stojanovic J, Vladimirov S, Marinkovic V, Velickovic D, Sibinovic P. Monitoring of the photochemical stability of carvedilol and its degradation products by the RP-HPLC method. J Serb Chem Soc. 2007;72:37–44.
23. Mazzarino M, De La Torre X, Mazzei F, Botre F. Rapid screening of beta-adrenergic agents and related compounds in human urine for anti-doping purpose using capillary electrophoresis with dynamic coating. J Sep Sci. 2009;32:3562–70.
24. Xiao Y, Wang HU, Han J. Simultaneous determination of carvedilol and ampicillin sodium by synchronous fluorimetry. Spectrochim Acta, Part A. 2005;61:567–73.
25. Gannu R, Yamsani VV, Rao YM. New RP-HPLC method with UV-detection for the determination of carvedilol in human serum. J Liq Chromatogr Rel Technol. 2007;30:1677–85.

16

Synthesis and psychobiological evaluation of modafinil analogs in mice

Arezou Lari[1], Isaac Karimi[2], Hadi Adibi[3], Alireza Aliabadi[3], Loghman Firoozpour[4] and Alireza Foroumadi[4,5*]

Abstract

Background and the purpose of the study: Modafinil, a novel wake-promoting agent with low potential for abuse and dependence, has a reliable structure to find some novel derivatives with better activity and lower potential for abuse and risk of dependency. This study was designed to evaluate psychobiological activity of some novel *N*-aryl modafinil derivatives.

Methods: Seven novel *N*-aryl modafinil derivatives were synthesized through three reactions: a) preparation of benzhydrylsulfanyl acetic acid through reaction of benzhydrol with thioglycolic acid, b) formation of desired amide by adding the substituted aniline to activated acid with EDC (1-ethyl-3-(3-dimethyl amino propyl) carbodiimide). This reaction was catalyzed by HOBt (*N*- hydroxylbenzotriazole), and c) oxidation of sulfur to sulfoxide group with H_2O_2. Then, their psychobiological effect on the performance of male albino mice were compared to that of modafinil as following: wakefulness by determining the effects of derivatives on phenobarbital-induced loss of the righting reflex (LOPR); exploratory activity by measuring activity in the open field test (OFT); depression by measuring immobility time (IT) during forced swimming test (FST) and the anxiogenic and anxiolytic like effects by using elevated plus-maze test (EPM). All tests were videotaped and analyzed for the frequency and duration of the behaviors during the procedures.

Conclusions: 2-(Benzhydrylsulfonyl)-*N*-(4-chlorophenyl)acetamide (**4c**) showed comparable result in LOPR test. However, all analogs were found to be stimulant except 2-(benzhydrylsulfinyl)-*N*-phenylacetamide (**4a**). Also **4c** led the most exploratory activity in mice among derivatives. FST results showed that 4a had the longest IT while modafinil, 2-(benzhydrylsulfinyl)-*N*-(3-chlorophenyl) acetamide (**4b**) and 2-(benzhydrylsulfinyl)-*N*-(4-ethylphenyl) acetamide (**4d**) had the shortest IT. In EPM, all derivatives showed anxiogenic-like behavior since they decreased open arms time and open arms entries and simultaneously increased close arms time.

Keywords: Modafinil, Wake-promoting agent, Narcolepsy

Introduction

Narcolepsy is a neurological sleep disorder that is estimated to affect as many as 200,000. It is as widespread as multiple sclerosis and more prevalent than cystic fibrosis, but it is less well known [1,2].

The main treatment of narcolepsy is using of central nervous system (CNS) stimulants such as amphetamine, methylphenidate and modafinil which is widely regarded as the first-line medication for narcolepsy (Figure 1) [1,3]. Amphetamine and methylphenidate are associated with a significant abuse potential while modafinil which has lower abuse potential [4,5]. Surprisingly, modafinil is used sometimes to treat methamphetamine dependency; however this type of therapy has not been authoritized [6].

In one study, some modafinil analogs were evaluated for their CNS activity [7]. Most of the derivatives of nitrogen group like $NHCH_3$, NHCH $(CH_3)_2$, HCN $(CH_3)_3$ were stimulant, although some analogs with piperidine or morpholine groups were sedative. Here, synthesis and psychobiological evaluation of novel modafinil derivatives with different *N-Aryl* moieties were reported. These analogs with suitable Log *P* were chosen due to their easy transfer across the blood brain barrier. The tilted compounds were prepared according to Scheme 1. The key intermediate 2-(benzhydrylthio) acetic acid (**2**) was prepared from benzhydrol and thioglycolic acid. Amidation of appropriate

* Correspondence: aforoumadi@yahoo.com
[4]Drug Design and Development Research Center, Tehran University of Medical Sciences, Tehran, Iran
[5]Neuroscience Research Center, Institute of Neuropharmacology, Kerman University of Medical Sciences, Kerman, Iran
Full list of author information is available at the end of the article

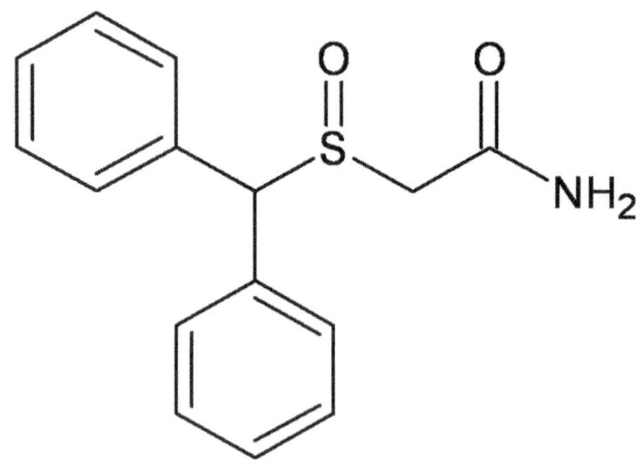

Figure 1 Chemical structure of modafinil.

aniline with 2-(benzhydrylthio)acetic acid yielded the corresponding amide (**3a-3g**). The obtained amides (**3a-3g**) gently oxidized by H_2O_2 to form the corresponding sulfoxide derivatives (**4a-4g**).

Material and methods

Chemistry

All chemical reagents and solvents used in this study were purchased from Merck AG (Darmstadt, Germany). Melting points were determined by Kofler hot stage apparatus and are not corrected. The IR spectra were obtained on a Shimadzu 470 spectrophotometer (potassium bromide disks). NMR spectra were appropriately recorded using a Bruker 400 spectrometer (Bruker Bioscience, Billerica, MA, USA), and chemical shifts were expressed as δ (ppm) with tetramethylsilane as internal standard. The mass spectra were run on a Finigan TSQ-70 spectrometer (Finigan, USA) at 70 eV. Merck silica gel 60 F_{254} plates were used for analytical TLC.

Synthesis of 2-(benzhydrylthio)acetic acid (2)

A mixture of benzhydrol (50.0 g, 271.4 mmol) and thioglycolic acid (25.0 g, 271.4 mmol) in trifluoroacetic acid (300 mL) was stirred at room temperature for 3 h. The solvent was removed under reduced pressure to afford a crude solid. Water (300 ml) was added and the resulting precipitate collected by filtration. The solid was washed with *n*-hexane (400 ml) and dried to afford a white solid (69.2 g).

Yield: 99%, mp: 126–129°C. IR (KBr, cm^{-1}); ῡ: 3071, 2570, 1941, 1860, 1809, 1689, 1596, 1491, 1301, 1203, 1137, 1209, 1021, 804. ^{1}H-NMR ($CDCl_3$, 400 MHz) δ (ppm): 3.1 + .3699 (s, 2H, $-SCH_2CO-$), 5.5 (s, 1H, Ph-CH-Ph), 7.13 (t, $J = 7.6$ Hz, aromatic), 7.22-7.25 (m, aromatic), 7.25 (m, aromatic), 7.33 (m, aromatic), 7.45 (m, aromatic) [8].

General procedure for the synthesis of compounds 3a-3g

The mixture of 2-(benzhydrylthio) acetic acid **(2)**, EDC (1-ethyl-3-(3-dimethylaminopropyl) carbodiimide) (1 mol) and HOBt (hydroxybenzotriazole) (1 mol) in acetonitrile solvent was kept under stirring for 30 min in order to activate acid group. Afterwards, appropriate aniline derivative was added and the mixture was stirred at room temperature for 24 h. The solvent was evaporated and

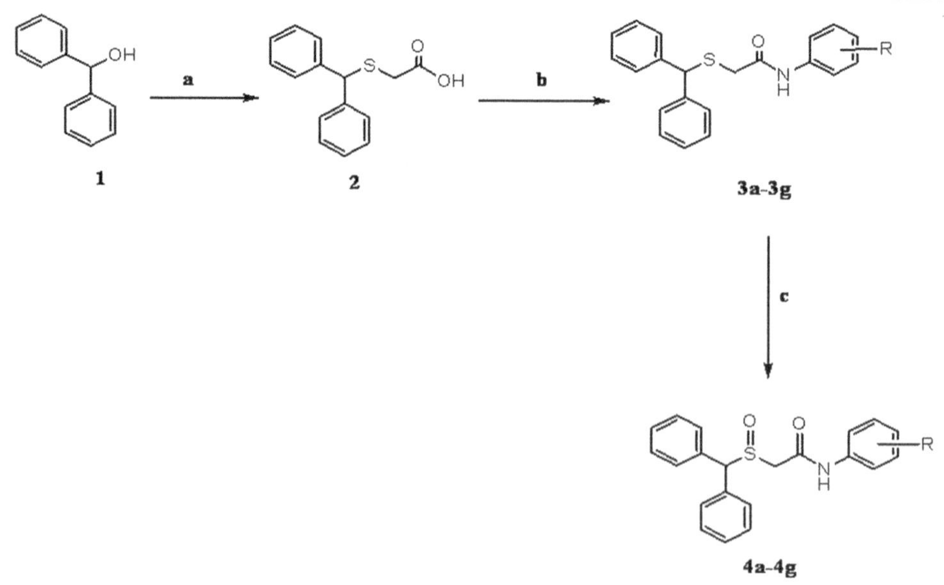

Scheme 1 **Synthesis of target compounds 4a-4g (R: (a) = H, (b) = 3-Cl, (c) = 4-Cl, (d) = 4-Et, (e) = 3,4-Cl, (f) = 4-NO_2, (g) = 4-Br), Reagents and conditions: (a) Thioglycolic acid, TFA, 3 h; (b) appropriate amine, EDC, HOBt; (c) appropriate amide, H_2O_2, acetic acid.**

ethyl acetate was added to the residue. The organic phase was washed with sulfuric acid 5%, sodium bicarbonate and brine. Then, the organic layer was dried over anhydrous sodium sulfate, filtered and evaporated to dryness. The residue was chromatographed on silica gel plate eluting with ethyl acetate/petroleum [9].

2-(benzhydrylthio)-N-phenylacetamide (3a)
Yield: 81%, mp: 90°C. IR (KBr, cm^{-1}); ū: 3431, 3243, 3060, 2959, 2854, 1655, 1597, 1547, 1491, 1443, 1325, 754, 696. ^{1}H-NMR ($CDCl_3$, 400 MHz) δ (ppm): 3.26 (s, 2H, -SCH_2CO-), 5.18 (s, 1H, Ph-CH-Ph), 7.13 (t, J=7.6 Hz, aromatic), 7.22-7.25 (m, aromatic), 7.30-7.35 (m, aromatic), 7.41 (d, J=8 Hz, aromatic), 7.48 (d, J=8 Hz, aromatic), 8.41 (brs, 1H, NH).

2-(benzhydrylthio)-N-(3-chlorophenyl) acetamide (3b)
Yield: 73%, mp: 60°C. IR (KBr, cm^{-1}); ū: 3426, 3329, 3229, 3064, 2923, 1665, 1641, 1593, 1525, 1421, 1310, 1240, 1129, 1074, 878, 775, 698. ^{1}H-NMR ($CDCl_3$, 400 MHz) δ (ppm): 3.27 (s, 2H, -SCH_2CO-), 5.18 (s, 1H, PhCHPh), 7.15 (m, aromatic), 7.25-7.41 (m, aromatic), 8.42 (brs, 1H, NH).

2-(benzhydrylthio)-N-(4-chlorophenyl) acetamide (3c)
Yield: 78%, mp: 90°C. IR (KBr, cm^{-1}); ū: 3430, 3121, 3067, 2923, 2853, 1646, 1549, 1490, 1400, 1093, 1034, 823, 700. ^{1}H-NMR ($CDCl_3$, 400 MHz) δ (ppm): 3.27 (s, 2H, -SCH_2CO-), 5.15 (s, 1H, PhCHPh), 7.25-7.41 (m, 14H, aromatic), 8.41 (s, 1H, NH).

2-(benzhydrylthio)-N-(4-ethylphenyl) acetamide (3d)
Yield: 72%, mp: 87°C. IR (KBr, cm^{-1}); ū: 3258, 3060, 2962, 2925, 2873, 1638, 1599, 1535, 1449, 1410, 1321, 1124, 1073, 1025, 971, 825, 743, 697. ^{1}H-NMR ($CDCl_3$, 400 MHz) δ (ppm): 1.22 (t, 3H, CH_3), 2.62 (q, 2H, CH_2), 3.25 (s, 2H, -SCH_2CO-), 5.19 (s, 1H, PhCHPh), 7.15-7.42 (m, 14H, aromatic), 8.40 (s, 1H, NH).

2-(benzhydrylthio)-N-(3, 4-dichlorophenyl) acetamide (3e)
Yield: 75%, mp: 85°C. IR (KBr, cm^{-1}); ū: 3400, 3268, 3087, 2922, 1710, 1650, 1591, 1528, 1480, 1376, 1318, 1118, 1027, 870, 811, 748, 697. ^{1}H-NMR ($CDCl_3$, 400 MHz) δ (ppm): 3.28 (s, 2H, -SCH_2CO-), 5.14 (s, 1H, PhCHPh), 7.65 (s, 1H, H_2-Dichlorophenyl) and 7.24-7.40 (m, 12H, aromatic), 8.37 (brs, 1H, NH).

2-(benzhydrylthio)-N-(4-nitrophenyl) acetamide (3f)
Yield: 68%, mp: 80-84°C. IR (KBr, cm^{-1}); ū: 3313, 3087, 3017, 2923, 1675, 1616, 1596, 1552, 1500, 1334, 1307, 1255, 1117, 853, 748, 696. ^{1}H-NMR ($CDCl_3$, 400 MHz) δ (ppm): 3.34 (s, 2H, -SCH_2CO-), 5.16 (s, 1H, PhCHPh), 7.24 (d, J= 8Hz, aromatic), 7.31 (t, J=4Hz, aromatic), 7.4 (d, J= 8Hz, aromatic), 7.61 (d, 2H, J=8Hz, *p*-Nitrophenyl), 8.19 (d, 2H, J= 8.8Hz, *p*-Nitrophenyl), 8.64 (brs, 1H, NH).

2-(benzhydrylthio)-N-(4-bromophenyl) acetamide (3g)
Yield: 84%, mp: 92°C. IR (KBr, cm^{-1}); ū: 3237, 3027, 2927, 1714, 1641, 1593, 1533, 1490, 1396, 1314, 1125, 1072, 1008, 818, 746, 696. ^{1}H-NMR ($CDCl_3$, 400 MHz) δ (ppm): 3.28 (s, 2H, -SCH_2CO-), 5.17 (s, 1H, PhCHPh), 7.32-7.48 (m, 14H, aromatic), 8.42 (brs, 1H, NH).

General procedure for the synthesis of 2-(benzhydrylsulfinyl)-N-phenylacetamide (4a-4g)
2-(benzhydrylthio)-*N*-phenylacetamide (3.46 g, 0.013 mol) was taken in glacial acetic acid (14 ml) with stirring. 1.34 ml of 30% H_2O_2 was added with chilling in ice water. The mixture was left in the refrigerator for 4 h and thereafter worked up by treating with 70 ml of ice-cold water. The precipitated material was filtered under suction and washed with ice-cold water to give 1.5 g of white crystals (43%), mp: 159-160°C [10].

2-(benzhydrylsulfinyl)-N-phenyl acetamide (4a)
Yield: 70%, mp: 98°C. IR (KBr, cm^{-1}); ū: 3426, 3056, 2924, 2854, 1673, 1600, 1551, 1493, 1446, 1325, 1112, 1033, 755, 698.

^{1}H-NMR (d ppm, $CDCl_3$, 400 MHz): 3.23 (d, 1H, -SCH_2CO-, J = 12Hz), 3.66 (d, 1H, -SCH_2CO-, J = 12Hz), 5.25 (s, 1H, PhCHPh), 7.12 (t, J = 8Hz, aromatic), 7.26 (s, 1H, aromatic), 7.31 (t, J = 8Hz, aromatic), 7.36-7.52 (m, aromatic), 9.21 (brs, 1H, NH). ^{13}C-NMR (125 MHz, $CDCl_3$): δ 51.95 (S-CH_2), 71.54 (S-CH), 120.15 ($C_{2,\ 6}$ aniline), 124.64 (C_4 aniline), 128.77 ($C_{3,\ 5}$ aniline), 128.87 ($C_{3,5}$ phenyl), 128.97 (C_4 phenyl), 129.51 ($C_{2,6}$ phenyl), 133.78 (C_1 phenyl), 134.29 (C_1 aniline), 175.00 (C = O). MS (m/z): 349 (M^+), 309, 167, 119, 104, 93, 77, 65, 57, 43.

2-(benzhydrylsulfinyl)-N-(3-chlorophenyl) acetamide (4b)
Yield: 68%, mp: 160°C. IR (KBr, cm^{-1}); ū: 3441, 3250, 3184, 3066, 3026, 2923, 2856, 1682, 1596, 1546, 1480, 1430, 1372, 1320, 1035, 794, 700. ^{1}H-NMR ($CDCl_3$, 400 MHz) δ (ppm): 3.23 (d, 1H, -SCH_2CO-, J= 12Hz), 3.67 (d, 1H, -SCH_2CO-, J= 12Hz), 5.27 (s, 1H, PhCHPh), 7.08-7.50 (m, 13H, aromatic), 7.69 (s, 1H, H_2-*m*-Chlorophenyl), 9.35 (brs, 1H, NH). ^{13}C-NMR (125 MHz, $CDCl_3$): δ 52.34 (S-CH_2), 71.38 (S-CH), 117.88 (C_3 aniline), 120.04 (C_2 aniline), 124.55 (C_4 aniline), 128.84 ($C_{3,\ 5}$ phenyl), 128.90 (C_4 phenyl), 128.99 ($C_{2,6}$ phenyl), 129.51 (C_6 aniline), 131.94 (C_5 aniline), 133.67 (C_1 phenyl), 134.37 (C_1 aniline), 162.16 (C=O). MS (m/z): 385 (M^++2), 383 (M^+), 293, 201, 167, 153, 127, 111, 91, 64, 47.

2-(benzhydrylsulfinyl)-N-(4-chlorophenyl) acetamide (4c)
Yield: 73%, mp: 170°C. IR (KBr, cm^{-1}); ū: 3444, 3248, 2920, 1684, 1597, 1541, 1489, 1398, 1320, 1246, 1037, 743, 701.

^{1}H-NMR ($CDCl_3$, 400 MHz) δ (ppm): 3.26 (d, 1H, -SCH_2CO-, $J = 16Hz$), 3.66 (d, 1H, -SCH_2CO-, $J = 16Hz$), 5.26 (s, 1H, PhCHPh), 7.24 (d, 2H, $J = 8Hz$, *p*-Chlorophenyl), 725–7.50 (m, 12H, aromatic), 9.33 (brs, 1H, NH). ^{13}C-NMR (125 MHz, $CDCl_3$): δ 52.21 (S-CH_2), 71.52 (S-CH), 121.19 (C-Cl), 128.85 ($C_{2,\ 6}$ aniline), 128.91 ($C_{3,5}$ phenyl), 128.98 (C_4 phenyl), 129.52 ($C_{2,6}$ phenyl), 129.56 ($C_{3,5}$ aniline), 134.29 (C_1 phenyl), 136.18 (C_1 aniline), 162.08 (C=O). MS (m/z): 385 (M^++2), 383 (M^+), 167, 153, 127, 111.

2-(benzhydrylsulfinyl)-N-(4-ethylphenyl) acetamide (4d)

Yield: 74%, mp: 158°C. IR (KBr, cm^{-1}) ῡ: 3253, 3185, 3058, 2957, 2923, 2858, 1679, 1540, 1412, 1322, 1043, 957, 832, 747, 701.

^{1}H NMR ($CDCl_3$, 400 MHz) δ (ppm): 1.23 (t, 3H, CH_3), 2.63 (q, 2H, CH_2), 3.23 (d, 1H, $J = 12Hz$, -SCH_2CO-), 3.66 (d, 1H, -SCH_2CO-, $J = 12Hz$), 5.21 (s, 1H, PhCHPh), 7.16-7.48 (m, 14H, aromatic), 9.21 (brs, 1H, NH). ^{13}C-NMR (125 MHz, $CDCl_3$): δ 15.66 (CH_3), 28.33 (CH_2), 36.97 (S-CH_2), 55.09 (S-CH), 120.22 (C_4 aniline), 127.53 ($C_{2,\ 6}$ aniline), 128.25 ($C_{3,5}$ phenyl), 128.34 (C_4 phenyl), 128.46 ($C_{2,6}$ phenyl), 128.84 ($C_{3,5}$ aniline), 135.02 (C_1 phenyl), 140.10 (C_1 aniline), 166.28 (C = O). MS (m/z): 377 (M^+), 284, 279, 191, 167, 149, 105, 85, 71, 57.

2-(benzhydrylsulfinyl)-N-(3, 4-dichlorophenyl) acetamide (4e)

Yield: 63%, mp: 140°C. IR (KBr, cm^{-1}); ῡ: 3293, 3258, 3101, 3052, 2912, 1711, 1686, 1587, 1383, 1312, 1224, 1146, 1036, 878, 820, 742, 698. ^{1}H NMR ($CDCl_3$, 400 MHz) δ (ppm): 3.24 (d, 1H, J =16Hz, -SCH_2CO-), 3.67 (d, 1H, $J = 16Hz$, -SCH_2CO-), 5.32 (s, 1H, PhCHPh), 7.23-7.48 (m, 12H, aromatic), 7.77 (s, 1H, H_2-*m*-Chlorophenyl), 9.45 (brs, 1H, NH). ^{13}C-NMR (125 MHz, $CDCl_3$): δ 52.13 (S-CH_2), 71.41 (S-CH), 118.99 (C_4 aniline), 121.48 (C_2 aniline), 121.56 (C_6 aniline), 128.87 ($C_{3,5}$ phenyl), 129.04 (C_4 phenyl), 129.50 ($C_{2,\ 6}$ phenyl), 129.56 (C_3 aniline), 131.94 (C_5 aniline), 133.64 (C_1 phenyl), 134.19 (C_1 aniline), 162.14 (C=O). MS (m/z): 421 (M^+4), 419 (M^++2), 417 (M^+), 199, 184, 167, 149, 105.

2-(benzhydrylsulfinyl)-N-(4-nitrophenyl) acetamide (4f)

Yield: 76%, mp: 198°C. IR (KBr, cm^{-1}); ῡ: 3448, 3202, 3078, 2922, 2852, 1702, 1618, 1598, 1566, 1497, 1335, 1251, 1159, 1039, 859, 748, 698. ^{1}H NMR ($CDCl_3$, 400 MHz) δ (ppm): 3.47 (d, 1H, -SCH_2CO-, $J = 12Hz$), 3.76 (d, 1H, -SCH_2CO-, $J = 12Hz$), 5.42 (s, 1H, PhCHPh), 7.35-7.41 (m, 8H, aromatic), 7.53 (d, 2H, $J = 8.4Hz$, aromatic), 7.78(d, 2H, $J = 8Hz$, *p*-Nitrophenyl), 8.16 (d, 2H, $J = 8Hz$, *p*-Nitrophenyl), 10.40 (brs, 1H, NH). MS (m/z): 394 (M^+), 279, 257, 236, 167, 149, 69, 57, 43.

2-(benzhydrylsulfinyl)-N-(4-bromophenyl) acetamide (4g)

Yield: 66%, mp: 155°C. IR (KBr, cm^{-1}); ῡ: 3430, 2923, 2853, 1741, 1663, 1630, 1454, 1379, 1240, 1155, 1034, 837, 743, 700. ^{1}H NMR ($CDCl_3$, 400 MHz) δ (ppm): 3.24 (d, 1H, -SCH_2CO-, $J = 16Hz$), 3.65 (d, 1H, -SCH_2CO-, $J = 16Hz$), 5.33 (s, 1H, PhCHPh), 7.26-7.49 (m, 14H, aromatic), 9.44 (s, 1H, NH). ^{13}C-NMR (125 MHz, $CDCl_3$): δ 51.68 (S-CH_2), 71.76 (S-CH), 117.24 (C-Br), 121.82 ($C_{2,\ 6}$ aniline), 128.82 ($C_{3,5}$ phenyl), 129.00 (C_4 phenyl), 129.43 ($C_{2,\ 6}$ phenyl), 129.55 ($C_{3,\ 5}$ aniline), 131.94 (C_1 phenyl), 136.61 (C_1 aniline), 162.19 (C=O). MS (m/z): 429 (M^++2), 428 (M^++1), 368, 362, 167, 152, 69, 57, 43.

Psychobiological activity

Animals

This study approved by the Laboratory Animal Care Committee of School of Veterinary Medicine, Razi University, Kermanshah, Iran. The experiments were carried out on male albino mice weighing 20–25 g at the beginning of the experiments. The animals were maintained under standard laboratory conditions (12-h light/dark cycle, room temperature 21 ± 1°C) with free access to tap water and laboratory chow (Dan-e-pars Co., Kermanshah, Iran) except during brief periods of experiments, and were adapted to the laboratory conditions for at least 1 week. Each experimental group consisted of 5–6 animals.

Drugs

The compounds tested were: modafinil (Modiodal®, Cephalon, France), Phenobarbital (Chemi darou product, Iran) and our made modafinil derivatives. All agents were diluted to an adequate concentration using dimethyl sulfoxide (DMSO). They were administered intraperitoneally (i.p.) 30 min prior to each behavioral test. Control groups received DMSO injection at the same volume and by the same route. The doses of modafinil and its derivatives (100 mg/kg) employed in the present study was adopted from previous study [11]. The dose of phenobarbital (50 mg/kg) was chosen according to that commonly used dose reported in the literature [12]. In all tests, each mouse was tested once.

Phenobarbital-induced loss of righting reflex

Phenobarbital (50 mg/kg i.p.) was administered to each mouse. The loss of righting reflex (LORR) was measured as the time interval between losing and recovery of the righting reflex after phenobarbital administration. Recovery of the righting reflex was defined as the ability of the animal to return to its feet 3 times within 60 sec when placed on its back [13]. Mice received modafinil or its derivatives (100 mg/kg, i.p.) 30 min before i.p. injection of phenobarbital. The ethological room was illuminated with a soft light and external noise was attenuated.

Open field test (OFT)

The open field consisted of a square arena (60 × 60 cm^2), with a white floor divided into 36 squares (10 × 10 cm^2), enclosed by continuous, 25-cm-high walls made of glass. The test was initiated by placing a single mouse in the middle of the arena and letting him move freely for 5 min. The mice had not been pre-exposed to the arena. Mouse behavior was continuously videotaped by a video camera placed over the apparatus and the arena was carefully cleaned with alcohol and rinsed with water after every test to eliminate olfactory cues. Decrease of the latency to enter the central part was considered as an indicator of anxiolysis and locomotor activity was evaluated by counting the number of segments crossed with a 4-paw as described previously [14].

Forced swimming test (FST)

Mice were individually forced to swim in a plastic cylinder ($25 \times 25 \times 40$ cm^3) containing 18 cm of water at 22°C. This volume of water precluded mice touching the bottom with their feet or tails. Mice were submitted to the procedure for 15 min on the first day (pretest) and for 5 min on the second day test, 24 h later. Each mouse i.p. received the tested derivatives 30 min before forced swimming paradigm. At the end of the swimming exposition, the animals were removed from the water and gently dried. The initial 5 min of both swimming sessions were videotaped for behavioral analysis. The immobility time (IT) was recorded only during the last 4 min of these periods, and was defined as the sum of time that the animal was floating, with the face above the water surface and making only slight movements with the front paws to keep from submerging as described previously [15]. The frequency of alternation between mobility and immobility behaviors gradually decreased as time lapsed, the animals tending to remain much more immobile. The decrease and increase of immobility time were interpreted as antidepressive or depressive actions, respectively [16].

Elevated plus maze (EPM)

Behavioral effect of modafinil and its derivatives were elevated in the mouse EPM paradigm. The experimental apparatus is shaped like a "plus" sign and consists of a central platform (5×5 cm), two open arms ($30 \times 15 \times 5$ cm) and two equal-sized closed arms opposite to each other. The maze is made of wood, elevated to a height of 50 cm above the floor. A video camera was mounted vertically about 1meter above the plus-maze for recording behavioral responses. The test consisted of placing a mouse in the central platform facing an enclosed arm and allowed it to freely explore the maze for 5 min. Entry into one arm was defined as the animal placing all four paws into that arm. The test arena was wiped with a damp cloth after each trial. The number of entries into the open and closed arms and the time spent in open arms were measured in the offline condition. Anxiolytic activity was indicated with increase of time spent in open arms or with number of open arms entries while anxiogenic effects are characterized with decrease of these measures.

For the purpose of analysis, open-arm activity was quantified as the amount of time that the rat spent in the open arms relative to the total amount of time spent in open arm (open/total × 100), and the number of entries into the open arms was quantified relative to the total number of entries into open arm (open/total × 100) [17].

Statistics

The data are expressed as mean ± S.E.M. The statistical analyses were performed using one-way analyses of variance (ANOVA). Post-hoc comparison of means was carried out with the Tukey's test for multiple comparisons, when appropriate. All data were analyzed using the General Linear Models Procedure of SPSS ver.16 (SPSS Inc., Chicago, IL, USA). The confidence limit of $P < 0.05$ was considered as statistically significant.

Results and discussion

Chemistry

Our synthetic route to target compounds **4a-4g** (Table 1) is shown in Scheme 1. The key intermediate 2-(benzhydrylthio) acetic acid **2** was prepared from benzhydrol and thioglycolic acid in trifluoroacetic acid (TFA). 1-Ethyl-3-(3-dimethylaminopropyl) carbodiimide (EDC) was treated with 2-(benzhydrylthio) acetic acid **2** in the presence of hydroxybenzotriazole (HOBt) and stirred for 30 min in acetonitrile. Then, appropriate amine derivative was added and stirring was continued overnight. Thereafter the mixture was washed sequentially with %5 $NaHCO_3$ and saturated NaCl solutions, and then dried over Na_2SO_4. Removal of the solvent under reduced pressure afforded the amide derivatives **3a-3g**. The obtained amide derivatives **3a-3g** were gently oxidized by H_2O_2 to form the corresponding sulfoxide derivatives **4a-4g** (Table 1) and analyzed by ^1H NMR, infrared, mass spectroscopy and melting point.

^1H NMR spectrum of intermediate **2** showed the benzylic hydrogen was more deshielded (5.50 ppm) than benzylic hydrogen of benzhydrol. Based on ^1H NMR analysis of intermediates **3a-3g**, the corresponding signals of protons CH benzylic, methylene group adjacent to carbonyl substituent, and NH were appeared within 5.0-5.2 ppm as a singlet, 3.2-3.5 ppm as a singlet, 8.40-8.65 ppm as a broad singlet respectively. Broad singlet peak of the NH proton is a good sign for formation of the amidic bond in this series. The aromatic hydrogens of the phenyl rings are generally appeared in the range between 7.0-8.0 ppm. The ^1H NMR spectra of compounds **4a-4g** corresponding to the methylene group between carbonyl and sulfoxide substituents showed a doublet of doublet splitting pattern. This behavior is due to existence of two diastereotopic hydrogens of the

Table 1 Effects of *N*-aryl derivatives of modafinil on behavior of albino mice in the elevated plus-maze

Compound	Open arms entries (O.E)	Open arms time spend (O.T)	Close arms entries (C.E)	Close arms time spend (C.T)
Modafinil	8.25(2.17)	71.7(10.5)	11.75(3.88)	228.2(10.5)
4a	1.00(1.00)[a]	1.5(1.5)[aab]	8.00(3.82)	221.2(23.8)[aa]
4b	7.25(1.25)	84.5(19.3)	6.25(0.47)	215.5(19.3)
4c	0.00(0.00)[aab]	0.0(0.0)[aab]	2.00(0.00)	285.0(6.4)[aa]
4d	3.50(1.50)	57.5(17.5)	4.50(1.50)	242.5(17.5)
4e	0.00(0.00)[a]	0.0(0.0)[aa]	1.50(0.50)	300.0(0.0)[aa]
4f	6.00(1.00)	120.0(10.0)	6.50(1.50)	180.0(10.0)
4g	2.50(1.190) [a]	16.75(10.0)[aa]	8.25(2.59)	216.2(26.7)[aa]
Control	12.25(2.86)	123.5(19.5)	10.50(3.92)	175.5(19.1)

Data are presented as mean ± S.E.M.
[a]$P < 0.05$ *vs.* control group, [aa]$P < 0.001$ *vs.* control group, [b]$P < 0.05$ *vs.* modafinil group.

methylene group. In addition, mass spectrometry analysis of the synthesized compounds **4a-4g** showed expectable fragmentation and hence established the structure of modafinil derivatives. Potassium bromide (KBr) disk was used to obtain the infra red (IR) spectrum related to each compound. The peak related to the carbonyl group appeared in <1700 cm^{-1} is a sign of the amidic carbonyl group in IR spectrum and it is a confirmation for the formation of the amidic moiety in these compounds.

Psychobiological activity

LORR

For comparability of data, we had to use same doses of derivatives. Based on previous study [10], 100 mg/kg of modafinil could be a suitable dose. In this dose, some analogs like **4c** made mice subconscious after i.p. administration of phenobarbital. On the other hand, some mice which received compound **4a**, died. This may be due to more sedative activity of this analog.

In comparison with control animals, compound **4a** significantly increased phenobarbital-induced LORR while other compounds demonstrated a decrease in the duration of LORR.

The experiment showed that compound **4c** was the best CNS stimulant among our synthetic derivatives however it was a slightly weaker than modafinil. Stimulant activity of used compounds is ranged in the following order:

Modafinil > **4c** > **4g** > **4d** > **4f** > **4b** > **4e** > DMSO (control) > **4a**

OFT

The results of the duration of active exploration in the OFT are presented in Figure 2. Mean square crossing of compound **4c**, **4d** and **4f** did not show significant differences when compared to the respective control and modafinil groups. Compound **4a**, **4b** and **4g** were recognized to significantly reduce square crossing compared to control (**4a**, **4g**: $p < 0.05$, **4b**: $p < 0.001$). Furthermore, the square crossing of compounds **4a**, **4b**, **4e** and **4g** were significantly decreased compared to modafinil (**4a**, **4b** and **4g**: $P < 0.001$, #5: $P < 0.05$, respectively).

The results in Figure 3 showed that all compounds except compound **4f** failed to reach the statistically significant level in measuring the latency to enter the central part compared to control and modafinil groups. Compound **4f** showed had a reliable decrease in the latency to enter the central part compared to the both groups ($P < 0.05$).

FST

The effects of derivatives and modafinil on IT during trials were depicted in Figure 4. The control animals showed 45 ± 3 sec immobility duration during FST. Compounds **4a** and **4e** increased IT and showed considerable differences when compared to the respective control groups ($P < 0.001$). Compound **4g** also lengthened IT in comparison to control ($P < 0.05$). In addition,

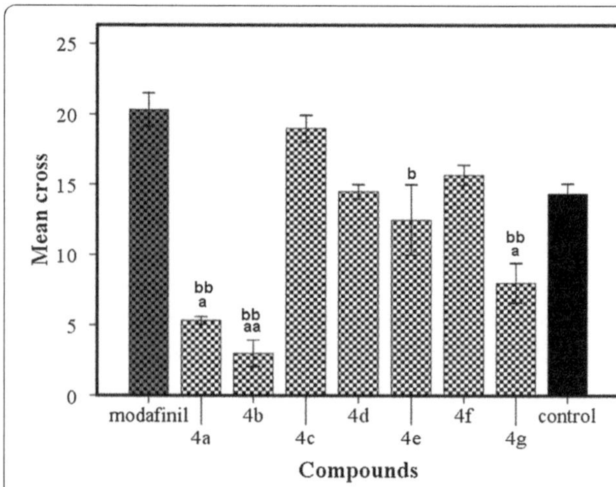

Figure 2 Exploratory activity (mean ± S.E.M.) in albino mice in the open field test. [a]$P < 0.05$, [aa]$P < .001$ *vs.* control and [b]$P < 0.05$, [bb]$P < 0.001$ *vs.* modafinil groups.

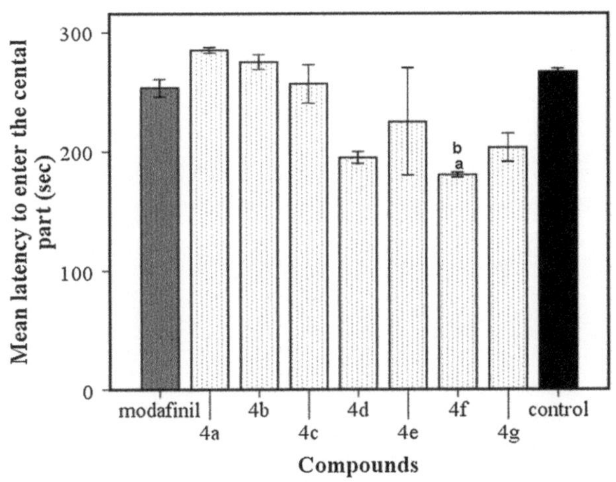

Figure 3 Effects of different derivatives in open field test in mice. Data are expressed as mean ± SEM of the latency to enter the central part. [a]P < 0.05 *vs.* control, [b]P < 0.05 *vs.* modafinil.

compounds **4a**, **4e**, **4g** and control showed a significant increase in IT compared to modafinil group (P < 0.001).

The rest of the compounds significantly decreased IT in comparison to control (P < 0.001).

EPM

Mice exposed to compounds **4a**, **4c**, **4e** and **4g** showed decline in open arms entries and open arms spent time in comparison to control mice (P < 0.05). However, modafinil, compounds **4b**, **4d** and control (DMSO) showed similar results (P > 0.05). (See Table 1.)

The percent of close arms entries revealed that all derivatives showed a non-significantly decrease in this parameter compared to those of control and modafinil groups.

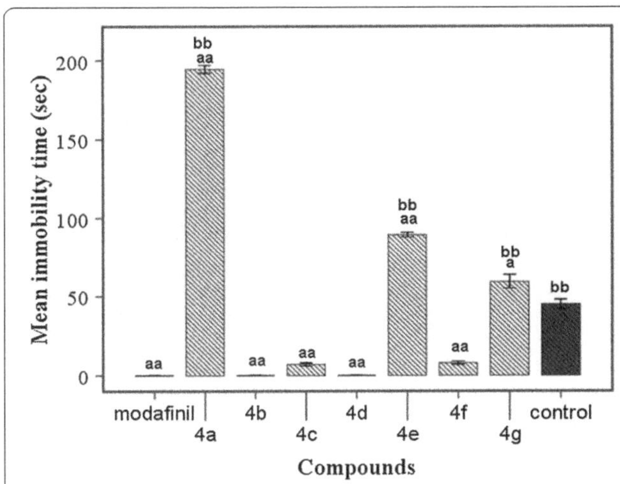

Figure 4 Effect of different derivatives of modafinil on the immobility response in forced swimming test ([a]P < .05, [aa]P < .001 *vs.* control and [bb]P < 0.001 *vs.* modafinil groups).

Compound **4a**, **4c**, **4e** and **4g** produced a reliable increase of close time spend (P < 0.05) than control group.

Conclusions

We have described a novel series of modafinil analogs (**4a-4g**) that displayed some kind of CNS activities. From our psychobiological results, compounds **4a**, **4c**, **4e** and **4g** decreased frequencies of open arms entries and duration of open arms spent times, suggesting an anxiogenic-like effect and as well as these derivatives increased close arms time significantly. Compounds **4a**, **4e** and **4g** also lengthened IT in FST, indicating that the derivatives exerted a depressive action, while other derivatives shortened IT and would be considered to have antidepressant effects. The square crossing numbers of compounds **4a**, **4b** and **4g** showed a significant reduction compared to modafinil and control groups which suggest this compound may be putative sedative. Compound **4f** induced an anxiolytic-like effect because it decreased the latency to enter the central part compared to other derivatives. The results of EPM also roughly confirmed the anxiolytic-like effect of compound **4f**. Based on LORR test, it is evident that most of the analogs exhibited stimulant activity in LORR test and compound **4c** is the most potent ones. Only compound **4a** (aniline substitution) was recognized as sedative analog. Finally, little discrepancies among results obtained from different psychobiological tests in this study may be related to the different mechanisms of actions of these derivatives and future studies are highly requested to exploit the structure-function relationships of these derivatives in more details.

Competing interests

The authors declare that they have no competing interests.

Authors' contributions

AL: Synthesis of target compounds and performing the biological tests. IK: supervision of the psychobiological part. HA: collaboration in identifying of the structures of target compounds and manuscript preparation. AA: collaboration in identification of synthesized compounds. LF: collaboration in synthesis of target compound and manuscript preparation. AF: Design of target compounds and supervision of the synthetic part. All authors read and approved the final manuscript.

Author details

[1]Students Research Committee, Faculty of Pharmacy, Kermanshah University of Medical Sciences, Kermanshah, Iran. [2]Laboratory of Molecular and Cellular Biology, School of Veterinary Medicine, Razi University, Kermanshah, Iran. [3]Novel Drug Delivery Research Center, Faculty of Pharmacy, Kermanshah University of Medical Sciences, Kermanshah, Iran. [4]Drug Design and Development Research Center, Tehran University of Medical Sciences, Tehran, Iran. [5]Neuroscience Research Center, Institute of Neuropharmacology, Kerman University of Medical Sciences, Kerman, Iran.

References

1. Hublin C: **Narcolepsy: current drug treatment options.** *CNS Drugs* 1996, **5**:426–436.

2. U.S. Modafinil in Narcolepsy Multicenter Study Group: **Randomized trial of modafinil as a treatment for excessive daytime somnolence of narcolepsy.** *Neurology* 2000, **54:**1166–1175.
3. Thorpy M: **Therapeutic advances in narcolepsy.** *Sleep Med* 2007, **8:**427–440.
4. Mitler MM, Harsh J, Hirshkowitz M, Guilleminaultd C: **Long-term efficacy and safety of modafinil (PROVIGIL) for the treatment of excessive daytime sleepiness associated with narcolepsy.** *Sleep Med* 2000, **1:**231–243.
5. Willie JT, Renthal W, Chemelli RM, Miller MS, Scammell TE, Yanagisawa M, *et al*: **Modafinil more effectively induces wakefulness in orexin-null mice than in wild-type littermates.** *Neuroscience* 2005, **130:**983–995.
6. Mehrjerdi ZA: **Crystal in Iran: methamphetamine or heroin kerack.** *Daru* 2013, **15:**21–22.
7. De Risi C, Ferraro L, Pollini GP, Tanganelli S, Valente F, Veronese AC: **Efficient synthesis and biological evaluation of two modafinil analogs.** *Bioorg Med Chem* 2008, **16:**9904–9910.
8. Prisinzano T, Podobinski J, Tidgewell K, Luo M, Swenson D: **Synthesis and determination of the absolute configuration of the enantiomers of modafinil.** *Tetrahedron* 2004, **15:**1053–1058.
9. Aliabadi A, Shamsa F, Ostad SN, Emami S, Shafiee A, Davoodi J, *et al*: **Synthesis and biological evaluation of 2-Phenylthiazole-4-carboxamide derivatives as anticancer agents.** *Eur J Med Chem* 2010, **11:**5384–5389.
10. Chatterjie N, Stables JP, Wang H, Alexander GJ: **Anti-narcoleptic agent modafinil and its sulfone: a novel facile synthesis and potential anti-epileptic activity.** *Neurochem Res* 2004, **29:**1481–1486.
11. Cao J, Prisinzano TE, Okunola OM, Kopajtic T, Shook M, *et al*: **SARs at the monoamine transporters for a novel series of modafinil analogues.** *ACS Med Chem Lett* 2011, **2:**48–52.
12. Yadav AV, Nade VS: **Anti-dopaminergic effect of the methanolic extract of Morus alba L. leaves.** *Indian J Pharmacol* 2008, **40:**221–226.
13. Wu CF, Zhang HL, Liu W: **Potentiation of ethanol-induced loss of the righting reflex by ascorbic acid in mice: interaction with dopamine antagonists.** *Pharmacol Biochem Behav* 2000, **66:**413–418.
14. Lalonde R, Strazielle C: **The relation between open-field and emergence tests in a hyperactive mouse model.** *Neuropharmacology* 2009, **57:**722–724.
15. Ferigolo M, Barros H, Marquadt A, Tannhauser M: **Comparison of behavioral effects of moclobemide and deprenyl during forced swimming.** *Pharmacol Biochem Behav* 1998, **60:**431–437.
16. Enríquez-Castillo A, Alamilla J, Barral J, Gourbière S, Flores-Serrano AG, *et al*: **Differential effects of caffeine on the antidepressant-like effect of amitriptyline in female rat subpopulations with low and high immobility in the forced swimming test.** *Physiol Behav* 2008, **94:**501–509.
17. Miraghaee S, Karimi I, Becker LA: **Psychobiological assessment of smoke of agarwood (Aquilaria spp.) in male rats.** *J Appl Biol Sci* 2011, **5:**45–53.

17

Unraveling the cytotoxic potential of Temozolomide loaded into PLGA nanoparticles

Darshana S Jain[1], Rajani B Athawale[1*], Amrita N Bajaj[2], Shruti S Shrikhande[1], Peeyush N Goel[3], Yuvraj Nikam[3] and Rajiv P Gude[3*]

Abstract

Background: Nanotechnology has received great attention since a decade for the treatment of different varieties of cancer. However, there is a limited data available on the cytotoxic potential of Temozolomide (TMZ) formulations. In the current research work, an attempt has been made to understand the anti-metastatic effect of the drug after loading into PLGA nanoparticles against C6 glioma cells.
Nanoparticles were prepared using solvent diffusion method and were characterized for size and morphology. Diffusion of the drug from the nanoparticles was studied by dialysis method. The designed nanoparticles were also assessed for cellular uptake using confocal microscopy and flow cytometry.

Results: PLGA nanoparticles caused a sustained release of the drug and showed a higher cellular uptake. The drug formulations also affected the cellular proliferation and motility.

Conclusion: PLGA coated nanoparticles prolong the activity of the loaded drug while retaining the anti-metastatic activity.

Keywords: C6 cell line, Gliomas, PLGA nanoparticles, Temozolomide

Background

Glioblastoma multiforme is WHO classified grade IV type of brain tumors depicting pleomorphism and atypical nuclei [1]. The current therapeutic modality for the treatment includes surgery followed by chemotherapy and radiation. Despite the progress in understanding of molecular basis in the gliomas, the prognosis of tumors remains dismal [2]. The main reason for the poor prognosis is the complexity of the brain and presence of Blood Brain Barrier (BBB). This comprises of endothelial cells that does not allow entry of exogenous material, bacteria, viruses and chemotherapeutic agents. Further, the expression of the efflux transporters adds to its complexity [3].

However, BBB allows the passage of small sized particles that are hydrophobic in nature [4]. Nanoparticles viz. solid lipid nanoparticles, polymeric nanoparticles, nano emulsions have been fabricated and used against gliomas [5-7]. Small sized particles are better permeated though the barrier with the target ability to the cancerous cells. TMZ has been a drug of choice and is used as a first line agent for the treatment of gliomas after its surgical resection. However, due to a very short half life of 1.8 h and protein binding of 15% [8,9] repeated administration of the drug is required. In addition, less site specificity is demonstrated by the drug and thus the amount of the drug reaching the tumor site becomes limited. The probability of aiming the cancerous cells with sustained release of the loaded drugs/agents by nanoparticles prompted us to undertake the present work. Nanoparticles loaded with doxorubicin, daunorubicin, epirubicin, temozolomide, methotrexate and many other such chemotherapeutic agents have been prepared and characterized for various physico-chemical properties [10-14].

Polymeric nanoparticles are amongst the most preferred delivery system for treatment of cancers due to higher penetrability, sustainability, degradability and better payload. The reason for selecting PLGA is based on its tunable properties and biodegradability. Biodegradability leads to formation of lactic acid and glycolic acid that are readily cleared form the body as by products

* Correspondence: rajani.athawale@gmail.com; rgude@actrec.gov.in
[1]Department of Pharmaceutics, C.U. Shah College of Pharmacy, SNDT Women's University, Juhu Tara Road, Santacruz (West), Mumbai 400 049, India
[3]Gude Lab, Advanced Centre for Treatment, Research & Education in Cancer (ACTREC), Tata Memorial Centre, Kharghar, Navi Mumbai 410 210, India
Full list of author information is available at the end of the article

[15]. There are no reports for the *in vitro* performance of TMZ encapsulated in nanoparticulate formulations till date.

In this purview, we had decided to fabricate PLGA nanoparticles loaded with anti cancer agent TMZ for targeting glial cells. The prepared nanoparticles could thus reach the target cells by passage though the BBB and demonstrate better penetrability though the cancerous cells. Further, we have evaluated the performance index of both the free and encapsulated drug. The results clearly suggest the applicability of PLGA coated nanoparticles for the management of gliomas.

Methods

Cell lines

The C6 glioma cell line was procured from NCCS, Pune, India. It was maintained in HAM's 12 medium (GIBCO) supplemented with 10% heat inactivated fetal bovine serum, FBS (GIBCO) and primocin (100 μg/mL). Cultures were maintained at 37°C in 5% CO_2 humidified atmosphere.

Materials

Temozolomide was a generous gift sample from Cipla Pvt. Ltd. Vikhroli, Mumbai. PLGA was obtained as a gift sample from PURAC (PDLG 50:50 grade). Poloxamer 188 (Lutrol F 68) was obtained as a gift sample from BASF Ltd. Mumbai. All the other chemicals/reagents used were either of analytical grade or the highest purity commercially available.

Preparation of nanoparticles

PLGA nanoparticles were prepared by a method principally involving solvent diffusion technique [15]. Briefly, 50 mg of PLGA was solubilised in 4 mL of acetonitrile. To the same solution 30 mg of the drug was added and solubilised. The above solution was emulsified with an aqueous solution (4 mL) comprising of 0.5% poloxamer 188 using IKA -18 Ultraturrax. Emulsified organic solvent was carefully poured into 8 mL of prechilled 0.5% poloxamer 188 solution kept stirring over a magnetic stirrer. Solvent was allowed to slowly diffuse leaving behind homogenous nanoparticles. Particle size and zeta potential for the developed particles were noted using Malvern Zetasizer 90S.

Particle size analysis and polydispersity index measurements

Particle size and polydispersity index for the developed nanoparticles were noted using Malveren Zetasizer instrument 90S (Ver 6.12.). Particle size indicates the average size acquired by the nanoparticles when dispersed in water whereas the polydispersity index depicted the homogeneity in distribution of these particles. In our study, 20 μL of the nanoparticulate suspension was suitably diluted with HPLC grade water in the polystyrene cuvette. The cuvette was then placed in the pathway of scattered light to record the fluctuations in the intensity of the light due to the presence of the particles. The intensity of the scattered light was measured at 90° using Malvern software to give the hydrodynamic diameter and the polydispersity index [16].

Zeta potential and diffusion coefficient measurements

Zeta potential measurements enable to determine surface charge acquired by the particles in solution. Samples were diluted using the procedure discussed for particle size measurement. A dip cell with electrode was inserted into the cuvette and then placed in Malvern Zetasizer 90 S. Diffusion coefficients and the particle mobility was noted for each sample. An average of approximately 15 runs was measured at 90° at the stationery level in the cylindrical cell. Auto correlated software depicted the zeta potential values for each sample depending upon the mobility of the particles towards the electrode.

In- vitro dissolution study

Diffusion though dialysis membrane was assessed to determine the diffusion and further dissolution of the drug in the dissolution medium. Quantification of the drug from the withdrawn aliquots during *in-vitro* dissolution was performed using developed and prevalidated UV method (JASCO). Pure Drug and nanoparticle batches equivalent to 20 mg of drug were weighed and transferred to dialysis membrane {cut off 6-8 KDa and diameter of 21.5 mm (Hi media dialysis membrane no. 50) sealed at one end by thread. Approximately, 1 mL of dissolution medium (sodium acetate buffer pH 5) was added in these bags, and another end was sealed. Prepared dialysis bags were dialyzed by suspending in 500 mL of pH 5 sodium acetate buffer placed in dissolution flask (Apparatus: Dissolution tester: Electrolab 6 T). Dissolution was performed in pH 5 sodium acetate buffer dissolution medium at rotation speed of 100 rpm. Intermittently aliquots were withdrawn at prefixed time intervals. Each time 1 mL was withdrawn and replenished with the same amount of dissolution medium during the study. Volume of the aliquots was made to 10 mL with dissolution medium and absorbance was measured at λmax of 255 nm on a UV spectrophotometer. Calculation for % drug release was performed at each time point and graphs indicating % drug released vs. time were plotted and are represented in Figure 1.

Cellular proliferation using MTT cytotoxicity assay

Cytotoxicity was determined using MTT assay as previously reported [17,18]. Briefly, 2500 and 1500 cells/well were seeded in a 96-well plate respectively. After 24 h

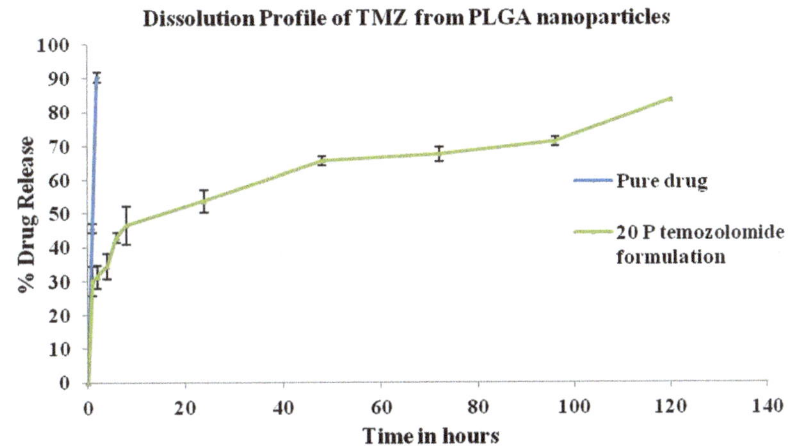

Figure 1 ***In vitro*** **Dissolution profile of pure drug and TMZ- PLGA nanoparticles.** An immediate release of 30% fraction of drug (unentrapped drug) in initial 2 h is seen, followed by sustained release of drug up to 120 h indicating the biphasic release pattern for the drug which is typical of PLGA nanoparticles.

cells were treated with pure drug TMZ, PLGA blank nanoparticles and PLGA nanoparticles loaded with TMZ at varying doses of (1,500-0.01 μg/mL). Plates were then incubated at 37°C for 72 h and 96 h in CO_2 incubator. The drug was discarded and the wells were washed twice with PBS at respective time points. MTT (1 mg/mL) was added to all the wells and incubated overnight. The plates were later centrifuged and the supernatant was finally discarded. The formazon crystals formed were dissolved in DMSO and the readings were taken using ELISA plate reader at dual wavelengths of 540/690 nm respectively. IC_{50}, the concentration required to kill 50% of the cells by TMZ was calculated. The graph was plotted on a logarithmic scale as percentage viability versus drug concentration and is represented in Figure 2.

Colony formation assay

Clonogenic assay was done to assess the long term cytotoxicity of different formulations. 600 cells were seeded in a 35 mm plate and after stabilization [19] treated with developed formulations: PLGA formulations (Drug loaded and blank) and pure drug. These were removed after an incubation period of 24 h, and the plates were washed with PBS to remove traces of the drug. Cells were later incubated in the presence of complete media for a period of 8–10 days. Fixation was done using 70% chilled methanol followed by staining using 1% crystal violet. Colonies containing 50 or more cells were counted and the results were plotted as number of colonies versus drug/formulation (Figure 3).

Wound scratch assay

Wound scratch assay was performed as per the earlier reports [18,20,21]. Approximately, 0.6 million cells were seeded into 35 mm plates. On the following day, cells were treated with 2 μg/mL mitomycin C for 1 h. The cells in the centre of the plates were later scraped using a sterile tip so as to form a wound. Sub-toxic doses of TMZ (75 μg/mL and 150 μg/mL), TMZ loaded formulations and PLGA formulations (equivalent to pure drug) were then added and incubated for 24 h. Drug formulations were removed and the plates were fixed using 70% methanol. The wound width was measured using the AxioVision Rel 4.8 imaging software, and the results were plotted as percent wound closure with respect to control. The controls were considered to be covered 100%. Results are represented in Figure 4.

Cellular morphology in presence of TMZ loaded in nanoparticulate formulation

Haematoxylin-Eosin (HE) staining was performed to observe the morphological changes upon drug treatment as described previously [17,18]. Sub-confluent cells were allowed to be grown on coverslips. Cells were then treated with TMZ, PLGA blank formulations and TMZ loaded into nanoparticulate formulations (concentration equivalent to 75 μg/mL) as done earlier and fixed using 70% chilled methanol. The cover slips were then stained using haematoxylin and eosin subsequently. Mounting was done on the glass slides using DPX mountant. Cells were later observed under Zeiss upright microscope. The results are shown in Figure 5.

Cellular uptake using confocal microscopy

The uptake of nanoparticles was performed using particles loaded with FITC, a hydrophilic dye. Sub-confluent cultures of C6 glioma were treated with only FITC and

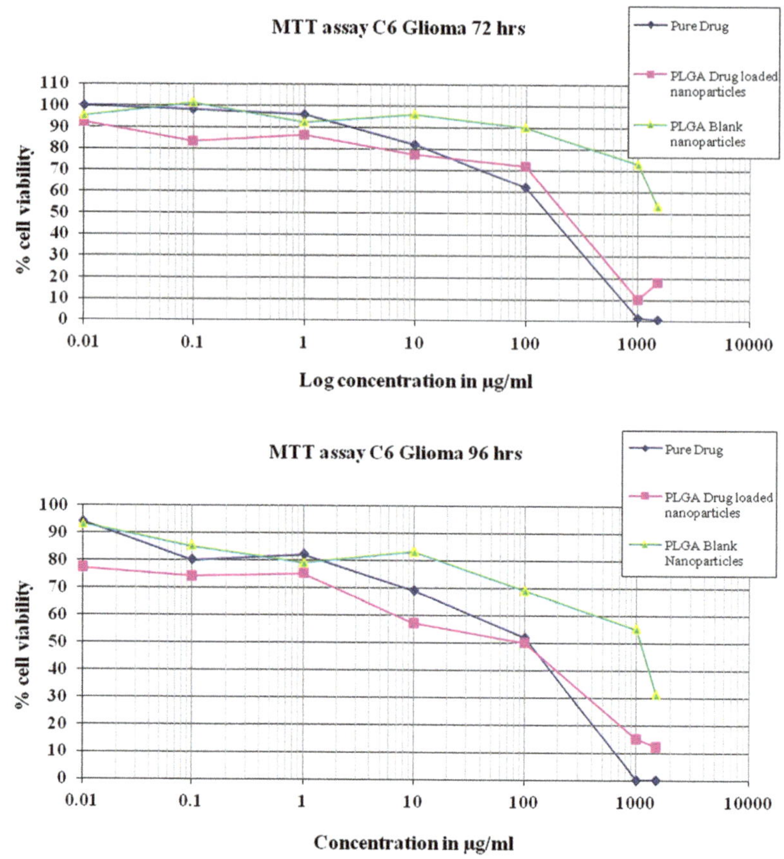

Figure 2 MTT assay performed for the pure drug and drug loaded PLGA nanoparticles. The observed IC_{50} was 150 µg/mL TMZ in pure form on C6 glioma irrespective of the time. However, the same drug when loaded into nanoparticles demonstrated an IC_{50} of 200 µg/mL and 150 µg/mL after 72 h and 96 h, respectively.

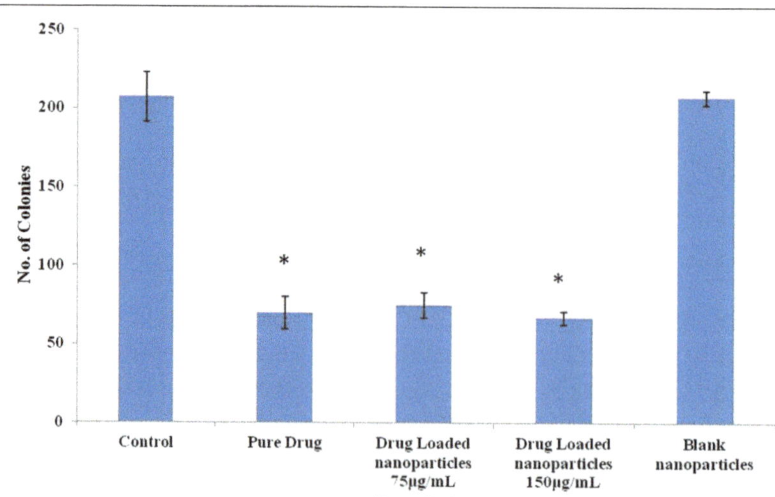

Figure 3 Clonogenic assay for pure drug, TMZ loaded PLGA nanoparticle formulations and placebo PLGA nanoparticles. The numbers of colonies for untreated and pure drug treated cells were found to be 221.00 ± 15.56 and 67.00 ± 10.26 respectively. However, in case of drug loaded nanoparticles the number of colonies were 75.00 ± 8.00, 70.66 ± 4.00 at concentrations of 75 µg/mL and 150 µg/mL respectively. (*$P < 0.05$).

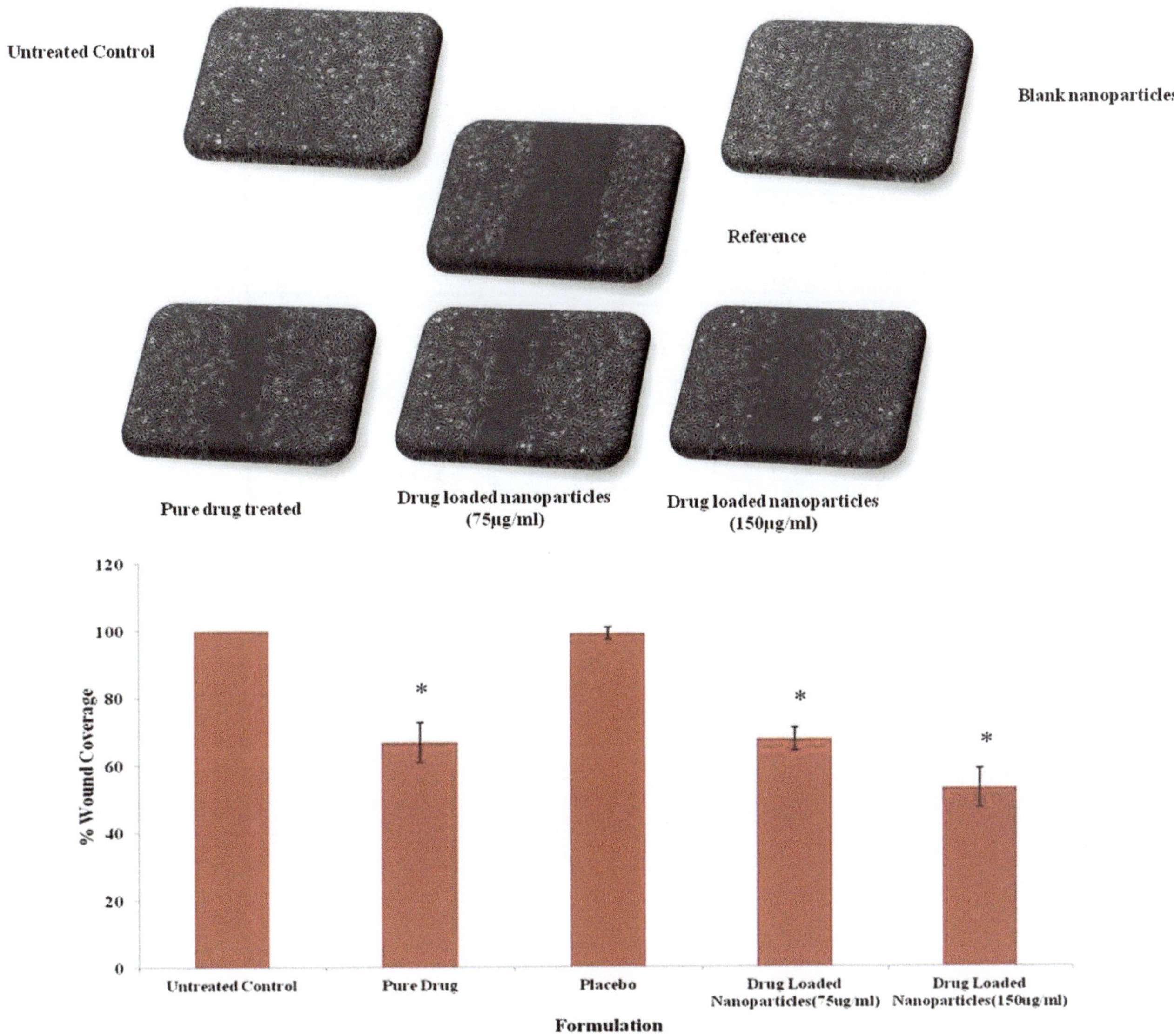

Figure 4 Wound Scratch assay to assess the role of developed nanoformulations on cellular motility. The wound coverage was found to be 66.84 ± 5.81, 67.59 ± 3.39 for TMZ and loaded nanoparticles at 75 µg/mL dose compared to the control (100%). A significant decrease in wound coverage at 150 µg/mL of nanoparticles concentration i.e 53.00 ± 5.82 is observed. However, no significant difference between placebo and control groups was observed (*$P < 0.05$).

FITC loaded nanoparticles for 2 h respectively. Cells were later washed with PBS and fixed using 1% paraformaldehyde (PFA). The cells were then treated with DAPI and then washing was done thrice with PBS. Mounting of coverslips was done using 2.5% DABCO on glass slides and then sealed with nail paint. Acquisition was done on LSM 510 confocal microscope from Zeiss at 63X. LSM image browser software was used for data analysis (Figure 6).

Cellular uptake using flow cytometry

Flow cytometric analysis was done to confirm our previous findings. Sub-confluent cultures of C6 glioma were treated with FITC and its loaded nanoparticles as done earlier [22]. Cells were thereafter harvested and fixed using 1% PFA. Cells were then washed using PBS and later suspended in the same. Acquisition was done using FACS Calibur and the results were analysed by CellQuest software (Figure 7).

Statistical analysis

All the experiments had been performed at least thrice. The results are indicated as Mean ± SD. One way ANOVA was used for the purpose of statistical significance. The results were considered to be statistically significant where *$P < 0.05$.

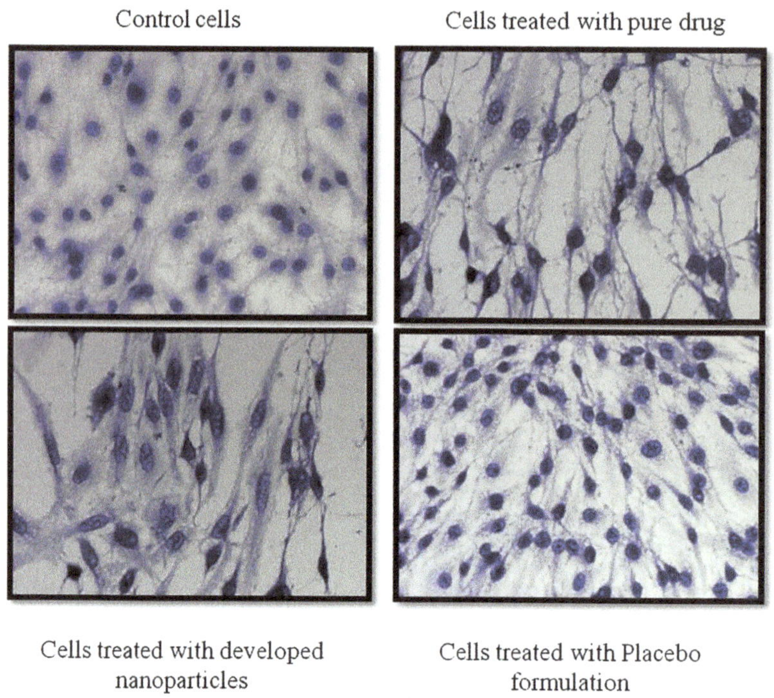

Figure 5 Changes in cellular morphology using HE staining. The spindle shape cells of C6 glioma is distorted after treatment with free TMZ and TMZ loaded formulations. Further, stress on the spindle fibres with further rounding up of the cells is being observed.

Results and discussion

Fabrication of nanoparticles

Solvent diffusion method was used for the fabrication of nanoparticles. Developed nanoparticles were subjected to particle size and zeta potential assessment. The particle size for the pure drug was found to be 1256 ± 82 nm (Approximately 1.3 μm crystalline structure particles). A size range of 150-160 nm was found for the developed nanoparticles with poly dispersity index values suggesting that the developed nanoparticles were monodisperse. The developed nanoparticles were then lyophilized and the assessment of the size was performed post lyophilisation. The developed lyophilized nanoparticulate formulation maintained the particle size even after reconstitution indicating stability and robustness of the developed nanoparticles. Zeta potential for the pure drug was found to be 17.40 ± 0.256 mV and for the developed nanoparticles was found to be – 20.50 ± 0.069 mV.

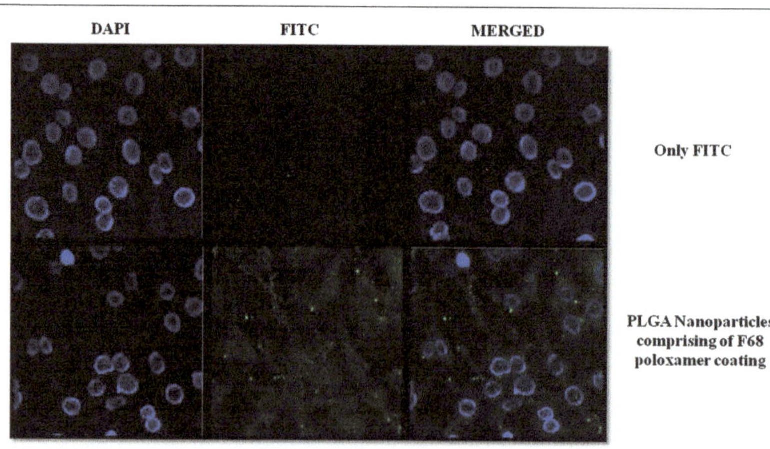

Figure 6 Immunofluorescence studies for cellular uptake of developed nanoparticles. Cells treated with FITC showed almost negligible fluorescence indicating absence of its uptake. However, cells treated with FITC loaded nanoparticles exhibited strong green fluorescence. Nucleus is stained with DAPI represented in dark blue colour.

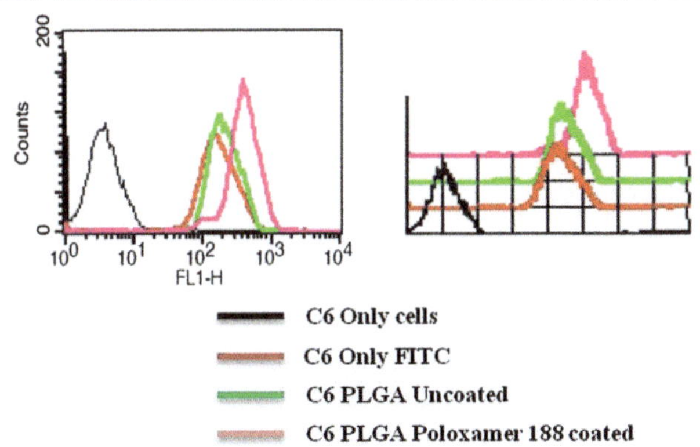

Figure 7 Cellular uptake using flow cytometry. Uptake of PLGA-poloxamer coated nanoparticles is higher (pink color) than the uncoated nanoparticles (green color) and cell treated with only FITC (red color). Black colour indicates background fluorescence because of only cells. Both 2D and 3D representations are shown.

There are numerous methods to design PLGA nanoparticles viz. solvent evaporation, microfluidisation, solvent diffusion, nanoprecipitation and salting out. The designed nanoparticles were developed successfully with solvent diffusion technique with acetonitrile as organic solvent. As the particles were designed for treatment of glioblastoma multiforme, the major obstacle to the delivery of particles would be passage though the BBB. However, BBB permit passage of small size entities (below 200 nm) which are hydrophobic in nature and hence particle size is an important parameter for entities aiming to pass the blood brain barrier. As the particle size range of our designed nanoparticles was below 200 nm better permeation can be expected though the barrier. The surface charge on the particle could be determined by the zeta potential. Negative values for the pure drug indicate that the charge on the surface is negative. The negatively charged drug particles are taken up the liver and further phagocytosized, thus only a small fraction of the drug remains in the circulation [23,24]. With the designed nanoparticles negative charge of the particles was maintained with the readings at the higher end of the negative charge. Higher values of the zeta potential determine the stability of the particle. Further, transmission electron microscopy images depicted formation of roughly round PLGA drug loaded nanoparticles. Poloxamer 188 layer with the thickness of around 6-10 nm was found using transmission electron microscopy [15].

In vitro dissolution profile

Dissolution was performed in sodium acetate buffer pH 5, considering the stability of the drug. TMZ is unstable at physiological pH and rapidly undergoes hydrolysis to form MTIC and AIC as metabolites. Pure drug diffuses out of the dialysis bag within 2 h as indicated in the graph plotted for TMZ. This reading can be correlated with the half life of the drug being 1.8 h that means the drug is readily available for its action *in vivo*. However, the developed nanoparticles demonstrated a slow release pattern of the drug when loaded into PLGA nanoparticles. The half life of the drug is extended as indicated from dissolution profile. An immediate release of 30% fraction of drug (unentrapped drug) in initial 2 h is seen, followed by sustained release of drug up to 120 h indicating the biphasic release pattern for the drug which is typical of PLGA nanoparticles. The developed nanoparticles could sustain the drug release and extend the half life of drug. The data warrants the avoidance of repeated administration of TMZ and this would be of clinical significance because the developed formulation avoids repeated administration of the active component *in vivo*. This action was further confirmed and correlated with performed *in vitro* cell line study.

Nanoparticles exert anti-proliferative effects in a dose and time dependent manner

Time and dose-dependent based MTT studies were performed to determine the IC_{50} of TMZ (72 h and 96 h). The observed IC_{50} for pure TMZ was found out to be 150 μg/mL against C6 glioma irrespective of the time. However, the same drug when loaded into nanoparticles demonstrated an IC_{50} of 200 μg/mL and 150 μg/mL after 72 h and 96 h, respectively. As the time of exposure of formulations to the cells was increased, IC_{50} showed a significant decrease. This further correlated with the dose. As the dose of the pure drug and drug loaded formulation was increased IC_{50} of the compound decreased. However, for pure drug IC_{50} was concentration but not time dependent. The developed formulations released the drug at a very slow rate and hence a small proportion of drug is available to exhibit action each time (drug release profile in Figure 2). The obtained results can be correlated with the dissolution profile of the drug. The diffusion of the drug from the formulation continued for more than 120 h. Hence, even after 96 h IC_{50} for pure drug and drug loaded nanoparticles did not match, confirming slow release of the drug from the developed formulation, as well as time and concentration dependent cytotoxicity of developed formulations. Further, to confirm the absence of cytotoxic action of the excipients used in the developed formulation, MTT assay was also performed for the blank formulation. High IC_{50} (> 1000 μg/mL after 96 h exposure) value of the blank formulation depicts the safety of the polymer and other excipients used for fabricating the nanoparticles. Based on these observations, 75 μg/mL and 150 μg/mL of TMZ in free and loaded form were selected for performing the subsequent experiments with 24 h exposure.

Effect of nanoparticles on the clonogenic potential

Anti-proliferative activity of the cells was performed using clonogenic assay. The numbers of colonies for untreated and pure drug treated cells were found to be 221.00 ± 15.56 and 67.00 ± 10.26. The number of colonies for drug loaded nanoparticles was found to be 75.00 ± 80, 70.66 ± 40 at concentrations of 75 µg/mL and 150 µg/mL respectively ($P < 0.05$). Cancer cells show a self sufficiency towards growth signals [25]. These results indicate that the cells lose the ability to replicate in the presence of drug and its formulations. The possible mechanism might be due to inhibition of EGFR and MAPK pathways by TMZ as reported earlier, that play key roles in the process of proliferation [26,27].

Nanoparticles affect motility of C6 glioma cells

Both pure TMZ and its nanoparticles formulations at dosage of 75 µg/mL showed a similar reduction in motility. The wound coverage was found out to be 66.84 ± 5.81, 67.59 ± 3.39 for pure and nanoparticles at 75 µg/mL dose compared to the control (100%). However, there was a significant decrease in wound coverage at 150 µg/mL of nanoparticles concentration i.e 53.00 ± 5.82 ($P < 0.05$). There was no significant difference between placebo and control groups respectively. The differences in migration between pure drug and drug loaded nanoparticles formulation (150 µg/mL) can be attributed to the slower diffusion of the drug from the nanoparticles. The effect of TMZ on Rho GTPase signaling might be the possible reason for hindering migration as earlier reported [27].

Changes in cellular morphology upon TMZ and PLGA nanoparticles treatment

C6 glioma cells exhibits atypical nuclei with pleomorphism characteristic of human glioma cancer. The spindle shape cells of C6 glioma is distorted after treatment with free TMZ and TMZ loaded formulation. Stress on the spindle fibres with further rounding up of the cells is being observed. Further, there is a decrease in cell volume and number with both the regimens, demonstrating equal efficacy of the developed drug loaded nanoparticles.

Immuno fluorescence showed a higher uptake of developed nanoparticles

C6 glioma cells were treated with FITC loaded into PLGA nanoparticles. Images for the uptake are depicted in Figure 6. Cells treated with pure dye showed almost negligible or background fluorescence indicating no uptake of the dye by the cells. However, cells treated with FITC loaded nanoparticles exhibited strong green fluorescence. The nucleus of the cells is stained with DAPI represented in blue colour. These results indicated that the developed nanoparticles are able to modulate the uptake of hydrophilic dye after its encapsulation in the particle. PLGA being a hydrophobic polymer with tunable properties masks the entity of FITC, a hydrophilic agent not readily permeating into the cells. Thus, it can be concluded that the uptake of hydrophilic/amphipathic agent will be enhanced by using PLGA designed nanoparticles.

Flow cytometric analysis showed an increase in uptake of developed nanoparticles

To further corroborate our earlier findings using confocal microscopy, we had performed the cellular uptake of the developed nano formulations in C6 glioma cells by flow cytometry. As can be seen in Figure 7, uptake of PLGA-poloxomer is high (pink color) than the uncoated (green color) and cell treated with only FITC (red color). These observations further substantiate our earlier findings.

Conclusions

The present study was performed to develop effective formulations targeting across the BBB. TMZ loaded nanoparticles were successfully prepared using solvent evaporation method. The developed nanoparticles exhibited slow release of the drug with prolongation of its half life. Further, cellular uptake of the nanoparticles was enhanced as confirmed using confocal and flow cytometry. These properties certainly enhance the safety profile of the drug with reducing its toxicity. Hence, it may be concluded Poly Lactic glycolic acid (PLGA) nanoparticles sustain the cytotoxic action of TMZ in C6 Glioma cells.

Competing interests

The authors declare that they have no competing interests.

Authors' contributions

DJ collected data, performed experiments such as fabrication of nanoparticles and manuscript writing. RA, AB also helped in writing the manuscript and correcting the manuscript. SS helped in collecting the information and data related to nanoparticulate formulations. PG performed uptake studies, drafting manuscript and performing cell line experiments along with YN. RG is project collaborator and provided technical expertise in correcting and drafting the manuscript. All authors read and approved the final manuscript.

Acknowledgements

The authors are thankful to DST-INSPIRE and CSIR for providing financial assistance to Ms. Darshana S. Jain and Mr. Peeyush N Goel respectively. The authors are also thankful to Cipla Pvt. Ltd and BASF, Mumbai for providing gift sample of temozolomide and poloxamer 188 respectively financially supporting the project. The authors also thank both the Confocal and flow cytometry facilities at ACTREC.

Author details

[1]Department of Pharmaceutics, C.U. Shah College of Pharmacy, SNDT Women's University, Juhu Tara Road, Santacruz (West), Mumbai 400 049, India. [2]SVKM's Dr. Bhanuben Nanavati College of Pharmacy, Vileparle, Mumbai 400 056, India. [3]Gude Lab, Advanced Centre for Treatment, Research & Education in Cancer (ACTREC), Tata Memorial Centre, Kharghar, Navi Mumbai 410 210, India.

References

1. Doolittle ND: **State of the science in brain tumor classification.** *Semin Oncol Nurs* 2004, **20:**224–230.
2. Gurney JG, Kadan-Lottick N: **Brain and other central nervous system tumors: rates, trends, and epidemiology.** *Curr Opin Oncol* 2001, **13:**160–166.
3. Laquintana V, Trapani A, Denora N, Wang F, Gallo JM, Trapani G: **New strategies to deliver anticancer drugs to brain tumors.** *Expert Opin Drug Deliv* 2009, **6:**1017–1032.
4. Begley DJ, Brightman MW: **Structural and functional aspects of the blood–brain barrier.** *Prog Drug Res* 2003, **61:**39–78.
5. Wang C-X, Huang L-S, Hou L-B, Jiang L, Yan Z-T, Wang Y-L, Chen Z-L: **Antitumor effects of polysorbate-80 coated gemcitabine polybutylcyanoacrylate nanoparticles *in vitro* and its pharmacodynamics *in vivo* on C6 glioma cells of a brain tumor model.** *Brain Res* 2009, **1261:**91–99.
6. Koziara JM, Lockman PR, Allen DD, Mumper RJ: **Paclitaxel nanoparticles for the potential treatment of brain tumors.** *J Control Release* 2004, **99:**259–269.
7. Sanchez De Juan B, Von Briesen H, Gelperina SE, Kreuter J: **Cytotoxicity of doxorubicin bound to poly (butyl cyanoacrylate) nanoparticles in rat glioma cell lines using different assays.** *J Drug Target* 2006, **14:**614–622.
8. Newlands E, Stevens M, Wedge S, Wheelhouse R, Brock C: **Temozolomide: a review of its discovery, chemical properties, pre-clinical development and clinical trials.** *Cancer Treat Rev* 1997, **23:**35–61.
9. Tentori L, Graziani G: **Recent approaches to improve the antitumor efficacy of temozolomide.** *Curr Med Chem* 2009, **16:**245–257.
10. Tian X-H, Lin X-N, Wei F, Feng W, Huang Z-C, Wang P, Ren L, Diao Y: **Enhanced brain targeting of temozolomide in polysorbate-80 coated polybutylcyanoacrylate nanoparticles.** *Int J Nanomedicine* 2011, **6:**445–452.
11. Gao K, Jiang X: **Influence of particle size on transport of methotrexate across blood brain barrier by polysorbate 80-coated polybutylcyanoacrylate nanoparticles.** *Int J Pharm* 2006, **310:**213–219.
12. Ying X, Wen H, Lu W-L, Du J, Guo J, Tian W, Men Y, Zhang Y, Li R-J, Yang T-Y: **Dual-targeting daunorubicin liposomes improve the therapeutic efficacy of brain glioma in animals.** *J Control Release* 2010, **141:**183–192.
13. Tian W, Ying X, Du J, Guo J, Men Y, Zhang Y, Li R-J, Yao H-J, Lou J-N, Zhang L-R: **Enhanced efficacy of functionalized epirubicin liposomes in treating brain glioma-bearing rats.** *Eur J Pharm Sci* 2010, **41:**232–243.
14. Friedman HS, Kerby T, Calvert H: **Temozolomide and treatment of malignant glioma.** *Clin Cancer Res* 2000, **6:**2585–2597.
15. Jain D, Athawale R, Bajaj A, Shrikhande S, Goel PN, Gude RP: **Studies on stabilization mechanism and stealth effect of Poloxamer 188 onto PLGA nanoparticles.** *Colloids Surf B Biointerfaces* 2013, **109:**59–67.
16. Nerkar N, Bajaj A, Shrikhande S, Jain D: **Fabrication of lipospheres for paclitaxel and assessment of *in vitro* cytotoxicity against U373 cancer cell lines.** *Thai J Pharm Sci* 2012, **36:**117–130.
17. Dua P, Gude RP: **Antiproliferative and antiproteolytic activity of pentoxifylline in cultures of B16F10 melanoma cells.** *Cancer Chemother Pharmacol* 2006, **58:**195–202.
18. Goel PN, Gude R: **Unravelling the antimetastatic potential of pentoxifylline, a methylxanthine derivative in human MDA-MB-231 breast cancer cells.** *Mol Cell Biochem* 2011, **358:**141–151.
19. Franken NA, Rodermond HM, Stap J, Haveman J, Van Bree C: **Clonogenic assay of cells *in vitro*.** *Nat Protoc* 2006, **1:**2315–2319.
20. Pichot C, Hartig S, Xia L, Arvanitis C, Monisvais D, Lee F, Frost J, Corey S: **Dasatinib synergizes with doxorubicin to block growth, migration, and invasion of breast cancer cells.** *Br J Cancer* 2009, **101:**38–47.
21. Lee HS, Seo EY, Kang NE, Kim WK: **[6]-Gingerol inhibits metastasis of MDA-MB-231 human breast cancer cells.** *J Nutr Biochem* 2008, **19:**313–319.
22. Jain D, Athawale R, Bajaj A, Shrikhande S, Goel PN, Nikam Y, Gude RP: **Poly lactic acid (PLA) nanoparticles sustain the cytotoxic action of temozolomide in C6 Glioma cells.** *Biomed Aging Path* 2013. doi:10.1016/j.biomag.2013.08.003.
23. Chen H, Wang L, Yeh J, Wu X, Cao Z, Wang YA, Zhang M, Yang L, Mao H: **Reducing non-specific binding and uptake of nanoparticles and improving cell targeting with an antifouling PEO-b-PgammaMPS copolymer coating.** *Biomaterials* 2010, **31:**5397–5407.
24. Frohlich E: **The role of surface charge in cellular uptake and cytotoxicity of medical nanoparticles.** *Int J Nanomedicine* 2012, **7:**5577–5591.
25. Hanahan D, Weinberg RA: **Hallmarks of cancer: the next generation.** *Cell* 2011, **144:**646–674.
26. Ramis G, Thomas-Moya E, de Mattos SF, Rodriguez J, Villalonga P: **EGFR inhibition in glioma cells modulates rho signaling to inhibit cell motility and invasion and cooperates with temozolomide to reduce cell growth.** *PLoS One* 2012, **7:**e38770.
27. Chen M, Rose AE, Doudican N, Osman I, Orlow SJ: **Celastrol synergistically enhances temozolomide cytotoxicity in melanoma cells.** *Mol Cancer Res* 2009, **7:**1946–1953.

18

Silymarin improved 6-OHDA-induced motor impairment in hemi-parkisonian rats: behavioral and molecular study

Rasool Haddadi[1,3], Alireza Mohajjel Nayebi[2,3*], Safar Farajniya[2], Shahla Eyvari Brooshghalan[2] and Hamdolah Sharifi[4]

Abstract

Background: Neuroinflammation and oxidative stress has been shown to be associated with the development of Parkinson disease (PD). In the present study, we investigated the effect of intraperitoneal (i.p.) administration of silymarin, on 6-OHDA-induced motor-impairment, brain lipid per-oxidation and cerebrospinal fluid (CSF) levels of inflammatory cytokine in the rats.

Results: The results showed that silymarin is able to improve motor coordination significantly ($p < 0.001$) in a dose dependent manner. There was a significant ($p < 0.001$) increase in MDA levels of 6-OHDA-lesioned rats whereas; in silymarin (100, 200 and 300 mg/kg, i.p. for 5 days) pre-treated hemi-parkinsonian rats MDA levels was decreased markedly ($p < 0.001$). Furthermore the CSF levels of IL-1β was decreased ($p < 0.001$) in silymarin (100, 200 and 300 mg/kg) pre-treated rats up to the range of normal non-parkinsonian animals.

Conclusion: We found that pre-treatment with silymarin could improve 6-OHDA-induced motor imbalance by attenuating brain lipid per-oxidation as well as CSF level of IL-1β as a pro-inflammatory cytokine. We suggest a potential prophylactic effect for silymarin in PD. However, further clinical trial studies should be carried out to prove this hypothesis.

Keywords: Silymarin, Catalepsy, MDA, IL-1β, 6-OHDA, Rotarod, Rat

Introduction

Parkinson's disease (PD) is the second most common and progressive neurodegenerative disorder worldwide with a prevalence of approximately 1% in people over age 60. Clinically, the disease is characterized by resting tremor, rigidity, bradykinesia and postural instability [1-3]. Progression of these symptoms is secondary to the selective loss of dopaminergic (DA) neurons in the substantia nigra pars compacta (SNpc) [4]. The primary cause of PD is still unknown although aging appears to be a major risk factor. Indeed, mitochondrial impairment and elevated oxidative stress have been linked to the PD pathogenesis [5]. It is well agreed that chronic neuro-inflammation has part in the pathogenesis of the disease [6,7]. For the first time in 1988, McGeer et al. reported increase of activated microglia in the SNc of parkinsonian patients, which was showed the involving of neuroinflammation in PD [8]. Chronic neuro-inflammation causes to damage of neural cells through generation of reactive oxygen species (ROS). In the brain, activated microglia are a major origin of cytokines and oxidizing radicals which are produced subsequent to activation of intracellular peroxidases and oxidative processes [9]. ROS can activate pro-inflammatory pathways and subsequently cause to damage of vulnerable neurons. Several studies showed that both oxidative stress and neuro-inflammation play a role in the neurodegeneration of SNc observed in PD [10,11]. The dopaminergic neurons (DA-neurons) of SNc are highly vulnerable to oxidative stress due to the high oxygen demand of this brain region together with the low levels of antioxidant enzymes [12]. Previous studies have demonstrated increase of activated microglia in the SNc of parkinsonian patients [8]. It has been found that microglial activation result in the

* Correspondence: nayebia@tbzmed.ac.ir
[2]Drug Applied Research Center, Tabriz University of Medical Sciences, Tabriz, Iran
[3]Department of Pharmacology and Toxicology, Faculty of Pharmacy, Tabriz University of Medical Sciences, Tabriz, Iran
Full list of author information is available at the end of the article

decrease of DA-neurons in patients suffering from PD [13,14]. Furthermore, the levels of proinflammatory cytokines such as tumor necrosis factor alpha (TNF-α), interleukin-1beta (IL-1β) and IL-6 that expressed by glial cells, increased markedly in the serum, brain and cerebrospinal fluid (CSF) of patients with PD [8,15,16]. To present, no effective therapies have been developed to treat PD; however, modulation of neuroinflammation is important to modify disease progression.

Silymarin (SM), is a polyphenolic flavonoid derived from the seeds and fruits of the milk thistle plant (*Silybum marianum*), routinely used to treat liver diseases and have antioxidative [17], anti-apoptotic [18], anti-inflammatory [19,20], and neuroprotective properties [21]. The anti-oxidative activity of SM is due to the scavenging of free radicals and activation of superoxide dismutase [22]. SM inhibits microglia activation and decreases inflammatory mediators; the mechanisms by which it protects dopaminergic neurons from lipopolysaccharide induced neurotoxicity [23]. Furthermore, several studies demonstrated protective effects of SM in several experimental models of neuronal injury, particularly in focal cerebral ischemia and cerebral ischemia–reperfusion-induced brain injury in rats [24,25]. However, less information is available about its effect on motor deficits associated with Parkinson disease. Therefore, the present study aims to investigate the effect of SM on 6-hydroxydopamine (6-OHDA)-induced motor imbalance and modification of cerebral levels of IL-1β and MDA as indicators of neuro-inflammation and oxidative damage.

Material and methods

Chemicals

All chemicals were purchased from Sigma Chemical Co. (USA). Solutions were made freshly on the days of experimentation by dissolving drugs in physiological saline (0.9% NaCl) except for silymarin which was dissolved in 50% polyethylene glycol (PEG). The drugs were injected intraperitoneally (i.p.) except for 6-hydroxydopamine (6-OHDA) which was injected into right substantia nigra pars compacta (SNc).

Animals

Male Wistar rats (220 ± 20 g) were used in this study. The animals were given food and water ad libitum and were housed in standard polypropylene cages, four per cage at a ambient temperature of 25 ± 2°C under a 12-h light/12-h dark cycle. Animals were habituated to the testing conditions including being transferred to the experimental environment, handled, weighed, and trained on the test platform for 10 min 2 days before the behavioral investigations were conducted. The present study was carried out in accordance with the ethical guidelines for the Care and Use of Laboratory Animals of Tabriz University of Medical Sciences, Tabriz, Iran (National Institutes of Health Publication No. 85–23, revised 1985).

Experimental protocol

In the beginning of study only the rats that showed normal walking on rotarod (700 ± 20 sec) were subjected to further experimentation. The healthy animals were randomized into 8 groups each consisting of eight rats. Rats in group 1 (control or intact) received no injection and were left untreated for the entire period of the experiment. Rats in group 2 (sham operated) were injected with saline containing 0.2% (w/v) ascorbic acid into SNc. Rats in group 3 received only 6-OHDA (8 μg/2 μl/rat; intra-SNc). Rats in group 4 pre-treated with vehicle PEG (i.p.) daily for 5 consecutive days and then were received intra-SNc injection of 6-OHDA in the same way as group 3. Rats in group 5 (positive control) pre-treated with i.p. administration of silymarin 200 mg/kg once daily (9 a.m.). Rats in groups 6 to 8 pre-treated with i.p. administration of silymarin (100, 200 and 300 mg/kg) once daily (9 a.m.) for 5 days and then were received intra-SNc injection of 6-OHDA in the same way as group 3 and then, after 3 weeks as recovery period, all animals were tested by rotarod.

At the end of experiments, the animals were anesthetized by i.p. injection of ketamine (80 mg/kg) and xylazine (10 mg/kg) and their cerebro-spinal fluid (CSF) were collected (as described below) and prepared for further analysis of IL-1β. Then animals were euthanized by an overdose of ether and the striatal tissue samples prepared for MDA assay.

Surgical procedures

The animals were anesthetized by i.p. injection of ketamine (80 mg/kg) and xylazine (10 mg/kg). After the rats were deeply anaesthetized (loss of corneal and toe pad reflexes), they were fixed in a stereotaxic frame (Stoelting, Wood Lane, IL, USA) in the flat position. The scalp hairs were completely shaved, swabbed with povidone iodine 10% and a central incision made to reveal skull. The coordinates for this position were determined according to the rat brain in stereotaxic coordinates [26] anteroposterior from bregma (AP) = −5.0 mm, mediolateral from the midline (ML) = 2.1 mm and dorsoventral from the skull (DV) = −7.7 mm. Desipramine (25 mg/kg, i.p.) was injected 30 min before intra-nigral injection of 6-OHDA to avoid degeneration of noradrenergic neurons. Then 6-OHDA (8 μg/per rat in 2 μl saline with 0.2% ascorbic acid) was infused by infusion pump at the flow rate of 0.2 μl/min into the right substantia nigra. At the end of injection, cannula was kept for an additional 2 min and then slowly was withdrawn. Sham-operated animals were submitted to the same procedure except 2 μl vehicle of 6-OHDA

(0.9% saline containing 0.2% (w/v) ascorbic acid) was infused into the SNc.

Cannula verification

For confirmation of placement of the cannula in the SNc of the brain, at the end of experiments all rats with guide cannula were euthanized by a high dose of ether and decapitated. The brains were removed and placed in a formaldehyde (10%) solution. After 1 week, the tissues were then embedded in paraffin. Then serial sections (3 µm) were cut with a microtome (Leitz, Germany), and as shown in (Figure 1), the placement of the tip of the cannula in the SNc, AP from bregma = −5.0 mm, was microscopically controlled (Figure 1). Data from rats with an incorrect placement of injecting cannula were excluded from the analysis.

Rotarod assay test

Animals were transferred to the experimental room at least 1 h before the test in order to let them habituate to the test environment. Assessment of motor coordination and balance was done by a commercially available rat rotarod apparatus on the day of 21 after 6-OHDA injection (Figure 2). Rat was mounted on the rotarod (18 RPM) and the time latency to fall from the rod was automatically recorded. All observations were made between 9 AM and 4 PM by an observer who was blind to the entity of treatments. All rats were pre-trained for 2 days in order to reach a stable performance. The latency to fall from the apparatus was recorded. Motor balance was assessed three weeks after neurotoxin injection in four consecutive times, each lasting 720 s (with one hour interval). Values were expressed as retention time on the rotarod in the four test trails.

CSF sampling

At the end of experiments, the anesthetized rats were mounted in a stereotaxic frame. The surface of the neck region were shaved and swabbed with ethanol (70%). The position of the animal's head was sustained downward at almost 45°. A needle (scalp vein-23) which connected to a draw syringe was put horizontally and centrally into the cisterna magna for CSF collection with no incision at this region. The colorless CSF sample was slowly drawn into the syringe in a volume of 100 µl. The CSF samples were kept frozen at −70°C until assessment by enzyme-linked immunosorbent assay (ELISA) method.

Malondialdehyde (MDA) assay

For MDA assessment, rats (n = 8) were euthanized, and selected brain regions (midbrain) were rapidly removed, cleaned, and immediately frozen in liquid nitrogen. Subsequently, tissue samples were weighed and homogenized (IKA Homogenizer, Staufen, Germany) in ice-cold buffer phosphate (50 mM, pH 6.0 at 4-8°C) and then were centrifuged at 10000 rpm for 20 min at 4°C. The supernatant was aliquot and stored at −80°C for further analysis. The MDA concentration in the supernatant was measured as described before [27]. Briefly, trichloroacetic acid and TBARS reagent were added to

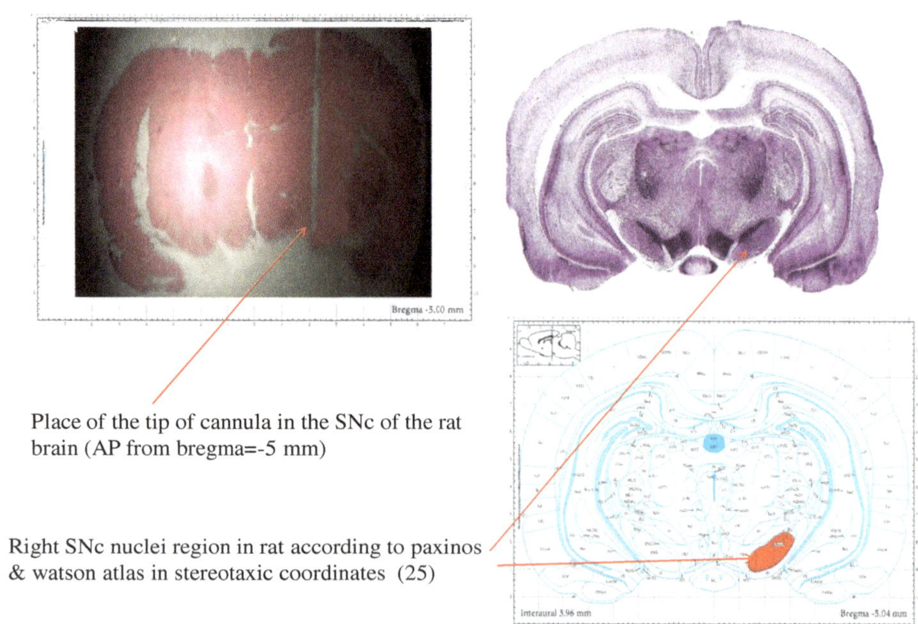

Figure 1 Photomicrograph section of rat brain. Placement of the cannula is shown according to the paxinos & Watson atlas in stereotaxic coordinates (25). Anteroposterior from bregma (AP) = −5.0 mm. Gomeri's one-step Trichrom method (10 M).

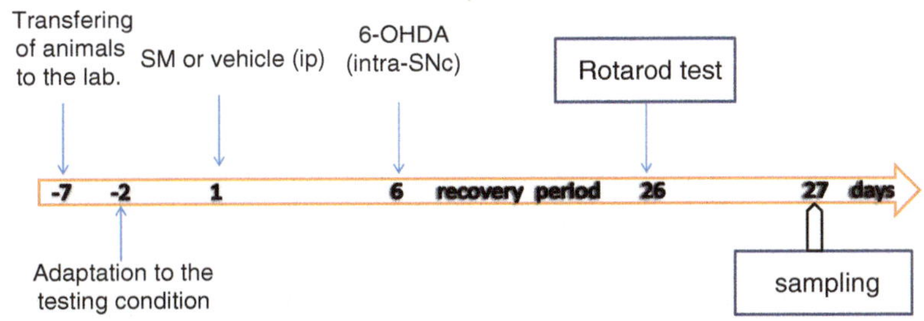

Figure 2 Schematic representation of the experimental procedure; see text for details.

supernatant, then mixed and incubated at 100°C for 80 min. After cooling on ice, samples were centrifuged at 1000 × g for 20 min and the absorbance of the supernatant was read at 532 nm. TBARS results were expressed as MDA equivalents using tetraethoxypropane as standard. The protein content of the supernatant was measured using Bradford Protein Assay kit (Sigma Chemical, St. Louis, MO).

IL-1β assay

The CSF level of IL-1β was determined by using commercial ELISA kits (Rat IL-1β kits, IBL, Hamburg, Germany) according to the manufacture's instruction. Conditions were the same for all assays. Briefly, the frozen CSF samples were diluted, added into the wells and incubated at room temperature for 120 min on a microplate shaker. After washing, diluted Streptavidin-Horseradish peroxidase-conjugated anti-mouse IL-1β was reacted for 60 min at room temperature (on microplate shaker set at 200 rpm). After washing again, the wells were developed with tetramethyl benzidine (TMB) for 10 min and the optical densities were read at 450 nm with an ELISA reader. The concentration of the IL-1β was expressed as pg/ml of CSF.

Statistical analysis

Data were expressed as the mean ± SEM, and were analyzed by one-way ANOVA in each experiment. In the case of significant variation ($p < 0.05$), the values were compared by Tukey test.

Results

The effect of intra-SNc-injection of 6-OHDA on motor- balance

The effect of intra-SNc injection of 6-OHDA on motor-coordination was evaluated by rotarod test. The duration of time to fall from rotating rod was evaluated in three groups of rats: normal, sham operated and 6-OHDA (8 μg/2 μl/rat)-lesioned rats. Drugs and vehicle were injected into the SNc through the implanted guide canula. As shown in Figure 3, 6-OHDA was able to induce significant ($p < 0.001$) motor imbalance in comparison with both normal and sham-operated rats so that 6-OHDA- lesioned rats fail to maintain their equilibrium

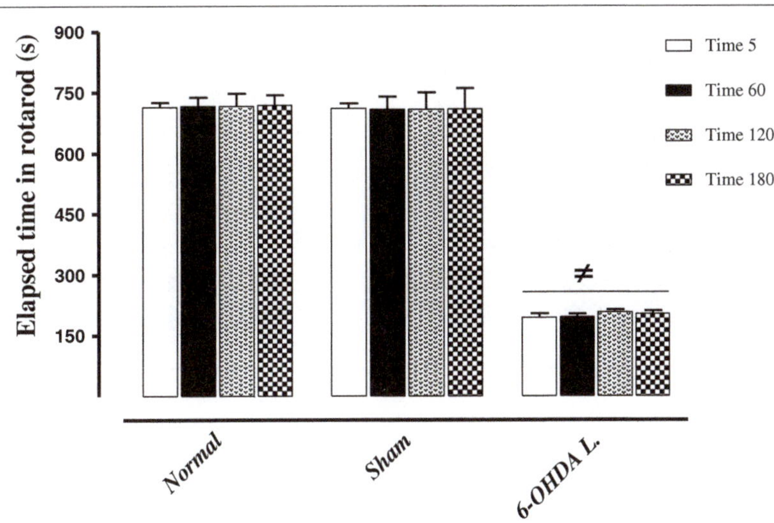

Figure 3 The rotarod results of normal, sham-operated and 6-OHDA-lesioned (8 μg/2 μl/rat) rats. Each bar represents the mean ± SEM of elapsed time on the rod (s); n = 8 rats for each group; ≠p < 0.001 as compared with normal and sham-operated groups. (L = .Lesioned).

on rotarod and a significant decrease (367% in compare with normal group) in retention time on rotarod was observed in these animals (Figure 3).

Effect of silymarin on 6-OHDA induced motor-incoordination

The effect of pre-treatment with silymarin (100, 200 and 300 mg/kg, i.p.) and its vehicle for 5 days, on 6-OHDA induced motor-incoordination was assessed 3 weeks after injection of 6-OHDA. In these groups motor balance was tested on 21 days after surgery for 4 repeated times (5, 60, 120 and 180 min). The results indicated that silymarin (in all 3 doses) significantly ($p < 0.001$) improved motor balance in 6-OHDA lesioned rats in a dose dependent manner (Figure 4A) so that the latency time to fall off increased (198%, 287% and 304%) in lesioned rats pre-treated with 100, 200 and 300 mg/kg of SM with respect to rats treated with vehicle, respectively. No alteration was observed on rotarod elapsed time in vehicle pre-treated rats (Figure 4B).

Effects of 6-OHDA and silymarin on the brain level of MDA

To investigate the possible involvement of MDA as a marker of the oxidative stress in PD we appraised the level of MDA in the ventral midbrain (brain region

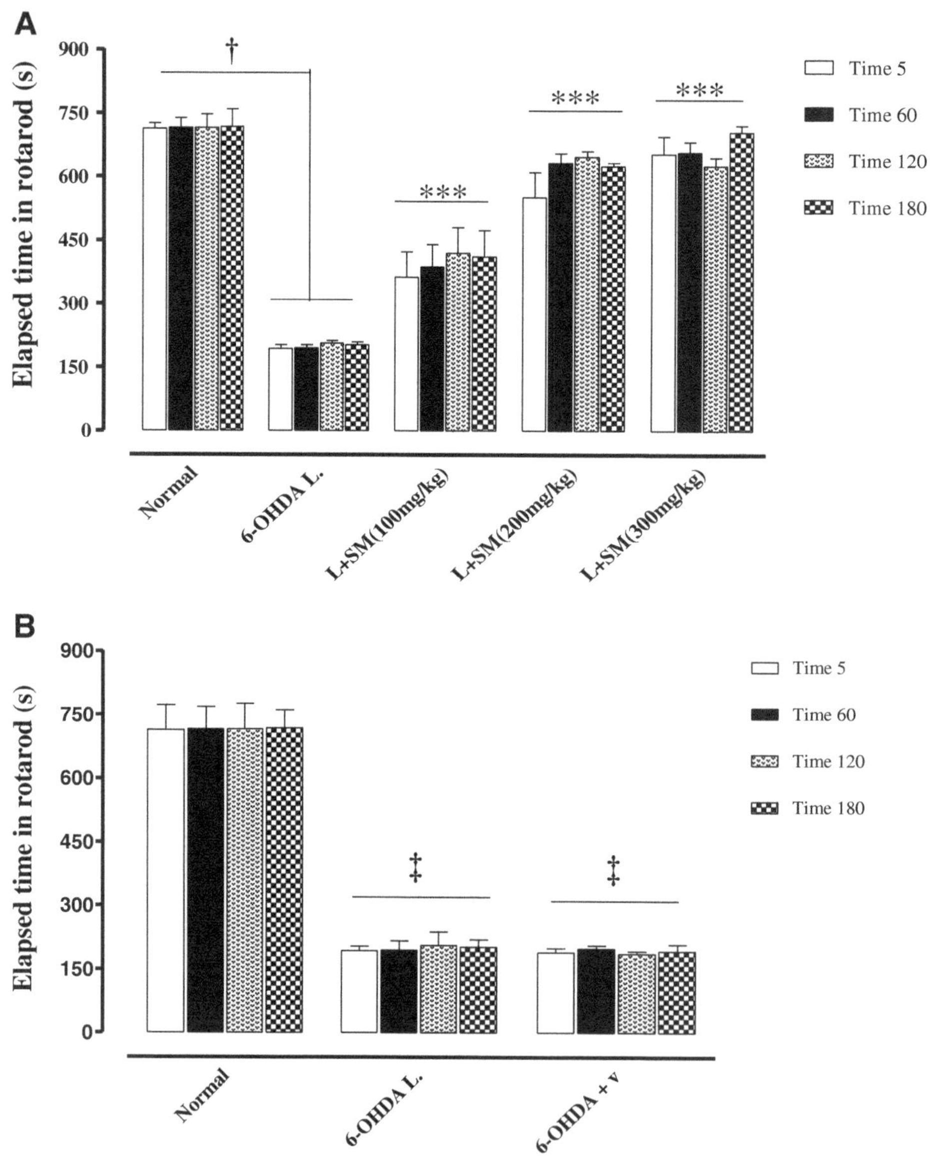

Figure 4 The rotarod test results of 6-OHDA (8 μg/2 μl/rat)-lesioned rats that pre-treated with silymarin (100, 200 and 300 mg/kg, i.p. for 5 days) (A) and silymarin vehicle (B). Each bar represents the mean ± SEM of elapsed time (s) on the rod; n = 8 rats for each group; $^{\dagger}p < 0.001$ between normal and 6-OHDA groups; $^{***}p < 0.001$ when compared with 6-OHDA lesioned rats; $^{\ddagger}p < 0.001$ when compared with normal rats. (SM = Silymarin); (V = Vehicle of silymarin); (L = .Lesioned).

containing the SNc dopaminergic neurons). In the present study 6-OHDA injection given to the rats resulted in a significant ($p < 0.001$ vs. control) increase in lipid peroxidation in brain tissue, as measured by an increase in the level of MDA in the brain (Figure 5). The MDA level in the brain was found to reduce from 11.4 ± 1.1 nm/mg protein in 6-OHDA group to 6.62 ± 0.51, 6.25 ± 0.48 and 5.6 ± 0.63 ($p < 0.001$) nm/mg pr., in SM (100, 200, and 300 mg/kg/day) pre-treated groups, in a dose dependent manner, respectively (Figure 5).

Effect of silymarin on the CSF level of IL-1β

To further explore on the protection against 6-OHDA induced Parkinson disease by silymarin, the potential effect of silymarin on the level of IL-1β, which is a key pro-inflammatory cytokine released following microglia activation, was investigated in the present study. The results showed that 6-OHDA markedly increased the IL-1β level by 286.5% ($P < 0.001$ vs. control) (Figure 6). Pretreatment with silymarin with all three doses (100, 200, and 300 mg/kg/day) significantly attenuated the level of IL-1β from 332.8 ± 52 pg/ml of CSF in the 6-OHDA group to 129.5 ± 26 ($P < 0.001$), 113.2 ± 11 ($P < 0.001$), and 86.16 ± 7 ($P < 0.001$) pg/ml respectively, in a dose-dependent manner (Figure 6).

Discussion

We have previously reported that short-term administration of silymarin at induction of PD by 6-OHDA prevents from catalepsy and reduces myeloperoxidase activity and inflammatory cytokines [28]. In the present study it has been indicated that SM improves motor impairment following intra-SNc injection of 6-OHDA in rats and amends the neuroinflammation and oxidative stress factors.

Different beneficial effects of silymarin have been reported in several in vitro and in vivo studies. Recently, the beneficial effect of silymarin has been reported in an Alzheimer's disease rat model [29]. However, less information is available about its effect on motor impairment in experimental models of PD. Behavioral assessment is a strong hallmark in evaluation of neuroprotection. Particularly, in rodents, motor-incoordination which is a reliable marker of the nigrostriatal neurodegeneration, is one symptoms of PD that can be created by unilateral intra-SNc injection of 6-OHDA and assessed by rotarod as a common standard motor-balance test [30]. In the 6-OHDA-induced PD model used in the present study, 6-OHDA caused a significant motor-imbalance, so that walking of rats on the rotating drum was lesser in 6-OHDA lesioned group compared to the control group. This is in accordance to previous studies reported that 6-OHDA (8-12 μg/2 μl/rat) induces motor-imbalance as an early symptom of PD by decreasing number of SNc neurons [30,31]. Indeed unilateral lesion of SNc compels a rat to put its weight abnormally on the both sides of its body for movement and equilibrium; hence this cause to motor disorders and motor asymmetry [31,32].

According to the results, silymarin (in all three doses) improved motor-incoordination induced by 6-OHDA. Baluchnejadmojarad et al. reported that silymarin attenuates the rotational behavior in 6-OHDA-lesioned rats and protects nigrostriatal neurons against 6-OHDA-induced neurodegenerative process [21]. 6-OHDA has pro-oxidant activity which causes to neurotoxicity. This toxin subsequent of auto-oxidation in the extracellular space, produce reactive oxygen species (ROS) [33]. Furthermore, it has been reported that 6-OHDA induce DA cells degeneration selectively by generation of free radicals and subsequently induction of oxidative stress and

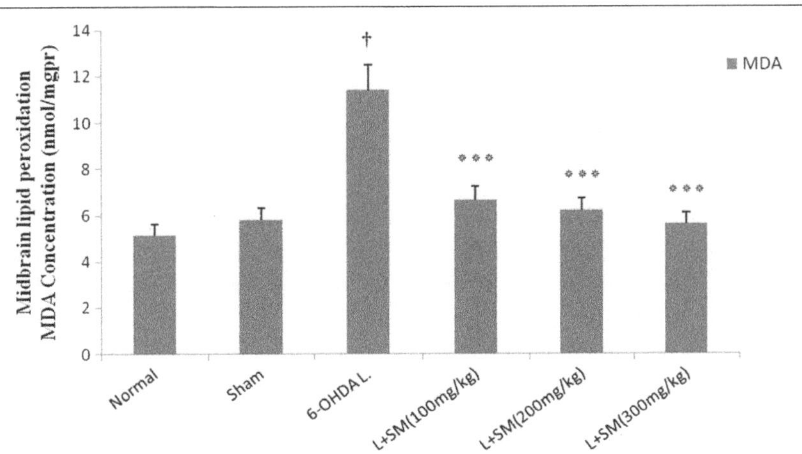

Figure 5 The effect of i.p. administration of silymarin (SM) at the doses of 100, 200, and 300 mg/kg/day (for 5 days) on lipid peroxidation in midbrain as measured by MDA concentration. Values are mean ± SEM (n = 8). †P < 0.001 from respective normal value; ***P < 0.001 as compared with 6-OHDA injected group using one way ANOVA with Tukey post hoc test. (L = .Lesioned).

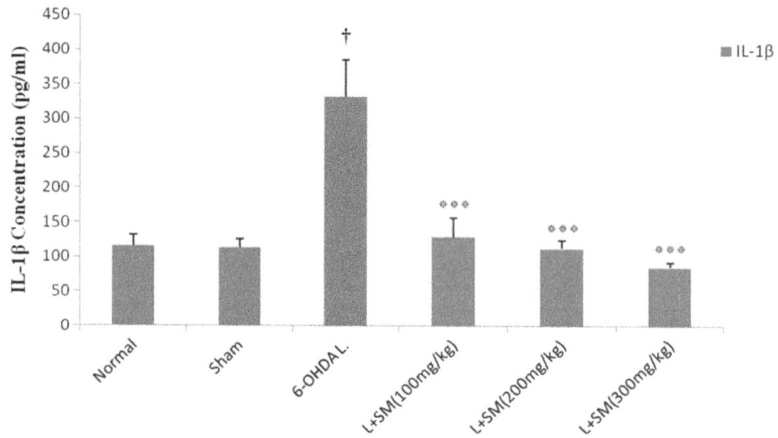

Figure 6 The effect of i.p. administration of silymarin (SM) at the doses of 100, 200, and 300 mg/kg/day (for 5 days) on IL-1β concentration in CSF (Figure 6). Values are mean ± SEM (n = 8). †P < 0.001 from respective normal value; ***P < 0.001 as compared with 6-OHDA injected group using one way ANOVA with Tukey post hoc test. (L = .Lesioned).

mitochondrial respiration dysfunction [34]. Additionally, oxidative stress result in microglia activation which leads to neurotoxicity of DA-neuron [14]. We suggest that the observed enhancement of motor balance in silymarin pre-treated hemi-parkinsonian rats in this study may be due to its possible neuroprotective effect. This effect may be exerted through counteracting oxidative stress process [35] maybe through regulating antioxidant defense system as well as inhibition of free radical generation [35].

To investigation of this issue, we also evaluated brain levels of MDA as lipid peroxidation marker in silymarin pre-treated hemi-parkinsonian rats. Malondialdehyde, a thiobarbiturate reactive substance, which formed as an end product of the peroxidation of lipids, served as an index of the intensity of oxidative stress. Our result showed a marked increase in midbrain lipid peroxidation as evidenced by elevation of MDA concentration in 6-OHDA-lesioned rats whereas, silymarin prevented dose-dependently from increase of MDA levels and restored it to the range of intact animals. According to these finding, we thought that silymarin attenuates the severity of oxidative stress through inhibition of lipid peroxidation. Also, it has been reported that the level of brain superoxide dismutase (SOD) and glutathione reductase (GR) as antioxidant enzymes decreased in parkinsonian rats and SM restored their levels in parkinsonian animals [21,36], which are totally in agreement with our findings.

Another key finding of the present study was that the reduction of brain MDA levels in silymarin pre-treated parkinsonian rats was associated with a significant decrease in pro-inflammatory cytokine. Our results showed that hemi-parkinsonian rats have a significant increase in CSF level of IL-1β, whereas its level was restored up to the normal range of intact animals by silymarin. This is in accordance with other previous studies which show that 6-OHDA- neurotoxicity induced by microglia activation and subsequent increase of TNF-α, IL-6 and IL-1β levels in both substantia nigra (SN) and striatum [8,37-39]. DA neurons in SNc are vulnerable to inflammatory affront as a major exciter of neurodegenerative disease because of high density of microglia in SNc [40]. Pro-inflammatory cytokines such as TNF-α, IL-6 and IL-1β are released by activated microglia in striatum and SN [41], which have an important role in neurotoxicity [42]. It was noted that SM reduced the levels of IL-6 and TNF-α as well as suppression of MPO activity in hemi-parkinsonian rats [28]. Furthermore silymarin inhibit nuclear factor kappa B (NF-kB) activation in DA neurons [23], and down-regulate cyclooxygenase-2 (COX-2) in brain [25], which could subsequently decrease release of IL-1β.

The anti-oxidant activity can be considered as a possible neuroprotective mechanism of silymarin in PD. It can be postulated that neuroprotective and anti-neuroinflammatory effects of silymarin, in 6-OHDA induced hemi-parkinsonian rats, are almost due to reduction of pro-inflammatory cytokines and suppression of oxidative stress.

Conclusion

In conclusion, we found that short-term pre-treatment with silymarin improved 6-OHDA-induced motor-imbalance and protected animals against neurotoxicity of 6-OHDA. Furthermore silymarin decreased CSF levels of IL-1β and decreased lipid peroxidation as evidenced by striatal level of MDA in 6-OHDA-lesioned rats. We suggest a possible protective role for SM against neuroinflammation and oxidative damages induced in PD. More clinical investigations should be done to prove its therapeutical application in PD.

Competing interest
The authors declare that they have no competing interest.

Authors' contributions
RH involved in doing behavioral experiments and drafting. MNA the supervisor of the study participated and involved in concept, design, support of study, interpretation of data and final check of the draft. SF has made contribution in study as an advisor. SEB and HS involved in doing behavioral experiments. All authors read and approved the final manuscript.

Acknowledgement
We wish to thank the Director of Drug Applied Research Center, Tabriz University of Medical Sciences for supporting this study.

Author details
[1]Student Research Committee, Tabriz University of Medical Sciences, Tabriz, Iran. [2]Drug Applied Research Center, Tabriz University of Medical Sciences, Tabriz, Iran. [3]Department of Pharmacology and Toxicology, Faculty of Pharmacy, Tabriz University of Medical Sciences, Tabriz, Iran. [4]Urmia University of Medical Science, Urmia, Iran.

References

1. Jankovic J, Stacy M: **Medical management of levodopa-associated motor complications in patients with Parkinson's disease.** *CNS Drugs* 2007, **21:**677–692.
2. Smeyne RJ, Jackson-Lewis V: **The MPTP model of Parkinson's disease.** *Mol Brain Res* 2005, **134:**57–66.
3. Warner TT, Schapira AHV: **Genetic and environmental factors in the cause of Parkinson's disease.** *Ann Neurol* 2003, **53:**S16–S25.
4. Rodriguez-Oroz MC, Jahanshahi M, Krack P, Litvan I, Macias R, Bezard E, Obeso JA: **Initial clinical manifestations of Parkinson's disease: features and pathophysiological mechanisms.** *Lancet Neurol* 2009, **8:**1128–1139.
5. Obeso JA, Rodriguez-Oroz MC, Goetz CG, Marin C, Kordower JH, Rodriguez M, Hirsch EC, Farrer M, Schapira AH, Halliday G: **Missing pieces in the Parkinson's disease puzzle.** *Nat Med* 2010, **16:**653–661.
6. Hirsch EC, Hunot S: **Neuroinflammation in Parkinson's disease: a target for neuroprotection?** *Lancet Neurol* 2009, **8:**382–397.
7. Lee J-K, Tran T, Tansey MG: **Neuroinflammation in Parkinson's disease.** *J Neuroimmune Pharmacol* 2009, **4:**419–429.
8. McGeer P, Itagaki S, Boyes B, McGeer E: **Reactive microglia are positive for HLA-DR in the substantia nigra of Parkinson's and Alzheimer's disease brains.** *Neurology* 1988, **38:**1285–1285.
9. Block M, Hong J: **Chronic microglial activation and progressive dopaminergic neurotoxicity.** *Biochem Soc Trans* 2007, **35:**1127–1132.
10. Hirsch EC, Vyas S, Hunot S: **Neuroinflammation in Parkinson's disease.** *Parkinsonism Relat Disord* 2012, **18:**S210–S212.
11. Varçin M, Bentea E, Michotte Y, Sarre S: **Oxidative stress in genetic mouse models of Parkinson's disease.** *Oxid Med Cell Longev* 2012, **2010:**624925. doi:10.1155/2012/624925.
12. Floyd RA: **Antioxidants, oxidative stress, and degenerative neurological disorders.** *Exp Biol Med* 1999, **222:**236–245.
13. Kim WG, Mohney RP, Wilson B, Jeohn GH, Liu B, Hong JS: **Regional difference in susceptibility to lipopolysaccharide-induced neurotoxicity in the rat brain: role of microglia.** *J Neurosci* 2000, **20:**6309–6316.
14. Cicchetti F, Brownell A, Williams K, Chen Y, Livni E, Isacson O: **Neuroinflammation of the nigrostriatal pathway during progressive 6-OHDA dopamine degeneration in rats monitored by immunohistochemistry and PET imaging.** *Eur J Neurosci* 2002, **15:**991–998.
15. Mogi M, Harada M, Riederer P, Narabayashi H, Fujita K, Nagatsu T: **Tumor necrosis factor-α (TNF-α) increases both in the brain and in the cerebrospinal fluid from parkinsonian patients.** *Neurosci Lett* 1994, **165:**208–210.
16. Brodacki B, Staszewski J, Toczyłowska B, Kozłowska E, Drela N, Chalimoniuk M, Stępien A: **Serum interleukin (IL-2, IL-10, IL-6, IL-4), TNFα, and INFγ concentrations are elevated in patients with atypical and idiopathic parkinsonism.** *Neurosci Lett* 2008, **441:**158–162.
17. Mandegary A, Saeedi A, Eftekhari A, Montazeri V, Sharif E: **Hepatoprotective effect of silyamarin in individuals chronically exposed to hydrogen sulfide; modulating influence of TNF-α cytokine genetic polymorphism.** *Daru* 2013, **21:**28.
18. Manna SK, Mukhopadhyay A, Van NT, Aggarwal BB: **Silymarin suppresses TNF-induced activation of NF-κB, c-Jun N-terminal kinase, and apoptosis.** *J Immunol* 1999, **163:**6800–6809.
19. Gupta O, Sing S, Bani S, Sharma N, Malhotra S, Gupta B, Banerjee S, Handa S: **Anti-inflammatory and anti-arthritic activities of silymarin acting through inhibition of 5-lipoxygenase.** *Phytomedicine* 2000, **7:**21–24.
20. Esmaily H, Vaziri-Bami A, Miroliaee AE, Baeeri M, Abdollahi M: **The correlation between NF-κB inhibition and disease activity by coadministration of silibinin and ursodeoxycholic acid in experimental colitis.** *Fundam Clin Pharmacol* 2011, **25:**723–733.
21. Baluchnejadmojarad T, Roghani M, Mafakheri M: **Neuroprotective effect of silymarin in 6-hydroxydopamine hemi-parkinsonian rat: involvement of estrogen receptors and oxidative stress.** *Neurosci Lett* 2010, **480:**206–210.
22. Muzes G, Deak G, Lang I, Nekam K, Gergely P, Feher J: **Effect of the bioflavonoid silymarin on the in vitro activity and expression of superoxide dismutase (SOD) enzyme.** *Acta Physiol Hung* 1991, **78:**3–9.
23. Wang MJ, Lin WW, Chen HL, Chang YH, Ou HC, Kuo JS, Hong JS, Jeng KCG: **Silymarin protects dopaminergic neurons against lipopolysaccharide-induced neurotoxicity by inhibiting microglia activation.** *Eur J Neurosci* 2002, **16:**2103–2112.
24. Raza SS, Khan MM, Ashafaq M, Ahmad A, Khuwaja G, Khan A, Siddiqui MS, Safhi MM, Islam F: **Silymarin protects neurons from oxidative stress associated damages in focal cerebral ischemia: A behavioral, biochemical and immunohistological study in Wistar rats.** *J Neurol Sci* 2011, **309:**45–54.
25. Hou Y-C, Liou K-T, Chern C-M, Wang Y-H, Liao J-F, Chang S, Chou Y-H, Shen Y-C: **Preventive effect of silymarin in cerebral ischemia–reperfusion-induced brain injury in rats possibly through impairing NF-κB and STAT-1 activation.** *Phytomedicine* 2010, **17:**963–973.
26. Paxinos G, Watson C: *The rat brain in stereotaxic coordinates.* UK: Academic press, Elsevier Inc.; 2007.
27. Kaya H, Sezik M, Ozkaya O, Dittrich R, Siebzehnrubl E, Wildt L: **Lipid peroxidation at various estradiol concentrations in human circulation during ovarian stimulation with exogenous gonadotropins.** *Horm Metab Res* 2004, **36:**693–695.
28. Haddadi R, Mohajjel Nayebi A, Brooshghalan SE: **Pre-treatment with silymarin reduces brain myeloperoxidase activity and inflammatory cytokines in 6-OHDA hemi-parkinsonian rats.** *Neurosci Lett* 2013, **555:**106–111.
29. Yaghmaei P, Azarfar K, Dezfulian M, Ebrahim-Habibi A: **Silymarin effect on amyloid-β plaque accumulation and gene expression of APP in an Alzheimer's disease rat model.** *Daru* 2014, **22:**24.
30. Nayebi AM, Rad SR, Saberian M, Azimzadeh S, Samini M: **Buspirone improves 6-hydroxydopamine-induced catalepsy through stimulation of nigral 5-HT (1A) receptors in rats.** *Pharmacol Rep* 2010, **62:**258–264.
31. Carvalho MM, Campos FL, Coimbra B, Pêgo JM, Rodrigues C, Lima R, Rodrigues AJ, Sousa N, Salgado AJ: **Behavioral characterization of the 6-hydroxidopamine model of Parkinson's disease and pharmacological rescuing of non-motor deficits.** *Mol Neurodegene* 2013, **8:**14.
32. Meredith GE, Sonsalla PK, Chesselet M-F: **Animal models of Parkinson's disease progression.** *Acta Neuropathol* 2008, **115:**385–398.
33. Hanrott K, Gudmunsen L, O'Neill MJ, Wonnacott S: **6-hydroxydopamine-induced apoptosis is mediated via extracellular auto-oxidation and caspase 3-dependent activation of protein kinase Cδ.** *J Biol Chem* 2006, **281:**5373–5382.
34. Barnum CJ, Tansey MG: **Modeling neuroinflammatory pathogenesis of Parkinson's disease.** *Prog Brain Res* 2010, **184:**113–132.
35. Nencini C, Giorgi G, Micheli L: **Protective effect of silymarin on oxidative stress in rat brain.** *Phytomedicine* 2007, **14:**129–135.
36. Fabiana M, Andrea T, Giulia S, Cecilia B, Manuel ZMJ, Giorgio C-F, Patrizia H: **Neuroprotective effect of sulforaphane in 6-hydroxydopamine-lesioned mouse model of Parkinson's disease.** *Neurotoxicology* 2013, **36:**63–71.
37. Mogi M, Togari A, Tanaka K, Ogawa N, Ichinose H, Nagatsu T: **Increase in level of tumor necrosis factor (TNF)-α in 6-hydroxydopamine-lesioned striatum in rats without influence of systemic L-DOPA on the TNF-α induction.** *Neurosci Lett* 1999, **268:**101–104.
38. Nagatsu T, Mogi M, Ichinose H, Togari A: **Changes in cytokines and neurotrophins in Parkinson's disease.** *J Neural Transm Suppl* 2000, **36:**277–290.

39. Mogi M, Harada M, Kondo T, Riederer P, Inagaki H, Minami M, Nagatsu T: **Interleukin-1β, interleukin-6, epidermal growth factor and transforming growth factor-α are elevated in the brain from parkinsonian patients.** *Neurosci Lett* 1994, **180:**147–150.
40. Qin L, Wu X, Block ML, Liu Y, Breese GR, Hong JS, Knapp DJ, Crews FT: **Systemic LPS causes chronic neuroinflammation and progressive neurodegeneration.** *Glia* 2007, **55:**453–462.
41. Shadrina M, Slominsky P, Limborska S: **Molecular mechanisms of pathogenesis of Parkinson's disease.** *Int Rev Cell Mol Biol* 2010, **281:**229–266.
42. Sawada M, Imamura K, Nagatsu T: **Role of cytokines in inflammatory process in Parkinson's disease.** *J Neural Transm Suppl* 2006, **70:**373–381.

19

Pharmacological evaluation of the semi-purified fractions from the soft coral *Eunicella singularis* and isolation of pure compounds

Monia Deghrigue[1*], Carmen Festa[2], Lotfi Ghribi[3], Maria Valeria D'auria[2], Simona de Marino[2], Hichem Ben Jannet[3], Rafik Ben Said[4] and Abderrahman Bouraoui[1]

Abstract

Background: Gorgonians of the genus *Eunicella* are known for possessing a wide range of pharmacological activities such as antiproliferative and antibacterial effect. The aim of this study was to evaluate the anti-inflammatory and gastroprotective effect of the organic extract and its semi-purified fractions from the white gorgonian *Eunicella singularis* and the isolation and identification of pure compound(s) from the more effective fraction.

Methods: Anti-inflammatory activity was evaluated, using the carrageenan-induced rat paw edema test and in comparison to the reference drug Acetylsalicylate of Lysine. The gastroprotective activity was determined using HCl/EtOH induced gastric ulcers in rats. The purification of compound(s) from the more effective fraction was done by two chromatographic methods (HPLC and MPLC). The structure elucidation was determined by extensive spectroscopic analysis (^{1}H and ^{13}C NMR, COSY, HMBC, HMQC and NOESY) and by comparison with data reported in the literature.

Results: The evaluation of the anti-inflammatory activity of different fractions from *Eunicella singularis* showed in a dependent dose manner an important anti-inflammatory activity of the ethanol fraction, the percentage of inhibition of edema, 3 h after carrageenan injection was 66.12%, more effective than the reference drug (56.32%). In addition, this ethanolic fraction showed an interesting gastroprotective effect compared to the reference drugs, ranitidine and omeprazol. The percentage of inhibition of gastric ulcer induced by HCl/ethanol in rats was 70.27%. The percentage of the reference drugs (ranitidine and omeprazol) were 65 and 87.53%, respectively. The purification and structure elucidation of compound(s) from this ethanolic fraction were leading to the isolation of five sterols: cholesterol (5α-cholest-5-en-3β-ol) **(1)**; ergosterol (ergosta-5,22-dien-3β-ol) **(2)**; stigmasterol (24-ethylcholesta-5, 22-dien-3b-ol) **(3)**; 5α,8α-epidioxyergosta 6,22-dien-3β-ol **(4)** and 3β-hydroxy-5α,8α-epidioxyergosta-6-ene **(5)**; and one diterpenoid: palmonine D **(6)**.

Conclusion: Based on data presented here, we concluded that diterpenoids and sterols detected in the ethanolic fraction can be responsible for its pharmacological activity.

Keywords: *Eunicella singularis*, Anti-inflammatory activity, Gastroprotective effect, Marine natural product, Diterpenoid, Sterols

* Correspondence: monia.deghrigue@laposte.net
[1]Laboratoire de développement chimique, galénique et pharmacologique des médicaments (LR12ES09). Equipe de Pharmacologie marine, Faculté de pharmacie de Monastir, Université de Monastir, Monastir, Tunisie
Full list of author information is available at the end of the article

Background

Nature has developed an enormous diversity during several billion years of evolution. The Mediterranean Area represents one of the world's major centers of animal diversity; with around 20 gorgonian species, four belong to the genus *Eunicella*: *E. verrucosa*, *E. filiformis*, *E. cavolini* and *E. singularis* [1].

Although natural compounds have been replaced by synthetic chemistry as the main source of new drugs, marine invertebrates remain an unequalled source of biochemical diversity. The studies on gorgonian have great importance in the research of marine resources of active compounds mainly by the pharmaceutical industry or for other uses. In fact, the gorgonians (Anthozoa, Gorgonacea) are known for possessing a wide range of pharmacologic and health promoting properties including antibacterial [2], antiviral [3], antiplasmodial [4], antifouling [5], antiproliferative [6], cytotoxic [7] and insecticidal [8] effects. The gorgonian of the genus *Eunicella* has been demonstrated to contain a wide variety of natural products as steroids and diterpenes [9,10]. These compounds posses anticancer, gastroprotective and anti-inflammatory activities [11]. For many years, our marine pharmacological group in Tunisia has been involved in an accurate research program on gorgonian constituents in order to define both their chemical composition and their biological activities. On the other hand, the use of non-steroidal anti-inflammatory drugs (NSAID) for the treatment of inflammatory diseases is associated with adverse effects as peptic ulcer [12]. Therefore, the research of potent anti-inflammatory drugs from natural sources and with fewer side effects had become necessary. This study has yielded the anti-inflammatory and gastroprotective effects of the organic extract and its semi-purified fractions of the white gorgonian *Eunicella singularis* (Esper, 1791). The structure elucidation of the isolated compounds from the active fraction was done by 1D and 2D NMR experiments and by comparison with literature data.

Methods

General procedures

HPLC was performed using a Waters model 510 pump equipped with Waters Rheodine injector and a differential refractometer, model 401. Medium pressure liquid chromatography (MPLC) was performed on a Buchi apparatus using a silica gel (230–400 mesh) column.

NMR spectra were obtained on Varian Inova 400 and Varian Inova 500 NMR spectrometers (^{1}H at 400 and 500 MHz, ^{13}C at 100 and 125 MHz, respectively) equipped with a Sun hardware, δ (ppm), *J* in hertz, and spectra referred to CD_3Cl_3 (δH=7.27; δC= 70.0) as internal standard. High-resolution ESIMS spectra were performed with a Micromass QTOF Micro mass spectrometer. All reagents were commercially obtained (Aldrich, Fluka) at the highest commercial quality and used without further purification except where noted. All reactions were monitored by TLC on silica gel plates (Macherey–Nagel). Carrageenan (BDH Chemicals Ltd Poole England), Acetylsalicylate of Lysine (ASL) were purchased from Sigma Chemical (Berlin, Germany). Ranitidine was obtained from Medis (Tunis, Tunisia), omeprazole was obtained from AstraZeneca (Monts).

Collection and extraction

E. singularis was collected from the Mediterranean Sea in various areas of the coastal region of Tabarka (Tunisia), in June 2010, at a depth between 20 and 30 m. Identification of specimens was carried out in the National Institute of Marine Sciences and Technologies (Salamboo, Tunisia) where a voucher specimen of *E. singularis* was deposited under the following reference 1132. After maceration of 600 g of the powdered material with methanol and dichloromethane (1:1, v/v) for 48h three times, the organic extract (40 g) was purified, using C18 cartridges (Sep-pack, Supelco), by gradient elution with different organic solvents in the order of decreased polarity: ethanol, acetone and methanol/CH_2Cl_2 (1:1) to give three semi-purified fractions: ethanol (F-EtOH), acetone (F-Ac) and methanol/CH_2Cl_2 (F-MeOH/CH_2Cl_2) fractions. Organic solvents were removed from recuperated fractions using rotating evaporator at 40°C.

Purification, isolation and structure elucidation

F-EtOH (15 g) was fractionated according to the Kupchan partitioning procedure [13] as follow: the ethanolic fraction was dissolved in a mixture of MeOH/H_2O containing 10% H_2O and partitioned against *n*-hexane to give 10.3 g of the crude extract. The water content (% v/v) of the MeOH extract was adjusted to 30% and partitioned against $CHCl_3$ to give 3.9 g of the crude extract. The aqueous phase was concentrated to remove MeOH and then extracted with *n*-BuOH (268 mg of crude extract) (Figure 1). The *n*-hexane extract (5 g) was fractioned by silica gel MPLC using a solvent gradient system from CH_2Cl_2 to MeOH. Fraction eluted with CH_2Cl_2: MeOH 99:1 (307 mg) was purified by HPLC on a Nucleodur 100–5 C18 (5 μm; 10 mm i.d. × 250 mm) with 99% MeOH: H_2O as eluent (flow rate 3mL/min) to give 1.3 mg of 5α-cholest-5-en-3β-ol (**1**) (t_R=55 min) and 2.4 mg of 24-ethylcholesta-5, 22-dien-3β-ol (**3**) (t_R=83min) (Figure 1).

Fraction eluted with CH_2Cl_2:MeOH 95:5 (288 mg) was purified by HPLC on a Nucleodur 100–5 C18 (5 μ, 4.6 mm i.d. × 250 mm) with 95% MeOH:H_2O as eluent (flow rate 1 mL/min) to give 0.1 mg of ergosta-5,22-dien-3β-ol (**2**) (t_R=74 min) (Figure 1).

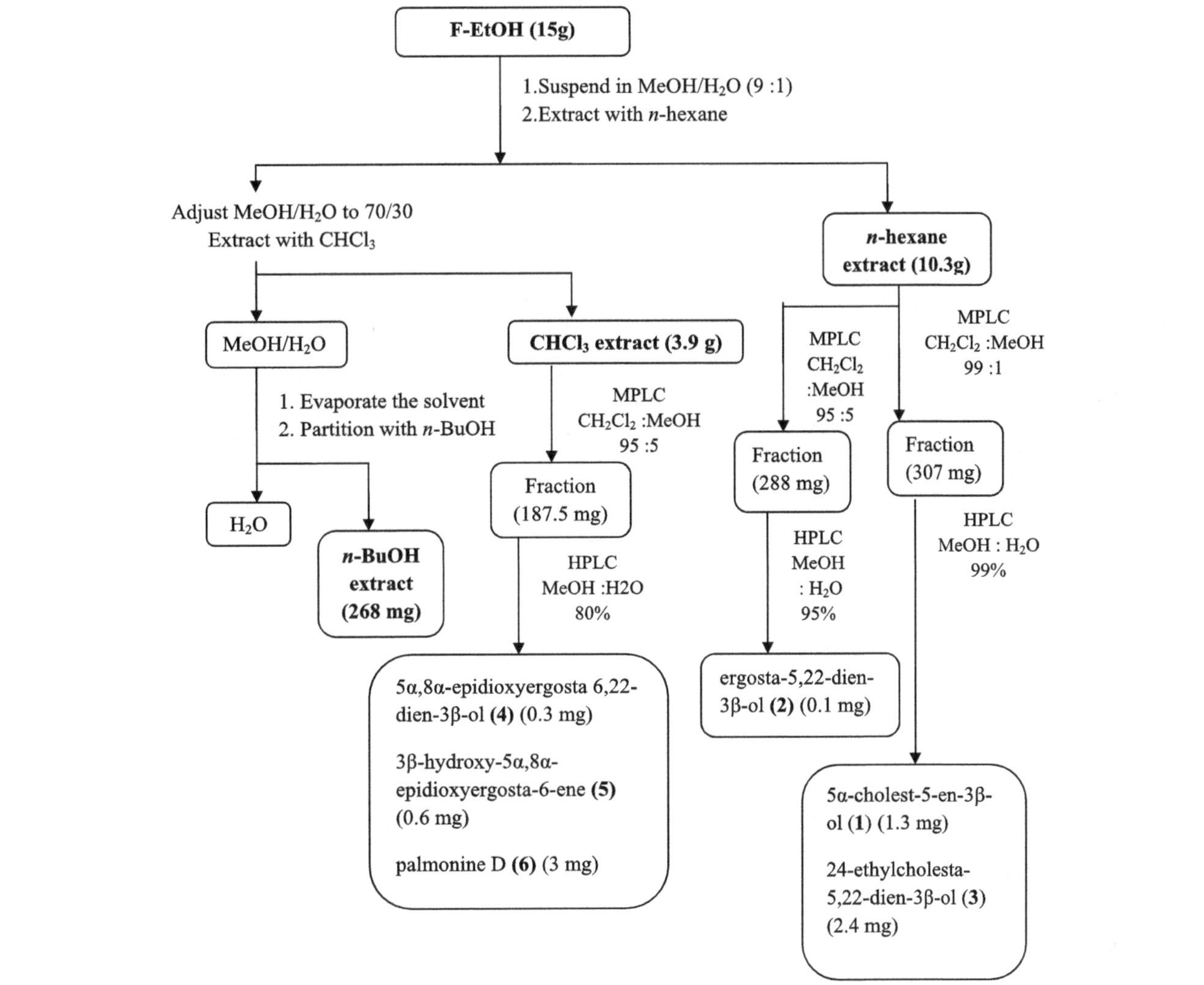

Figure 1 Purification and separation process of the isolation of six compounds from the ethanolic fraction from *E. singularis*.

The $CHCl_3$ extract (3.9 g) was chromatographed by silica gel MPLC using a solvent gradient system from CH_2Cl_2 to CH_2Cl_2: MeOH 1:1.

Fraction eluted with CH_2Cl_2: MeOH 95:5 (187.5 mg) was further purified by HPLC on a Nucleodur 100–5 C18 (5 μ, 4.6 mm i.d. × 250 mm) with 80% MeOH:H_2O as eluent (flow rate 1 mL/min) to give 0.3 mg of 5α,8α-epidioxyergosta 6,22-dien-3β-ol (**4**) (t_R=29 min), and 0.6 mg of 3β-hydroxy-5α,8α-epidioxyergosta-6-ene (**5**) (t_R=2 min) and 3 mg of palmonine D (**6**) (t_R=3 min) (Figure 1).

The purities of compounds were determined to be greater than 95% by HPLC and NMR. Furthermore, HPLC chromatograms and spectroscopic data of each compound were reported (Additional file 1).

Pharmacological evaluation

Animals

Wistar rats of either sex, weighing 150–200 g were obtained from Pasteur Institute (Tunis, Tunisia). Housing conditions and *in vivo* experiments were approved according to the guidelines established by the European Union on Animal Care (CCE Council 86/609).

Carrageenan-Induced Rat Paw Edema

The anti-inflammatory activity of the organic extract and its semi-purified fractions on carrageenan-induced paw edema was determined according to Winter et al. [14]. The animals were divided into eleven groups of six rats each. The control group received an intraperitoneal (i.p.) dose of saline solution (NaCl 9g/L, 2.5 mL/kg), the reference group received Acetylsalicylate of Lysine (ASL) (300 mg/kg, i.p.), and the test groups received the organic extract of *E. singularis* (50, 100 and 200 mg/kg, i.p.) and its semi-purified fractions F-EtOH, F-Ac and F-MeOH/CH_2Cl_2 (25 and 50 mg/kg, i.p.). After 30 min, 0.05mL of a 1% carrageenan suspension was injected into the left hind paw. The paw volume up to the tibiotarsal articulation was measured using a plethysmometer (model

7150, Ugo Basile, Italy). The measures were determined at 0 h (V_0) (before carrageenan injection) and 1, 3 and 5 h later (V_T) (after carrageenan injection). Paw swelling was determined for each rat and the difference between V_T and V_0 was taken as the edema value. The percentages of inhibition were calculated according to the following formula:

$$\% \text{ inhibition} = \left[(V_T - V_0)_{control} - (V_T - V_0)_{treated\ group} / (V_T - V_0)_{control}\right] \times 100$$

Gastric lesions induced by HCl/ethanol

The gastroprotective activity of the organic extract of *E. singularis* and its semi-purified fractions F-EtOH, F-Ac and F-MeOH/CH_2Cl_2 was studied in 150 mM HCl/EtOH induced gastric ulcer [15]. Rats were divided into fifteen groups, fasted for 24 h prior receiving an intraperitoneal doses of vehicle (NaCl 9g/L, 2.5 mL/kg) for the control group, organic extract (50, 100 and 200 mg/kg, i.p.) and its semi-purified fractions F-EtOH, F-Ac and F-MeOH/CH_2Cl_2 (5, 10 and 25 mg/kg, i.p.) for the twelve test groups. Two other groups received ranitidine (60 mg/kg, i.p.) and omeprazole (30 mg/kg, i.p.) as reference drugs. After 30 min, all groups were orally treated with 1mL of 150 mM HCl/EtOH solution for gastric ulcer induction. Animals were killed 1 h after the administration of ulcerogenic agent, their stomachs were excised and opened along the great curvature, washed and stretched on cork plates. The surface was examined for the presence of lesions and the extent of the lesions was measured. The summative length of the lesions along the stomach was recorded (mm) as lesion index.

Statistical analysis

Data are presented as the mean±standard error (s.e.m). Statistical analysis was performed using Student's t-test. The significance of difference was considered to include values of $P<0.05$.

Results and discussion

The current study was carried out to determine the in *vivo* anti-inflammatory and gastroprotective activities of the organic extract of *E. singularis* and its semi-purified fractions. The chemical composition of the more effective fraction was determined by both 1D and 2D NMR experiments.

As shown in Figure 2, 1D and 2D NMR analysis of the ethanolic fraction (F-EtOH) from the gorgonian *E. singularis* resulted in the identification of six compounds.

Compound **1** was isolated as colorless powder. The molecular formula was determined to be $C_{27}H_{46}O$. Analysis of ^1H and ^{13}C NMR data evidenced a Δ^5 dihydroxysteroid structure with a saturated C8 cholestane side chain. Comparison with literature data allowed assigning the 5α-cholest-5-ene-3β-ol (cholesterol) structure [16].

Compound **2** has a molecular formula of $C_{28}H_{46}O$ as determined by HRESIMS. Compound **2** was identified as ergosta-5,22-dien-3β-ol (ergosterol) [17] (Figure 2). This compound was also isolated from the soft coral *Tubastraea coccinea* and *T. tagusensis* [17].

Compound **3** was isolated as colorless powder. The molecular formula was determined to be $C_{28}H_{46}O$. Its identity was determined by 1D and 2D NMR data as 24-ethylcholesta-5,22-dien-3b-ol (stigmasterol) earlier isolated from the halophyte *Salicornia herbacea* [18] and then reported also from the plant *Aglaia eximia* [19].

Compound **4** was isolated as white powder. The molecular formula was determined to be $C_{28}H_{44}O_3$ by HRESIMS data. NMR data disclosed the 5α,8α-epidioxyergosta 6,22-dien-3β-ol structure. This compound was also isolated from the fungus *Sporothrix schenckii* [20] and the fungus *Cryptoporus volvatus* [21].

Compound **5** has a molecular formula of $C_{28}H_{46}O_3$ as determined by HRESIMS. ^1H and ^{13}C NMR indicated that compound **5** is the Δ^{22} derivative of compound **4**. Therefore compound **5** was identified as 3β-hydroxy-5α,8α-epidioxyergosta-6-ene [21].

Compound **6** was isolated as colorless oil. The molecular formula was determined to be $C_{24}H_{36}O_6$ by HRESIMS. The analysis of ^1H NMR spectrum clearly revealed an eunicellin diterpenoid structure. The ^{13}C NMR spectrum revealed 24 carbon signals. ^1H- and ^{13}CNMR assignments were carried out with the aid of the detailed 2D analyses (COSY, HMQC, NOESY, and HMBC) and the resulting NMR evidence revealed **6** to be defined as palmonine D [22]. Three sterols named 5α, 8α-epidioxysterols, pregnanes and 9,11-secosterols were separated from *E. cavolini*, another specie of the genus *Eunicella* [10,11]. The five sterols identified in our study were isolated for the first time from *E. singularis* and were not yet found with another specie from this genus.

Palmonine D is also purified from *E. labiata*, another specie of the genus *Eunicella* [22]. Other researchers reported the isolation of five diterpenoids from the gorgonian *E. labiata*, labiatamide A, labiatamide B, labiatin A, labiatin B and labiatin C [23] but these compounds were not yet separated from *E. singularis*. Massileunicellin A, was obtained from *E. cavolini* [24] but also was not identified from *E.singularis*.

The results reported in Figures 3 and 4 showed the anti-inflammatory effects of organic extract and its semi-purified fractions from *E. singularis* administered intraperitoneally.

E. singularis organic extract presented a dose- related, statistically significant anti-inflammatory activity on carrageenan induced paw edema which was comparable with the reference drug, Acetylsalicylate of Lysine (ASL),

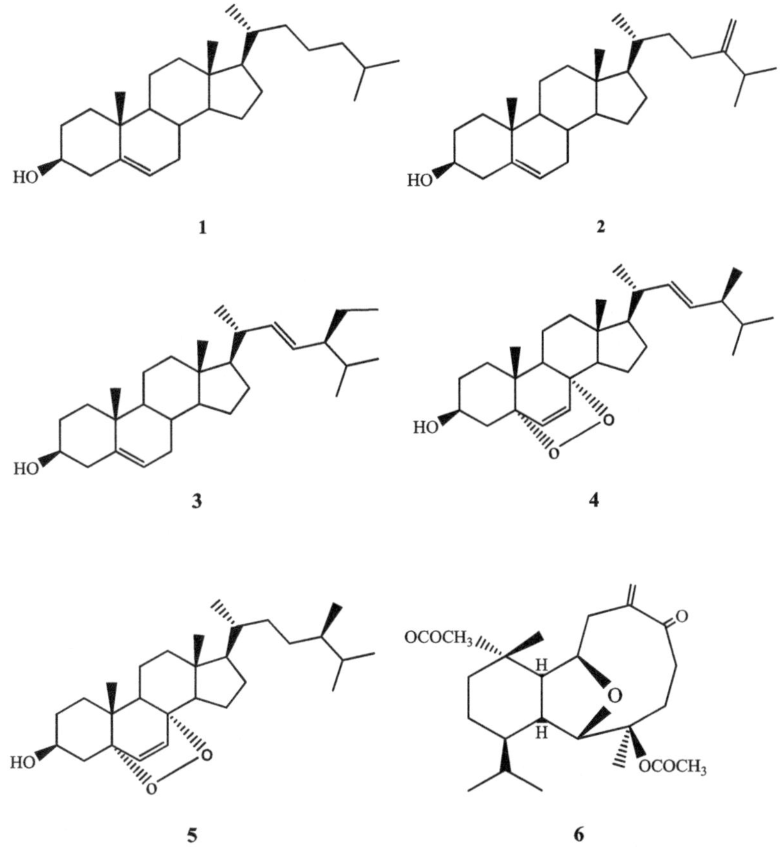

Figure 2 Chemical structures of six compounds isolated from the white gorgonian *E. singularis*. Five sterols **(1-5)**: 5α-cholest-5-en-3β-ol **(1)**; ergosta-5,22-dien-3β-ol **(2)**; 24- ethylcholesta-5,22-dien-3b-ol **(3)**; 5α,8α-epidioxyergosta 6,22-dien-3β-ol **(4)** and 3β-hydroxy- 5α,8α-epidioxyergosta-6-ene **(5)**; and one diterpenoid: palmonine D **(6)**.

a potent inhibitor of cyclooxygenase-2. The percent inhibition of edema at dose levels of 50, 100 and 200 mg/kg were 42.61%, 56.47% and 64.31% (at 3 h), respectively (Table 1). The semi-purified fractions (F-Ac, F-EtOH, F-MeOH/CH_2Cl_2) were assessed for anti-inflammatory effect at 25 and 50 mg/kg. A dose-related anti-inflammatory property was observed for the three fractions with highly significant activity of F-EtOH at dose 50 mg/kg with a percentage of inhibition of 66.12% at 3 h. While F-Ac and F-MeOH/CH_2Cl_2 at a dose of 50 mg/kg reduced

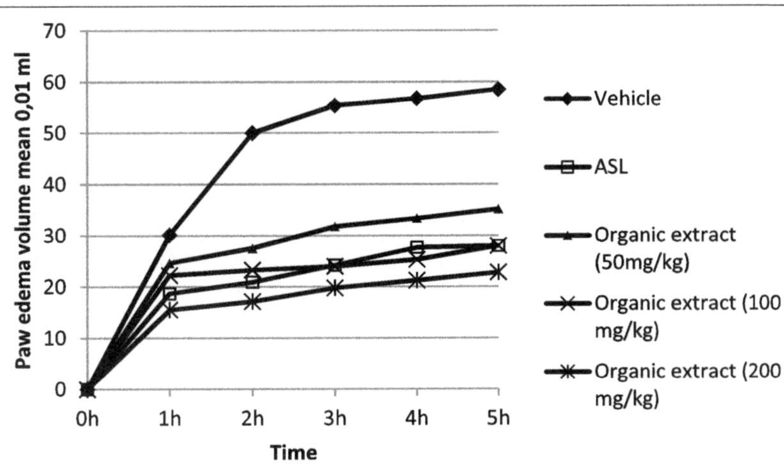

Figure 3 Effect of intraperitoneal administration of the organic extract from *E. singularis* on the carrageenan-induced rat paw edema. Values are mean ± SEM.

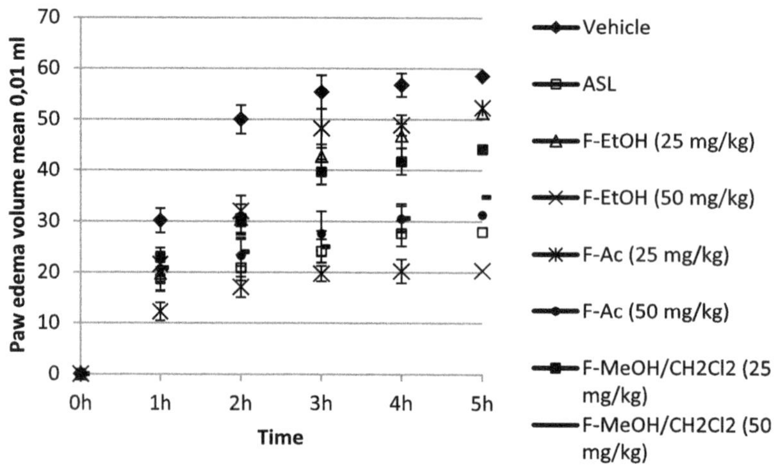

Figure 4 Effect of intraperitoneal administration of semi-purified fractions (F-Ac, F-EtOH and F-MeOH/CH2Cl2 from *E. singularis* on the carrageenan-induced rat paw edema. Values are mean ± SEM.

edema with a percentage of 50.22 and 54.78% (at 3 h), respectively. ASL as a reference standard drug inhibited the edema formation due to carrageenan to an extent of 56.32% (at 3 h) at the dose of 300 mg/kg. The development of edema induced by carrageenan corresponds to the events in the acute phase of inflammation mediated by histamine, bradykinin and prostaglandins produced under an effect of cyclooxygenase-2 (COX-2) [25]. This enzyme is an inducible cyclooxygenase which boosts the inflammatory response by COX-2 mediated prostaglandin E_2 (PGE_2) [26]. Hence, it is probably that the organic extract and its semi-purified fractions from the gorgonian *E. singularis* reduced inflammation by blocking the cyclooxygenase2 (COX-2). Morever, several studies reported that steroids isolated from other species of the genus *Eunicella* have anti-inflammatory activity such as secosteroids [11]. The high anti-inflammatory activity of the fraction F-EtOH can be related with the presence of its main steroid constituents. The chemical analysis of this fraction (F-EtOH) revealed the presence of five sterols: 5α-cholest-5-en-3β-ol (cholesterol) **(1)**; ergosta-5,22-dien-3β-ol (ergosterol) **(2)**; 24-ethylcholesta-5,22-dien-3b-ol (stigmasterol) **(3)**; 5α,8α-epidioxyergosta 6,22-dien-3β-ol **(4)** and 3β-hydroxy-5α,8α-epidioxyergosta-6-ene **(5)**.

The gastroprotective effect of *E. singularis* organic extract and its semi-purified fractions against HCl/EtOH induced gastric damage in rats is shown in (Table 2) and the results are comparable to that of the reference drugs ranitidine, histamine H_2 receptor antagonist, and omeprazole, a proton pump inhibitor [27]. Oral administration of

Table 1 Anti-inflammatory effect of the intraperitoneal administration of *E. singularis* organic extract and its semi-purified fractions (F-EtOH, F-Ac and F-MeOH/CH_2Cl_2) and of reference drug (Acetylsalicylate of Lysine; ASL) in carrageenan-induced rat paw edema test

Treatment	Dose (mg/kg)	Edema (10^{-2}ml) (mean±s. e. m)			Edema inhibition (%)		
		1 h	3 h	5 h	1 h	3 h	5 h
Vehicle	-	30.12±2.38	55.35±3.3	58.5±4.69	-	-	-
Organic extract	50	24.62±2.8	31.76±3.6**	35.14±4.1*	18.26	42.61	39.92
	100	22.22±2.9	23.94±4.1**	27.95±1.5**	32.84	56.47	52.21
	200	15.5±3.2*	19.75±2.4**	22.75±3.6**	48.53	64.31	61.11
F-EtOH	25	19.73±1.6	42.74±2.7	51.26±2.6	34.49	22.78	12.36
	50	12.25±1.5**	18.75±2**	20.37±2.4**	59.32	66.12	65.17
F-Ac	25	21.55±2.6	48.24±2.4	52.33±3.5	28.42	12.84	10.53
	50	20.63±2.4	27.55±3.2**	31.27±2.7*	31.48	50.22	46.54
F-MeOH/CH_2Cl_2	25	22.85±3.2	39.67±2.6	44.2±4.8	24.12	28.32	24.43
	50	20.82±2.4	25.02±2.9**	34.79±3.4*	30.86	54.78	40.52
ASL	300	19.66±3.4	24.17±2.7**	27.95±3.1**	34.71	56.32	52.22

Values are expressed as mean±SEM; n=6 animals. *P<0.01, **P<0.001.

Table 2 Effect of *E. singularis* organic extract and its semi-purified fractions (F-EtOH, F-Ac, F-MeOH/CH_2Cl_2), and of reference drugs (ranitidine and omeprazol) on gastric ulcer induced by HCl/ethanol in rats

Treatment	Dose (mg/kg)	Ulcer index (mm)	Inhibition (%)
Vehicle	-	78.5±3,49	-
Organic extract	50	31.52±2,42**	59.84
	100	24.46±2,48**	68.84
	200	19.49±3,48**	75.16
F-EtOH	5	43.36±1,52*	44.76
	10	37.20±3,05**	52.61
	25	23.33±1**	70.27
F-Ac	25	61.97±0,7	21.05
F-MeOH/CH_2Cl_2	5	66.59±2,33	15.17
	10	58.78±2,82	25.11
	25	29.17±4,04**	62.84
Ranitidine	60	27.47±2.3**	65
Omeprazol	30	9.78±0,81*	87.53

Values are expressed as mean±SEM; n=6 animals. *P<0.01, **P<0.001.

HCl/EtOH produced gastric mucosal damage with severe hemorrhage with lesion index of 78.5 mm in the untreated group. Treatment of rats by organic extract of *E. singularis* produced a significant decrease in gastric hemorrhage and the lesion index was inhibited by 60, 68 and 75% at doses of 50, 100 and 200 mg/kg, respectively. The semi-purified fractions were assessed for gastroprotective activity at 5, 10 and 25 mg/kg. A dose-related gastroprotective effect was observed for the fractions F-EtOH and F-MeOH/CH_2Cl_2 with highly significant activity for the ethanolic fraction (F-EtOH) at 25 mg/kg. The lesion index was inhibited by 44, 52 and 70% at doses of 5, 10 and 25 mg/kg, respectively; while in the ranitidine treated animals (60 mg/kg) the inhibition was 65%. F-Ac failed to protect stomach tissues from mucosal damage. The two classical ulcer drugs ranitidine and omeprazole showed a significant activity with a percentage of inhibition of gastric lesions of 65 and 87%, respectively. Some reports on the gastroprotective effect of diterpenes belonging to different structural skeletons are published [28]. In addition, another studies demonstrated that several terpenes or their derivatives posses gastroprotective activity in different models of induced gastric lesions in animals [29]. This gastroprotective effect seems to be related with an increase of the defensive mechanisms of the stomach, such as prostaglandin synthesis and mucus production [30]. Therefore, the involvement of diterpenoids palmonine D **6** isolated from the active fraction F-EtOH is hypothesized and can be responsible for its high activity.

Furthermore, various phenolic compounds (alkaloids, glycosides, and saponins) detected in *E. singularis* organic extract and fractions [6] may be responsible for its activity. Several studies reported that alkaloids have anti-inflammatory and gastroprotective effects [31]. Also, Glycosides, terpenoids and steroids detected in our samples are known to have anti-inflammatory and gastroprotective properties [10,32] The synergic effect of different compounds of *E. singularis* ethanolic fraction may be responsible for its higher anti-inflammatory and gastroprotective activities. Furthermore, the high free radical scavenging activity of F-EtOH in the DPPH test [6] suggests that the antioxidant activity may be one of the mechanisms of its gastroprotective and anti-inflammatory properties, because both ulcerous and inflammatory processes are related to an increase of free radicals [33].

Conclusion

In conclusion, the obtained results demonstrated that the ethanolic fraction of *E. singularis* had the highest activity in the two tests (anti-inflammatory and gastroprotective). The structure elucidation of compounds isolated from this fraction revealed the presence of five sterols and a eunicellan-based diterpenoid which may be responsible for its activity.

Additional file

Additional file 1: HPLC chromatograms and spectroscopic data of six compounds isolated from the white gorgonian *E. singularis*.

Competing interests

The authors declare that they have no competing interests.

Authors' contributions

AB and HBJ were the supervisors and designed the study. MD carried out pharmacological activities. CF and LG contribute to the chemical study. SDM and MVDA carried out the structure elucidation. RBS made contribution to preparation of organic extract and fractions from *E. singularis*. All authors read and approved the final manuscript.

Author details

[1]Laboratoire de développement chimique, galénique et pharmacologique des médicaments (LR12ES09). Equipe de Pharmacologie marine, Faculté de pharmacie de Monastir, Université de Monastir, Monastir, Tunisie. [2]Department of Pharmacy, University of Naples "Federico II", via D. Montesano 49, I- 80131 Napoli, Italy. [3]Laboratoire de chimie hétérocyclique, produits naturels et réactivité. Equipe de chimie médicinale et produits naturels (LR11ES39), Faculté des sciences de Monastir, Université de Monastir, Monastir, Tunisie. [4]Institut National des Sciences et Technologie de la Mer (INSTM), Salambo, Tunis, Tunisie.

References

1. Gori A, Bramanti L, Lopez-Gonzalez P, Thoma JN, Gili GM, Grinyo J, Uceira V, Rossi S: **Characterization of the zooxanthellate and azooxanthellate morphotypes of the Mediterranean gorgonian *Eunicella singularis*.** *Mar Biol* 2012, **159:**1485-1496.
2. McEnroe FJ, Fenical W: **Structures and synthesis of some new antibacterial sesquiterpenoids from the gorgonian coral *Pseudopterogorgia rigida*.** *Tetrahedron* 1978, **34:**1661-1664.

3. Groweiss A, Look S, Fenical W: **Solenolides, new antiinflammatory and antiviral diterpenoids from a marine octocoral of the genus *Solenopodium*.** *J Org Chem* 1988, **53**:2401-2406.
4. Wei X, Rodriguez AD, Baran P, Raptis RG, Sanchez JA, Ortega-Barria E, Gonzalez J: **Antiplasmodial cembradiene diterpenoids from a Southwestern Caribbean gorgonian octocoral of the genus *Eunicea*.** *Tetrahedron* 2004, **60**:11813-11819.
5. Qi SH, Zhang S, Qian PY, Xiao ZH, Li MY: **Ten new antifouling briarane diterpenoids from the South China Sea gorgonian *Junceella juncea*.** *Tetrahedron* 2006, **62**:9123-9130.
6. Deghrigue M, Dellai A, Bouraoui A: **In vitro antiproliferative and antioxidant activities of the organic extract and its semi-purified fractions from the Mediterranean gorgonian *Eunicella singularis*.** *Int J Pharm Pharm Sci* 2013, **5**:432-439.
7. Sheu JH, Sung PJ, Cheng MC, Liu HY, Fang LS, Duh CY, Chiang MY: **Novel Cytotoxic Diterpenes, Excavatolides A-E, Isolated from the Formosan Gorgonian *Briareum excavatum*.** *J Nat Prod* 1998, **61**:602-608.
8. Grode SH, James TR, Cardellina JH, Onan KD: **Molecular structures of the briantheins, new insecticidal diterpenes from *Briareum polyanthes*.** *J Org Chem* 1983, **48**:5203-5207.
9. Berrue F, Kerr RG: **Diterpenes from gorgonian corals.** *Nat Prod Rep* 2009, **26**:681-710.
10. Ioannou E, Abdel-Razik AF, Alexi X, Vagias C, Alexis MN, Roussis V: **Pregnanes with antiproliferative activity from the gorgonian *Eunicella cavolini*.** *Tetrahedron* 2008, **64**:11797-11801.
11. Ioannou E, Abdel-Razik AF, Alexi X, Vagias C, Alexis MN, Roussis V: **9,11-Secosterols with antiproliferative activity from the gorgonian *Eunicella cavolini*.** *Bioorg Med Chem* 2009, **17**:4537-4541.
12. Hossain H, Al-Mansur A, Akter S, Sara U, Ahmed MR, Jahangir AA: **Evaluation of anti-inflammatory activity and total tannin content from the leaves of *Bacopa monnieri* (Linn.).** *IJPSR* 2014, **5**(4):1246-1252.
13. Kupchan SM, Britton RW, Ziegler MF, Sigel CW: **Bruceantin, a new potent antileukemic simaroubolide from *Brucea antidysenterica*.** *J Org Chem* 1973, **38**:178-179.
14. Winter CA, Risley EA, Nuss GW: **Carrageenan induced edema hind paw of the rat as an easy for anti-inflammatory drugs.** *Proc Soc Exp Biol Med* 1962, **3**:544-547.
15. Mizui T, Doteuchi M: **Effect of polyamines on acidified ethanol-induced gastric lesions in rats.** *Japanese J Pharmacology* 1983, **33**:939-945.
16. Acimovic J, Rozman D: **Steroidal triterpenes of cholesterol synthesis.** *Molecules* 2013, **18**:4002-4017.
17. Lages BG, Fleury BG, Hovell AMC, Rezende CM, Pinto AC, Creed JC: **Proximity to competitors changes secondary metabolites of non-indigenous cup corals, *Tubastraea* spp., in the southwest Atlantic.** *Mar Biol* 2012, **159**:1551-1559.
18. Wang X, Zhang M, Zhao Y, Wang H, Liu T, Xin Z: **Pentadecyl ferulate, a potent antioxidant and antiproliferative agent from the halophyte *Salicornia herbacea*.** *Food Chem* 2013, **141**:2066-2074.
19. Harneti D, Supriadin A, Ulfah M, Safari A, Supratman U, Awang K, Hayashi H: **Cytotoxic constituents from the bark of *Aglaia eximia* (Meliaceae).** *Phytochem Lett* 2014, **8**:28-31.
20. Sgarbi DBG, da Silva AJR, Carlos IZ, Silva CL, Angluster J, Alviano CS: **Isolation of ergosterol peroxide and its reversion to ergosterol in the pathogenic fungus *Sporothrix schenckii*.** *Mycopathologia* 1997, **139**:9-14.
21. Wei-Guang M, Xing-Cong L, De-Zu W, Chong-Ren Y: **Ergosterol peroxides from *Cryptoporus volvatus*.** *Acta Bot Yunnanica* 1994, **16**(2):196-200.
22. Ortega MJ, Zubia E, Salva J: **A new cladiellane diterpenoid from *Eunicella labiata*.** *J Nat Prod* 1997, **60**:485-487.
23. Roussis V, Fenical W, Vagias C, Kornprobst JM, Miralles J: **Labiatamides A, B, and other eunicellan diterpenoids from the Senegalese gorgonian *Eunicella labiata*.** *Tetrahedron* 1996, **52**:2735-2742.
24. Hanson JR: **Diterpenoids.** *Nat Prod Rep* 2001, **18**:88-94.
25. Borgi W, Ghedira K, Chouchane N: **Antiinflammatory and analgesic activities of Zizyphus lotus root barks.** *Fitoterapia* 2007, **78**:16-19.
26. Inoue H, Ohshima H, Kono H, Yamanaka M, Kubota T, Aihara M, Hiroi T, Yago N, Ishida H: **Supressive effects of tranilast on the expression of inducible cyclooxygenase (COX-2) in interleukin-1-β-stimulated fibroblasts.** *Biochem Pharmacol* 1997, **53**:1941-1944.
27. Ishihara M, Ito M: **Influence of aging on gastric ulcer healing activities of cimetidine and omeprazole.** *Eur J Pharmacol* 2002, **444**:209-215.
28. Schmeda-Hirschmann G, Astudillo L, Rodriguez J, Theoduloz C, Yanez T: **Gastroprotective effect of the Mapuche crude drug Araucaria araucana resin and its main constituents.** *J Ethnopharmacol* 2005, **101**:271-276.
29. Farina C, Pinza M, Pifferi G: **Synthesis and anti-ulcer activity of new derivatives of glycyrrhetic, oleanolic and ursolic acids.** *Il Farmaco* 1998, **53**:22-32.
30. Hiruma-Lima CA, Gracioso JS, Toma W, Paula ACB, Almeida ABA, Brasil DD, Muller AH, Souza-Brito AR: **Evaluation of the gastroprotective activity of cordatin, a diterpene isolated from Aparisthmium cordatum (Euphorbiaceae).** *Biol Pharm Bull* 2000, **23**:1465-1469.
31. Moulin M, Coquerel A: *Pharmacologie, connaissance et pratique.* 2èmeth edition. Paris: Masson; 2002:845.
32. Radjasa OK, Vaske YM, Navarro G, Vervoort HC, Tenney K, Linington RG, Crews P: **Highlights of marine invertebrate-derived biosynthetic products: their biomedical potential and possible production by microbial associants.** *Bioorg Med Chem* 2011, **19**:6658-6674.
33. Pedernera AM, Guardia T, Guardia Calderon C, Rotelli AE, de la Rocha NE, Di Genaro S, Pelzer LE: **Anti-ulcerogenic and anti-inflammatory activity of the methanolic extract of *Larrea divaricata* Cav. In rats.** *J Ethnopharmacol* 2006, **105**:415-420.

A comparative study on the physicochemical and biological stability of IgG_1 and monoclonal antibodies during spray drying process

Vahid Ramezani[1,2], Alireza Vatanara[1*], Abdolhossein Rouholamini Najafabadi[1], Mohammad Ali Shokrgozar[3], Alireza Khabiri[4] and Mohammad Seyedabadi[5]

Abstract

Background: The main concern in formulation of antibodies is the intrinsic instability of these labile compounds. To evaluate the physicochemical stability of antibody in dry powder formulations, physical stability of IgG_1 and a monoclonal antibody (trastuzumab) during the spray drying process was studied in a parallel study and the efficacy of some sugar based excipients in protection of antibodies was studied.

Results: The SDS-PAGE analysis showed no fragmentation of antibodies after spray drying in all formulations. The secondary structure of antibodies contained 40.13 to 70.19% of β structure in dry state. Also, CD spectroscopy showed the similar secondary structure for trastuzumab after reconstitution in water. ELISA analysis and cell culture studies were conducted in order to evaluate bioactivity of monoclonal antibody. Formulations containing combination of excipients provided maximum tendency of trastuzumab to attach to the ELISA antigen (86.46% ± 2.3) and maximum bioactivity when incubated with $SKBr_3$ cell line (the cell viability was decreased to 65.99% ± 4.6). Incubation of formulations with L929 cell line proved the biocompatibility of the excipients and non-toxic composition of formulations.

Conclusion: The IgG_1 and trastuzumab demonstrated similar behavior in spray drying process. The combination of excipients containing trahalose, hydroxypropyl beta cyclodextrin and beta cyclodextrin with proper ratio improved the physical and chemical stability of both IgG_1 and monoclonal antibody.

Keywords: Antibody, Trastuzumab, Spray drying, Trehalose, Hydroxypropyl beta cyclodextrin, Beta cyclodextrin

Background

Monoclonal antibodies as an important part of therapeutic proteins are approved for treatment of various chronic and life threatening diseases. Their specific action and relatively low side effects have contributed to vast application of antibodies in many diseases [1]. The majority of antibodies are administrated by injection ordinarily; however, new antibodies and new administration routes such as inhalation [2], transdermal [3], vaginal [4], oral [5] and nasal [6] are investigated broadly as new delivery systems.

The main concern in formulation of antibodies is the intrinsic instability of these labile compounds. Generally, proteins are sensitive molecules to various physical instabilities like denaturation, aggregation, fragmentation and chemical reactions such as deamination, oxidation and isomerization [7,8]. Embedding of protein in dry matrix improves the stability versus physical and chemical degradation by various mechanisms [9-11].

Spray drying as a one-step process has been widely studied in production of dry powders containing proteins [12]. As a limitation, proteins as like as antibodies could be destabilized due to the high temperature and pressures in this process. In this way, the effects of various excipients [9,12] and process variables [12,13] have been investigated in lots of studies [9,10,12,13]. In our previous study, D-optimal design was conducted to optimize IgG_1 formulation in the presence of sugars and cyclodextrins in order to understand how the spray drying affects the antibody. But as like as many other

* Correspondence: vatanara@tums.ac.ir
[1]Department of Pharmaceutics, Faculty of Pharmacy, Tehran University of Medical Sciences, Tehran, Iran
Full list of author information is available at the end of the article

researches, these efforts have been focused on the processing of IgG as a model antibody and extension of the results of a general antibody to the monoclonal antibodies remains as a challenge. To the extent of our knowledge, no systematic study has been reported as a comparison between these two categories of antibodies. In the present work, trastuzumab as a monoclonal antibody was formulated parallel to the IgG_1 in the presence of sugar based excipients and the physical stability were compared. Trastuzumab is an important humanized monoclonal antibody that is approved in treatment of breast cancer with over-expressed HER2 receptor [14,15]. So, assessment of the biological activity of trastuzumab is supportive to evaluate the conformational stability of protein during the process.

Material and methods

Materials

Hydroxypropyl beta cyclodextrin (HPβCD) was obtained from Acros (Belgium) and Beta cyclodextrin (βCD) was purchased from Sigma (USA). Trehalose dehydrate, potassium phosphate dibasic and disodium sulfate were acquired from Merck (Germany). Trastuzumab (Herceptin®) was purchased from Roche Ltd (Hungary) and the chemicals were from sigma (USA). Human IgG_1 (with molecular weight of about 150 KD) was supplied by Kedrion (Italy). Prior to each investigation, low molecular weight additive of antibody solution was removed by dialysis with deionized water (cut off: 15 kDa).

Spray drying of antibody formulations

Spray drying was performed on various aqueous solutions of antibody with different excipients according to Table 1. The design of study was in accordance with the findings of previous studies on IgG_1. A lab scale Buchi-191 spray dryer (Buchi, Switzerland) was employed to obtain the dry antibody powder. The inlet temperature of 100°C, air flow rate of 700 L/h, liquid feed rate of 1.7 mL/min, and aspiration rate of 100% were selected. The resulted dry powders were collected in dry and well closed glass vials and stored at 4°C.

Table 1 Composition of various formulations of IgG_1 and trastuzumab

Formulation	IgG_1	Trastuzumab	HPβCD	βCD	Trehalose
F_1	-	1	-	-	-
F_2	-	1	1	-	-
F_3	-	1	-	1	-
F_4	-	1	-	-	1
F_5	-	1	1	1	0.26
F_6	1	-	-	-	-
F_7	1	-	1	-	-
F_8	1	-		1	-
F_9	1	-	-		1
F_{10}	1	-	1	1	0.26

Size exclusion chromatography

Size exclusion chromatography (SEC) was conducted to evaluate the percentage of soluble IgG aggregations as one of the most important physical instabilities. In order to separate the monomer from aggregated antibody, a 300 mm TSK 3000 SWXL column (Tosoh Biosep, Germany) was employed. Approximately, 20 μL of each sample containing 2.5 mg/mL was injected. The mobile phase consisted of 0.1 M disodium hydrogen phosphate and 0.1 M sodium sulfate (pH 6.8) with flow rate of 0.5 mL/min. The antibody concentration was measured by a UV detector (Waters, USA) at 280 nm. All experiments were performed in triplicate.

Sodium dodecyl sulfate polyacrylamide gel electrophoresis (SDS-PAGE)

In order to determine the antibody fragmentation, non-reducing sodium dodecyl sulphate-poly (acrylamide) gel electrophoresis (SDS-PAGE) was performed. Polyacrylamide gel 10% was prepared and diluted sample with concentration of 100 μg/mL was loaded. The samples were mixed with equal volumes of sample buffer before loading. Protein molecular weight marker of Fermentas® (Germany) was used to estimate the sample molecular weight.

Fourier transformation infrared spectroscopy (FT-IR)

Nicolet Magna spectrometer (USA) was applied to record the infrared spectra. Briefly, 2 mg of each sample was pressed with 200 mg KBr to make a clear tablet. The Jasco Spectra Manager® software (Japan) was used to deconvolution the spectra and detect the changes in secondary structure of antibody. Second derivative spectrum of amide I region (1600–1700 cm^{-1}) is a useful indicator to

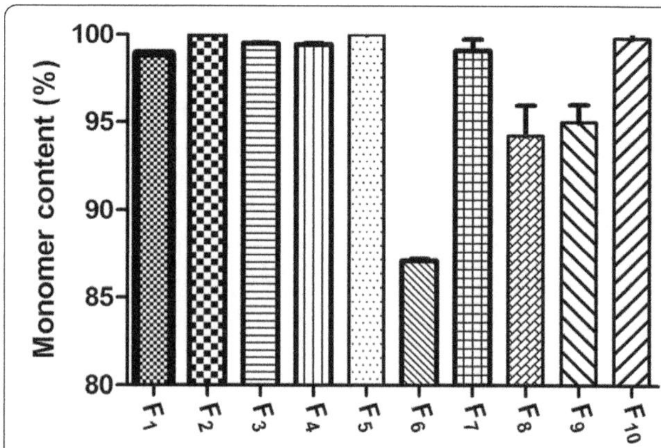

Figure 1 The percent of antibody monomer in microparticles immediately after spray drying analyzed by size exclusion chromatography (SEC).

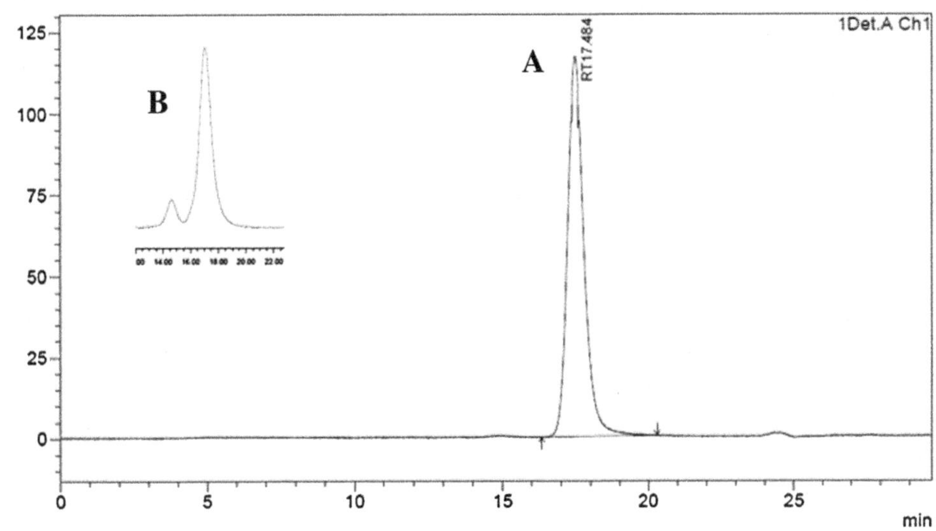

Figure 2 Size exclusion chromatography of F_5 (A); as shown, the aggregation related pick (B) has been disappeared in this formulation.

understand the protein structure. The percent of β sheet, α helix and turn was calculated by mixed Gaussian/ Lorentzian function considering β sheet structure absorption in 1640 cm^{-1} and 1695–1690 cm^{-1}, α helix in 1660–1650 cm^{-1} and turns from 1690 to1665 cm^{-1}.

Circular dichroism (CD)

Circular dichroism spectroscopy (AVIV, USA) was applied to analysis the secondary structure of monoclonal antibody after reconstitution. Proper amounts of processed powder were dissolved in purified water to make 250 μg/mL solutions. Measurement of buffer and antibody samples were performed in far-UV spectrophotometer at 20°C from 195 to 260 nm with the interval of 1 nm. Buffer spectra were substracted from the relevant protein solutions and converted to mean residual ellipticity. Deconvolution was performed to estimate the secondary structure of trastuzumab spectra. The secondary structure was calculated considering the molecular weight of 148 kDa for trastuzumab and a total number of 1328 amino acids.

Enzyme-linked Immunosorbent Assay (ELISA)

Direct ELISA was performed in order to determine the in-vitro activity of spray dried trastuzumab. Briefly, a 96 wells plate from Nunc (USA) was coated with 6 μg/mL of recombinant human HER_2 protein in carbonate/bicarbonate buffer over-night. The plate was blocked with 2% w/v BSA for 1 h at 37°C after three times of washing. About 100 μL of samples were added and incubated for 2 h at 37°C. After washing, 100 μL of the goat anti human antibody conjugated with horse radish peroxidase (HRP) was added and incubated at room temperature for 1 h. The bounded antibody was determined with tetramethyl benzemidine (TMB) as the proxidase substrate for 15 min and the concentration was determined at 650 nm by a STAT FAX 4700 ELISA reader (USA).

Cell culture studies

The human breast cancer cell line $SKBr_3$ and human fibroblast L929 were obtained from cell culture collection of Pasteur institute of Iran. $SKBr_3$ was cultured in RPMI medium supplemented with 10% of fetal bovine albumins

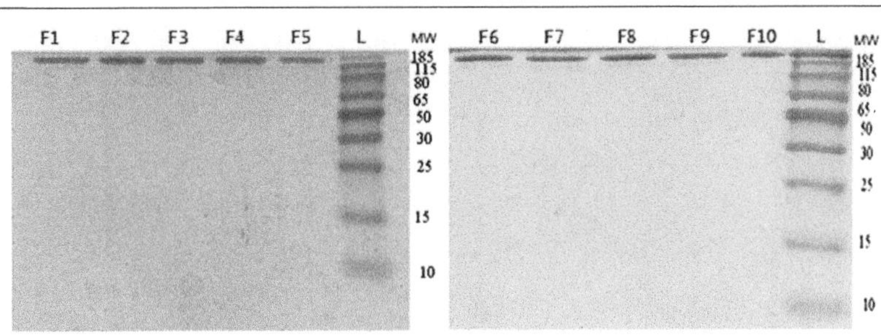

Figure 3 SDS-PAGE of formulations contained trastuzumab and IgG_1. The standard molecular weights were run in the left of gel.

and the L929 cell line was cultured in Dulbecco's modified Eagle's medium with 5% of fetal bovine albumin. Both culture mediums contained 1% of L-glutamine, 100 UI/mL of penicillin G and 100 mg/mL of streptomycin and maintained at 37°C in a humid atmosphere of 5% CO_2. For the experiment, the cells were harvested after brief incubation with trypsin (0.05%, w/v) and EDTA (0.02%, w/v).

Primarily, the cells were incubated with various concentrations of trastuzumab in the range of 10^1 to 10^6 ng/mL and the dose–response of trastuzumab on SKBr3 cells was determined. Further examinations were performed on the samples in concentrations of 10^5 ng/mL. To evaluate the biological activity of monoclonal antibody in various spray dried samples, the proper amount of each sample were dissolved in 100 mL of medium and added to 96-well plates in triplicate with 2×10^2 cells/well. Cell viability was assayed with mono tetrazolium 3-[4,5-dimethylthiazol-2-yl]-2,5-diphenyl tetrazolium bromide (MTT) colorimetric method. Briefly, the cells were exposed to tetrazolium after 48 h incubation with trastuzumab samples. Living cells were able to metabolized tetrazolium to non-soluble formazan, the formazan salts was dissolved and quantified using spectrophotometer plate reader (BioTek, USA) at 540 nm. The negative control was medium without trastuzumab and the positive control included unprocessed standard trastuzumab with determined concentration.

Statistical analysis

Data are presented as means ± SD and LSD-test was performed to evaluate the differences between groups. The statistical significancy of results is considered with a P value less than 0.05. The graphs have been drawn by GraphPad® Prism 5and Microsoft® Excel 2007.

Results and discussion

Similar to other proteins, antibodies can undergo degradation pathways during the spray drying process. Protein degradation can reduce the efficient binding of protein to the receptors and decrease the bioactivity. So it is very impotent to ensure the physical stability as well as biological activity of monoclonal antibodies after spray drying or other processes. In our previous study, optimization and characterization of IgG_1formulations led to use a combination of trehalose, HPβCD and βCD which resulted in protection of antibody structure up to 99.81 ± 0.7%. In the present study, as shown in Table 1, these excipients were employed in order to evaluate the stability of trastuzumab as a monoclonal antibody in comparison with IgG_1.

Physical stability of antibody

The percent of antibody aggregates after spray drying are presented in Figure 1. The pattern of aggregation in IgG_1 and trastuzumab was similar; however, the percent of aggregations were different. As seen, the pure IgG_1 contained 87.1% monomer and pure trastuzumab contained 98.9% monomer after process. Application of excipients successfully decreased the aggregation in both of antibodies. In this way, the efficacy of HPβCD was greater than βCD and trehalose. Combination of trehalose, HPβCD and βCD in the F_5 showed the highest effectiveness in protection of the trastuzumab monomer. As seen in Figure 2, the pick related to the trastuzumab dimmer in SEC chromatogram has been disappeared. This point implicates the synergistic effect of sugars in protection of antibody monomer. Similar observations have demonstrated the synergism effect of various sugars in preservation of proteins by water substitution mechanism [10].

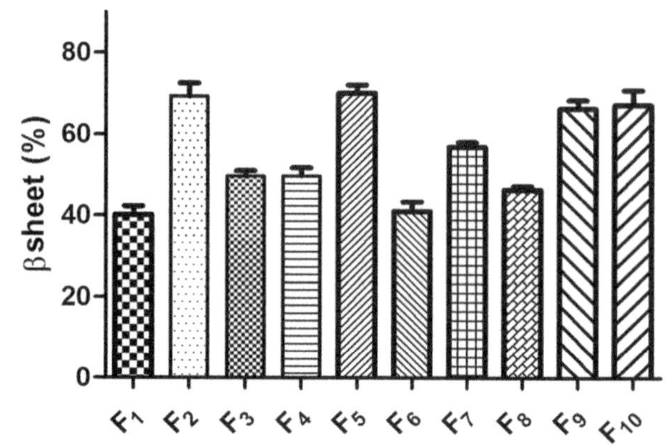

Figure 4 Amount of β structure in dry state analyzed by FTIR in various samples.

Non reducing SDS-PAGE was performed in order to reveal fragmentation of antibodies during the spray drying. In this type of SDS-PAGE, reducing agents are not used and consequently, evaluation of protein structure is possible without reduction of di-sulfide bounds. Therefore,

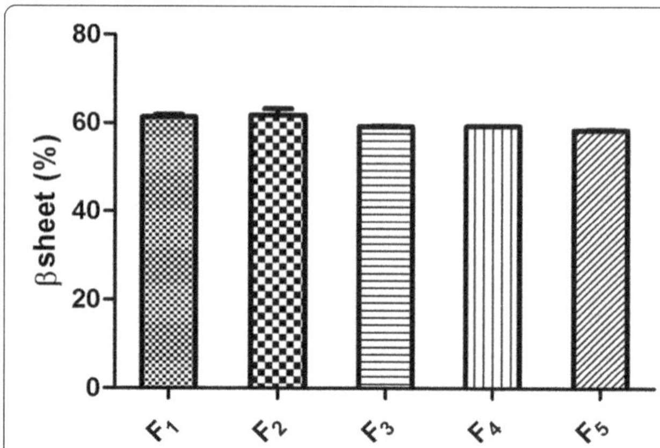

Figure 5 Amount of β structure of spray dried trastuzumab after reconstitution in water analyzed by CD.

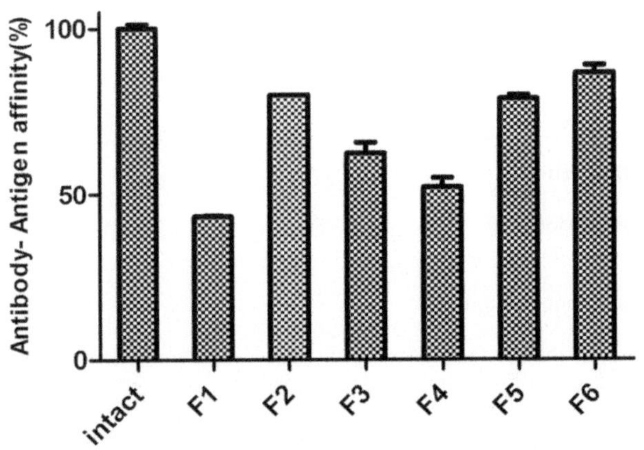

Figure 6 The Affinity of trastuzumab to Her_2 antigen in various spray dried formulations by ELISA study.

detection and quantification of process-related fragmentation would be possible. As shown in Figure 3, all formulations of both trastuzumab and IgG_1 present bonds just in 150 kDa and there is no distinct bond in lower molecular weight regions. Amphlett G et al. (1996) showed that the bonds such as Asp-Gly and Asp-Pro are more sensitive to cleavage in proteins backbone. So the proteins are prone to cleavage and fragmentation in these places [16]. Moreover, disulfide bonds cleavage lead to formation of antibody fragments of 25 and 50 kDa. If fragmentation took place during the spray drying process, we expected to observe the distinct bonds in SDS-PAGE gel, but the results suggested that process stresses did not affect the trastuzumab backbone. So the data implicated that the short time exposure of antibodies to harsh conditions of spray drying did not induce antibody fragmentation.

The secondary structure of antibody samples was evaluated by FTIR spectroscopy in dry state. As presented in Figure 4, the lowest ratio of β structures (40.13 ± 2.1%) was perceived when pure antibodies were processed by spray drying and presence of excipients in the formulations of antibody increased the β structures content; Where, F_2 provided 69.35% and F_5 contained 70.19% of β structure. Processing of pure IgG_1 lead similarly to 41.01% of β structures and F_{10} as the formulation containing the composition of excipients, preserved the high amounts of β structure after spray drying (67.21%).

The secondary structure of monoclonal antibody, after reconstitution in water, was assessed using far-UV CD spectrophotometer. The amounts of β sheet and β turns in the processed trastuzumab were about 60%. Comparison of FTIR and CD data revealed that dehydration of trastuzumab resulted in substantial and measurable conformational changes and it emphasize that protein structure is highly depended on protein type and formulation conditions, but these changes can be reversible or irreversible. According to the Figure 5, results indicated that trastuzumab reforms to the native structure after reconstitution in water. In agreement, similar studies showed that selection of proper stabilizers minimize the structural changes of proteins such as poly-L-lysine [17], acetate dehydrogenase and phosphor fructokinase [18].

Biological activity

The biological activity of trastuzumab depends on its ability to target the extracellular domain of human epidermal growth factor receptor protein in tumor cells. Trastuzumab therapy reduces the tumor cells proliferation by several mechanisms. On the one hand, it promotes cell cycle arrest and apoptosis in tumor or metastatic cells and on the other hand, it activates an antibody-dependent cellular cytotoxicity (ADCC) response with the aid of natural killer (NK) cells. The NK cells induce cell death by attaching to the Fc domain of antibody and the activity of trastuzumab highly depends on the ability to contact with HER_2 antigen as well as NK cells receptors.

ELISA is an appropriate method for simultaneous evaluation of both F_c and F_{ab} fragments of antibody; since, in this analysis method, the structural changes in the antibody are exaggerated. Any change in the F_{ab} or F_c can affect the affinity of antibody to the antigen or secondary antibody. Direct ELISA was applied to evaluate the stability of trastuzumab during the spray drying

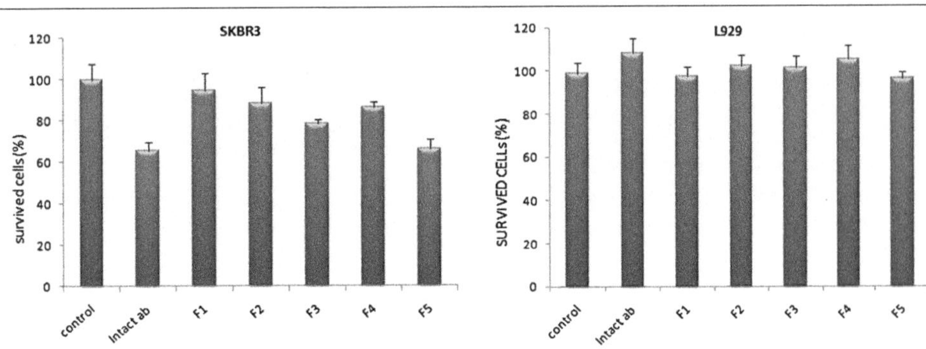

Figure 7 The survived $SKBr_3$ and L929 cell line after incubation with 10^5 ng/mL of trastuzumab in various formulations.

in comparison with unprocessed antibody as positive controls. As presented in Figure 6, just 43.2 ± 0.2% of the pure antibody was quantified after processing; whereas, presence of excipients in F_2 and F_5 enhanced the affinity of antibody to the antigen up to 79.9 ± 0.1% and 86.5 ± 2.3%, respectively.

Furthermore, bioactivity of monoclonal antibody was evaluated by means of HER_2-over-expressing breast cancer cell line ($SKBr_3$). The cells were incubated in the presence of 10^5 ng/mL of spray dried samples and unprocessed standard trastuzumab as positive control. The cells viability was evaluated by MTT assay after 48 hours. Statistical comparison of survived cells after incubation showed that the ability of F_1 containing processed pure trastuzumab to kill the cells was the minimum (Figure 7). The 2-side dunnett test indicated no difference between F_1 and negative control. However, the unprocessed trastuzumab presented a great activity to kill the $SKBr_3$ cells (with the minimum cell viability of 65.88 ± 3.95% after incubation). The ANOVA with the aid of post doc (LSD) test among spray dried formulations indicated the equal ability of F_2, F_3, F_4 with F_5, which showed the greatest ability to preserve the antibody activity (65.99 ± 4.6%). Also, LSD test indicated no difference between F_5 and positive control. As a result, it could be deduced that combination of various excipients with different properties led to inhibition of aggregation and preservation of antibody structure as well as protection of amino acids in the protein backbone.

Some previous studies indicated the citotoxicity of cyclodextrine and other derivatives on the body cells or on red blood cells [19,20]. The L929 is a fibroblast cell line L929 without any HER_2 antigen on the surface that is suitable for evaluation of toxicity and biocompatibility of formulations. The same concentration of trastuzumab was incubated with this cell line and analysis of cell viability in the presence of different formulations showed no toxic effect at concentrations of 10^5 ng/mL and the 100% of cells were alive after incubation with various formulations after 48 hr (Figure 7). Consequently, we concluded that the death in $SKBr_3$ cells were due to the active trastuzumab rather than formulation excipients. Also the biocompatibility of formulations was confirmed in this experiment.

Conclusion

This report focused on physicochemical stability and biological activity of antibodies after spray-drying. Combination of HPβCD, βCD and trehalose provided the maximum efficacy in protection of the IgG_1 as a general antibody and trastuzumab as a monoclonal antibody. Coexistence of these excipients in the formulations preserved monomers up to 99.1% and 99.9% for IgG and trastuzumab, respectively.

The conformational changes of processed antibodies in dry structure were reversible and it could reform to the native stricter after reconstitution in water. The activity of trastuzumab in best formulation was detected up to 86.46% in ELISA test and it was confirmed by cell culture studies.

Competing interests

The authors declare that they have no competing interests.

Authors' contributions

VR performed the experiment and prepared the manuscript; AV and ARN supervised the project and helped in study design; MASH gave consultation on cell culture and analyzing the antibody bioactivity; AKH gave consultation on ELISA assay, MS helped in statistical analysis and preparation of the manuscript. All authors read and approved the final manuscript.

Acknowledgement

This study (was/has been) funded and supported by Tehran university of medical sciences (TUMS).

Author details

[1]Department of Pharmaceutics, Faculty of Pharmacy, Tehran University of Medical Sciences, Tehran, Iran. [2]Department of Pharmaceutics, Faculty of Pharmacy, Shahid Sadoughi University of Medical Sciences, Yazd, Iran. [3]National Cell Bank of Iran, Pasteur Institute of Iran, Tehran, Iran. [4]Department of Mycology, Pasteur Institute of Iran, Tehran, Iran. [5]Department of Molecular Imaging, The Persian Gulf Biomedical Sciences Research Institute, Bushehr University of Medical Sciences, Bushehr, Iran.

References

1. An Z: **Monoclonal antibodies-a proven and rapidly expanding therapeutic modality for human diseases.** *Protein Cell* 2010, **1**:319–330.
2. Hacha J, Tomlinson K, Maertens L, Paulissen G, Rocks N, Foidart JM, Noel A, Palframan R, Gueders M, Cataldo DD: **Nebulized anti-IL-13 monoclonal antibody Fab' fragment reduces allergen-induced asthma.** *Am J Respir Cell Mol Biol* 2012, **47**:709–717.
3. Li G, Badkar A, Nema S, Kolli CS, Banga AK: **In vitro transdermal delivery of therapeutic antibodies using maltose microneedles.** *Int J Pharm* 2009, **368**:109–115.
4. Castle PE, Karp DA, Zeitlin L, Garcia-Moreno EB, Moench TR, Whaley KJ, Cone RA: **Human monoclonal antibody stability and activity at vaginal pH.** *J Reprod Immunol* 2002, **56**:61–76.
5. Reilly R, Domingo R, Sandhu J: **Oral delivery of antibodies.** *Clin-Pharmacokinet* 1997, **32**:313–323.
6. Kaye RS, Purewal TS, Alpar OH: **Development and testing of particulate formulations for the nasal delivery of antibodies.** *J Control Release* 2009, **135**:127–135.
7. Wang W, Singh S, Zeng DL, King K, Nema S: **Antibody structure, instability, and formulation.** *J Pharm Sci* 2007, **96**:1–26.
8. Daugherty AL, Mrsny RJ: **Formulation and delivery issues for monoclonal antibody therapeutics.** *Adv Drug Deliv Rev* 2006, **58**:686–706.
9. Schule S, Schulz-Fademrecht T, Garidel P, Bechtold-Peters K, Frieb W: **Stabilization of IgG1 in spray-dried powders for inhalation.** *Eur J Pharm Biopharm* 2008, **69**:793–807.
10. Chang LL, Pikal MJ: **Mechanisms of protein stabilization in the solid state.** *J Pharm Sci* 2009, **98**:2886–2908.
11. Maury M, Murphy K, Kumar S, Mauerer A, Lee G: **Spray-drying of proteins: effects of sorbitol and trehalose on aggregation and FT-IR amide I spectrum of an immunoglobulin G.** *Eur J Pharm Biopharm* 2005, **59**:251–261.
12. Ramezani V, Vatanara A, Rouholamini Najafabadi A, Gilani K, Nabi-Meybodi M: **Screening and evaluation of variables in the formation of antibody particles by spray drying.** *Powder Technol* 2013, **233**:341–346.
13. Costantino HR, Andya JD, Nguyen PA, Dasovich N, Sweeney TD, Shire SJ, Hsu CC, Maa YF: **Effect of mannitol crystallization on the stability and aerosol performance of a spray-dried pharmaceutical protein,**

recombinant humanized anti-IgE monoclonal antibody. *J Pharm Sci* 1998, **87:**1406–1411.

14. Hortobagyi GN: **Trastuzumab in the treatment of breast cancer.** *N Engl J Med* 2005, **353:**1734–1736.
15. Montemurro F, Valabrega G, Aglietta M: **Trastuzumab-based combination therapy for breast cancer.** *Expert Opin Pharmacother* 2004, **5:**81–96.
16. Amphlett G, Cacia J, Callahan W, Cannova-Davis E, Chang B, Cleland JL, Darrington T, DeYoung L, Dhingra B, Everett R, Foster L, Frenz J, Garcia A, Giltinan D, Gitlin G, Gombotz W, Hageman M, Harris R, Heller D, Herman A, Hershenson S, Hora M, Ingram R, Janes S, Watanabe C: **A compendium and hydropathy/flexibility analysis of common reactive sites in proteins: reactivity at Asn, Asp, Gln, and Met motifs in neutral pH solution.** *Pharm Biotechnol* 1996, **9:**1–140.
17. Prestrelski SJ, Tedeschi N, Arakawa T, Carpenter JF: **Dehydration-induced conformational transitions in proteins and their inhibition by stabilizers.** *Biophys J* 1993, **65:**661–671.
18. Prestrelski SJ, Arakawa T, Carpenter JF: **Separation of freezing-and drying-induced denaturation of lyophilized proteins using stress-specific stabilization. II. Structural studies using infrared spectroscopy.** *Arch Biochem Biophys* 1993, **303:**465–473.
19. Kiss T, Fenyvesi F, Kovacsne BI, Feher P, Leposane KR, Varadi J, Szente L, Fenyvesi E, Ivanyi R, Vecsernyes M: **Cytotoxic examinations of various cyclodextrin derivatives on Caco-2 cells.** *Acta Pharm Hung* 2007, **77:**150–154.
20. Kiss T, Fenyvesi F, Bacskay I, Varadi J, Fenyvesi E, Ivanyi R, Szente L, Tosaki A, Vecsernyes M: **Evaluation of the cytotoxicity of beta-cyclodextrin derivatives: evidence for the role of cholesterol extraction.** *Eur J Pharm Sci* 2010, **40:**376–380.

Improved anticancer delivery of paclitaxel by albumin surface modification of PLGA nanoparticles

Mehdi Esfandyari-Manesh[1,2], Seyed Hossein Mostafavi[2,3,4], Reza Faridi Majidi[4], Mona Noori Koopaei[2], Nazanin Shabani Ravari[1,2], Mohsen Amini[5], Behrad Darvishi[1,4], Seyed Nasser Ostad[6], Fatemeh Atyabi[1,2] and Rassoul Dinarvand[1,2*]

Abstract

Background: Nanoparticles (NPs) play an important role in anticancer delivery systems. Surface modified NPs with hydrophilic polymers such as human serum albumin (HSA) have long half-life in the blood circulation system.

Methods: The method of modified nanoprecipitation was utilized for encapsulation of paclitaxel (PTX) in poly (lactic-co-glycolic acid) (PLGA). Para-maleimide benzoic hydrazide was conjugated to PLGA for the surface modifications of PLGA NPs, and then HSA was attached on the surface of prepared NPs by maleimide attachment to thiol groups (cysteines) of albumin. The application of HSA provides for the longer blood circulation of stealth NPs due to their escape from reticuloendothelial system (RES). Then the physicochemical properties of NPs like surface morphology, size, zeta potential, and in-vitro drug release were analyzed.

Results: The particle size of NPs ranged from 170 to 190 nm and increased about 20–30 nm after HSA conjugation. The zeta potential was about -6 mV and it decreased further after HSA conjugation. The HSA conjugation in prepared NPs was proved by Fourier transform infrared (FT-IR) spectroscopy, faster degradation of HSA in Differential scanning calorimetry (DSC) characterization, and other evidences such as the increasing in size and the decreasing in zeta potential. The PTX released in a biphasic mode for all colloidal suspensions. A sustained release profile for approximately 33 days was detected after a burst effect of the loaded drug. The in vitro cytotoxicity evaluation also indicated that the HSA NPs are more cytotoxic than plain NPs.

Conclusions: HSA decoration of PLGA NPs may be a suitable method for longer blood circulation of NPs.

Keywords: PLGA, Surface modified nanoparticles, Drug delivery, Albumin, Paclitaxel

Background

Different scientists including pharmaceutics, chemists, biologist, and nanotechnologist have been working indefatigably to defeat cancer. A major interest in this area is to improve drug targeting towards tumor cells and decrease the unwilling effects of chemotherapeutics [1-3]. Nanotechnology is very promising in this field and increases the efficacy of targeting by introducing passive and active targeting [4,5].

The interest on utilizing NPs formulated from biodegradable and biocompatible polymers such as the most commonly used PLGA are rising rapidly [6]. These NPs are broadly studied as anticancer delivery systems since it has special characteristics such as controlled release and biocompatibility [6].

A new approach to evade the short half-life of the conventional drug and allow targeted delivery to tumor cells is drug targeting achieved by size engineering and surface modification [7,8]. Vasculatures in tumor presents several irregularities in contrast with normal vessels resulting in enhanced permeation and retention (EPR) effect [9,10] and this will cause the nanoparticles with diameters less than 100 nm being selectively taken up by

* Correspondence: dinarvand@tums.ac.ir
[1]Nanotechnology Research Centre, Faculty of Pharmacy, Tehran University of Medical Sciences, Tehran, Iran
[2]Novel Drug Delivery Lab, Department of Pharmaceutics, Faculty of Pharmacy, Tehran University of Medical Sciences, Tehran, Iran
Full list of author information is available at the end of the article

tumor Vasculatures [8,11]. However, the drug biodistribution profile of the cytotoxic drugs change massively while they are incorporated with NPs, because the modified particles are swiftly opsonised and massively cleared by mono nuclear phagocytes system (MPS) [10-12]. Surface modification of particles with hydrophilic polymers like polyethylene glycol (PEG) and albumin leading to the development of long-circulating and stealth particles for delivery of anticancer drugs [13,14]. Furthermore, the lack of lymph vessels and higher interstitial fluid pressure in the most tumors than normal ones causes inefficient removal of interstitial fluid and soluble macromolecules [15]. Therefore, the NPs mount up in the interstitium which retards their uptake (EPR effect), unless those particles are degraded [16,17].

The HSA coated NPs were prepared in two ways. First, non-covalent interactions where HSA molecules only saturate the surface without any covalent linkage [11] and second, albumin conjugated particles were synthesised via reaction between ξ-amino groups of lysine residues and the protein ligand with aldehyde functional or carboxylic acid [18,19]. The second method is more common.

Accordingly, we have developed a novel strategy that benefit from high efficiency and selectivity of the thiol. In this study we did a site-specific conjugation on the HSA that in spite of the fact that it minimize a loss in biological activity of it but meanwhile decrease immunogenicity. It happens because reagents that specifically react with the thiol group of cysteines, and the number of free cysteines on the surface of a protein is much less [15]. HSA conjugation to surface of NPs was done through the disulphide bonds between the HSA and the paramaleimido benzoic hydrazid (PMBH) derivative of PLGA. The encapsulation efficiency (EE), drug release, and morphology of nanoparticles were then investigated. At last cyto-toxicity of PTX loaded NPs was studied using 3-(4,5-dimethyathiazol-2-yl)-2,5-diphenyltetrazoliumbromide (MTT) assay.

Materials and methods

Materials

PLGA (50:50, M_W: 48000 g/mol) with carboxyl end group and HSA were purchased from Sigma company. N, N'-dicyclohexylcarbodiimide (DCC), N–hydroxysuccinimide (NHS), and 3-(4,5-dimethyathiazol-2-yl)-2,5-diphenyltetrazoliumbromide (MTT) were purchased from Sigma-Aldrich (St. Louis, MO, USA). PMBH, Na_3PO_4, NaH_2PO_4, NaOH, sodium bicarbonate and also NaCl was obtained from Merck. PTX purchased from Cipla Company. Dulbecco's modified eagle's medium (DMEM), penicillin, streptomycin antibiotic mixture and fetal bovine serum (FBS) were obtained from Life technologies (grand Island, NY, USA). Polyvinyl alcohol (PVA) was acquired from Acros (Geel, Belgium). 2-(N-morpholino ethane sulfonic acid) (MES) was purchased from Fluka (St. Louis, MO, USA). All other solvents and reagents which are not stated were from Merck (Darmstadt, Germany).

Methods

Synthesis of PLGA with functional group of maleimide

Maleimide-functionalized copolymer PLGA was synthesized using the conjugation between paramaleimido benzoic hydrazid (PMBH) and PLGA–COOH. PLGA–COOH (5 g, 0.1 mmol) in 10 ml of methylene chloride was changed to PLGA–NHS with surfeit of N-hydroxysuccinimide (NHS, 135 mg, 1.1 mmol) in the presence of N, N'-dicyclohexylcarbodiimide (230 mg, 1.1 mmol). Then, 0.42 mol PMBH was added to the solution of activated PLGA and the reaction was allowed to proceed overnight on magnetic stirrer. The mixture was evaporated using rotary evaporator and the prepared film of PLGA-PMBH polymer was washed properly using de-ionized water and dried naturally for about two weeks. The synthesized polymer was assessed using H-NMR and FT-IR spectroscopy.

Preparation of PTX-loaded NPs

The method of modified nanoprecipitation was utilized for the preparation of drug encapsulated into particles of PLGA-PMBH [20-22]. In brief, 20 mg of polymer and 1.4 mg of PTX were dissolved in 4 ml of acetone and then injected (rate = 0.5 ml/min) into 16 ml of aqueous phase containing 0.5% PVA as surfactant and emulsified by probe sonication (Misonix, USA) for 5 min with amplitude of 10. Subsequently, the organic solution was evaporated gently on magnetic stirrer (600 rpm) for 9 hours. The NPs were washed and recovered using centrifuge process 25,000 rpm for 30 min (Sigma 3K30, Germany) and then lyophilized at – 40°C for 48 h (Christ Alpha 1–4; Germany). It should be mentioned that during the procedure, Several parameters in NPs preparation such as surfactant concentration, ratio of organic to aqueous, ratio of drug to polymer, and applied external energy witch have critical effects on the eventual size of NPs and drug loading were assessed in this experiment to obtain optimize situation.

HSA conjugation on the surface of PLGA NPs

5 mg of NPs was dispersed in 4 ml of degassed deionized water using bubbling nitrogen. HSA (10 mg/ml) were dissolved in 5 ml of degassed deionized water which have NaCl 0.15 M (pH 6.2–6.5) instantly before injecting it into the suspension. 1 ml of degassed solution contained ethylene diamine tetra acetic acid (EDTA) 4 mM and NaCl 0.3 M (pH 6.2–6.5) then were added to the suspension under the nitrogen pressure. The mixture was put a side overnight for the conjugation to perform

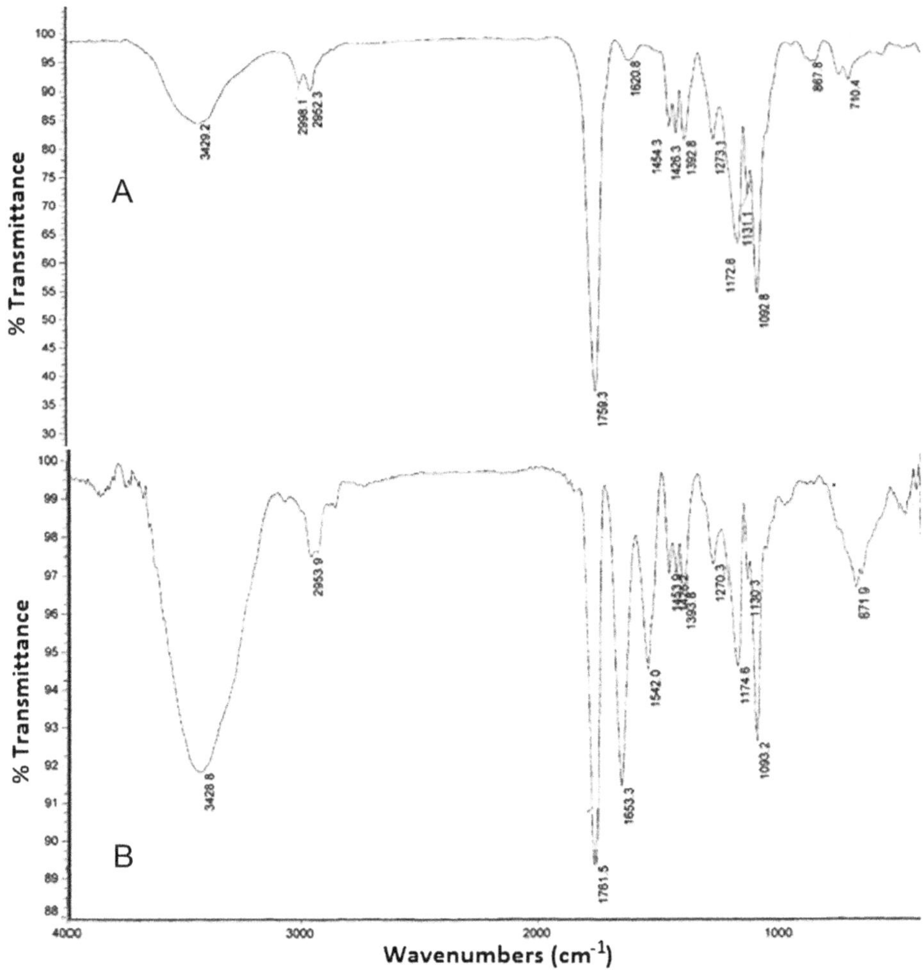

Figure 1 FT-IR spectrum. **(A)** PLGA NPs **(B)** PLGA-HSA NPs.

on the stirrer. The HSA conjugated PLGA NPs was purified and the unreacted HSA was removed using centrifuge (18000 rpm, 30 min, 3 times).

Measurement of size and zeta potential of NPs

Nearly 1 mg of NPs was suspended in 2 ml deionized water using bath sonicator. Mean size and polydispersity index (PDI) of NPs were evaluated using dynamic light scattering (DLS) instrument (Nano ZS, Malvern Instruments, UK). Afterward, samples were placed in an electrophoretic cell and zeta potential was determined.

Surface morphology

Scanning electron microscopy (SEM, Philips XL 30, Philips, The Netherlands) was used to determine the shape and surface morphology of the produced NPs. NPs were coated with gold under vacuum before scanning electron microscopy.

FT-IR analysis

To examine the conjugation was done correctly IR analysis. To perform this procedure we prepared a uniform mixture of lyophilized PLGA and PLGA-HSA NPs (separately) and KBr.

Differential scanning calorimetry (DSC)

Different ratio of physical mixture of raw materials included PLGA, HSA, PTX and also PLGA NPs and PLGA-HSA NPs were weighted equivalently (7 mg) and then sealed in standard aluminum pans. The experiment carried out using

Table 1 Particle size, zeta potential, encapsulation, and loading of NPs before and after conjugation

NPs	Size (nm)	Zeta (mV)	Encapsulation %	Loading
PLGA	187.0 ± 10.0	-6.7 ± 1.5	80.1 ± 11.0	10.7 ± 2.6
PLGA-HSA	207.0 ± 5.2	-13.6 ± 1.4	75.4 ± 12.0	8.2 ± 1.3

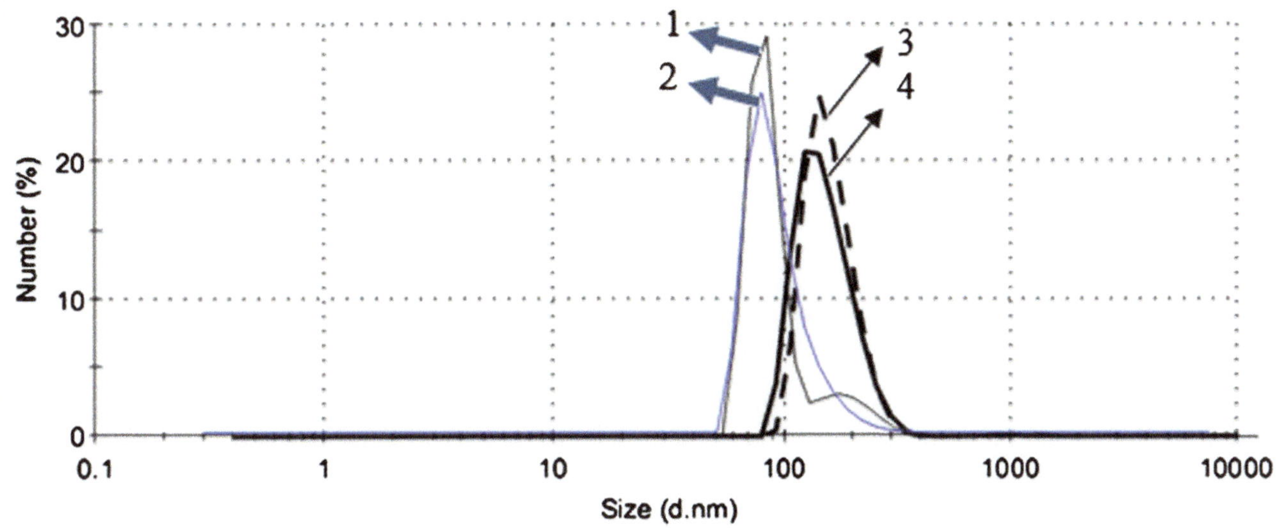

Figure 2 Nanoparticle size increase after HSA conjugation. 1 and 2 are PLGA NPs before HSA conjugation, and 3 and 4 are PLGA-HSA NPs after HSA conjugation.

(Mettler Toledo, GmbH, Switzerland) in ascending mode (10°C min/min) started from 40°C to 600°C.

Drug loading and encapsulation efficiency

To determine the drug loading and encapsulation efficiency, PTX entrapped in the NPs was measured by HPLC (Agilent LC1100, Agilent, Tokyo, Japan) at room temperature. The column was C18 column (25 cm × 0.46 cm internal diameter, pore size 5 μm; Teknokroma, Barcelona, Spain). The mobile phase consisted of acetonitrile/water (1/1 v/v). Lyophilized NPs (2.5 mg) were dissolved in acetonitrile (1 ml) (a common solvent for PLGA and drug) and shaken lightly followed by sonication for 6 min. Then, 2 ml of methanol was added to precipitate the polymer. The sample was filtered and drug quantity in filterant was determined by HPLC analysis.

$$Drug\,Loading\ \% = \left(\frac{weight\ of\ drug\ in\ NPs}{weight\ of\ NPs}\right) \times 100$$

$$Encapsulation\ Efficiency\ \% = \left(\frac{weight\ of\ drug\ in\ NPs}{weight\ of\ feed\ NPs}\right) \times 100$$

In vitro drug release

In order to evaluate in vitro release profile of PTX from PLGA and PLGA-HSA NPs, 2.5 mg of lyophilized samples were dispersed in 5 ml phosphate buffer saline solution (PBS, 0.01 M) containing 5% w/v of sodium dodecyl sulphate (SDS) with different pH (5 and 7.4) [21]. Afterward, suspensions poured into dialysis bags (cut off molecular weight 12000 g/mol) and immersed into the 50 ml of PBS with similar pH to the PBS in the bags. Subsequently, beakers placed on a shaker pre-set its temperature on 37°C

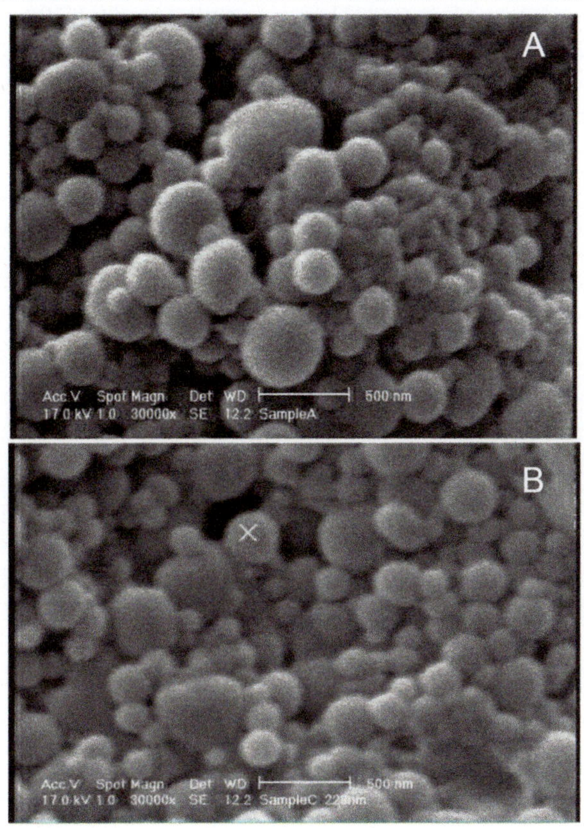

Figure 3 SEM micrographs of NPs with 30,000 times magnification. **(A)** PLGA NPs **(B)** PLGA-HSA NPs.

and 100 cycles per minute for during 33 days because of slow degradation proses of PLGA. For further assessments, all 50 ml of media (PBS) replaced with a same amount of new PBS at predetermined time intervals. The amount of released PTX was determined by HPLC in wavelength of 228 nm.

In vitro cell viability

MTT test was used to study the in vitro cytotoxicity of the subsequent PTX formulations on cell line of T47D: PTX loaded PLGA-HSA NPs, PTX loaded PLGA NPs, free PTX, and unloaded NPs.

T47D cells were seeded at the density of 1×10^4 viable cells/well in 96-well plates (Costar, Chicago, IL) and it is also incubated for 24 hours to providing enough time for cell attachments. Then the formulation (100 μL, 1–200 nM, and 48 h) was used to substitute the medium. A stock solution made in dimethyl sulfoxide (1 mg/ml PTX) for PTX. The concentration of dimethyl sulfoxide kept under 0.5% since at this concentration it has no effect on proliferation of cells and RPMI-1640 culture medium was used as diluents for preparing the working solution of free PTX drug and NPs. 20 μl MTT (5 mg/ml in phosphate-buffered saline) was added at specified periods of time to each well, and after 3 – 4 hours the culture medium containing MTT solution was eliminated. Then, micro plate reader (570 nm) used to read it after dissolve of formazan crystals in dimethyl sulfoxide (100 μL). At last following equation used to evaluate cell viability:

$$\text{Cell viability } (\%) = (\text{Ints}/\text{Intcontrol}) \times 100$$

In this equation Ints equal to the colorimetric intensity of cells which is incubated with the samples, and Intcontrol is the colorimetric intensity of cells that incubated with the phosphate-buffered saline only as positive control.

Results and discussion

Synthesis of polymer

PLGA functionalized with maleimide group was synthesized and characterized. 1H-NMR and FT-IR analysis was used for confirmation of the primary chemical structure of PMBH–PLGA.

There was overlapping doublets at 1.6 ppm which are a confirmation for the methyl groups of the lactic acid. The multiples peaks at 4.8 ppm and 5.2 ppm correspond to the $-CH_2$ of glycolic acid and -CH of lactic acid, respectively. The high complexity of the peaks at 4.8 ppm and 5.2 ppm resulting from different sequences of glycolic acid and lactic in the backbone of polymer. There are also some detectable proton signals from maleimide and phenyl groups. Peaks which were present the hydrogens of linker are very weak compered to peaks present

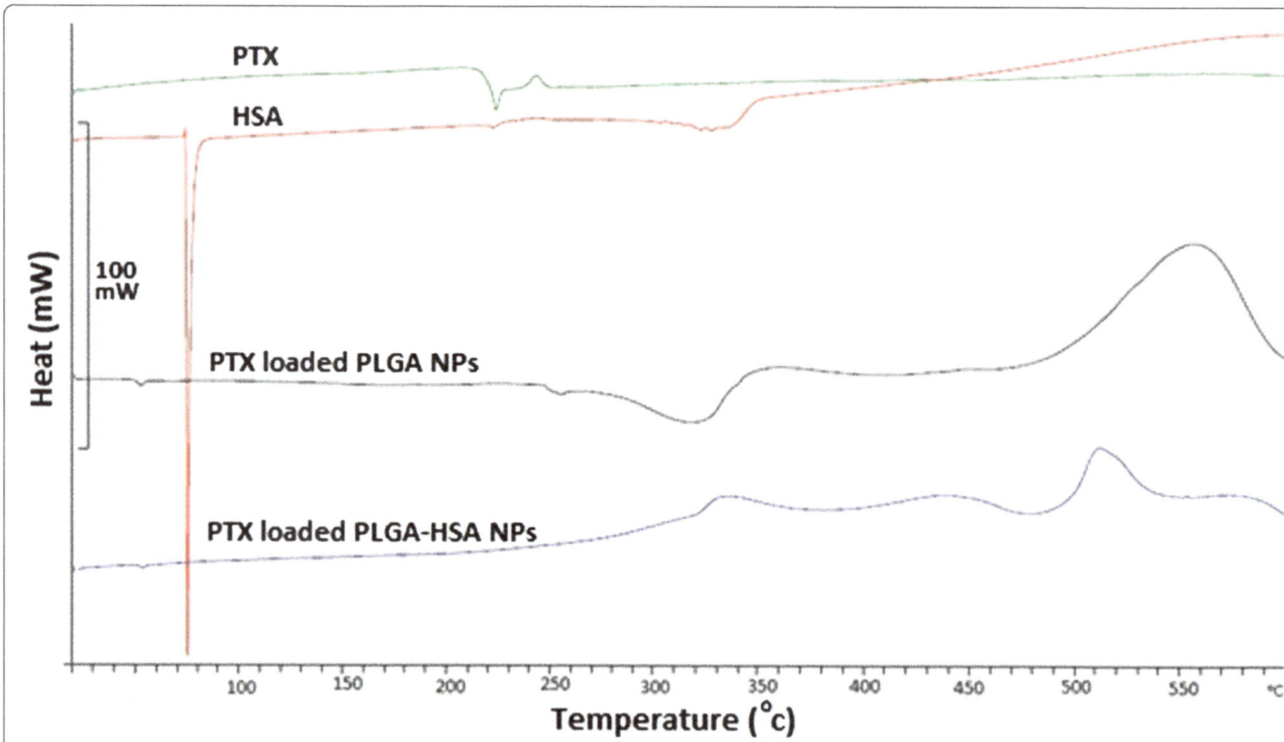

Figure 4 DSC thermograms of PTX, HSA, PLGA NPs, and PLGA-HSA NPs.

PLGA hydrogens because of the small ratio of linker to PLGA. A triplet peak on 7.2- 7.4 can be interoperating as benzoic hydrogens and a small peak found on 6.6 ppm shows the maleimide's hydrogens [22].

Conjugation of PLGA-PMBH was shown by FT-IR assessment (Figure 1). Formation of amide bonds are one of the most important reactions in synthesis of PLGA-PMBH. FTIR spectrum of synthesised polymer verified the amide group formation by some peaks, more specifically; the weak bands at 1620 cm^{-1} were assigned to amide bonds. These results verified the formation of PLGA-PMBH was done successfully.

Nanoparticles characterization

In the current study the modified nanoprecipitation method was chosen for NPs preparation. Several parameters in NPs preparation such as surfactant concentration, ratio of organic to aqueous, ratio of drug to polymer, and applied external energy have crucial effects on the eventual size of NPs and drug loading, so all of these parameters effects were assessed and the optimized formulations were used to prepare NPs to obtain optimized size [23]. Zeta potential, drug loading, and size of NPs were assessed using DLS and HPLC, respectively (Table 1). The evaluation of NPs size by DLS instrument revealed that the mean particle size of NPs was 190 ± 10 nm and when it was conjugated with HSA it increased about 20–30 nm and reached the mean size of 210 ± 10 nm. Theoretically if HSA with axial ratio of 2.66 nm and hydrodynamic radius of 3.7 nm conjugates in high amount around the surface of NPs, it should increase the size of each NPs roughly 19.7 nm and DLS assessment shows the predicted growth in dimension of each NPs (Figure 2). This phenomenon is clearly observed in SEM pictures that are shown in Figure 3. SEM pictures evaluation shows that NPs have spherical shape and mostly have monodispersed size distribution. The nanoparticle's zeta potential assessed by DLS display that PLGA NPs have negative charge (-6 mV) and the zeta potential reaches to -13 mV after HSA conjugation in PLGA-HSA NPs. HSA is also is a negative protein and conjugation will reduce the NPs charge [24].

DSC thermograms of pure PTX, pure HSA, and PTX loaded PLGA NPs and PTX loaded PLGA-HSA NPs demonstrated in Figure 4. In the drug diagram an endothermic peak observed around 220°C and the absence of that in NPs calorimetric curves proposes the lack of crystallinity after NPs preparation; this suggests that during NPs formation polymer hinders crystallization of PTX and the drug exist in the amorphous state. Other verifications, the differences between PLGA NPs and PLGA-HSA NPs peaks show the conjugation of HSA because of the faster degradation of HSA in PLGA-HSA NPs compared to PLGA NPs [25].

HSA conjugation

The infrared spectra of PLGA NPs and PLGA-HSA NPs were recorded by using the KBr pellet method (Figure 1). A very sharp peak at 1650 cm^{-1} in PLGA-HSA NPs that obviously point towards amide bonds existed in amino acids in HSA proved the conjugation take place correctly. FT-IR spectrum, faster degradation of HSA in DSC characterization, increasing the size of NPs, and decreasing the zeta potential are reasons which were proved the conjugation of HSA to PLGA-PMBH.

Drug release profile

In vitro drug release was evaluated in PBS with 2 different pH including 5.5 and 7.4 to assess how the different pH may affect the release profile. Acidic pH was chosen to simulate drug release behavior in the cancer cells. It also was examined before and after conjugation of HSA. In all NPs, 80% of loaded PTX released continuously in a sustained manner during 33 days when assessed in pH of 5.5 and about 70% drug released when experiment was carried out in neutral medium. This phenomena

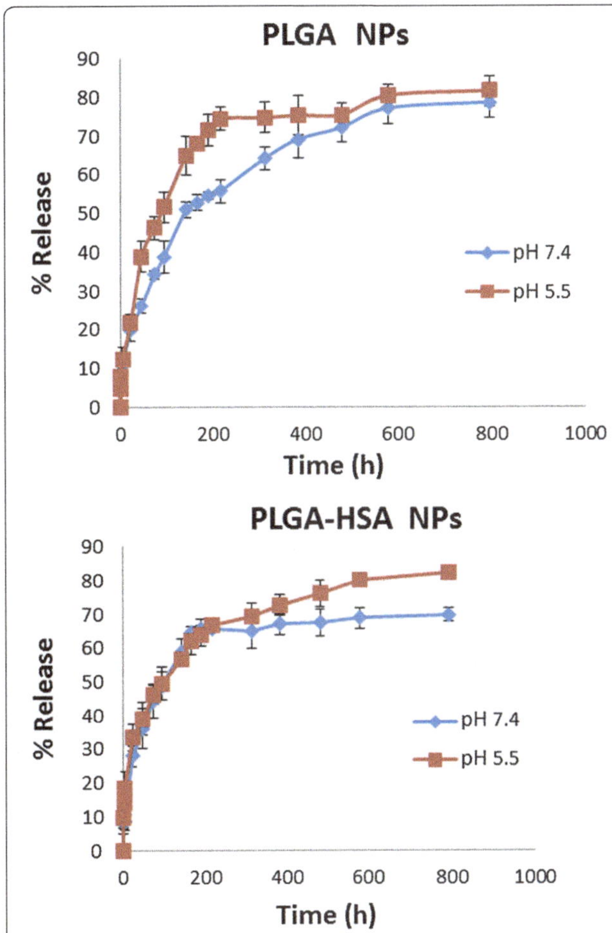

Figure 5 In vitro PTX release profile from PLGA NPs and PLGA-HSA NPs. Data points represent mean ± SD (n = 3).

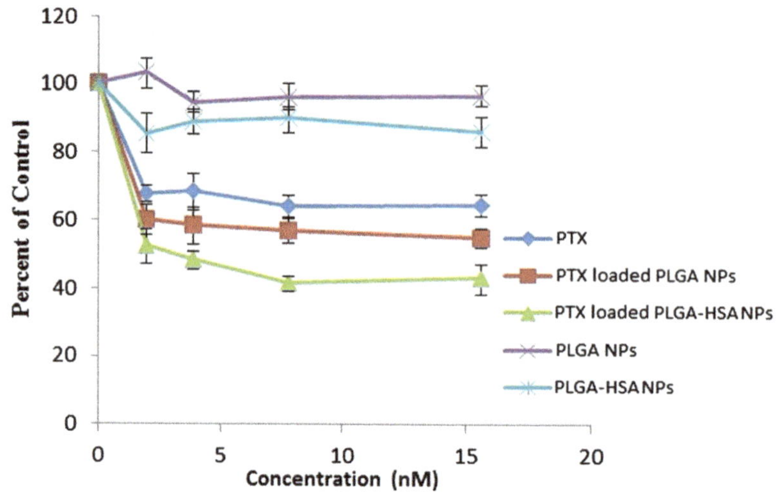

Figure 6 The in vitro cytotoxicity of free PTX, PTX loaded PLGA NPs, and PTX loaded PLGA-HSA NPs with different amount of PTX on T47D breast cancer cells. Data points represent mean ± SD (n = 3).

shows that drug disperse uniformly inside particles and it comes out of it by diffusion. Figure 5 shows that the drug release in acidic environment is faster than neutral ones for all NPs. Hence, this carrier can release drug faster in acidic surroundings of tumors. Acidic pH enhances hydrolization of ester linkage in PLGA and help encapsulated drug to release in control and sustain manner [24-27].

In vitro cytotoxicity

Figure 6 shows the in vitro cytotoxicity of free PTX, PTX loaded PLGA NPs, and PTX loaded PLGA-HSA NPs with different amount of PTX on breast cancer cells (T47D). Figure 6 illustrate that the cytotoxicity of PTX loaded PLGA-HSA NPs was significantly higher than the free PTX and PTX loaded PLGA NPs. Moreover, PTX loaded PLGA NPs have significantly more cytotoxic effect than free PTX. The percent viability of free PTX, PTX loaded PLGA NPs, and PTX loaded PLGA-HSA NPs were 64%, 54%, and 43% in 15 nM concentration, respectively. The enhancement of antitumor activity of PLGA-HSA NPs may be caused by gp60 (albondin) receptor and caveolar transport which both help these particles to increased transendothelial cell transportation of HSA [23,24]. First, HSA molecules bind to gp60 receptors and this binding activates caveolin. After caveolin configuration, HSA and other plasma constituents transfer transversely the endothelial cell to the interstitial space. Improved intratumor delivery of PTX may also other reason for the increased antitumor activity of PLGA-HSA NPs. Activated gp60 receptors which are specific for HSA help transportation of this molecule into tumor tissues by bypassing blood vessel wall barriers [25]. Unloaded NPs tested to evaluate the effect of polymerization and conjugation on cell viability and statistical analysis proved that these parameters do not affect cell viability.

Conclusions

Preparation of the PTX loaded PLGA NPs were done by modified nanoprecipitation method. The hydrophobic PLGA NPs were decorated by hydrophilic HSA as novel anticancer delivery system. The PMBH was used as linker for the conjugation of HSA on the surface of PLGA NPs. The drug loading and encapsulation efficiency were 13% and 80%, respectively. Our results demonstrated that by using PMBH as linker and this method of nanoprecipitation, HSA conjugated NPs would be obtained with desired size, morphological, and drug loading properties. The in vitro cytotoxicity also showed that the HSA decorated NPs are more cytotoxic when compared with plain NPs and free anticancer agent, so these NPs can be used successfully in drug delivery of anticancer agents.

Competing interests

The authors declare that they have no competing interests.

Authors' contributions

MEM conceived the study and drafted the manuscript. SHM carried out the experiments and assisted in preparation of the manuscript. RFM and MNK supervised the synthesis and characterization of nanoparticles. NSR reviewed and revised the manuscript, MA supervised the synthesis and characterization of nanoparticles, BD helped with the characterization tests. SNO supervised the cell culture study, FA co-supervised the study, and RD supervised and coordinated the study and is the corresponding author of the manuscript. All authors read and approved the final manuscript.

Authors' information

Mehdi Esfandyari-Manesh and Seyed Hossein Mostafavi are considered as first author with equal responsibility and rights.

Author details

[1]Nanotechnology Research Centre, Faculty of Pharmacy, Tehran University of Medical Sciences, Tehran, Iran. [2]Novel Drug Delivery Lab, Department of Pharmaceutics, Faculty of Pharmacy, Tehran University of Medical Sciences,

Tehran, Iran. [3]Department of Bioengineering, University of California, Riverside, CA, USA. [4]Medical Nanotechnology Department, School of Advanced Technologies in Medicine, Tehran University of Medical Sciences, Tehran, Iran. [5]Department of Medicinal Chemistry, Faculty of Pharmacy, Tehran University of Medical Sciences, Tehran, Iran. [6]Department of Toxicology and Pharmacology, Faculty of Pharmacy, Tehran University of Medical Science, Tehran, Iran.

References

1. Soppimath KS, Aminabhavi TM, Kulkarni AR, Rudzinski WE. Biodegradable polymeric nanoparticles as drug delivery devices. J Control Release. 2001;70:1–20.
2. Langer R. Drug delivery and targeting. Nature. 1998;392:5–10.
3. Koopaei MN, Khoshayand MR, Mostafavi SH, Amini M, Khorramizadeh MR, Jeddi Tehrani M, et al. Docetaxel loaded PEG-PLGA nanoparticles: optimized drug loading, in-vitro Cytotoxicity and in-vivo Antitumor Effect. Iran J Pharm Res. 2014;13:819–33.
4. Koo OM, Rubinstein I, Onyuksel H. Role of nanotechnology in targeted drug delivery and imaging: a concise review. Nanomed Nanotechnol, Biol Med. 2005;1:193–212.
5. Koopaei MN, Maghazei MS, Mostafavi SH, Jamalifar H, Samadi N, Amini M, et al. Enhanced antibacterial activity of roxithromycin loaded pegylated poly lactide-co-glycolide nanoparticles. Daru. 2012;20:92–9.
6. Sourabhan S, Kaladhar K, Chandra PS. Method to enhance the encapsulation of biologically active molecules in PLGA nanoparticles. Trends Biomater Artif Organs. 2009;22:211–5.
7. Mostafavi SH, Aghajani M, Amani A, Darvishi B, Noori Koopaei M, Pashazadeh AM, et al. Optimization of paclitaxel-loaded poly (D, l-lactide-co-glycolide-N-p-maleimido benzoic hydrazide) nanoparticles size using artificial neural networks. Pharm Dev Technol. 2014;1:1–9.
8. Danhier F, Feron O, Preat V. To exploit the tumor microenvironment: passive and active tumor targeting of nanocarriers for anti-cancer drug delivery. J Control Release. 2012;148:135–46.
9. Park K. Questions on the role of the EPR effect in tumor targeting. J Control Release. 2013;172:391.
10. Fang J, Sawa T, Maeda H. Factors and mechanism of "EPR" effect and the enhanced antitumor effects of macromolecular drugs including SMANCS. Adv Exp Med Biol. 2003;519:29–49.
11. Maeda H, Sawa T, Konno T. Mechanism of tumor-targeted delivery of macromolecular drugs, including the EPR effect in solid tumor and clinical overview of the prototype polymeric drug SMANCS. J Control Release. 2001;74:47–61.
12. Hirsjarvi S, Passirani C, Benoit JP. Passive and active tumour targeting with nanocarriers. Curr Drug Discov Technol. 2011;8:188–96.
13. Okamura Y, Fujie T, Maruyama H, Handa M, Ikeda Y, Takeoka S. Prolonged hemostatic ability of polyethylene glycol-modified polymerized albumin particles carrying fibrinogen gamma-chain dodecapeptide. Transfusion. 2007;47:1254–62.
14. Moghimi SM, Hunter AC, Murray JC. Long-circulating and target-specific nanoparticles: theory to practice. Pharmacol Rev. 2001;53:283–318.
15. He X, Ma J, Mercado AE, Xu W, Jabbari E. Cytotoxicity of Paclitaxel in biodegradable self-assembled core-shell poly (lactide-co-glycolide ethylene oxide fumarate) nanoparticles. Pharm Res. 2008;25:1552–62.
16. Marcucci F, Lefoulon FO. Active targeting with particulate drug carriers in tumor therapy: fundamentals and recent progress. Drug Discov Today. 2004;9:219–28.
17. Stylianopoulos T. EPR-effect: utilizing size-dependent nanoparticle delivery to solid tumors. Ther Deliv. 2013;4:421–3.
18. Manjappa AS, Chaudhari KR, Venkataraju MP, Dantuluri P, Nanda B, Sidda C, et al. Antibody derivatization and conjugation strategies: application in preparation of stealth immunoliposome to target chemotherapeutics to tumor. J Control Release. 2010;150:2–22.
19. Weber C, Reiss S, Langer K. Preparation of surface modified protein nanoparticles by introduction of sulfhydryl groups. Int J Pharm. 2000;211:67–78.
20. Fonseca C, Simões S, Gaspar R. Paclitaxel-loaded PLGA nanoparticles: preparation, physicochemical characterization and in vitro anti-tumoral activity. J Control Release. 2002;83:273–86.
21. Wang YM, Sato H, Adachi I, Horikoshi I. Preparation and characterization of poly (lactic-co-glycolic acid) microspheres for targeted delivery of a novel anticancer agent, Taxol. Chem Pharm Bull. 1996;44:1935–40.
22. Fessi H, Puisieux F, Devissaguet JP, Ammoury N, Benita S. Nanocapsule formation by interfacial polymer deposition following solvent displacement. Int J Pharm. 1989;55:R1–4.
23. Liu J, Meisner D, Kwong E, Wu XY, Johnston MR. A novel trans-lymphatic drug delivery system: Implantable gelatin sponge impregnated with PLGA "paclitaxel microspheres. Biomaterials. 2007;28:3236–44.
24. Tessmar J, Mikos A, Gopferich A. The use of poly (ethylene glycol)-block-poly (lactic acid) derived copolymers for the rapid creation of biomimetic surfaces. Biomaterials. 2003;24:4475–86.
25. Manchanda R, Fernandez-Fernandez A, Nagesetti A, McGoron AJ. Preparation and characterization of a polymeric (PLGA) nanoparticulate drug delivery system with simultaneous incorporation of chemotherapeutic and thermo-optical agents. Colloids Surf B: Biointerfaces. 2009;75:260–7.
26. Musumeci T, Ventura CA, Giannone I, Ruozi B, Montenegro L, Pignatello R, et al. PLA/PLGA nanoparticles for sustained release of docetaxel. Int J Pharm. 2006;325:172–9.
27. Gindy ME, Ji S, Hoye TR, Panagiotopoulos AZ, Prud'homme RK. Preparation of poly (ethylene glycol) protected nanoparticles with variable bioconjugate ligand density. Biomacromolecules. 2008;9:2705–11.

Artemia salina as a model organism in toxicity assessment of nanoparticles

Somayeh Rajabi[1], Ali Ramazani[1,2*], Mehrdad Hamidi[3] and Tahereh Naji[1]

Abstract

Background: Because of expanding presence of nanomaterials, there has been an increase in the exposure of humans to nanoparticles that is why nanotoxicology studies are important. A number of studies on the effects of nanomatrials in *in vitro* and *in vivo* systems have been published. Currently cytotoxicity of different nanoparticles is assessed using the 3-(4,5-dimethylthiazol-2-yl)-2,5-diphenyltetrazolium bromide (MTT) assay on different cell lines to determine cell viability, a tedious and expensive method. The aim of this study was to evaluate the *Artemia salina* test in comparison with the MTT assay in the assessment of cytotoxicity of nanostructures because the former method is more rapid and convenient and less expensive.

Methods: At the first stage, toxicity of different nanoparticles with different concentrations (1.56–400 μg/mL) was measured by means of the brine shrimp lethality test. At the second stage, the effect of nanoparticles on the viability of the L929 cell line was assessed using the MTT assay. Experiments were conducted with each concentration in triplicate.

Results: The results obtained from both tests (*A. salina* test and MTT assay) did not have statistically significant differences ($P > 0.05$).

Conclusions: These findings suggest that the *A. salina* test may expedite toxicity experiments and decrease costs, and therefore, may be considered an alternative to the *in vitro* cell culture assay.

Keywords: *Artemia salina*, Toxicity, Nanoparticle, Cell culture

Background

Nanoscience is a novel science that is being developed to probe and manipulate matter on the scale of single atoms and molecules. Physicist Richard P. Feynman was the first to mention molecular machines built with atomic precision at a meeting of the American Physical Society in 1959 [1], and Noro Taniguchi, a professor at the University of Tokyo, coined the term nanotechnology in 1979 [2]. Nanotechnology is the use of nanoscience to design NMs (nanomaterials) and NPs (nanoparticles), with structural components between 1 and 100 nanometers; it is thought to be one of the key technologies of the 21st century [3,4]. In the above range, physicochemical characteristics of NPs in biological systems can vary. Some potential hazards have been identified in the life cycle of NMs and NPs [5,6]. Growing research and development in nanotechnology have resulted in the identification of many unique properties of nanomaterials such as enhanced magnetic, catalytic, optical, electrical, and mechanical properties when compared to conventional formulations of the same materials [7]. While nanoparticles have a wide variety of functions, there has been increasing issues and debate amongst the regulatory and scientific community regarding the fate of nanoparticles in biological systems and associated side effects these agents might have on living organisms [8-12]. These materials are increasingly used for commercial purposes and leading to direct and indirect exposure of humans [13]. Any *in vivo* use of nanoparticles requires thorough understanding of the kinetics and toxicology of the particles, establishment of principles and test procedures to ensure safe manufacture and usage of nanomaterials, and comprehensive training of personnel in safety and potential hazards of nanotechnology [13]. Nanotoxicology research is applied

* Correspondence: ramazania@zums.ac.ir
[1]Cell and Molecular Biology Departments, Pharmaceutical Sciences Branch, Islamic Azad University, Tehran, Iran
[2]Biotechnology Departments, School of Pharmacy, Zanjan University of Medical Sciences, Zanjan, Iran
Full list of author information is available at the end of the article

to various fields including biology and pathology, but typically to pharmacology and to the use of NMs and nanodevices for diagnostic and therapeutic purposes. Therefore, a key goal for toxicologists is to identify *in vitro* and *in vivo* assays accurately reflecting the ability of NPs to induce toxic effects in the humans and in the environment. In addition, standardized tests for both *in vitro* and *in vivo* studies are needed to develop better and more rapid screening techniques and to predict toxicity [14,15]. The cytotoxicity effects of NPs were investigated in a multitude of animal models by means of *in vivo* tests employing the typical NP exposure routes, i.e., pulmonary, oral, dermal, and injection based [16]. The cost and labor intensiveness of the *in vivo* studies have led researchers to the use of *in vitro* methods for assessment of NPs cytotoxicity. In addition, animal rights advocates have criticized the use of animals in nanotechnology experiments. All *in vivo* studies must be conducted with the approval of regulatory bodies such as IACUC (an Institutional Animal Care and Use Committee) to ensure ethical treatment of animals [16]. For the above reasons, *in vitro* techniques are increasingly used for the analysis of cytotoxicity of NPs including cell culture, the WST-1 assay [17,18], XTT assay, MTT assay [19,20], LDH assay, BrdU assay, and fluorescence microscopy [21,22]. Currently, cytotoxicity testing of various NPs in cell culture involves the MTT assay, which determines cell viability based on mitochondrial function by measuring the activity of mitochondrial enzymes [23-27]. In this test, tetrazolium is reduced by mitochondrial succinate dehydrogenase of live cells to water-insoluble purple formazan crystals, which are subsequently solubilized using an organic solvent (e.g., dimethyl sulfoxide; DMSO) [28]. The cell viability is quantified based on absorbance of the solution at 570 nm. Therefore, the MTT assay requires solubilization steps with tetrazolium, which is toxic to cells and can interfere with some chemical reactions [28]. The cytotoxicity assays are often tedious and expensive, and there is a lack of a simple and rapid screening procedure. Nowadays, brine shrimp lethality assays are extensively used in research and applied toxicology [29]. There is a tendency to use an *Artemia salina* assay in toxicological tests that screen a large number of extracts for drug discovery in medicinal plants [30-33]. This is because in this case, aseptic techniques are not required, and thus *A. salina* assays could replace the more ethically challenging MTT assay that requires animal serum [34]. This assay was proposed by Michael and coworkers in 1959 and was later adopted by many laboratories as a method for preliminary estimation of toxicity [35]. *Artemia* is one of the most valuable test organisms available for ecotoxicity testing, and the available research suggests that several applications of *Artemia* to toxicology and ecotoxicology will continue to be used widely [36]. Because of the rapidity, convenience, and low cost of *Artemia*-based assays, we decided to evaluate the *A. salina* test in comparison with the MTT assay in the assessment of cytotoxicity of different classes of NPs.

Materials and methods

Materials

Fetal bovine serum (FBS), phosphate-buffered saline (PBS), trypsin, penicillin, streptomycin, DMSO, 3-[4,5-dimethylthiazol-2-yl]-2,5-diphenyl tetrazolium bromide (MTT), Triton X-100, and the RPMI-1640 medium supplemented with 10% heat inactivated FBS were purchased from Sigma–Aldrich. The mouse fibroblast cell line (L929) was provided by Pasteur Institute of Iran.

Synthesis of NPs

Sixteen NPs from different classes (Table 1) were prepared by the Nanotechnology Laboratory of School of Pharmacy of Zanjan University of Medical Sciences. The zeta potential and particle size distribution of the prepared nanoparticles were determined by photon correlation spectroscopy (PCS) using a Nano/zetasizer (Malvern Instruments, Nano ZS, Worcestershire, UK) working on the dynamic light scattering (DLS) platform.

Cell culture and determination of cytotoxicity by MTT assay

The effect of NPs on the viability of L929 cells was assessed by means of the MTT assay. After thawing, the cells were cultured in the RPMI 1640 medium containing 10% FBS, penicillin (100 units/mL), and streptomycin (100 mg/mL) at 37°C in a humidified 5% CO_2 incubator. The cells were seeded in a 96-well plate at a density of 5,000 cells per well (the cells were stained with trypan blue and counted with haemocytometer). These cells were incubated overnight at 37°C before the cell viability test. A stock suspension of each NP at 50 mg/mL in distilled water was prepared. After that, fresh suspensions of different concentrations of NPs (two fold serial dilutions from 1.56–400 μg/mL) were made using serial dilution of the stock suspensions of NPs in the RPMI 1640 medium, immediately before use. We added 200 μL of a suspension (different concentrations of NPs) to each well of the microtiter plates. The cells were incubated for 24 h under the same conditions. Wells without any NPs served as a negative control. The experiments were performed in triplicate for each concentration. To assess cell survival, 100 μL of an MTT solution (2 mg/mL in PBS) was added to each well and incubated for 3 h at 37°C to produce insoluble formazan. Then, 100 μL of DMSO was added to dissolve formazan crystals, and the absorbance was measured on an Infinite M200 microplate reader (Tecan) at 570 nm, with 630 nm as a reference wavelength. The percentage of cell viability

Table 1 Names and characteristics of NPs used in this study

NPs class	NPs name	Size NPs (nm)	Zeta potential (mV)
Inorganic nanoparticles	Magnetic	55	- 31
	Nanosfer	97	+8.9
Lipid-base nanoparticles	Liposome	139.3	- 28
	Coated SLNs	464.6	+20
	Uncoated SLNs	176.3	- 45
	Nanogele + SLN	376.6	+4
Polymeric nanoparticles	Nanogele	270	+22
	Micellar	97.9	- 1.10
	PAMAM (G5)	6	+36.8
	PAMAM-FA	55	+36.4
	PAMAM-PEG-FA	70	9.12
Drug nanoparticles	Nanosuspansion Atorvastatin	269.8	ND
	Nanosuspansion Ibuprofen	160.9	ND
	Nanosuspansion Repaglinide	260.6	ND
	Nanosuspansion Cyclosporin	220.5	ND
	Nanosuspansion Azitromycin	270	ND

ND; not determined.

was calculated using the formula $(A_{test}/A_{control}) \times 100$, where A_{test} is the mean absorbance of treated cells and $A_{control}$ is the mean absorbance of a negative control.

Toxicity testing by *A. salina*

A. salina eggs were purchased from the Aquatic Animal Research Center, Urmia University, Urmia, Iran. Dried cysts were placed in a bottle containing artificial sea water which was prepared by dissolving 35 g of sodium chloride in 1 L of distilled water. After 36–48 h incubation at room temperature (28–30°C) under conditions of strong aeration and continuous illuminations [33], the larvae (nauplii) hatched within 48 h.

The evaluation of cytotoxicity of NPs in *A. salina* was performed according to the previous methods [30,33,37,38]. The assay was carried out on larvae of brine shrimp (*A. salina* Leach.). A stock solution of 50 mg of nanoparticles in 1 mL of distilled water was prepared. Then, fresh suspensions with different concentrations of NPs (two fold serial dilutions from 1.56–400 μg/mL) were made by means of serial dilution of the stock suspensions of NPs in artificial sea water (35 g/L) immediately before use. We added 200 μL of a suspension (different concentrations of NPs) to each well of the 96-well microtiter plates. After that, 10 nauplii per well were added in the 96-well plates and incubated at room temperature for 24 h. The numbers of surviving nauplii in each well were counted under a stereoscopic microscope after 24 h. The experiments were conducted in triplicate for each concentration. The negative control wells contained 10 nauplii and artificial sea water only. The percentages of deaths were calculated by comparing the number of survivors in the test and control wells. The lethality was calculated using Abbott's formula as follows: % Lethality = [(Test – Control)/Control] × 100.

Statistical analysis

All experiments were done in triplicate and the results were calculated as a mean ± standard deviation (SD). The experimental data were processed using the paired sample *t*-test, Pearson correlation and linear regression analysis of the SPSS version 16.0 software for Windows. The toxicity of each nanoparticle was calculated from the 50% lethality dose (LD_{50}) by means of Finney's Probit analysis [39].

Results

Cytotoxicity of nanostructures by the MTT assay

The MTT assay is a viable method for assessing *in vitro* cytotoxicity of NPs. In this study, L929 cells were treated with different concentrations (0.78–200 μg/mL) of the 16 NPs (Table 1). Cell viability was determined 24 hours after the treatment. The results are presented in Table 2. Uncoated solid lipid nanoparticles (SLNs), Nanogel + SLN, Bare Nanogel, polyamidoamine (PAMAM; G5), and PAMAM-FA demonstrated moderate cytotoxicity. In contrast, the NPs with $IC_{50} > 200$ μg/mL were not toxic to the L929 cell line. The cytotoxicity was weak when the IC_{50} values were between 150 and 200 μg/mL.

Cytotoxicity of nanostructures in the brine shrimp assay

The brine shrimp lethality assay was also used to determine the cytotoxicity of NPs. According to the results

Table 2 NPs toxicity assay by *Artemia salina* and MTT assay

NPs name	*Artemia salina* assay, LC_{50} (μg/m)	95% confidence limits for concentration		MTT assay, IC_{50} (μg/ml)	95% confidence limits for concentration	
		Lower bound	Upper bound		Lower bound	Upper bound
Magnetic	698.710	431.764	2669.870	997.402	527.931	3340.601
Nanosfer	302.001	215.853	497.009	207.431	141.862	365.065
Liposome	751.249	432.851	6492.955	1002.666	543.931	4358.603
Coated SLNs	360.594	285.519	501.000	605.594	472.900	1248.021
Uncoated SLNs	239.040	192.979	310.917	149.018	90.886	328.486
Nanogele + SLN	19.656	15.141	24.908	113.903	58.153	380.573
Nanogele	40.440	8.221	95.196	130.171	77.672	285.277
Micellar	560.060	352.592	1801.667	686.002	263.396	1329.851
PAMAM (G5)	145.6	60.435	671.764	72.254	41.149	139.077
PAMAM-FA	213.316	185.467	839.316	99.783	61.360	130.925
PAMAM-PEG-FA	401.21	256.482	1002.310	270.585	129.042	496.556
Nanosuspansion Atorvastatin	417.349	272.658	1046.615	807.668	301.840	1080.114
Nanosuspansion Ibuprofen	373.526	285.877	559.357	156.433	117.536	244.043
Nanosuspansion Repaglinide	807.754	488.424	4335.993	297.756	221.995	527.574
Nanosuspansion Cyclosporin	531.961	368.036	1095.239	167.965	108.493	230.459
Nanosuspansion Azitromycin	110.316	57.555	231.560	162.512	168.114	249.652

(Table 2), of the 16 NPs that we screened for lethality in *A. salina*, only two NPs (Nanogel + SLN and Nanogel) showed strong toxicity (LC_{50} < 100 μg/mL). In contrast, NPs of Uncoated SLN, PAMAM (G5), Nanosuspension Ibuprofen, and Nanosuspension Azithromycin exhibited moderate cytotoxicity (LC_{50} ranged between 100 and 500 μg/mL), and the other NPs showed weak cytotoxicity in *A. salina* (LC_{50} range 500–1000 μg/mL) [37,40]. Comparison between the results of two methods is indicated in Figure 1. As shown in Figure 1, the trend lines and the direction of the graphs are in same direction.

Discussion

Several assays for eco-toxicological testing of nanomaterials have been developed. Different model systems such as bacteria [41], fathead minnows [42], zebrafish embryos [43], copepod [44], Daphnia [45,46], and rainbow trout [47,48] have been reported [49]. In addition to standard tests, there is a need to establish better, rapid and convenient methods to predict the toxic effects of nanomaterials. Till now, A few studies have reported the toxicity effect of nanomaterials on *A. salina* [38,50-52]. These studies were investigated on metal nanoparticles

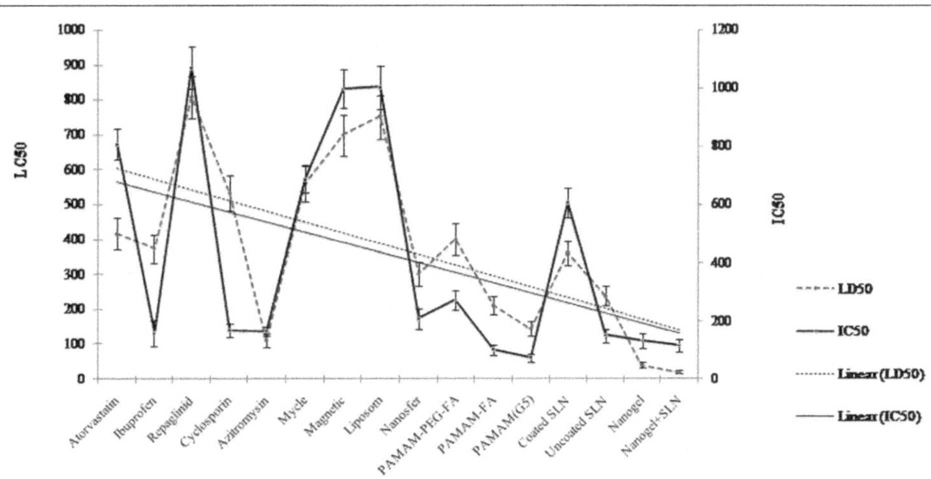

Figure 1 Comparison of *Artemia salina* and MTT assay results

and we want develop the *A. salina* assay for toxicity assessment of different class of nanomaterials especially those used for drug deliveries.

In this work, cytotoxicity of 16 NPs was assessed using two methods: the brine shrimp lethality assay and the MTT assay in L929 cells. According to the results (Figure 1) the correlation between the LC_{50} and IC_{50} values is significant ($R^2 = 0.72$, $P = 0.000$). This mean that 72% variability noted in MTT method could be accounted for by brine shrimp lethality assay and 28% is unaccounted for due to measurement error. There was not statistically significant difference between two assays when the results were compared with paired t test ($P = 0.402$). Also the comparison between LC_{50} and IC_{50} mean values statistically analyzed by chi square test and the result showed that there is no differences between two assay methods ($P = 0.235$). This mean that results obtained by brine shrimp lethality assay is comparable with MTT results. Both the ranking and the degree of cytotoxicity were similar between the brine shrimp lethality assay and the MTT assay. As it has been shown in Table 2, the ranges of 95% confidence limit are wide. The width of the confidence interval for an individual study depends to a large extent on the sample size. Larger studies tend to give more precise estimates of effects (and hence have narrower confidence intervals) than smaller studies. In order to obtain a more reliable estimate of the confidence interval it may be necessary to perform several independent assays and to combine these into one single confidence interval [53]. The results demonstrate the ability of the brine shrimp lethality assay to accurately quantify cytotoxicity of NPs and to replace the MTT assay, which is expensive and tedious. In this field, cytotoxicity assays and experimental procedures often lack a simple, convenient, and rapid screening method. On the other hand, the brine shrimp lethality assay has been used in toxicology research routinely for over thirty years [36]. The genus *Artemia* has a several advantages that make it ideal for general toxicity assays including wide geographical distribution, adaptability to extreme conditions, capability to use several nutrient resources, and availability of their cysts for collection [36]. The brine shrimp assay is convenient because it is rapid (24 h), economical, and simple. The eggs of *A. salina* are readily available at low cost and remain viable for years in dry storage. The assay easily accommodates a large number of nauplii for statistical validation and no special equipment is needed. Moreover, this assay does not require animal serum and thereby it prevents unnecessary use of animals in scientific experiments. In summary, it is possible to measure cytotoxicity of NPs using the brine shrimp lethality assay instead of the common *in vitro* cell culture assays.

Conclusion

This work shows that the brine shrimp lethality assay can be used to study toxicity of nanostructures. Self-sufficiency and rapid results are important advantages of this method. *Artemia*-based toxicity assay of NPs are cheap, continuously available, simple and reliable and are thus an important answer to routine needs of toxicity screening, for industrial monitoring requirements or for regulatory purposes. Our data are expected to facilitate pharmacological and nanotoxicological research.

Competing interests

The authors declare that they have no competing interests.

Authors' contributions

SR carried out the experiments and drafted the manuscript. AR designed the study and participated in data analysis. MH participated in study design. TN helped in study design and manuscript preparation. All authors read and approved the final manuscript.

Acknowledgments

We thank the research deputy of Zanjan University of Medical Sciences (ZUMS) for financial support of this project.

Author details

[1]Cell and Molecular Biology Departments, Pharmaceutical Sciences Branch, Islamic Azad University, Tehran, Iran. [2]Biotechnology Departments, School of Pharmacy, Zanjan University of Medical Sciences, Zanjan, Iran. [3]Zanjan Pharmaceutical Nanotechnology Research Center, Zanjan University of Medical Sciences, Zanjan, Iran.

References

1. Toumey CP. Reading Feynman into nanotechnology. Techné: Res Philos Technol. 2009;12:133–68.
2. Singh M, Manikandan S, Kumaraguru A. Nanoparticles: a new technology with wide applications. Res J Nanosci Nanotechnol. 2011;1:1–11.
3. Lloyd SM, Lave LB, Matthews HS. Life cycle benefits of using nanotechnology to stabilize platinum-group metal particles in automotive catalysts. Environ Sci Technol. 2005;39:1384–92.
4. Yadav A, Ghune M, Jain DK. Nano-medicine based drug delivery system. J Advanced Pharm Educ Res. 2011;1:201–13.
5. Drobne D. Nanotoxicology for safe and sustainable nanotechnology. Arh Hig Rada Toksikol. 2007;58:471–8.
6. Ikramullah A, Salve D, Pai G, Rathore M, Joshi D. In vitro cytotoxicity testing of silver nano-particals in lymphocyte and sperm cells. Ind J Fund Appl Life Sci. 2013;3:44–7.
7. Arora S, Rajwade JM, Paknikar KM. Nanotoxicology and in vitro studies: the need of the hour. Toxicol Appl Pharmacol. 2012;258:151–65.
8. Sharma A, Madhunapantula SV, Robertson GP. Toxicological considerations when creating nanoparticle-based drugs and drug delivery systems. Expert Opin Drug Metab Toxicol. 2012;8:47–69.
9. Hsieh SF, Bello D, Schmidt DF, Pal AK, Rogers EJ. Biological oxidative damage by carbon nanotubes: fingerprint or footprint? Nanotoxicology. 2012;6:61–76.
10. Wessels A, Van Berlo D, Boots AW, Gerloff K, Scherbart AM, Cassee FR, et al. Oxidative stress and DNA damage responses in rat and mouse lung to inhaled carbon nanoparticles. Nanotoxicology. 2011;5:66–78.
11. Mogharabi M, Abdollahi M, Faramarzi M. Toxicity of nanomaterials; an undermined issue. Daru. 2014;22:59.
12. Mostafalou S, Mohammadi H, Ramazani A, Abdollahi M. Different biokinetics of nanomedicines linking to their toxicity; an overview. Daru. 2013;21:14.
13. Nel A, Xia T, Madler L, Li N. Toxic potential of materials at the nanolevel. Science. 2006;311:622–7.
14. Dhawan A, Sharma V. Toxicity assessment of nanomaterials: methods and challenges. Anal Bioanal Chem. 2010;398:589–605.
15. Maccormack TJ, Clark RJ, Dang MK, Ma G, Kelly JA, Veinot JG, et al. Inhibition of enzyme activity by nanomaterials: potential mechanisms and implications for nanotoxicity testing. Nanotoxicology. 2012;6:514–25.

16. Suh WH, Suslick KS, Stucky GD, Suh YH. Nanotechnology, nanotoxicology, and neuroscience. Prog Neurobiol. 2009;87:133–70.
17. Dechsakulthorn F, Hayes A, Bakand S, Joeng L, Winder C. In vitro cytotoxicity assessment of selected nanoparticles using human skin fibroblasts. AATEX. 2007;14:397–400.
18. Gonzales M, Mitsumori LM, Kushleika JV, Rosenfeld ME, Krishnan KM. Cytotoxicity of iron oxide nanoparticles made from the thermal decomposition of organometallics and aqueous phase transfer with Pluronic F127. Contrast Media Mol Imaging. 2010;5:286–93.
19. Zanette C, Pelin M, Crosera M, Adami G, Bovenzi M, Larese FF, et al. Silver nanoparticles exert a long-lasting antiproliferative effect on human keratinocyte HaCaT cell line. Toxicol In Vitro. 2011;25:1053–60.
20. Sauer UG, Vogel S, Hess A, Kolle SN, Ma-Hock L, van Ravenzwaay B, et al. In vivo-in vitro comparison of acute respiratory tract toxicity using human 3D airway epithelial models and human A549 and murine 3T3 monolayer cell systems. Toxicol In Vitro. 2013;27:174–90.
21. Decker T, Lohmann-Matthes ML. A quick and simple method for the quantitation of lactate dehydrogenase release in measurements of cellular cytotoxicity and tumor necrosis factor (TNF) activity. J Immunol Methods. 1988;115:61–9.
22. Korzeniewski C, Callewaert DM. An enzyme-release assay for natural cytotoxicity. J Immunol Methods. 1983;64:313–20.
23. Alley MC, Scudiero DA, Monks A, Hursey ML, Czerwinski MJ, Fine DL, et al. Feasibility of drug screening with panels of human tumor cell lines using a microculture tetrazolium assay. Cancer Res. 1988;48:589–601.
24. Campling BG, Pym J, Baker HM, Cole SP, Lam YM. Chemosensitivity testing of small cell lung cancer using the MTT assay. Br J Cancer. 1991;63:75–83.
25. Fisichella M, Dabboue H, Bhattacharyya S, Saboungi ML, Salvetat JP, Hevor T, et al. Mesoporous silica nanoparticles enhance MTT formazan exocytosis in HeLa cells and astrocytes. Toxicol In Vitro. 2009;23:697–703.
26. Silva GA. Introduction to nanotechnology and its applications to medicine. Surg Neurol. 2004;61:216–20.
27. Wang H, Cheng H, Wang F, Wei D, Wang X. An improved 3-(4,5-dimethyl-thiazol-2-yl)-2,5-diphenyl tetrazolium bromide (MTT) reduction assay for evaluating the viability of Escherichia coli cells. J Microbiol Methods. 2010;82:330–3.
28. Berridge MV, Herst PM, Tan AS. Tetrazolium dyes as tools in cell biology: new insights into their cellular reduction. Biotechnol Annu Rev. 2005;11:127–52.
29. Costa-Lotufo LV, Khan MT, Ather A, Wilke DV, Jimenez PC, Pessoa C, et al. Studies of the anticancer potential of plants used in Bangladeshi folk medicine. J Ethnopharmacol. 2005;99:21–30.
30. Kheiri Manjili H, Jafari H, Ramazani A, Davoudi N. Anti-leishmanial and toxicity activities of some selected Iranian medicinal plants. Parasitol Res. 2012;111:2115–21.
31. Ramazani A, Sardari S, Zakeri S, Vaziri B. In vitro antiplasmodial and phytochemical study of five Artemisia species from Iran and in vivo activity of two species. Parasitol Res. 2010;107:593–9.
32. Ramazani A, Zakeri S, Sardari S, Khodakarim N, Djadidt ND. In vitro and in vivo anti-malarial activity of Boerhavia elegans and Solanum surattense. Malar J. 2010;9:124.
33. Sangian H, Faramarzi H, Yazdinezhad A, Mousavi SJ, Zamani Z, Noubarani M, et al. Antiplasmodial activity of ethanolic extracts of some selected medicinal plants from the northwest of Iran. Parasitol Res. 2013;112:3697–701.
34. Mclaughlin JL, Rogers LL, Anderson JE. The use of biological assays to evaluate botanicals. Drug Inf J. 1998;32:513–24.
35. Insanu M, Anggadiredja J, Kayser O. Curcacycline A and B–new pharmacological insights to an old drug. Int J Appl Res Nat Prod. 2012;5:26–34.
36. Nunes BS, Carvalho FD, Guilhermino LM, Van Stappen G. Use of the genus Artemia in ecotoxicity testing. Environ Pollut. 2006;144:453–62.
37. Meyer BN, Ferrigni NR, Putnam JE, Jacobsen LB, Nichols DE, McLaughlin JL. Brine shrimp: a convenient general bioassay for active plant constituents. Planta Med. 1982;45:31–4.
38. Ashtari K, Khajeh K, Fasihi J, Ashtari P, Ramazani A, Vali H. Silica-encapsulated magnetic nanoparticles: enzyme immobilization and cytotoxic study. Int J Biol Macromol. 2012;50:1063–9.
39. Finney DJ. The adjustment for a natural response rate in probit analysis. Ann Appl Biol. 1949;36:187–95.
40. Padmaja R, Arun PC, Prashanth D, Deepak M, Amit A, Anjana M. Brine shrimp lethality bioassay of selected Indian medicinal plants. Fitoterapia. 2002;73:508–10.
41. Lyon DY, Fortner JD, Sayes CM, Colvin VL, Hughe JB. Bacterial cell association and antimicrobial activity of a C60 water suspension. Environ Toxicol Chem. 2005;24:2757–62.
42. Zhu S, Oberdorster E, Haasch ML. Toxicity of an engineered nanoparticle (fullerene, C60) in two aquatic species, Daphnia and fathead minnow. Mar Environ Res. 2006;62(Suppl):S5–9.
43. Zhu X, Zhu L, Li Y, Duan Z, Chen W, Alvarez PJ. Developmental toxicity in zebrafish (Danio rerio) embryos after exposure to manufactured nanomaterials: buckminsterfullerene aggregates (nC60) and fullerol. Environ Toxicol Chem. 2007;26:976–9.
44. Templeton RC, Ferguson PL, Washburn KM, Scrivens WA, Chandler GT. Life-cycle effects of single-walled carbon nanotubes (SWNTs) on an estuarine meiobenthic copepod. Environ Sci Technol. 2006;40:7387–93.
45. Hund-Rinke K, Simon M. Ecotoxic effect of photocatalytic active nanoparticles (TiO2) on algae and daphnids. Environ Sci Pollut Res Int. 2006;13:225–32.
46. Roberts AP, Mount AS, Seda B, Souther J, Qiao R, Lin S, et al. In vivo biomodification of lipid-coated carbon nanotubes by Daphnia magna. Environ Sci Technol. 2007;41:3025–9.
47. Smith CJ, Shaw BJ, Handy RD. Toxicity of single walled carbon nanotubes to rainbow trout, (Oncorhynchus mykiss): respiratory toxicity, organ pathologies, and other physiological effects. Aquat Toxicol. 2007;82:94–109.
48. Fraser TW, Reinardy HC, Shaw BJ, Henry TB, Handy RD. Dietary toxicity of single-walled carbon nanotubes and fullerenes (C60) in rainbow trout (Oncorhynchus mykiss). Nanotoxicology. 2011;5:98–108.
49. Ambrosone A, Marchesano V, Mazzarella V, Tortiglione C. Nanotoxicology using the sea anemone Nematostella vectensis: from developmental toxicity to genotoxicology. Nanotoxicology. 2014;8:508–20.
50. Cornejo-Garrido H, Kibanova D, Nieto-Camacho A, Guzman J, Ramirez-Apan T, Fernandez-Lomelin P, et al. Oxidative stress, cytoxicity, and cell mortality induced by nano-sized lead in aqueous suspensions. Chemosphere. 2011;84:1329–35.
51. Ates M, Daniels J, Arslan Z, Farah IO. Effects of aqueous suspensions of titanium dioxide nanoparticles on Artemia salina: assessment of nanoparticle aggregation, accumulation, and toxicity. Environ Monit Assess. 2013;185:3339–48.
52. Pretti C, Oliva M, Pietro RD, Monni G, Cevasco G, Chiellini F, et al. Ecotoxicity of pristine graphene to marine organisms. Ecotoxicol Environ Saf. 2014;101:138–45.
53. Hong W, Meier P, Deininger R. Estimation of a single probit line from multiple toxicity test data. Aquat Toxicol. 1988;12:193–202.

23

A randomized controlled trial of gonadotropin-releasing hormone agonist versus gonadotropin-releasing hormone antagonist in Iranian infertile couples: oocyte gene expression

Fatemeh Sadat Hoseini[1], Seyed Mohammad Hossein Noori Mugahi[2], Firoozeh Akbari-Asbagh[3], Poopak Eftekhari-Yazdi[4], Behrouz Aflatoonian[5], Seyed Hamid Aghaee-Bakhtiari[6], Reza Aflatoonian[7] and Nasser Salsabili[8*]

Abstract

Background: The main objective of the present work was to compare the effects of the gonadotropin-releasing hormone agonist (GnRH-a) and GnRH antagonist (GnRH-ant) on the gene expression profiles of oocytes obtained from Iranian infertile couples undergoing in vitro fertilization (IVF).

Methods: Fifty infertile couples who underwent IVF between June 2012 and November 2013 at the Infertility Center of Tehran Women General Hospital, Tehran University of Medical Sciences, were included in this study. We included women that had undergone IVF treatment because of male factor, tubal factor, or unexplained infertility. The women randomly underwent controlled ovarian stimulation (COS) with either the GnRH-a ($n = 26$) or the GnRH-ant ($n = 24$). We obtained 50 germinal vesicle (GV) oocytes donated by women in each group. After the sampling, pool of 50 GV oocytes for each group was separately analyzed by quantitative polymerase chain reaction (qPCR).

Result: The expression levels of Adenosine triphosphatase 6 (ATPase 6), Bone morphogenetic protein 15 (BMP15), and Neuronal apoptosis inhibitory protein (NAIP) genes were significantly upregulated in the GnRH-ant group compared to the GnRH-a group, with the fold change of 3.990 (SD ± 1.325), 6.274 (SD ± 1.542), and 2.156 (SD ± 1.443), respectively, ($P < 0.001$). Growth differentiation factor 9 (GDF9) mRNA did not have any expression in the GnRH-a group; however, GDF9 mRNA was expressed in the GnRH-ant group. Finally, it was found that the genes involved in the DNA repairing and cell cycle checkpoint did not have any expression in either group.

Conclusion: The present study showed, for the first time, the expression levels of genes involved in the cytoplasmic maturity (BMP15, GDF9), adenosine triphosphate production (ATPase 6), and antiapoptotic process (NAIP), in human GV oocytes were significantly higher in the GnRH-anta group than in the GnRH-a group in COS. Higher expression level of these genes when GnRH-ant protocol is applied, this protocol seems to be a more appropriate choice for women with poly cystic ovarian syndrome, because it can probably improve the expression of the aforementioned genes.

Trial registration: Current Controlled Trials: IRCT 2014031112307 N3.

Keywords: Gene expression, Controlled ovarian stimulation, GnRH antagonist, GnRH agonist

* Correspondence: nsalsabili56@yahoo.com
[8]Department of Physiotherapy, School of Rehabilitation of Tehran University of Medical Sciences, Tehran, Iran; Lab director Assisted Conception Unit, Tehran Women General Hospital, Tehran University of Medical Sciences, Tehran, Iran
Full list of author information is available at the end of the article

Background

Controlled ovarian stimulation (COS) is an important part of reproductive medicine; it also plays a vital role in inducing a pregnancy through assisted reproductive technology (ART). Higher pregnancy and implantation rates, compared to natural cycles, can be achieved using COS. Currently, three objectives are commonly followed when using COS for ART: ovulation induction, suppression of hypophyseal activity, and the growth stimulation of multiple follicles. For this purpose, two kinds of drugs are commonly used: gonadotropin releasing hormone agonists (GnRH-a) and gonadotropin releasing hormone antagonists (GnRH-ant). Multi-follicular recruitment causes a rapid increase in serum 17-beta estradiol (E2) levels during stimulated cycles, which in turn results in an untimely release of LH. The use of GnRH analogs can prevent the luteinizing hormone (LH) surge, which in turn improves the oocyte yield with more embryos and allows for better selection and therefore an increased pregnancy rate [1].

GnRH-a have been the most widely used drug for women undergoing COS, either for ICSI or for IVF [2]. GnRH-ant, on the other hand, has been introduced in clinical practice as a valid alternative in the last decade. In contrast to GnRH-a that decrease the number of receptors, GnRH-ant competitively inhibit endogenous GnRH from binding to its receptors. Consequently, they induce a direct, dose-dependent block of GnRH-receptors that are quickly reversible, which help avoid a flare effect [1].

Since 2001, several studies have compared the efficacy of the two GnRH analogs [2,3]. A recent Cochrane review indicated no evidence of a statistically significant difference in the rates of live births or ongoing pregnancies of the two GnRH analogs. In addition, the incidence of ovarian hyperstimulation syndrome (OHSS) in GnRH-ant treatment was lower than that of the GnRH-a treatment [3-5]. Furthermore, the following characteristics of the two protocols have also been compared: the number of oocytes retrieved and embryos transferred, the quality of oocyte morphology, implantation rate, the cycle cancellation rate, endometrial receptivity, follicular microenvironment, the percentage of granulosa cells with positive DNA fragmentation and apoptosis, genes expression in cumulus cells, and the distribution pattern and activity of human mature oocyte mitochondria [6-9].

It should be noted that the quality of oocytes obtained following controlled ovarian stimulation (COS) may vary significantly. Most oocytes are capable of being fertilized; however, nearly half of the fertilized ones can complete preimplantation development and even fewer ones can still implant. It has been shown that defects or variations in the ovulation or maturation processes have significant associations with gene expression alterations in oocytes and their supporting cells [10].

As mentioned earlier, although different clinical and molecular studies have been conducted to compare the efficacy of GnRH-a and GnRH-ant in assistant reproductive technique (ATR), results have been mostly inconsistent; Microarray studies conducted on human oocytes have indicated that some genes are expressed in both GV and MII stages, though with different levels. In fact, the more the oocytes move towards the maturity, the expression level of these genes increases [10-28]. These genes include those involved in the maturity of human oocytes (BMP15 and GDF9, both from the TGF beta category) [29,30], those involved in the cellular cycle and meiosis (BUB1, MAD2L1, CDC20, ATR, and ATM) [10-28,31], the energy-producing, mitochondrial gene (ATPase6) [27], and NAIP, which indicates oocytes viability [32-34]. Additionally, it is reported that COS can affect the gene expression level of oocytes [10]. During ovulation, mature and immature oocytes are obtained at the same time; however, the mature oocyte is used to treat patients. If differences are observed in the expression levels of the above mentioned genes in the cytoplasm of the GV oocytes due to different COS protocols (i.e. GnRH-ant or GnRH-a), the same conditions are expected to exist in the cytoplasm of mature oocytes. In other words, if increased levels of cytoplasmic maturity factors are observed following a COS protocol compared to the other, it highly likely to observe the same conditions in the cytoplasm of mature oocytes (MII) which co-exist with the GV oocytes in the same cycle. Therefore, for the first time, we decided to investigate the expression levels of nine genes involved in the cytoplasmic maturity, antiapoptotic process, cell cycle checkpoint, DNA repairing, and adenosine triphosphate production in germinal vesicle oocytes regarding the type of controlled ovarian stimulation in human. No studies have so far compared the genes expression in oocytes of women undergoing IVF/ICSI cycles between the GnRH-a and GnRH-ant protocols.

Materials

Subjects

Fifty infertile couples who underwent IVF/intracytoplasmic sperm injection (ICSI) between June 2012 and November 2013 at the Infertility Center of Tehran Women General Hospital, Tehran University of Medical Sciences, were included in this study. They were in good physical and mental conditions. We included the women that had undergone IVF treatment because of male factor, tubal factor, or unexplained infertility. These women did not have ovulatory dysfunction, were aged ≤40 years, and had a normal baseline follicle stimulating hormone (FSH) and luteinizing hormone (LH) (<10 mIU/mL).

Methods

Ovarian Stimulation and Oocyte Collection

The women underwent controlled ovarian stimulation with either the GnRH-a long protocol (n = 26) or the GnRH-ant fixed multi-dose protocol (n = 24), which was randomly assigned by the statistician [11,12].

The mean age (SD) of the participants was 31.7 (±5.7) years. In the GnRH-a long protocol group (n = 26), the treatment started by administering oral contraception pill (OCP) on the 2nd or the 3rd day of the pervious menstrual cycle. The daily administration of Buserelin acetate 500 μg (Suprefact, Aventis, Germany) was started preceding the IVF cycle from day 21 until pituitary down-regulation (serum E2 < 50 pg/ml in the absence of follicular structures larger than 10 mm). The Buserelin dose was reduced to 250 μg/d until the day of human chorionic gonadotropin (hCG) injection when pituitary down-regulation was achieved.

In the GnRH-ant fixed multi-dose protocol group (n = 24), Cetrorelix acetate 0.25 mg/day (Cetrotide, Serono, Switzerland) was initiated on the sixth day of the gonadotropin stimulation.

Ovarian stimulation was started on the 3rd day of the current menstrual cycle by injection of rFSH Follitropin alfa (Gonal F, Serono, Italy) at a daily dose of 150 to 225 IU in each group.

Administration of Buserelin and Cetrorelix was continued until hCG was injected. When at least 3 follicles with a mean diameter of 17 mm were developed (evaluated by transvaginal sonography), hCG 5000 IU/2/IM (Choriomon, IBSA Institut Biochimique S.A., Switzerland) was injected. About 34–36 h later, ultrasound-guided transvaginal oocyte retrieval was performed [13]. One hundred morphologically normal germinal vesicle oocytes were donated by 50 healthy women with normal ovarian reserve functions. The oocytes were aspirated transvaginally after COS. All the women had mature oocytes for ICSI, but they donated immature ones to our study. We obtained 50 germinal vesicle oocytes from 26 women aged 30.4 ± 5.5 years in the GnRH-a long protocol group and 50 germinal vesicle oocytes from 24 women aged 33.8 ± 5.6 years in the GnRH-ant protocol group. The oocytes were collected in a Quinn's Advantage Medium with HEPES (Sage, USA) supplemented with 20 % human serum albumin and then granulosa cells were removed from oocytes using mechanical and chemical (Hyaluronidase type 4, Sigma Aldrich, USA) methods.

After stripping off granulosa cells, we used an inverted microscope (Nikon, Tokyo, Japan) to monitor the maturity of the oocytes.

In the COS cycles, immature oocytes constitute up to 10-15 % of the retrieved oocytes. Germinal vesicle (GV) oocytes are immature oocytes whose maturation process have been stopped in the prophase of the first meiotic stage and are characterized by enlarged nucleus and absent of polar body. Germinal vesicle oocytes were individually transferred into RNase-free micro centrifuge tubes. Then, 30 μl of RLT buffer (Ambion, Austin, USA) was added to them. All samples were kept in a refrigerator at a temperature of −80°C until the time of the analysis. After the sampling, the pools of 50 germinal vesicle oocytes from the GnRH-a long protocol group and 50 germinal vesicle oocytes from the GnRH-ant protocol group were separately analyzed by qPCR.

RNA isolation, cDNA production and qPCR

ALLELEID 6.0 software was used for designing Exon-Junction primers. Molecular evolutionary genetics analysis (MEGA 4) software was also used for conducting sequence alignment. Oligo 6 Software was employed for the final assessment (Temperature/ Formation/False priming sites). Finally, we assessed primers in NCBI BLAST, as presented in Table 1.

Before isolating the RNA, the germinal vesicle oocytes were thawed within RLT buffer at room temperature and then pooled. To separate the RTL buffer from the pooled oocytes, they were then centrifuged at 12000 g for 3 minutes in order to extract total RNA, based on the standard protocol suggested by the manufacturer (Trizol, Invitrogen, USA). In order to remove genomic DNA contamination from the samples, the total RNA obtained from both groups was treated with DNase I (Fermentas, Sanktleon-rot, Germany). The total RNA concentration of the pooled germinal vesicle oocytes after treatment was 594 μg/ml for the GnRH-a long protocol group and 672 μg/ml for the GnRH-ant protocol group, determined by a Thermo Scientific Nano Drop 2000 Spectrophotometer. cDNA was synthesized according to manufacturer's instructions (Fermentas, Sanktleon-rot, Germany) using random hexamer primers.

We performed qPCR on the cDNA obtained from the pooled of germinal vesicle oocytes. Relative gene expression was calculated as the abundance ratio of each target gene to β-actin.

Quantitative real time PCR reactions were conducted in duplicates using a Roto- Gene Q instrument (Qiagen, German) with SYBR® Premix Ex Taq™ II master mix according to the procedure suggested by the manufacturer's instructions (Takara, Japan). The protocol for qPCR was initiated with a denaturizing step at 95°C for 30 seconds, followed by 50 cycles of 2-step, real-time PCR under the following conditions: 5 seconds at 95°C for denaturation and 30 seconds at 59–60°C for annealing and extension.

No template control (NTC) was used as the negative control. The specificity of the PCR fragments was determined using melting curve analysis. All melting curves produced one peak for each of the PCR products.

Table 1 Oligonucleotide primer sequences used for qPCR in the present study

Gene name	Primer	Accession no.	T°C	Product size (bp)
GDF9		NM_005260.4	60	162
Sense	CCAGGTAACAGGAATCCTTC			
Antisense	GGCTCCTTTATCATTAGATTG			
BMP15		NM_005448.2	60	129
Sense	CCTCACAGAGGTATCTGGC			
Antisense	GGAGAGATTGAAGCGAGTTAG			
ATPase 6		YP_003024031.1	60	123
Sense	CTGTTCGCTTCATTCATTG			
Antisense	GGTGGTGATTAGTCGGTTG			
NAIP		NM_004536.2	60	184
Sense	GGAGTATTTGGATGACAGAAAC			
Antisense	TAGATTACCACTGGAGTCTTCC			
BUB1		NM_001278616.1	59	100
Sense	AAGGTCCGAGGTTAATCC			
Antisense	CACTGGTGTCTGCTGATAGG			
MADL2		NM_002358.3	60	169
Sense	CTTCTCATTCGGCATCAAC			
Antisense	ACACTTGTATAACCAATCTTTCAG			
CDC20		NM_001255.2	60	202
Sense	GATGTAGAGGAAGCCAAGATC			
Antisense	CCACAAGGTTCAGGTAATAGTC			
ATR		NM_001184.3	60	150
Sense	GATGCCACTGCTTGTTATG			
Antisense	CCACTCGGACCTGTTAGC			
ATM		NM_000051.3	60	107
Sense	GCATTACGGGTGTTGAAG			
Antisense	ATATAGAAGGACCTCTACAATG			
β.actin		NM_001101.3	60	90
Sense	CAAGATCATTGCTCCTCCTG			
Antisense	ATCCACATCTGCTGGAAGG			

Ethical considerations

The present study was approved by the ethics committee of Tehran University of Medical Sciences. The study was completely explained to the women, and informed consent was obtained before collecting germinal vesicles oocytes. The study was formally registered with the following code: IRCT 2014031112307 N3.

Statistical analysis

We used One-way ANOVA to compare quantitative variables between the two groups and chi-square for qualitative variables by SPSS version 16 (Chicago, IL, USA). The significance level was set at 0.05. The efficiency values given by the Linreg software and relative expression were calculated using the REST 2009 software (Qiagen, Hilden, Germany) [14], which is a standalone software tool used for estimating up and down regulation for gene expression studies. The ΔΔCT was obtained by finding the difference between the groups. The fold change was calculated as $FC = 2^{-\Delta\Delta CT}$. For this purpose, β.actin was used as the reference gene for expression normalization.

Results

There were no significant differences in the age, hormonal profile, number of oocytes retrieved, infertility duration, and cause of infertility between the two groups ($P > 0.05$). However, the serum level of 17-beta estradiol on the day of hCG administration was higher in the GnRH-ant protocol group than in the GnRH-a long protocol group; however, this difference was not statistically significant, as presented in Tables 2 and 3.

Table 2 Mean (standard deviation) age, duration of infertility, number of oocytes retrieved, serum LH, FSH, TSH, PRL, AMH, and serum 17-beta estradiol in the GnRH-a protocol vs. GnRH-ant protocol group

Variable	GnRH-a long protocol (*n* = 26)	GnRH-ant protocol (*n* = 24)	Total (*n*=50)	*P* value
Age (yrs)	30.4 ± 5.5	33.8 ± 5.6	31.7 ± 5.7	0.100
Duration of infertility (yrs)	6.8 ± 3.5	4.6 ± 5.1	5.8 ± 4.5	0.086
Retrieved oocytes no.	11.0 ± 5.8	12.8 ± 8.3	11.8 ± 7.1	0.372
MII	6.2 ± 6.2	8.3 ± 6.3	7.2 ± 7.2	0.157
MI	1.8 ± 1.7	1.5 ± 1.6	1.6 ± 1.7	0.579
GV	2.1 ± 1.8	2.3 ± 1.8	2.2 ± 1.8	0.671
Deg.	0.8 ± 2.1	0.6 ± 2.1	0.7 ± 2.0	0.762
Serum 17 beta-estradiol (Pg/ml)*	5007.9 ± 8105	5988.3 ± 8110.6	5478.5 ± 8040.8	0.671
Serum LH (IU/L)	6.5 ± 2.9	5.5 ± 2.5	6.0 ± 2.8	0.256
Serum FSH (IU/L)	6.5 ± 2.5	6.3 ± 2.2	6.4 ± 2	0.706
Serum TSH (μIU/L)	3.0 ± 2.1	2.4 ± 1.1	2.7 ± 1.7	0.213
Serum PRL (ng/ml)	113.3 ± 186.2	107.0 ± 173.0	110.0 ± 178.2	0.902
Serum AMH (ng/ml)	5.0 ± 4.8	5.9 ± 5.6	5.4 ± 5.2	0.535

*On the day of hCG administration.
LH: luteinising hormone; FSH: follicle-stimulating hormone; TSH: thyroid-stimulating hormone; PRL: prolactin; AMH: anti-mullerian hormone.
MII: mature oocyte (Meiosis II); MI: immature oocyte (Meiosis I); GV: immature oocyte (Germinal Vesicle); Deg.: degenerative oocyte.

The present study showed that the expression levels of genes involved in the cytoplasmic maturity (*BMP15* and *GDF9*), antiapoptotic process *(NAIP)*, and adenosine triphosphate production *(ATPase 6)* in human GV oocytes were significantly higher in the GnRH-ant group versus in the GnRH-a group. ATPase 6, BMP15, and NAIP were significantly upregulated in the GnRH-ant group compared to the GnRH-a group with the fold change of 3.990 (SD ± 1.325), 6.274 (SD ± 1.542), and 2.156 (SD ± 1.443), respectively, (P value < 0.001). *GDF9* mRNA did not have any expression in the GnRH-a group; however, *GDF9* mRNA was expressed in the GnRH-ant group. These results are shown in Figure 1.

Finally, it was found that the genes involved in the DNA repairing, i.e. Ataxia telangiectasia and Rad3-related protein *(ATR),* and Ataxia telangiectasia mutated *(ATM);* and those involved in the cell cycle checkpoint, i. e. Bone morphogenetic protein 15 (*BUB1),* Mitotic arrest deficient-like 1 (*MAD2L1),* and Cell division cycle 20 (*CDC20),* did not have any expression in either group, as presented in Table 4.

Table 3 Distribution of the causes of infertility in the GnRH-a protocol vs. GnRH-ant protocol group

Variable	GnRH-a (%)	GnRH-ant (%)	*P* value
Cause of infertility			
• Male factor	16 (61.5)	9 (37.5)	
• Tubal factor	8 (30.8)	11 (45.58)	
• Unexplained	2 (7.7)	4 (16.7)	
Total	26.0 (100.0)	24.0 (100.0)	0.220

Discussion

Clinical studies have suggested similar pregnancy and live birth rates for both GnRH-a and GnRH-ant protocols [1,3,15-21], which has been further supported by some molecular studies [6-9]. Additionally, no significant morphological difference has been observed in the oocytes of the two groups after COS [22].

However, several advantages have been observed for the GnRH-ant protocol, including the fact that under this protocol, the endometrial receptivity is more similar to the natural cycle receptivity (in terms of endometrial chemokines and growth factors) [23]. In addition, when

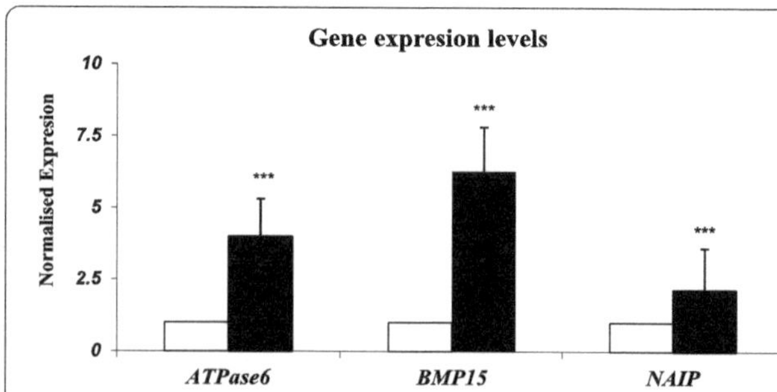

Figure 1 Results of the gene expression analysis with REST when using β.actin as the reference gene. Fold change (*Y* axis) represents the relative expression of *ATPase 6, BMP15, NAIP* mRNA in the pooled GV oocytes of the GnRH-ant protocol group (as tested group) versus the pooled GV oocytes of the GnRH-a long protocol group (as control group). ATPase 6, BMP15, and NAIP significantly were upregulated in GnRH-ant group in compared to GnRH-a group with the fold change of 3.990 (SD ± 1.325), 6.274 (SD ± 1.542), and 2.156 (SD ± 1.443), respectively, *** P < 0.001. Agonist protocol group □. Antagonist protocol group ■.

Table 4 The genes expression of germinal vesicle oocyte in GnRH agonist group compared with GnRH antagonist group

Gene symbol	Gene title	GnRH-a group		GnRH-anta group	
		Exist	Not exist	Exist	Not exist
Transforming growth factors					
GDF9	Growth differentiation factor 9		+	+	
BMP15	Bone morphogenetic protein 15	+		+	
Mitochondria					
ATPase6	Adenosine triphosphatase 6	+		+	
Antiapoptotic					
NAIP	Neuronal apoptosis inhibitory protein	+		+	
Cell cycle checkpoint markers					
BUB1	Budding uninhibited by benzimidazoles 1		+		+
MAD2L1	Mitotic arrest deficient-like 1		+		+
CDC20	Cell division cycle 20		+		+
DNA repair markers					
ATR	Ataxia telangiectasia and Rad3		+		+
ATM	Ataxia telangiectasia mutated		+		+
Reference gene					
B.actin	beta actin	+		+	

comparing GnRH-ant protocol and GnRH-a long protocols, the time of the appearance of the endometrial triple layer is statistically significant for the pregnancy rate only for the former protocol [24]. In addition to its safety and effectiveness, GnRH-ant allows for the flexibility of treatment in a wider range of women populations, including poor responders, women undergoing first-line controlled ovarian stimulation, and women diagnosed with polycystic ovarian syndrome. Therefore, the GnRH-ant protocol can be considered as a suitable alternative to the long agonist protocol, due mainly to its shorter duration of treatment and the need for fewer injections. Consequently, this leads to a significantly lower amount of administered gonadotropins, which most probably leads to improved women compliance [25]. We observed, for the first time, that the expression levels of genes involved in the cytoplasmic maturity, antiapoptotic process, and ATP production in human GV oocytes were significantly higher in the GnRH-anta group than in the GnRH-a group in COS.

As with other studies, in the present work, the same ovulation-triggering drug was used in the COS cycle for both groups; the only difference was the type of GnRH used for the two groups, which makes the present work different from the study of Hass et al. [26], in which oocyte cells were used for genetic evaluations.

The present study showed that the expression levels of genes involved in the cytoplasmic maturity, antiapoptotic process, and adenosine triphosphate production were significantly higher in the pooled oocytes of the women in the GnRH antagonist group versus those of the women in the GnRH agonist group ($P < 0.001$). These results are shown in Figure 1.

ATPase 6 gene plays a critical role in ATP production by mitochondria. Deficiencies in the production of mitochondrial ATP can be linked to impaired oocyte fertilization, incomplete development of the embryo at later stages, and several other cellular and chromosomal disorders including errors in chromosomal segregation, lethal cytoplasmic defects, non disjunction disorders resulting in aneuploidy, and development failure of the sperm derived mitotic apparatus [27]. Therefore, the higher expression level of *ATPase6* in the pooled oocytes of the women in the GnRH-ant protocol group vs. those of the women in the GnRH-a long protocol group suggests that under the antagonist protocol, the mitochondrial activity may be more appropriate. In other words, higher-quality mitochondrial respiration and oxidative phosphorylation cascade occur in the oocytes of GnRH-ant group. The higher expression level of this gene and, in turn, higher energy production cause cell division spindles to form under better conditions [27].

Transforming growth factors beta *(TGF-ß)* are important paracrine growth factors that are secreted by the ovarian stroma or follicles surrounding the ovary, converting primordial follicles to primary ones. During folliculogenesis stages, oocytes secretion of *TGF-ß*, such as *BMP15* and *GDF9* [28], can regulate female fertility in several mammals [5,29,30]. *GDF9* and *BMP15* are responsible for transformation. They also cause the reproduction of granulosa cells under the influence of FSH, which mainly secrete estradiol [35]. Estradiol is required for the maturation of oocytes and development of embryo in vivo. Additionally, follicular atresia and granulosa cell apoptosis are inhibited by *GDF9*. Moreover, the proliferation, apoptosis, metabolism, and expansion of the cumulus oocyte complex are organized by the secretion of *GDF9* and *BMP15* [29].

According to the results from the present study, *GDF9* and *BMP15* are expressed in the pooled GV oocytes of the women in the GnRH-ant protocol group. Our study also showed that the expression level of *GDF9* was higher than that of *BMP15* in the antagonist group, which is consistent with the results of previous studies [30]. *GDF9* gene was not expressed in the pooled GV oocytes of the women in the GnRH-a long protocol group. The higher expression of these genes in the pooled GV oocytes of the GnRH-ant protocol group could be due to the fact that in the GnRH-a long protocol, complete inhibition of gonadotropins occurs on the 2nd or the 3rd day of the current menstrual cycle. The study of Lainas et al. [36] indicated that the serum levels of E2, FSH, and LH hormones were significantly higher before administering OCP on the 2nd or the 3rd day of the pervious menstrual cycle when compared to the same day in the OCP plus GnRH-a long protocol, mainly due to the suppression of inner gonadotropin in this protocol (FSH: 5.8 vs. 3.6 IU/L; LH:5.6 vs. 1.2 IU/L; and E2: 30.5 vs. 12 pg/ml before and after using OCP/GnRH-a, respectively). This, however, does not occur in the GnRH-ant protocol. In the GnRH-ant protocol, the initial dose of GnRH-ant is administered on the 6th or the 7th day of the current menstrual cycle, which causes immediate inhibition of LH by influencing the GnRH receptors in the pituitary gland. Therefore, adequate follicle stimulation can be provided by a combination of exogenous FSH and endogenous LH secretion in early treatment [37]. In other words, administration of GnRH-ant protocol occurs in late follicular development (on the 5th or the 6th day of the gonadotropin stimulation when estradiol is increased).

NAIP is one of the members of the inhibitor of apoptosis protein (IAP) family. By regulating the caspase activity (inhibition of both caspase 3 and caspase 9), which is an important part of the apoptotic machinery, this gene can prevent apoptosis of granulosa cells during the ovarian folliculogenesis stages and can cause the follicles to develop from the primary stage to the graafian follicle [32]. In the oocyte, the expression of this gene can increase 2–4 times due to the effect of gonadotropin, which indirectly leads to oocyte survival [33,34]. After a thorough literature search, it was determined that the present study examined, for the first time, the expression level of *NAIP* in human oocytes. The higher level of the expression of this gene in the pooled oocytes in the GnRH-ant protocol versus the pooled oocytes in the GnRH-a long protocol most likely suggests that the oocyte survival is improved by applying the former protocol.

In addition, in the present study, *BUB1, MAD2L1, CDC20, ATR, and ATM* genes did not have any expression in either group, which is most likely because that the oocytes used in the present work were germinal vesicle oocytes whose growth is arrested in the diplotene stage of the first meiotic prophase, as presented in Table 4.

ATR and *ATM* are a type of serine/threonine protein kinase. DNA double-strand breaks recruit and activate this serine/threonine protein kinase. This leads to the phosphorylation of several key proteins that are responsible for the initiation of DNA damage checkpoint activation, which finally results in cell cycle arrest, DNA repair, or apoptosis. *ATM* and *ATR* prevent premature chromosome condensation (PCC) until the DNA replication is completed [31].

In order to prevent premature separation of sister chromatids, *MAD2L1* and *BUB1*, which in turn interact with *CDC20* at check point activation, inhibit *CDC20/APC* [10]. Previous studies indicated that during the meiosis, *BUB1*, *MAD2L1*, and *CDC20* had high expressions in the oocytes [28].

There are controversial findings regarding the difference in the serum levels of estradiol on the day of hCG administration between GnRH-ant and GnRH-a long protocols. Some studies have reported that the serum levels of estradiol on the day of hCG administration are significantly higher in the GnRH-a long protocol than in the GnRH-ant protocol [38]; other studies, however, have reported reverse findings [21,39-41]. In the present study, the serum levels of estradiol on the day of hCG administration were higher in the GnRH-ant protocol than the GnRH-a long protocol although the difference was not statistically significant, as presented in Tables 2. The serum level of estradiol is an indicator of the function of granulosa cells, suggesting that these cells have better performance in producing estradiol in the GnRH-ant protocol versus the GnRH-a long protocol.

Studies have indicated that the application of GnRH agonist protocol causes mid-cycle gonadotropine flares and ovarian hyperstimulation syndrome (OHSS), which is more observed in women with poly-cystic ovarian syndrome (PCOs). Therefore, the GnRH-ant protocol is a better choice than the GnRH-a protocol for ovarian stimulation in infertile women due to PCOs [1,4,25].

On the other hand, Li et al. [30] reported that the expression of GDF9 and BMP15 genes is necessary for the maturity of the oocyte cytoplasm; therefore, these two can be used as markers of oocyte quality in terms of its evolution. In addition, it was reported that in the oocytes of infertile women with PCOs, the expression level of GDF9 and BMP15 genes is lower than that of normal individuals, which can be the reason for the lowered quality of oocytes in these patients, which in turn leads to reduced fertility and the rate of success in IVF.

Therefore, since the results from the present study suggested higher expression level of these genes when GnRH-ant protocol is applied [Figure 1], this protocol seems to be a more appropriate choice for women with PCOs, because it can probably improve the expression of the aforementioned genes.

Although similar studies should be performed on the matured oocytes, but obtaining of donated mature oocytes (in vivo) is not ethically feasible for research purposes. On the other hand, the mature oocytes obtained from GV in vitro maturation is not appropriate for this purpose, mainly because studies have indicated that the in vitro culture conditions have adverse genetic and epigenetic impact on the growth of GV oocytes; therefore, this can prevent the researchers from observing the same findings. We suggest that future studies should be performed on donated mature oocytes which, together with the results of the present work, can help provide a broader molecular perspective in this field and make the most appropriate ovarian stimulation protocol.

Conclusions

Results from the present study indicated, for the first time, that in the germinal vesicle oocytes of women with normal ovarian function, the expression levels of genes involved in the cytoplasmic maturity (GDF9 and BMP15), antiapoptotic process (NAIP), and ATP production (ATPase 6) were significantly higher in the GnRH-anta protocol group than in the GnRH-a long protocol group. GDF9 mRNA did not have any expression in the GnRH-a group; however, GDF9 mRNA was expressed in the GnRH-ant group. Therefore, since the results from the present study suggested higher expression level of these genes when GnRH-ant protocol is applied, this protocol seems to be a more appropriate choice for women with PCOs, because it can probably improve the expression of the aforementioned genes.

Competing interest

The authors declare that they have no competing interests associated with this publication and there has been no significant financial support for this work that could have influenced its outcome.

Authors' contributions

FS H involving in the study design, data collection, and data analysis. N S, P E-Y, SMHN-M and F A-A involving in the study design. F A-A, B A and N S involving in data collection. SH A-B and R A involving in conducting the experiments, designing the primers, and analyzing the data. The manuscript was drafted by FS H, and all the other authors had intellectual contributions by critically reviewing the paper and leaving their comments. Finally, all the authors read and approved the final version of the manuscript.

Acknowledgments

The present study was funded by Deputy Ministry for Research, Tehran University of Medical Sciences (TUMS); grant no. 91-02-30-18324. The authors wish to thank all the oocyte donors. We would like to thank Dr. Masud Yunesian for helping with the study design and data analysis. We are also grateful to all the members of our ART team for their assistance during this study and to the staff of the Royan Institute for Reproductive Biomedicine and Stem Cell for carrying out the qPCR tests.

Author details

[1]Department of Anatomy and Reproductive Biology, School of Medicine, Tehran University of Medical Sciences, Tehran, Iran. [2]Departments of Histology, School of Medicine, Tehran University of Medical Sciences, Tehran, Iran. [3]Department of Obstetrics and Gynecology, Tehran Women General Hospital, School of Medicine, Tehran University of Medical Sciences, Tehran, Iran. [4]Department of Embryology at Reproductive Biomedicine Research Center, Royan Institute for Reproductive Biomedicine, ACECR, Tehran, Iran. [5]Lab director Assisted Conception Units, Laleh Hospital, Tehran, Iran and Madar Hospital, Yazd, Iran. [6]Department of Molecular Biology and Genetic Engineering, Stem Cell Technology Research Center, Tehran, Iran and Molecular Medicine Department, Biotechnology Research Center, Pasteur Institute of Iran, Tehran, Iran. [7]Department of Endocrinology and Female Infertility at Reproductive Biomedicine Research Center, Royan Institute for Reproductive Biomedicine, ACECR, Tehran, Iran. [8]Department of Physiotherapy, School of Rehabilitation of Tehran University of Medical Sciences, Tehran, Iran; Lab director Assisted Conception Unit, Tehran Women General Hospital, Tehran University of Medical Sciences, Tehran, Iran.

References

1. Marci R, Graziano A, Lo Monte G, Piva I, Soave I, Marra E, Lisi F, Moscarini M, Caserta D: **GnRH antagonists in assisted reproductive techniques: a review on the Italian experience.** *Eur Rev Med Pharmacol Sci* 2013, **17**:853–873.
2. Nardo LG, Bosch E, Lambalk CB, Gelbaya TA: **Controlled ovarian hyperstimulation regimens: a review of the available evidence for clinical practice. On behalf of the British Fertility Society P&P Committee.** *Hum Fertil (Camb)* 2013, **16**:144–150.
3. Johnston-MacAnanny EB, DiLuigi AJ, Engmann LL, Maier DB, Benadiva CA, Nulsen JC: **Selection of first in vitro fertilization cycle stimulation protocol for good prognosis patients: gonadotropin releasing hormone antagonist versus agonist protocols.** *J Reprod Med* 2011, **56**:12–16.
4. Al-Inany HG, Youssef MA, Aboulghar M, Broekmans F, Sterrenburg M, Smit J, Abou-Setta AM: **GnRH antagonists are safer than agonists: an update of a Cochrane review.** *Hum Reprod Update* 2011, **17**:435–435.
5. Orvieto R, Patrizio P: **GnRH agonist versus GnRH antagonist in ovarian stimulation: An ongoing debate.** *Reprod BioMed Online* 2013, **26**:4–8.
6. Devjak R, Fon Tacer K, Juvan P, Virant Klun I, Rozman D, Vrtacnik Bokal E: **Cumulus cells gene expression profiling in terms of oocyte maturity in controlled ovarian hyperstimulation using GnRH agonist or GnRH antagonist.** *PLoS One* 2012, **7**:e47106.
7. Kaya A, Atabekoglu CS, Kahraman K, Taskin S, Ozmen B, Berker B, Sonmezer M: **Follicular fluid concentrations of IGF-I, IGF-II, IGFBP-3, VEGF, AMH, and inhibin-B in women undergoing controlled ovarian hyperstimulation using GnRH agonist or GnRH antagonist.** *Eur J Obstet Gynecol Reprod Biol* 2012, **164**:167–171.
8. Lavorato HL, Oliveira JB, Petersen CG, Vagnini L, Mauri AL, Cavagna M, Baruffi RL, Franco JG Jr: **GnRH agonist versus GnRH antagonist in IVF/ICSI cycles with recombinant LH supplementation: DNA fragmentation and apoptosis in granulosa cells.** *Eur J Obstet Gynecol Reprod Biol* 2012, **165**:61–65.
9. Liu N, Ma Y, Li R, Jin H, Li M, Huang X, Feng HL, Qiao J: **Comparison of follicular fluid amphiregulin and EGF concentrations in patients undergoing IVF with different stimulation protocols.** *Endocrine* 2012, **42**:708–716.
10. Gasca S, Pellestor F, Assou S, Loup V, Anahory T, Dechaud H, De Vos J, Hamamah S: **Identifying new human oocyte marker genes: a microarray approach.** *Reprod Biomed Online* 2007, **14**:175–183.
11. Kahraman K, Berker B, Atabekoglu CS, Sonmezer M, Cetinkaya E, Aytac R, Satiroglu H: **Microdose gonadotropin-releasing hormone agonist flare-up protocol versus multiple dose gonadotropin-releasing hormone**

antagonist protocol in poor responders undergoing intracytoplasmic sperm injection–embryo transfer cycle. *Fertil Steril* 2009, **91**:2437–2444.
12. Roberto M, Donatella C, Vincenza D, Carla T, Antonio P, Massimo M: GnRH antagonist in IVF poor-responder patients: results of a randomized trial. *Reprod BioMed Online* 2005, **11**:189–193.
13. Ye H, Huang G-n, Zeng P-h, Pei L: IVF/ICSI outcomes between cycles with luteal estradiol (E2) pre-treatment before GnRH antagonist protocol and standard long GnRH agonist protocol: a prospective and randomized study. *J Assist Reprod Genet* 2009, **26**:105–111.
14. Pfaffl MW, Horgan GW, Dempfle L: Relative expression software tool (REST©) for group-wise comparison and statistical analysis of relative expression results in real-time PCR. *Nucleic Acids Res* 2002, **30**:e36–e36.
15. Luna M, Vela G, McDonald CA, Copperman AB: Results with GnRH antagonist protocols are equivalent to GnRH agonist protocols in comparable patient populations. *J Reprod Med* 2012, **57**:123–128.
16. Mekaru K, Yagi C, Asato K, Masamoto H, Sakumoto K, Aoki Y: Comparison between the gonadotropin-releasing hormone antagonist protocol and the gonadotropin-releasing hormone agonist long protocol for controlled ovarian hyperstimulation in the first in vitro fertilization-embryo transfer cycle in an unspecified population of infertile couples. *Reprod Med Biol* 2012, **11**:79–83.
17. Munoz M, Cruz M, Humaidan P, Garrido N, Perez-Cano I, Meseguer M: The type of GnRH analogue used during controlled ovarian stimulation influences early embryo developmental kinetics: a time-lapse study. *Eur J Obstet Gynecol Reprod Biol* 2013, **168**:167–172.
18. Nardo LG, Fleming R, Howles CM, Bosch E, Hamamah S, Ubaldi FM, Hugues JN, Balen AH, Nelson SM: Conventional ovarian stimulation no longer exists: Welcome to the age of individualized ovarian stimulation. *Reprod BioMed Online* 2011, **23**:141–148.
19. Prapas Y, Petousis S, Dagklis T, Panagiotidis Y, Papatheodorou A, Assunta I, Prapas N: GnRH antagonist versus long GnRH agonist protocol in poor IVF responders: a randomized clinical trial. *Eur J Obstet Gynecol Reprod Biol* 2013, **166**:43–46.
20. Pu D, Wu J, Liu J: Comparisons of GnRH antagonist versus GnRH agonist protocol in poor ovarian responders undergoing IVF. *Hum Reprod* 2011, **26**:2742–2749.
21. Yang S, Chen XN, Qiao J, Liu P, Li R, Chen GA, Ma CH: Comparison of GnRH antagonist fixed protocol and GnRH agonists long protocol in infertile patients with normal ovarian reserve function in their first in vitro fertilization-embryo transfer cycle. *Zhonghua Fu Chan Ke Za Zhi* 2012, **47**:245–249.
22. Cota A, Oliveira J, Petersen CG, Mauri AL, Massaro FC, Silva L, Nicoletti A, Cavagna M, Baruffi R, Franco JG Jr: GnRH agonist versus GnRH antagonist in assisted reproduction cycles: oocyte morphology. *Reprod Biol Endocrinol* 2012, **10**:33.
23. Haouzi D, Assou S, Dechanet C, Anahory T, Dechaud H, De Vos J, Hamamah S: Controlled ovarian hyperstimulation for in vitro fertilization alters endometrial receptivity in humans: protocol effects. *Biol Reprod* 2010, **82**:679–686.
24. Kuć P, Kuczyńska A, Topczewska M, Tadejko P, Kuczyński W: The dynamics of endometrial growth and the triple layer appearance in three different controlled ovarian hyperstimulation protocols and their influence on IVF outcomes. *Gynecol Endocrinol* 2011, **27**:867–873.25.
25. Copperman AB, Benadiva C: Optimal usage of the GnRH antagonists: A review of the literature. *Reprod Biol Endocrinol* 2013, **11**:20.
26. Haas J, Ophir L, Barzilay E, Yerushalmi GM, Yung Y, Kedem A, Maman E, Hourvitz A: Gnrh agonist vs hCG for triggering of ovulation–differential effects on gene expression in human granulosa cells. *PLoS One* 2014, **9**:e90359.
27. Lee SH, Han JH, Cho SW, Cha KE, Park SE, Cha KY: Mitochondrial ATPase 6 gene expression in unfertilized oocytes and cleavage-stage embryos. *Fertil Steril* 2000, **73**:1001–1005.
28. Assou S, Anahory T, Pantesco V, Le Carrour T, Pellestor F, Klein B, Reyftmann L, Dechaud H, De Vos J, Hamamah S: The human cumulus–oocyte complex gene-expression profile. *Hum Reprod* 2006, **21**:1705–1719.
29. Gode F, Gulekli B, Dogan E, Korhan P, Dogan S, Bige O, Cimrin D, Atabey N: Influence of follicular fluid GDF9 and BMP15 on embryo quality. *Fertil Steril* 2011, **95**:2274–2278.
30. Wei LN, Liang XY, Fang C, Zhang MF: Abnormal expression of growth differentiation factor 9 and bone morphogenetic protein 15 in stimulated oocytes during maturation from women with polycystic ovary syndrome. *Fertil Steril* 2011, **96**:464–468.
31. Sancar A, Lindsey-Boltz LA, Unsal-Kaçmaz K, Linn S: Molecular mechanisms of mammalian DNA repair and the DNA damage checkpoints. *Annu Rev Biochem* 2004, **73**:39–85.
32. Verhagen AM, Coulson EJ, Vaux DL: Inhibitor of apoptosis proteins and their relatives: IAPs and other BIRPs. *Genome Biol* 2001, **2**:3009.3001–3009.3010.
33. Beug ST, Cheung HH: *LaCasse EC*. Korneluk RG: Modulation of immune signalling by inhibitors of apoptosis. Trends in immunology; 2012.
34. Smolewski P, Robak T: Inhibitors of apoptosis proteins (IAPs) as potential molecular targets for therapy of hematological malignancies. *Curr Mol Med* 2011, **11**:633–649.
35. Carlson BM, Brudon MC: *Human embryology and developmental biology*. St. Louis: Mosby; 1994.
36. Lainas TG, Petsas GK, Zorzovilis IZ, Iliadis GS, Lainas GT, Cazlaris HE, Kolibianakis EM: Initiation of GnRH antagonist on Day 1 of stimulation as compared to the long agonist protocol in PCOS patients. A randomized controlled trial: effect on hormonal levels and follicular development. *Hum Reprod* 2007, **22**:1540–1546.
37. Filicori M, Cognigni GE, Samara A, Melappioni S, Perri T, Cantelli B, Parmegiani L, Pelusi G, DeAloysio D: The use of LH activity to drive folliculogenesis: exploring uncharted territories in ovulation induction. *Hum Reprod Update* 2002, **8**:543–557.
38. Kara M, Aydin T, Aran T, Turktekin N, Ozdemir B: Comparison of GnRH agonist and antagonist protocols in normoresponder patients who had IVF-ICSI. *Arch Gynecol Obstet* 2013, **288**:1413–1416.
39. Lai Q, Zhang H, Zhu G, Li Y, Jin L, He L, Zhang Z, Yang P, Yu Q, Zhang S, XU JF, Wang CY: Comparison of the GnRH agonist and antagonist protocol on the same patients in assisted reproduction during controlled ovarian stimulation cycles. *Int J Clin Exp Pathol* 2013, **6**:1903–1910.
40. Li Y, Lai Q, Zhang H, Zhu G, Jin L, Yue J: Comparison between a GnRH agonist and a GnRH antagonist protocol for the same patient undergoing IVF. *J Huazhong Univ Sci Technolog Med Sci* 2008, **28**:618–620.
41. Taskin EA, Atabekoglu CS, Musali N, Oztuna D, Sonmezer M: Association of serum estradiol levels on the day of hCG administration with pregnancy rates and embryo scores in fresh ICSI/ET cycles down regulated with either GnRH agonists or GnRH antagonists. *Arch Gynecol Obstet* 2014, **298**:399–405.

N-Substituted indole carbohydrazide derivatives: synthesis and evaluation of their antiplatelet aggregation activity

Seyedeh Sara Mirfazli[1], Farzad Kobarfard[2,3], Loghman Firoozpour[4], Ali Asadipour[5], Marjan Esfahanizadeh[2], Kimia Tabib[2], Abbas Shafiee[1] and Alireza Foroumadi[1,5*]

Abstract

Background: Platelet aggregation is one of the most important factors in the development of thrombotic disorders which plays a central role in thrombosis (clot formation). Prophylaxis and treatment of arterial thrombosis are achieved using anti-platelet drugs. In this study, a series of novel substituted indole carbohydrazide was synthesized and evaluated for anti-platelet aggregation activity induced by adenosine diphosphate (ADP), arachidonic acid (AA) and collagen.

Methods: Our synthetic route started from methyl 1H-indole-3-carboxylate (1) and ethyl 1H-indole-2-carboxylate (4) which were reacted with hydrazine monohydrate 99%. The aldol condensation of the later compound with aromatic aldehydes led to the formation of the title compounds. Sixteen indole acylhydrazone derivatives, **3d-m** and **6d-i** were tested for anti-platelet aggregation activity induced by adenosine diphosphate (ADP), arachidonic acid (AA) and collagen.

Results: Among the synthesized compounds, **6g** and **6h** with 100% inhibition, proved to be the most potent derivatives of the 2-substituted indole on platelet aggregation induced by AA and collagen, respectively. In 3-substituted indole **3m** with 100% inhibition and **3f** and **3i** caused 97% inhibition on platelet aggregation induced by collagen and AA, respectively.

Conclusion: In this study, compounds **6g, 6h, 3m, 3f** and **3i** showed better inhibition on platelet aggregation induced by AA and collagen among the title compounds. Quantitative structure–activity relationship (QSAR) analysis between the structural parameters of the investigated derivatives and their antiplatelet aggregation activity was performed with various molecular descriptors but, analysis of the physicochemical parameters doesn't show a significant correlation between the observed activities and general molecular parameters of the synthesized derivatives. Although, due to the existence of several receptors on the platelets surface which are responsible for controlling the platelet aggregation, the investigated compounds in the present study may exert their activities through binding to more than one of these receptors and therefore no straight forward SAR could be obtained for them.

Keyword: Anti-platelet aggregation, Indole, *N*-acylhydrazone

* Correspondence: aforoumadi@yahoo.com
[1]Department of Medicinal Chemistry, Faculty of Pharmacy and Pharmaceutical Sciences Research Center, Tehran University of Medical Sciences, Tehran, Iran
[5]Neuroscience Research Center, Institute of Neuropharmacology, Kerman University of Medical Sciences, Kerman, Iran
Full list of author information is available at the end of the article

Background

Cardiovascular diseases are responsible for the largest number of death and disability worldwide. Platelet adhesion and aggregation are key events in hemostasis and thrombosis which cause disrupted atherosclerotic plaques that is the initiator of most thrombotic disorders including heart attacks and strokes [1-3]. Platelets play the major role in the pathogenesis of thromboembolic disorders and activation of the platelets by complex biochemical pathways and mediators is the primary step in this process [4,5]. Endogenous agonists such as arachidonic acid (AA), adenosine 5′-diphosphate (ADP) that acts on purinergic receptors on the platelet-known as P_2Y receptors, thromboxane A_2 (TxA_2), thrombin, platelet activating factor (PAF), epinephrine (EPN) and collagen are among potent agonists that initiate the formation of stable platelet aggregates [6-8].

Clinical evidence has clearly proven that antiplatelet aggregation agents are useful for preventing thrombotic disorders. On the other hand, there are still some serious limitations to currently use agents which include weak inhibition of platelet function (aspirin), slow onset of action (clopidogrel), variable response to treatment among patients and high incidence of bleeding events which is dose dependent in both aspirin and clopidogrel drug therapy [9]. Considering the current situation, pursuit of finding novel scaffolds as new antiplatelet aggregation drugs which are more effective and safer with fewer side effects is very important [10].

A novel group of heterocyclic acylhydrazone derivatives with antiplatelet aggregation activity on rabbit platelet-rich plasma have been reported [11,12]. Furthermore, the *N*-acylhydrazone (NAH) moiety, have shown a series of biological activities such as analgesic, anti-inflammatory [13-20], protozoa proteases inhibition [21], HIV-1 reverse transcriptase dimmer destabilization [22], antibiotic and antifungal activities [23], and cardiovascular actions [24-28].

Indole ring is another structural moiety which has been reported to have antiplatelet aggregation activity [29]. Considering this background, a diverse group of derivatives have been synthesized in this study by molecular hybridization between indole and hydrazone moieties, to find the structure–antiplatelet activity relationship of the derivatives. The schematic structural backbone for these compounds which contain both indole and *N*-acylhydrazone is depicted in Figure 1.

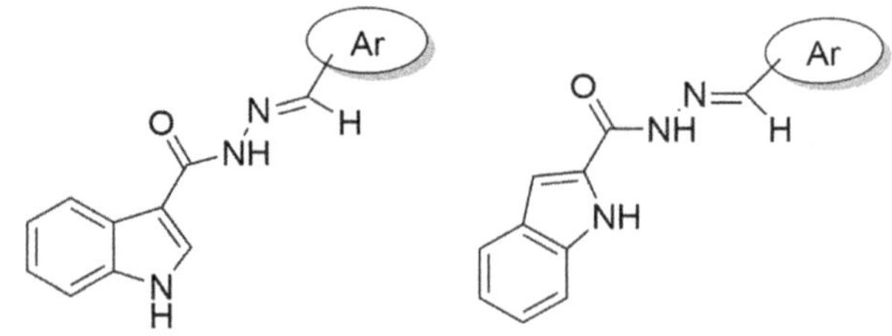

Figure 1 Schematic representation of the general hydrazone structural backbone with antiplatelet activity.

Chemistry

The synthetic procedure planned to obtain the desired indole *N*-acylhydrazone derivatives, is shown in Scheme 1. The key intermediates were obtained by hydrazinolysis of **1** and **4** in 96% and 91% yield, respectively, using hydrazine monohydrate 99% in ethanol. The final indole *N*-acylhydrazone derivatives were obtained by condensing the hydrazide intermediates with the proper aromatic aldehydes (ArCHO) in water and glacial acetic acid as the solvent, in good yields.

Material and methods

General

All commercial solvents, chemicals and reagents were purchased from either Merck or Sigma-Aldrich with the highest purity and used without further purification. Proton nuclear magnetic resonance (^1H NMR) spectra were recorded on a Bruker 500 MHz spectrometers (Bruker, Rheinstetten, Germany) and pick positions are illustrated in parts per million (δ) in DMSO-d_6 solution and tetramethylsilane (0.05% v/v) as internal standard and coupling constant values (J) are given in Hertz. Signal multiplicities are reported by: s (singlet), d (doublet), t (triplet), q (quadruplet), m (multiplet) and br (broad signal). For NMR spectral data assignments, the atom numbering of compounds is depicted in Table 1. Analytical thin layer chromatography (TLC) was performed with Merck silica gel plates and visualized with UV irradiation (254 nm) or iodine. Electrospray ionization mass spectra (ESI-MS) were obtained using Agilent 6410 Triple Quad. LC/MS. Melting points were obtained by an Electrothermal 9100 apparatus and are uncorrected. The IR spectra were taken by a Perkin-Elmer 843 spectrometer with KBr as diluent. The elemental analysis for C, H and N was performed by a Costech model 4010 and the percentage values agreed with the proposed structures within ±0.4% of the theoretical values. All described products showed ^1H NMR spectra according to the assigned structures. The physicochemical parameters including Clog P value, surface area, molecular volume, refractivity and polarizability were calculated by Hyperchem 8.0 software.

General procedure for the preparation of carbohydrazides (2, 5)

Compounds (**1** or **4**) (2.86 mmol) was added to a solution of hydrazine monohydrate 99% (2.14 mL; 2.18 g; 43.6 mmol) in ethanol (0.5 mL) and the reaction mixture

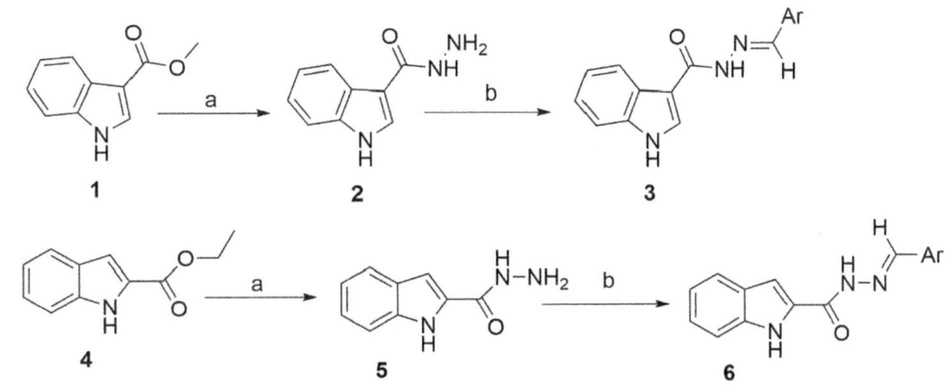

Scheme 1 The synthesis pathway for indoleN-acylhydrazones. Reagents and reaction condition: **a)** Hydrazine monohydrate 99% (NH_2NH_2), Ethanol (a few drop), reflux at 80°C, 3 h **b)** ArCHO, H_2O, Glacial acetic acid (a few drop), reflux at 100°C, 3 h.

was stirred at about 80°C temperature, for 2 h. TLC indicated the end of reaction. The mixture was cooled by addition of a water/ice mixture. The solid was filtered in excellent yield (Scheme 1) [30-32].

1*H*- indole-3-carbohydrazide (**2**) and 1*H*- indole-2-carbohydrazide (**5**) were prepared according to a literature method [30-32].

General procedure for the preparation of N-acylhydrazone derivatives

Equimolar amount of appropriate aromatic aldehyde was added to a solution of hydrazide compound (**2** or **5**) in 10 mL of water, in presence of catalytic amount of glacial acetic acid (0.4 mL). Reaction mixture was heated under reflux with stirring for about 2 h and poured into ice/water mixture. The precipitate was filtered and washed with cold water (Scheme 1).

N'-(4-hydroxybenzylidene)-1*H*-indole-3-carbohydrazide (**3i**), *N*'-(3-hydroxybenzylidene)-1*H*-indole-3-carbohydrazide (**3j**), *N*'-benzylidene-1*H*-indole-3-carbohydrazide (**3 m**), *N*'-(2-hydroxybenzylidene)-1*H*-indole-2-carbohydrazide (**6e**), *N*'-(2-methoxybenzylidene)-1*H*-indole-2-carbohydrazide (**6f**) and *N*'-benzylidene-1*H*-indole-2-carbohydrazide (**6i**) were prepared according to a literature method [30-32].

N'-(2-hydroxybenzylidene)-1H-indole-3-carbohydrazide (3d)

Yield: 92%, mp 256- 259°C. IR (KBr) cm^{-1}: 3365 (ν OH), 3283, 3041, 2927, 1660, 1614, 1596, 1577, 1564. ^1H NMR (500 MHz, DMSO): δ 11.79 (s, 1H, CONH), 11.71 (bs, 1H, Indole NH), 11.51 (bs, 1H, OH), 8.52 (s, 1H, —N=*CH*—) 8.21 (bs, 1H, —N=CH—C_6H_5, H_2), 8.20 (d, 1H, *J* = 7.85 Hz, —N=CH—C_6H_5 ,H_4), 7.52 (d, 1H, *J* = 7.5 Hz, —N=CH—C_6H_5, H_6), 7.50 (d, 1H, *J* = 7.8 Hz, —N=CH—C_6H_5, H_4), 7.29 (td, 1H, *J* = 7.0, 1.40 Hz, Indole H_7), 7.21 (td, 1H, *J* = 7.4, 1.45 Hz, Indole H_5), 7.17 (td, 1H, *J* = 7.0, 1.45 Hz, Indole H_6), 6.95- 6.91 (m, 2H, —N=CH—C_6H_5, H_3, H_5), ESI-Mass *m/z*: 280 $[M+H]^+$, 302 $[M+Na]^+$; Anal. Calcd. for $C_{16}H_{13}N_3O_2$: C, 68.81; H, 4.69; N, 15.05. Found: C, 68.64; H, 4.83; N, 14.92.

N'-(2-nitrobenzylidene)-1H-indole-3-carbohydrazide (3e)

Yield: 96%, mp 272- 274°C. IR (KBr) cm^{-1}: 3282, 3218, 3143, 3089, 1635, 1595, 1564, 1540 and 1353 (NO_2). ^1H NMR (500 MHz, DMSO): δ 11.83 (s, 1H, CONH), 11.81 (s, 1H, Indole NH), 8.72 (s, 1H, —N=CH—C_6H_5, H_2), 8.28 (bs, 1H, —N=*CH*—), 8.21 (d, 1H, J = 7.8 Hz, Indole H_4), 8.16 (d, 1H, J = 7.4 Hz, —N=CH—C_6H_5, H_6), 8.08 (dd, 1H, *J* = 7.20, 1.0 Hz, —N=CH—C_6H_5, H_3), 7.83 (t, 1H, *J* = 7.5 Hz, —N=CH—C_6H_5, H_5), 7.66 (td, 1H, *J* = 7.6, 1.35 Hz, —N=CH—C_6H_5, H_4), 7.49 (d, 1H, *J* = 7.9 Hz, Indole H_7), 7.23-7.16 (m, 2H, Indole H_5, H_6), ESI-Mass *m/z*: 309 $[M+H]^+$, 331 $[M+Na]^+$, 347 $[M+K]^+$; Anal. Calcd. for $C_{16}H_{12}N_4O_3$: C, 62.33; H, 3.92; N, 18.17. Found: C, 62.58; H, 4.08; N, 18.32.

N'-(2-methoxybenzylidene)-1H-indole-3-carbohydrazide (3f)

Yield: 69%, mp 229- 231°C. IR (KBr) cm^{-1}: 3300- 3200 (ν NH), 3112, 3076, 1622, 1601, 1578, 1540; ^1H NMR (500 MHz, DMSO): δ 11.73 (s, 1H, CONH), 11.41 (s, 1H, Indole-NH), 8.65 (bs, 1H, Indole H_2), 8.22 (bs, 2H, Indole H_4, —N=*CH*—), 7.87 (d, 1H, *J* = 6.70 Hz, —N=CH—C_6H_5, H_6), 7.48 (d, 1H, *J* = 7. 85 Hz, Indole H_7), 7.41 (td, 1H, *J* = 7.3, 1.35 Hz, —N=CH—C_6H_5, H_4), 7.20 (t, 1H, *J* = 7.0 Hz, —N=CH—C_6H_5, H_5), 7.15 (t, 1H, *J* = 7.4 Hz, Indole H_5), 7.12 (d, 1H, *J* = 8.3 Hz, —N=CH—C_6H_5, H_3), 7.04 (t, 1H, *J* = 7.4 Hz, Indole H_6), 3.89 (s, 3H, —OCH_3); ESI-Mass *m/z*: 294 $[M+H]^+$, 316 $[M+Na]^+$; Anal. Calcd. for $C_{17}H_{15}N_3O_2$: C, 69.61; H, 5.15; N, 14.33. Found: C, 69.46; H, 5.33; N, 14.12.

N'-(3-chlorobenzylidene)-1H-indole-3-carbohydrazide (3 g)

Yield: 78%, mp 288- 291°C. IR (KBr) cm^{-1}: 3545, 3390, 3320, 3263, 3068, 1635, 1580, 1558,1548; ^1H NMR (500 MHz, DMSO): δ 11.78 (s, 1H, CONH), 11.50 (s, 1H,

Table 1 Effect of 3-substituted indole (3d-m) and 2-substituted indole (6d-i) derivatives at 1 mM concentration on*in-vitro*platelet aggregation induced by AA, ADP and collagen

Derivative	Structure	AA	ADP	Collagen
		Inhibition (%)[b]		
3d	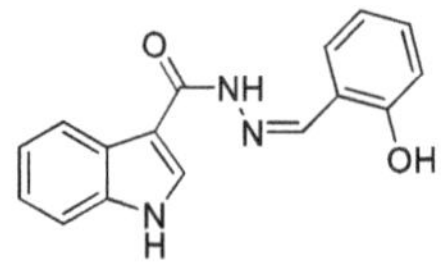	30.1 ± 3	31 ± 1.5	24.5 ± 2.1
3e	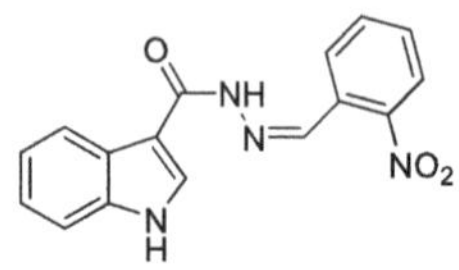	94 ± 5	20 ± 1.3	80 ± 4.3
3f	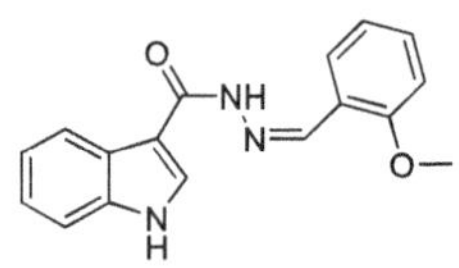	97 ± 4.9	41.5 ± 2.1	73.6 ± 2.9
3 g	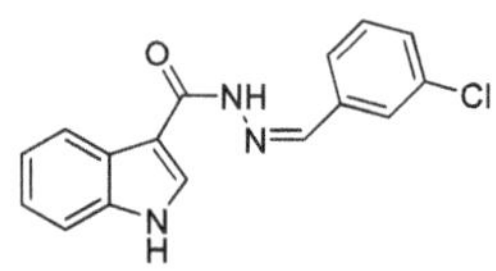	94 ± 2.5	46 ± 2.5	65.6 ± 3.1
3h	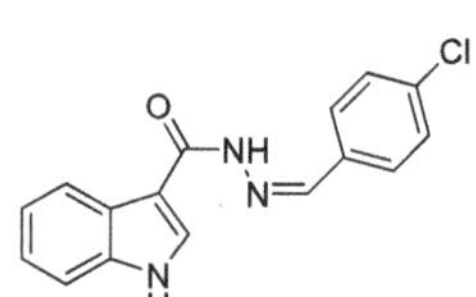	95 ± 3.9	21.3 ± 1	44.6 ± 2.1
3i	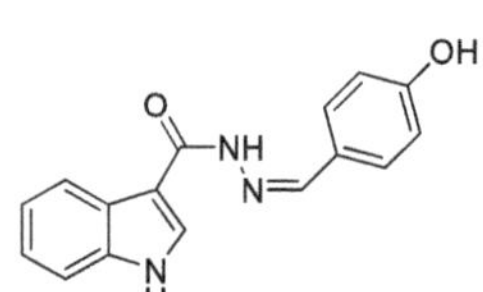	97 ± 5.1	47.5 ± 1.2	74 ± 3.9
3j	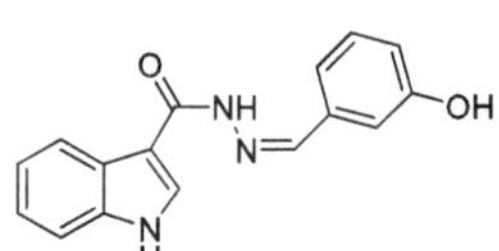	96 ± 4.6	42.8 ± 0.9	81 ± 1.9
3 k	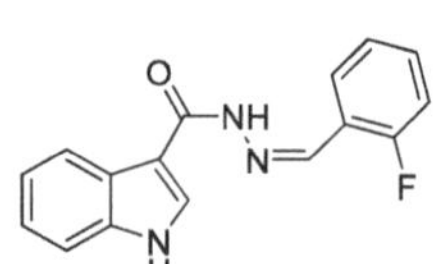	93 ± 1.9	55 ± 1.3	91 ± 2.7

Table 1 Effect of 3-substituted indole (3d-m) and 2-substituted indole (6d-i) derivatives at 1 mM concentration onin-vitroplatelet aggregation induced by AA, ADP and collagen *(Continued)*

3 l	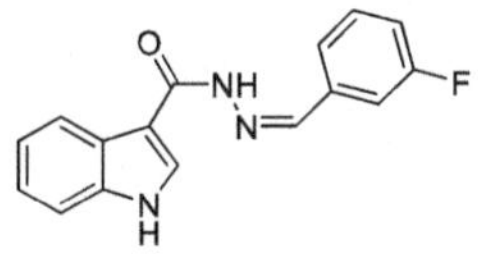	94 ± 3	53 ± 2.1	91 ± 0.9
3 m	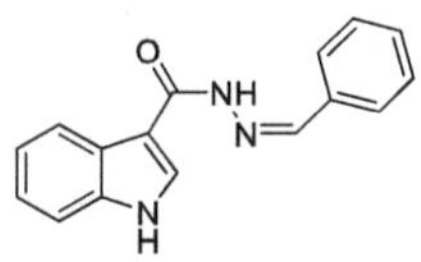	94 ± 2.8	35 ± 1.2	100 ± 2.0
6d	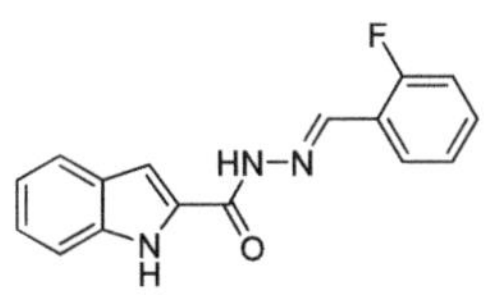	96 ± 4.1	31.4 ± 1.4	61.6 ± 3.2
6e	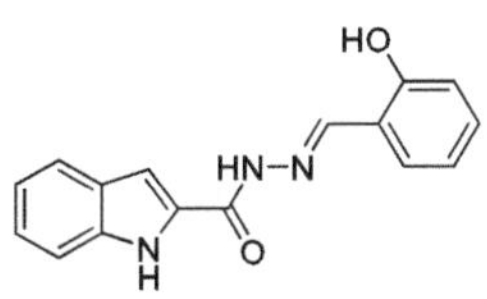	35 ± 2.5	66.8 ± 1.1	8 ± 0.9
6f	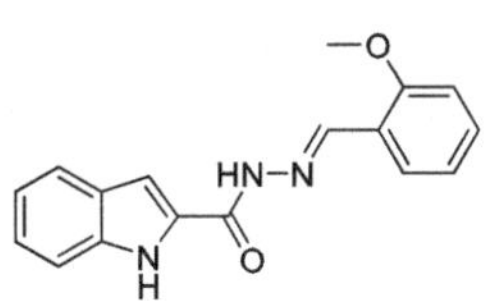	94.5 ± 3.1	25.9 ± 0.6	61 ± 3
6 g	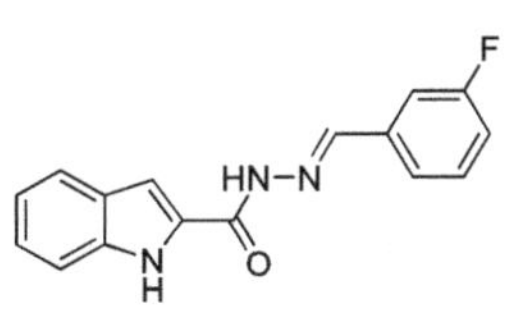	100 ± 3.8	26.8 ± 1	27.3 ± 1.2
6 h	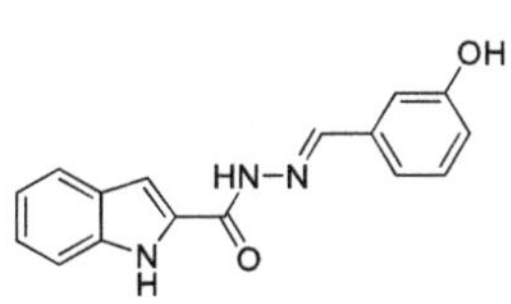	96 ± 2.9	24 ± 0.8	100 ± 3.4
6i	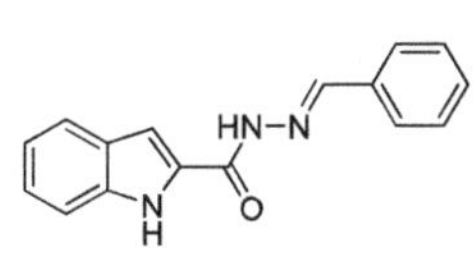	98 ± 1.4	51 ± 1.3	80 ± 2.5
Indomethacin[a]		100 ± 4.3	42 ± 1.1	100 ± 2.8
Aspirin[a]		100 ± 2.8	21 ± 0.6	100 ± 3.1

[a]Aspirin and Indomethacin were used as a positive control.
[b]Values are presented as mean ± S.E. of three separate determination.

Indole-NH), 8.27 (bs, 1H, —N=*CH*—), 8.21 (s, 1H, Indole H_2), 8.20 (s, 1H, Indole H_4), 7.78 (s, 1H, —N=CH—C_6H_5, H_2), 7.68 (d, 1H, $J = 7.0$ Hz, —N=CH—C_6H_5, H_6), 7.51- 7.47 (m, 3H, Indole H_7, —N=CH—C_6H_5, H_4, H_5), 7.22- 7.15 (m, 2H, Indole H_5, H_6); ESI-Mass *m/z*: 298 $[M + H]^+$, 320 $[M + Na]^+$; Anal. Calcd. for $C_{16}H_{12}ClN_3O$: C, 64.54; H, 4.06; N, 11.91. Found: C, 64.19; H, 4.24; N, 11.76.

N'-(4-chlorobenzylidene)-1H-indole-3-carbohydrazide (3 h)

Yield: 74%, mp 265- 267°C. IR (KBr) cm^{-1}: 3394, 3240, 3060, 1637, 1603, 1555, 1536; ^1H NMR (500 MHz, DMSO): δ 11.76 (s, 1H, CONH), 11.45 (s, 1H, Indole-NH), 8.35- 8.21 (m, 3H, —N=*CH*—, Indole H_2, H_4), 7.75 (d, 2H, $J = 8.5$ Hz, —N=CH—C_6H_5, H_2, H_6), 7.53 (d, 2H, $J = 8.5$ Hz, —N=CH—C_6H_5, H_3, H_5), 7.49 (d, 1H, $J = 8.0$ Hz, Indole H_7), 7.22- 7.15 (m, 2H, Indole H_5, H_6); ESI-Mass *m/z*: 298 $[M + H]^+$, 320 $[M + Na]^+$; Anal. Calcd. for $C_{16}H_{12}ClN_3O$: C, 64.54; H, 4.06; N, 11.91. Found: C, 64.43; H, 3.91; N, 12.16.

N'-(2-fluorobenzylidene)-1H-indole-3-carbohydrazide (3 k)

Yield: 90%, mp 239- 240°C. IR (KBr) cm^{-1}: 3299- 3073 (ν NH), 3032, 2956, 1636, 1614, 1586, 1555. ^1H NMR (500 MHz, DMSO): δ 11.77 (s, 1H, CONH), 11.50 (bs, 1H, Indole NH), 8.55 (bs, 1H, —N=*CH*—), 8.22 (d, 1H, $J = 7.5$ Hz, Indole H_4), 7.94 (t, 1H, $J = 6.8$ Hz, —N=CH—C_6H_5, H_4), 7.50- 7.45 (m, 3H, —N=CH—C_6H_5, H_6, Indole H_2, H_7), 7.33- 7.29 (m, 2H, —N=CH—C_6H_5, H_3, H_5), 7.21 (td, 1H, $J = 6.5$, 1.3 Hz, Indole H_5), 7.16 (td, 1H, $J = 6.5$, 1.3 Hz, Indole H_6); ESI-Mass *m/z*: 282 $[M + H]^+$, 304 $[M + Na]^+$; Anal. Calcd. for $C_{16}H_{12}FN_3O$: C, 68.32; H, 4.30; N, 14.94. Found: C, 68.64; H, 4.13; N, 14.62.

N'-(3-fluorobenzylidene)-1H-indole-3-carbohydrazide (3 l)

Yield: 87%, mp 278- 281°C. IR (KBr) cm^{-1}: 3319- 3200 (ν NH), 3139, 3089, 1647, 1591, 1558, 1500. ^1H NMR (500 MHz, DMSO): δ 11.76 (s, 1H, CONH), 11.50 (bs, 1H, Indole NH), 8.34- 8.27 (m, 3H, —N=*CH*—, Indole H_4, H_2), 7.57- 7.48 (m, 4H, —N=CH—C_6H_5 ,H_2, H_5, H6, Indole, H_7), 7.28- 7.24 (m, 1H, —N=CH—C_6H_5, H_4), 7.21 (td, 1H, $J = 6.8$, 1.2 Hz, Indole H_5), 7.16 (td, 1H, $J = 6.8$, 1.2 Hz, Indole H_6); ESI-Mass *m/z*: 282 $[M + H]^+$, 304 $[M + Na]^+$; Anal. Calcd. for $C_{16}H_{12}FN_3O$: C, 68.32; H, 4.30; N, 14.94. Found: C, 68.14; H, 4.03; N, 15.02.

N'-(2-fluorobenzylidene)-1H-indole-2-carbohydrazide (6d)

Yield: 98%, mp 186- 188°C. IR (KBr) cm^{-1}: 3450, 3227, 3038, 2922, 1643, 1621, 1612, 1593, and 1564. ^1H NMR (500 MHz, DMSO): δ 12.03 (s, 1H, CONH), 11.85 (s, 1H, Indole NH), 8.71 (s, 1H, —N=*CH*—), 7.98 (t, 1H, $J = 7.3$ Hz, —N=CH—C_6H_5 ,H_4), 7.70 (d, 1H, $J = 7.8$ Hz, —N=CH—C_6H_5,H_6), 7.52- 7.47 (m, 2H, Indole H_4, H_7), 7.35- 7.32 (m, 2H, Indole H_5, H_6), 7.24 (t, 1H, $J = 7.4$ Hz, —N=CH—C_6H_5, H_3), 7.08 (t, 1H, $J = 7.4$ Hz, —N=CH—C_6H_5, H_5); ESI-Mass *m/z*: 282 $[M + H]^+$; Anal. Calcd. for $C_{16}H_{12}FN_3O$: C, 68.32; H, 4.30; N, 14.94. Found: C, 68.14; H, 4.63; N, 15.12.

N'-(3-fluorobenzylidene)-1H-indole-2-carbohydrazide (6 g)

Yield: 88%, mp 171- 173°C. IR (KBr) cm^{-1}: 3448, 3313, 3264, 3126, 3071, 1629, 1597, 1577, 1529; ^1H NMR (500 MHz, DMSO): δ 12.02 (s, 1H, CONH), 11.84 (s, 1H, Indole NH), 8.47 (s, 1H, —N=*CH*—), 7.70 (d, 1H, $J = 8.0$ Hz, —N=CH—C_6H_5 ,H_2),7.61 (d, 1H, $J = 7.3$ Hz, Indole H_7), 7.58- 7.52 (m, 2H, —N=CH—C_6H_5 H_5, Indole, H_4), 7.48 (d, 1H, $J = 8.0$ Hz, —N=CH—C_6H_5, H_6), 7.34 (s, 1H, Indole H_3), 7.30 (t, 1H, $J = 8.5$ Hz, —N=CH—C_6H_5, H_6), 7.24 (t, 1H, $J = 7.5$ Hz, Indole H_6), 7.08 (t, 1H, $J = 7.5$ Hz, Indole H_5); ESI-Mass *m/z*: 282 $[M + H]^+$, 304 $[M + Na]^+$; Anal. Calcd. for $C_{16}H_{12}FN_3O$: C, 68.32; H, 4.30; N, 14.94. Found: C, 68.01; H, 4.33; N, 14.62.

N'-(3-hydroxybenzylidene)-1H-indole-2-carbohydrazide (6 h)

Yield: 89%, mp 278- 281°C. IR (KBr) cm^{-1}: 3412 (ν OH), 3227, 3185, 3048, 2924, 1624, 1599, 1583, 1564, 1507; ^1H NMR (500 MHz, DMSO): δ 12.05 (s, 1H, CONH), 11.84 (bs, 2H, Indole NH, OH), 8.44 (s, 1H, —N=*CH*—), 7.82 (s, 1H, —N=CH—C_6H_5, H_2), 7.74- 7.68 (m, 2H, Indole H_4, H_7), 7.53- 7.51 (m, 2H, —N=CH—C_6H_5, H_5, H_6), 7.47 (d, 1H, $J = 8.3$ Hz, —N=CH—C_6H_5, H_4), 7.34 (s, 1H, Indole H_3), 7.24 (t, 1H, $J = 7.1$ Hz, Indole H_6), 7.08 (t, 1H, $J = 7.1$ Hz, Indole H_5); ESI-Mass *m/z*: 280 $[M + H]^+$, 302 $[M + Na]^+$; Anal. Calcd. for $C_{16}H_{13}N_3O_2$: C, 68.81; H, 4.69; N, 15.05. Found: C, 69.04; H, 4.41; N, 14.92.

Biological assay

In vitro evaluation of anti-platelet aggregation activity

Human plasma used to measure the derivatives anti-platelet aggregation activity. Fresh blood was obtained from healthy volunteer with negative history of drug consumption from 15 days prior to the test. Platelet-rich plasma (PRP) was obtained from citrated whole blood (9:1 by volume) which centrifuged at 1,000 rpm for 8 min. The remained layer was centrifuged at 3,000 rpm for 15 min and the upper layer; PPP (Platelet poor plasma) was collected as the blank. The platelet count was adjusted to 250,000 plts/mL by diluting PRP with appropriate amount of PPP. To the PRP samples, test compounds previously dissolved in DMSO (at 0.05% final concentration) were added and samples were incubated for 5 min at 37°C. Then ADP (5 μM), collagen (1.25 mg/mL) or AA (1.25 mg/mL) was added and platelet shape change and aggregation were monitored for 5 min. DMSO (0.5% v/v) was used as negative control and aspirin and indomethacin were applied as standard drugs. The extent of platelet aggregation was calculated by the following formula:

$$\text{Inhibition\%} = [1\text{-}(D/S)] * 100$$

D = platelet aggregation in the presence of test compoundsS = platelet aggregation in the presence of solvent.

The platelet aggregation inhibitory activity was expressed as percent inhibition by comparison with that measured for the vehicle (DMSO) alone and IC_{50} values were obtained from log (concentration) – inhibition (%) diagram and was defined as the concentration of the test compound that inhibits the platelet aggregation by 50%. Data were presented as mean ± S.E.M. of three independent experiments performed in triplicate. IC_{50}values and inhibition data were analyzed with prism software.

Consent

The study was approved in the Institute Review Board with code number 93-6-10:1–1. Written informed consent was obtained from the patient for the publication of this report and any accompanying images.

Results

The synthetic pathway is disclosed in Scheme 1. Final desired derivatives were prepared by a two-step procedure. The structures were confirmed by spectroscopic techniques including IR, Mass and ^1H NMR. Molecular mass of all the derivatives was determined by Electronspray ionization mass spectrometry (ESI–MS) as M + 1 and/or M + 23 relating to hydrogen and sodium adducts of the intact molecules, respectively. All the synthesized compounds were evaluated for their ability to inhibit platelet aggregation of human platelet-rich plasma (PRP) induced by AA, ADP and collagen as potent aggregation inducers, and using indomethacin and aspirin were applied as standard drugs. The results of *in-vitro* antiplatelet aggregation activity for the title compounds were summarized in Table 1. All the derivatives were initially tested at 1 mM.

The physicochemical parameters of the derivatives were calculated and are listed in Table 2.

Table 2 General molecular parameters of the synthesized compounds

Compound	Clog P	R[a]	P[b]	V[c]	SA[d]	
					Approx.	Grid
3d	2.92	86.69	30.1	771.23	374.67	469.41
3e	-0.15	92.78	32.03	809.38	404.94	487.59
3f	3.35	88.16	30.83	781.07	373.02	472.72
3g	2.72	90.56	31.99	854.73	356.93	517.77
3h	3.85	91.28	32.12	807.06	402.79	488.39
3i	3.28	86.69	30.1	772.67	378.22	470.61
3j	2.72	88.16	30.83	784.59	381.64	474.45
3k	2.72	88.16	30.83	783.92	379.99	474.45
3l	3.85	91.28	32.12	807.9	403.8	488.87
3m	3.14	86.56	30.19	764.21	367.69	464.55
6d	3.26	87.96	30.1	775.75	381.25	476.6
6e	3.69	89.44	30.83	787.22	379.72	479.81
6f	3.06	94.21	32.66	844.8	422.2	515.34
6g	3.62	87.96	30.1	778.08	384.8	477.59
6h	3.06	89.44	30.83	791.05	387	482.43
6i	3.48	87.83	30.19	772.17	374	474.2

[a]Refractivity.
[b]Polarizability.
[c]Molecular volume.
[d]Surface area.

Discussion

Chemistry

All derivatives of 3-substituted indole and 2-substituted indole were obtained by the reaction of **2** and **5** with the proper aldehydes. *Synthesis of Schiff bases were* performed in ethanol with a few drops of glacial acetic acid. This reaction in the majority of the cases was straight forward; however, the products were soluble in ethanol and their separation was difficult. Therefore in another effort, the solvent was changed to water, a few drops of glacial acetic acid was added to the reaction mixture and heated for 10 min. After completion of reaction, the products were obtained in excellent yields.

In the ^1H NMR spectra of these compounds the existence of two singlet at 11.00 to 12.00 ppm was assigned to hydrazide NH and indole NH. Also, singlet signal at 8.20-8.80 ppm was assigned to H—C = N. The ^1H NMR and ESI-mass data of compounds approved the exact structures.

Antiplatelet aggregation activity

Platelet activation and thrombus formation are major causes of cardiovascular diseases and thrombosis. Thus, antiplatelet therapy is a useful way to prevent or treat these diseases; these diseases; thus, antiplatelet agents such as aspirin, ticlopidine and dipyridamole have been clinically used for thrombus-related diseases [9]. However, the side effects of mentioned agents frequently have been reported and a new group of compounds with greater efficacy and safety are desired. Therefore, in the present study, the inhibitory effects of synthesized compounds on platelet aggregation were evaluated by turbidimetric method reported by Born and Cross [33] using APACT 4004 aggregometer. The baseline value was set using PRP and maximal transmission using PPP. Compounds **3d-m** and **6d-i** were tested for anti-platelet aggregation activity induced by adenosine diphosphate (ADP), arachidonic acid (AA) and collagen using indomethacin and aspirin as standards.

Interestingly, most of the tested derivatives selectively inhibited platelet aggregation induced by AA and collagen with satisfactory percent inhibition values. According to the literature [15]; herein, antiplatelet aggregation activity of *N*-acylhydrazones is probably related to modulation of AA cascade enzymes.

Among the synthesized indole-2-carbaldehyde derivatives compound **6g** exhibited 100% inhibition of platelet aggregation at 1 mM when AA was used as agonist while this compound has no significant inhibitory activity against ADP and collagen induced platelet aggregation. Comparing the results obtained for indole derivatives, compounds **3m** and **6h** showed the best antiplatelet aggregation effect which induced by collagen. On the other hand, effects of the synthesized compounds on the platelet aggregation induced by ADP shows another pattern: all the compounds caused no significant inhibition on platelet aggregation except **6e** which showed 66.7% inhibition.

The IC_{50} values were calculated for more potent compounds (**3f, 3i, 3k, 3l, 3m, 6d, 6g, 6h** and **6i**) for the inhibition of AA and collagen-induced aggregation which are shown in Table 3.

However, the obtained results were compared with those reported by Kobarfard et al. on antiplatelet aggregation effect of some indole derivatives [4]. It was found that the insertion of acyl group to indole hydrazone moiety cannot improve platelet aggregation inhibitory activity.

In order to investigate the possible relationship between the structural parameters of the investigated derivatives and their antiplatelet aggregation activity, quantitative structure–activity relationship (QSAR) analysis was performed with various molecular descriptors. The calculated octanol–water partition coefficient (Clog P) has been considered as descriptor for the hydrophobic effect. The steric effect has been described by means of the surface area (SA: approx and grid) and molecular volume (V) refractivity (R) and polarizability (P) have been used as descriptors for both volume and electronic state (London dispersive forces) properties of the molecules. For each descriptor, the best multilinear regression equation was obtained. The calculated physicochemical parameters of the derivatives are listed in Table 2. Analysis of the physicochemical parameters doesn't show a significant correlation between the observed activities and general molecular parameters of the synthesized derivatives.

Table 3 IC_{50}values for the antiplatelet aggregation activity induced by collagen and AA[a]

Compound	Aryl	IC_{50} (μM)[b]	
		AA	Collagen
3f	2-methoxyphenyl	310±8.1	121.5±3.1
3i	4-hydroxyphenyl	290±5.3	188±2.8
3k	2-fluorophenyl	179±2.4	122±1.6
3l	3-fluorophenyl	321±3.9	120±4.0
3m	phenyl	182±5.2	21±0.9
6d	2-fluorophenyl	286±1.5	720±9.1
6g	3-fuorophenyl	140±4.3	>1000
6h	3-hydroxyphenyl	200±2.0	190±3.2
6i	phenyl	94±1.9	134±4.1
Indomethacin		3±0.2	1.2±0.1
Aspirin		30.3±2.6	9.7±0.6

[a]Data related to compounds 3 and 6 as shown in Scheme 1.
[b]IC_{50} values represent mean ± S.E. of triplicate measurements from one of three independent experiments.

Conclusion

In summary, we have synthesized sixteen *N*-acylhydrazone derivatives (**3d-m** and **6d-i**) and evaluated their antiplatelet aggregation activity against collagen, ADP and AA as the aggregation inducers. Compounds **3e, 3g, 3h, 3i, 3j, 3k, 3l, 3m, 6d, 6f, 6g, 6h** and **6i** showed significant antiplatelet aggregation (>90%) when arachidonic acid was used as the inducer. While, **3l, 3k, 3m** and **6h** exhibited best (>90%) platelet aggregation inhibition induced by collagen among other compounds.

Failure to extract a clear correlation between activities and general molecular parameters of the synthesized compounds could be related to the existence of several receptors on the platelets surface which are responsible for controlling platelet aggregation. Platelets are activated by variety of metabolic pathways. The mechanism of platelet aggregation pathway is very complex and involves multiple components and it can be controlled by heterogeneous group of endogenous compounds such as ADP, ATP, collagen, tryptophan, epinephrine, thromboxane A_2 and calcium. Each can independently and together begin the process leading to platelet aggregation. These compounds on platelets have specific receptors and the investigated compounds in the present study may exert their activities through binding to more than one of these receptors and therefore no straight forward SAR could be obtained. The findings of this study will be helpful for the development of new antiplatelet compounds providing some directions in the area of antiplatelet drug discovery.

Competing interests

The authors declare that they have no competing interests.

Authors' contributions

SSM: Synthesis of the title compounds and collaboration in the antiplatelet aggregation test. FK: Design of target compounds and supervision of the synthetic and pharmacological parts. LF: Collaboration in computational study. AA: collaboration in the synthetic part. ME: Performed the antiplatelet aggregation test. KT: collaborated in the antiplatelet aggregation test and identifying the structures of target compounds. AS: Design of target compounds and supervision of the synthetic part. AF: Design of target compounds and supervision of the synthetic part. All authors read and approved the final manuscript.

Acknowledgements
The authors are thankful for financial support from the Research Council of Tehran University of Medical Sciences and Iran National Science Foundation (INSF).

Author details
[1]Department of Medicinal Chemistry, Faculty of Pharmacy and Pharmaceutical Sciences Research Center, Tehran University of Medical Sciences, Tehran, Iran. [2]Department of Medicinal Chemistry, School of Pharmacy, Shahid Beheshti University of Medical Sciences, Tehran, Iran. [3]Phytochemistry Research Center, Shahid Beheshti University of Medical Sciences, Tehran, Iran. [4]Drug Design and Development Research Center, Tehran University of Medical Sciences, Tehran, Iran. [5]Neuroscience Research Center, Institute of Neuropharmacology, Kerman University of Medical Sciences, Kerman, Iran.

References

1. Mendis S, Puska P, Norrving B: **Global atlas on cardiovascular disease prevention and control.** 2011, [http://www.world-heart-federation.org/publications/books/global-atlas-on-cvd-prevention-and-control/]
2. Reddy MV, Tsai WJ, Qian K, Lee KH, Wu TS: **Structure–activity relationships of chalcone analogs as potential inhibitors of ADP- and collagen-induced platelet aggregation.** *Bioorg Med Chem* 2011, **19:**7711–7719.
3. Brito FCF, Kummerle AE, Lugnier C, Fraga CAM, Barreiro EJ, Miranda ALP: **Novel thienylacylhydrazone derivatives inhibit platelet aggregation through cyclic nucleotides modulation and thromboxane A_2synthesis inhibition.** *Eur J Pharmacol* 2010, **638:**5–12.
4. Mashayekhi V, Hajmohammad Ebrahim Tehrani K, Amidi S, Kobarfard F: **Synthesis of novel indole hydrazone derivatives and evaluation of their antiplatelet aggregation activity.** *Chem Pharm Bull* 2013, **61:**144–150.
5. DeCandia M, Liantonio F, Carotti A, De Cristofaro R, Altomare C: **Fluorinated benzyloxyphenyl piperidine-4-carboxamides with dual function against thrombosis: inhibitors of factor Xa and platelet aggregation.** *J Med Chem* 2009, **52:**1018–1028.
6. Maree AO, Fitzgerald DJ: **Variable platelet response to aspirin and clopidogrel in atherothrombotic disease.** *Circulation* 2007, **115:**2196–2207.
7. Meadows TA, Bhatt DL: **Clinical aspects of platelet inhibitors and thrombus formation.** *Circ Res* 2007, **100:**1261–1275.
8. Fathiazad F, Matlobi A, Khorrami A, Hamedeyazdan S, Soraya H, Hammami M, Maleki-Dizaji N, Garjani A: **Phytochemical screening and evaluation of cardioprotective activity of ethanolic extract of Ocimum basilicum L. (basil) against isoproterenol induced myocardial infarction in rats.** *DARU J Pharm Sci* 2012, **20:**87.
9. Eskandariyan Z, Esfahanizadeh M, Haj Mohammad Ebrahim Tehrani K, Mashayekhi V, Kobarfard F: **Synthesis of thioether derivatives of quinazoline-4-one-2-thione and evaluation of their antiplatelet aggregation activity.** *Arch Pharm Res* 2013, **37:**332–339.
10. Siwek A, Stączek P, Stefańska J: **Synthesis and structure activity relationship studies of 4-arylthiosemicarbazides as topoisomerase IV inhibitors with Gram-positive antibacterial activity. search for molecular basis of antibacterial activity of thiosemicarbazides.** *Eur J Med Chem* 2011, **46:**5717–5726.
11. Fraga AGM, Rodrigues CR, de Miranda ALP, Barreiro EJ, Fraga CAM: **Synthesis and evaluation of novel heterotricyclic acylhydrazones derivatives, designed as PAF antagonist candidates.** *Eur J Pharm Sci* 2000, **11:**285–290.
12. Cunha AC, Figueiredo JM, Tributino JLM, Miranda ALP, Castro HC, Zingali RB, Fraga CAM, de Souza MCBV, Ferreira VF, Barreiro EJ: **Antiplatelet properties of novel*N*-substituted-phenyl-1,2,3-triazole-4-acylhydrazone derivatives.** *Bioorg Med Chem* 2003, **11:**2051–2059.
13. Cunha AC, Tributino JLM, Miranda ALP, Fraga CAM, Barreiro EJ: **Synthesis and pharmacological evaluation of novel antinociceptive *N*-substituted-phenylimidazolyl- 4-acylhydrazone derivatives.** *Il Farmaco* 2002, **57:**999–1007.
14. Lima PC, Lima LM, da Silva KC, Le'da PH, de Miranda AL, Fraga CAM, Barreiro EJ: **Synthesis and analgesic activity of novel*N*-acylarylhydrazones and isosters, derived from natural safrole.** *Eur J Med Chem* 2000, **35:**187–203.
15. Silva GA, Costa LMM, Brito FCF, Miranda ALP, Barreiro EJ, Fraga CAM: **New class of potent antinociceptive and antiplatelet 10*H*-phenothiazine-1-acylhydrazone derivatives.** *Bioorg Med Chem* 2004, **12:**3149–3158.
16. Bezerra-Neto HJC, Lacerda DI, Miranda ALP, Alves HM, Barreiro EJ, Fraga CAM: **Design and synthesis of 3,4-methylenedioxy-6-nitrophenoxyacetylhydrazone derivatives obtained from natural safrole: new lead-agents with analgesic and antipyretic properties.** *Bioorg Med Chem* 2006, **14:**7924–7935.
17. Duarte CD, Tributino JLM, Lacerda DI, Martins MV, Alexandre-Moreira MS, Dutra F, Bechara EJH, De-Paula FS, Goulart MOF, Ferreira J, Calixto JB, Nunes MP, Bertho AL, Miranda ALP, Barreiro EJ, Fraga CAM: **Synthesis, pharmacological evaluation and electrochemical studies of novel 6-nitro-3,4-methylenedioxyphenyl-*N*-acylhydrazone derivatives: discovery of LASSBio-881, a new ligand of cannabinoid receptors.** *Bioorg Med Chem* 2007, **15:**2421–2433.
18. Lima LM, Frattani FS, dos Santos JL, Castro HC, Fraga CAM, Zingali RB, Barreiro EJ: **Synthesis and anti-platelet activity of novel arylsulfonateacylhydrazone derivatives, designed as antithrombotic candidates.** *Eur J Med Chem* 2008, **43:**348–356.
19. Tributino JLM, Duarte CD, Corre^a RS, Dorigetto AC, Ellena J, Romeiro NC, Castro NG, Miranda ALP, Barreiro EJ, Fraga CAM: **Novel 6-methanesulfonamide- 3,4-methylenedioxy-phenyl- *N*-acylhydrazones: orally effective anti-inflammatory drug candidates.** *Biorg Med Chem* 2009, **17:**1125–1131.
20. Maia RC, Silva LL, Mazzeu EF, Fumian MM, de Rezende CM, Doriguetto AC, Corrêa RS, Miranda ALP, Barreiro EJ, Fraga MCA: **Synthesis and analgesic profile of conformationally constrained N-acylhydrazone analogues: Discovery of novel N-arylideneamino quinazolin-4(3H)-one compounds derived from natural safrole.** *Bioorg Med Chem* 2009, **17:**6517–6525.
21. Chen R, Li X, Gong B, Selzer PM, Li Z, Davidson E, Kurzban G, Miller RE, Nuzum EO, McKerrow JH, Fletterick RJ, Gillmor SA, Craik CS, Kuntz ID, Cohen FE, Kenyon GL: **Structure-based design of parasitic protease inhibitors.** *Bioorg Med Chem* 1996, **4:**1421–1427.
22. Sluis-Cremer N, Arion D, Parniak MA: **Destabilization of the HIV-1 reverse transcriptase dimer upon interaction with N-acyl hydrazone inhibitors.** *Mol Pharmacol* 2002, **62:**398–405.
23. Dimmock JR, Baker GB, Taylor WG: **Arylhydrazones. Part II. The ultraviolet spectroscopy and antimicrobial evaluation of some substituted aroylhydrazones.** *Can J Pharm Sci* 1972, **7:**100–103.
24. Sudo RT, Zapata-Sudo G, Barreiro EJ: **The new compound, LASSBio 294, increases the contractility of intact and saponin-skinned cardiac muscle from Wistar rats.** *Br J Pharmacol* 2001, **134:**603–613.
25. Gonzalez-Serratos H, Chang R, Pereira EF, Castro NG, Aracava Y, Melo PA, Lima PC, Fraga CAM, Barreiro EJ, Albuquerque EX: **A novel thienylhydrazone, (2- thienylidene) 3,4-methylenedioxybenzoylhydrazine, increases inotropism and decreases fatigue of skeletal muscle.** *J Pharmacol Exp Ther* 2001, **229:**558–566.
26. Silva CLM, Noe LF, Barreiro EJ: **Cyclic GMP-dependent vasodilatory properties of LASSBio 294 in rat aorta.** *Br J Pharmacol* 2002, **135:**293–298.
27. Zapata-Sudo G, Sudo RT, Maronas PA, Silva GL, Moreira OR, Aguiar MI, Barreiro EJ: **Thienylhydrazone derivative increases sarcoplasmic reticulum Ca^{2+}release in mammalian skeletal muscle.** *Eur J Pharmacol* 2003, **470:**79–85.
28. Silva AG, Zapata-Sudo G, Kummerle AE, Fraga CAM, Barreiro EJ, Sudo RT: **Synthesis and vasodilatory activity of new*N*-acylhydrazone derivatives, designed as LASSBio-294 analogues.** *Bioorg Med Chem* 2005, **13:**3431–3437.
29. Park MK, Rhee YH, Lee HJ, Lee EO, Kim KH, Park MJ, Jeon BH, Shim BS, Jung CH, Choi SH, Ahn KS, Kim SH: **Antiplatelet and antithrombotic activity of indole-3-carbinol in vitro and in vivo.** *Phytother Res* 2008, **22:**58–64.
30. Alemany A, Bernabé M, Elorriaga C, Fernández AE, Lora-Tamayo M, Nieto O: **Patent; Patron, Invest. Cie. Tech.** *Bull Soc Chim Fr* 1966, **8:**2486–2497.

31. Bao XP, Zheng PC, Liu Y, Tan Z, Zhou YH, Song BA: **Salicylaldehyde-indole-2-acylhydrazone: a simple, colorimetric and absorption ratiometric chemosensor for acetate ion.** *Supramol Chem* 2013, **25**:246–253.
32. Wareth A, Sarhan AO: **On the synthesis and reactions of indole-2-carboxylic acid hydrazide.** *Monatsh Chem* 2001, **132**:753–763.
33. Born GVR: **Aggregation of blood platelets by adenosine diphosphate and its reversal.** *Nature* 1962, **194**:927–929.

Preparation and radiolabeling of a lyophilized (kit) formulation of DOTA-rituximab with ^{90}Y and ^{111}In for domestic radioimmunotherapy and radioscintigraphy of Non-Hodgkin's Lymphoma

Nazila Gholipour[1*], Amir Reza Jalilian[2], Ali Khalaj[3], Fariba Johari-Daha[2], Kamal Yavari[2], Omid Sabzevari[4], Ali Reza Khanchi[2] and Mehdi Akhlaghi[5]

Abstract

Background: On the basis of results of our previous investigations on ^{90}Y-DTPA-rituximab and in order to fulfil national demands to radioimmunoconjugates for radioscintigraphy and radioimmunotherapy of Non-Hodgkin's Lymphoma (NHL), preparation and radiolabeling of a lyophilized formulation (kit) of DOTA-rituximab with ^{111}In and ^{90}Y was investigated.

Methods: ^{111}In and ^{90}Y with high radiochemical and radionuclide purity were prepared by ^{112}Cd (p,2n)^{111}In nuclear reaction and a locally developed ^{90}Sr/^{90}Y generator, respectively. DOTA-rituximab immunoconjugates were prepared by the reaction of solutions of p-SCN-Bz-DOTA and rituximab in carbonate buffer (pH = 9.5) and the number of DOTA per molecule of conjugates were determined by transchelation reaction between DOTA and arsenaso yttrium(III) complex. DOTA-rituximab immunoconjugates were labeled with ^{111}In and ^{90}Y and radioimmunoconjugates were checked for radiochemical purity by chromatography methods and for immunoreactivity by cell-binding assay using Raji cell line. The stability of radiolabeled conjugate with the approximate number of 7 DOTA molecules per one rituximab molecule which was prepared in moderate yield and showed moderate immunoreactivity, compared to two other prepared radioimmunoconjugates, was determined at different time intervals and against EDTA and human serum by chromatography methods and reducing SDS-polyacrylamide gel electrophoresis, respectively. The biodistribution of the selected radioimmunoconjugate in rats was determined by measurement of the radioactivity of different organs after sacrificing the animals by ether asphyxiation.

Results: The radioimmunoconjugate with approximate DOTA/rituximab molar ratio of 7 showed stability after 24 h at room temperature, after 96 h at 4°C, as the lyophilized formulation after six months storage and against EDTA and human serum. This radioimmunoconjugate had a biodistribution profile similar to that of ^{90}Y-ibritumomab, which is approved by FDA for radioimmunotherapy of NHL, and showed low brain and lung uptakes and low yttrium deposition into bone.

Conclusion: Findings of this study suggest that further investigations may result in a lyophilized (kit) formulation of DOTA-rituximab which could be easily radiolabeled with ^{90}Y and ^{111}In in order to be used for radioimmunotherapy and radioscintigraphy of B-cell lymphoma in Iran.

Keywords: Rituximab, ^{90}Y, ^{111}In, Lymphoma-B, Biodistribution, Radioimmunotherapy

* Correspondence: gholipour@razi.tums.ac.ir
[1]Department of Radiopharmacy, Faculty of Pharmacy, Tehran University of Medical Sciences, P.O. Box: 14155–6451, Tehran, Iran
Full list of author information is available at the end of the article

Introduction

Non-Hodgkin's Lymphoma (NHL) also known as B and T cell lymphoma is a form of blood cancer originating in lymphatic system. Many investigations for treatment of NHL have been based on the development of antibody against CD-20 antigens which are expressed on the surface of B-cells [1]. Results of these investigations have led to drugs such as rituximab [2,3], a chimeric antibody for immunotherapy of CD20-positive low-grade NHL, and ibritumomab and tositumomab derived from immortalized mouse cells for the treatment of follicular lymphoma [4]. Since NHL is multifocal and radiosensitive [1,5,6], anti-CD20 monoclonal antibodies (mAbs) labeled with ^{111}In (^{111}In-ibritumomab) for imaging, ^{90}Y (^{90}Y- ibritumomab, Zevalin) for therapy and ^{131}I (^{131}I-tositumomab, Bexxar) for imaging and therapy have been approved for use in patients with NHL [4,7,8]. It has been shown that the response rate of NHL in radioimmunotherapy (RIT) with ^{90}Y-ibritumomab tiuxetan compared to rituximab immunotherapy is higher and unlike chemotherapy is not associated with severe mucositis, hair loss, or persistent nausea [1,5,8-10].

Radiolabeled Murine antibodies compared to those of humanized chimeric antibodies have shorter *in vivo* half-lives [1,5] and as a result lower toxicities due to non-specific body irradiation. However these antibodies as foreign proteins may induce immunologic and anaphylactic reactions [11] in patients because of development of human anti murine antibody (HAMA) response and have not been approved for re-injection or retreatment [5,7,12]. Consequently, considerable investigations have been carried out for the preparation of radioimmunoconjugates from rituximab, a chimeric antibody which induce distinctly less antibody responses and preparation of rituximab labeled with ^{90}Y [13,14], ^{111}In [15], ^{153}Sm [16], ^{177}Lu [17-19], ^{64}Cu [20], ^{149}Tb, ^{213}Bi, ^{227}Th and ^{225}Ac [11], through an additionally attached chelating agents such as different chemical forms of DTPA or DOTA [21,22] onto antibody, have been described. Due to high costs of commercially available radiolabeled anti CD20 monoclonal antibodies and on the basis of results of our previous investigations on ^{90}Y-DTPA-rituximab [14], where an unexpected high lung uptake was observed, and in the search for a radioimmunoconjugate of higher efficiency and lower toxicity, preparation of DOTA-rituximab which compared to DTPA-rituximab has higher stability appeared of interest. The aim of the present study was to develop a lyophilized formulation of DOTA-rituximab that could be labeled with ^{111}In and ^{90}Y in order to fulfil national demands to radioimmunoconjugates for radioscintigraphy and radioimmunotherapy of Non-Hodgkin's Lymphoma (NHL). While preparation of ^{90}Y-DOTA-rituximab has been reported [13], but characteristics, stability at different time intervals and different temperatures and biodistribution of the prepared radioimmunoconjugate have not been explained in details. This manuscript describes the synthesis, purification, and chemical characterization of a lyophilized (kit) DOTA-rituximab conjugate for labeling with ^{90}Y and ^{111}In and the radiochemical purity, in-vitro stability and biodistribution of the resulting radioimmunoconjugates.

Materials and methods

Materials

p-SCN-Bz-DOTA with %94 purity was obtained from Macrocyclics Inc. (NJ, USA). Rituximab (Reditux) was a pharmaceutical sample purchased from Cinnagen Co. (Tehran, Iran). Radio-TLC scanning was performed using a Bioscan AR-2000 radio TLC scanner instrument (Bioscan, Paris, France). A high purity germanium (HPGe) detector coupled with a Canberra™ (model GC1020-7500SL) multichannel analyzer and a dose calibrator ISOMED 1010 (Dresden, Germany) were used for counting radioactivity of organs of rats in biodistribution study. Analytical HPLC was performed by Shimadzu LC-10AT, armed with flow scintillation analyzer (Packard-150 TR) and UV-visible (Shimadzu) equipped with Whatman Partisphere C-18 column 250 × 4.6 mm, (Whatman Co. NJ, USA). Animal studies were performed in accordance with the United Kingdom Biological Council's Guidelines on the Use of Living Animals in Scientific Investigations, 2nd Edn. which was approved by Animal Ethics Committee of the Deputy of Research of Nuclear Science and Technology Research Institute (NSTRI) of Iran.

Preparation and quality control of ^{111}In-InCl$_3$

^{111}In-InCl^3 solution was produced by ^{112}Cd (p,2n)^{111}In nuclear reaction using a 30 MeV cyclotron in Agricultural, Medical and Industrial Research School (AMIRS) and purified by cation exchange chromatography on Dowex 50×8 resin. Gamma spectroscopy of the final sample was carried out by counting in an HPGe detector. Differential-pulsed anodic stripping polarography was used to ensure that the amount of cadmium, indium and copper ions in the sample are not higher than those of internationally accepted limits. The ^{111}In-InCl$_3$ solution was evaporated. The residue was dissolved in ultra-pure water and filtered under sterile condition. The radiochemical purity of the final ^{111}In solution was checked in 10 mM DTPA (pH = 5.0) solution (R_f of free $^{111}In^{3+}$ = 0.8) [15,23].

Preparation and quality control of ^{90}Y-YCl$_3$

^{90}Y-YCl$_3$ solution was prepared at Nuclear Science and Technology and Research Institute of Atomic Energy Organization of Iran by ion exchange chromatography technique through elution from an in-house made ^{90}Sr/^{90}Y generator which was developed for research purposes.

The radionuclidic purity of the solution for the presence of other radionuclides was tested by beta spectroscopy using liquid scintillation counter (LSC). The radiochemical purity of $^{90}YCl_3$ was checked by radio-TLC using 10 mM DTPA (pH = 5.0) solution (R_f of free $^{90}Y^{3+}$ = 0.8) [24].

Preparation of DOTA-rituximab immunoconjugates

DOTA-rituximab immunoconjugates were prepared according to the reported method [18] with only slight modifications. Briefly, one milliliter of rituximab solution (10 mg/ml) was freed from excipients first by ultrafiltration using Vivaspin-2 filter (30 kDa, Sartorius AG, 2 × 10 min at 2.684 g) and then by washing three times with carbonate buffer (1 ml, 0.2 M Na_2CO_3, pH = 9.5). The antibody was then removed from the upper part of filter using 3.5 ml of carbonate buffer (0.2 M Na_2CO_3, pH = 9.5). The final concentration of rituximab was determined by a biophotometer (Eppendorf) at OD = 280 nm and found to be 2.73 mg/ml. The structural integrity of the antibody was confirmed by reducing SDS-PAGE electrophoresis [13]. 1.1 ml aliquots of resulting rituximab (3 mg, 2×10^{-5} mmol/1.1 ml) solution in three sterile and pyrigen-free vials were treated with the solution of p-SCN-Bz-DOTA in carbonate buffer (0.2 M, pH = 9.5) in molar ratios of 5 (0.073 mg, 10^{-4} mmol), 15(0.22 mg, 3×10^{-4} mmol), and 25 (0.36 mg, 5×10^{-4} mmol), respectively. The solutions were gently mixed for 20 times by pipetting up and down and then incubated at room temperature for 24 h. The coupling reactions were terminated and unreacted p-SCN-Bz-DOTA were removed by adjustment of the pH of solutions to 7.0 using ammonium acetate buffer (0.25 M, pH = 5.5), followed by ultrafiltration and then washing three times with ammonium acetate buffer (0.25 M, pH = 5.5). The immunoconjugates were then removed from upper part of filters with 1 ml aliquots of ammonium acetate buffer (0.25 M, pH = 5.5). The concentration of the antibody in final immunoconjugate solutions were measured by a biophotometer and found to be around 2.84 mg/ml. The antibody solutions were dispensed in sterile vials at a quantity of 0.3 mg per vials and treated with 30 µl aliquots of mannitol solution (mannitol Ph Eur, 80 mg/ml in ultrapure water). Finally, the formulated immunoconjugate antibody solutions were freeze dried to obtain white pellets which were stored at −18°C.

Determination of the number of DOTA molecules per one rituximab molecule in DOTA-rituximab immunoconjugates

The DOTA to rituximab ratios were determined on the basis of a transchelation between DOTA and arsenaso yttrium (III) complex from a standard curve for absorbance of arsenaso yttrium (III) complex at 652 nm which was constructed for a series of solutions containing 8.1 µM AAIII, 3.9 µM Y(III) and different concentrations of p-SCN-Bz-DOTA (0–20 µM) in 0.15 M ammonium acetate buffer (pH = 7) [25].

Determination of the stability of the lyophilized (Kit) DOTA-rituximab immunoconjugates

Stability and degradation of the lyophilized DOTA-rituximab immunoconjugate kit (with selected DOTA: antibody ratio) was checked by integrity test using reducing SDS-polyacrylamide gel electrophoresis (reducing SDS-PAGE) at frequent monthly intervals (for 6 months) according to the method of Laemmli [26].

Radiolabeling and quality control of the radiolabeled immunoconjugates

Typically, 510 MBq of $^{111}InCl_3$ solution in 0.2 M HCl in conical vials were dried under a flow of nitrogen and residues were dissolved in 1500 µl of ammonium acetate buffer (pH = 5.5). 500 µl aliquots of ammonium acetate buffer were added to the vials containing lyophilized immunoconjugates (three different DOTA: antibody ratios) and the vials were mixed using pipetting up and down (10-20×) to dissolve immunoconjugates. Then 500 µl (170 MBq) aliquots of ^{111}In solution were added to vials and after mixing gently for 5 min by up and down pipetting, mixtures were incubated at 37°C for 1–2 h.

The radiochemical purity of the products was determined by ITLC on Whatman No.2, using 10 mM DTPA as mobile phase and HPLC on a C-18 column using a gradient system as a reported routine method in this laboratory [27]. To increase the radiochemical purity, the radioimmunoconjugates were purified by chromatography using PD-10 columns (GE healthcare) and ammonium acetate buffer (pH = 7.0) as eluting solvent. The final solutions were then passed through 0.22 micron biological filters for stability and biodistribution studies. Radiolabeling of the immunoconjugates with ^{90}Y and quality control of the resulting radioimmunoconjugate were carried out by the same method which was described for the preparation and quality control of ^{111}In-DOTA-rituximab.

Determination of the Immunoreactivity of radioimmunoconjugates

The immunoreactivity of radioimmunoconjugates were determined by the use of the cell-binding assay on Raji cell line, using 5 sequential dilutions of 10^6-10^7cells in exponential growth (microscopic determination generally indicated >90% viability). A known amount (6 ng) of antibody labeled with 2.54 MBq of ^{111}In and ^{90}Y, was incubated with cells in 200 µl of phosphate-buffered saline (0.15 molar NaCl and 0.01 molar phosphate buffer, pH = 7.0) containing 5% fetal calf serum and NaN_3

(0.02% w/v) for 2 h at 37°C. Nonspecific binding, generally less than 3%, was assessed by competition with 100 μg of unlabeled antibody and results were used for determination of specific binding which were analyzed at maximal observed binding on 10^7 cells by extrapolating to infinite antigen excess according to the reported method [28]. The Student T-test for paired samples was used for statistical comparison of results.

Determination of the stability of radiolabeled DOTA-rituximab against EDTA

A 0.1 ml aliquot of the radiolabeled product with approximate number of 7 molecules of DOTA per rituximab molecule was mixed with 0.1 ml of ethylenediaminetetraacetic acid (30 mM, pH = 7.4) and allowed to incubate for 4 h at room temperature. The radiochemical purity of incubated solution was evaluated by radio-TLC [15].

Determination of the stability of radiolabeled DOTA-rituximab in the presence of human serum

^{111}In- and ^{90}Y-DOTA-rituximab mixtures were incubated in freshly prepared human serum for 12 h at 37°C. Radiolabeling stability was assessed by size exclusion chromatography on a Sepharose column (1 × 30 cm) and using phosphate buffer solution as eluent at a flow rate of 0.5 ml/min. To obtain elution chromatogram, the incubated mixture was applied on the column and 1 ml fractions were collected and their radioactivities were determined. To calibrate the column, the control samples including free ^{111}In and ^{90}Y, radiolabeled human serum albumin and radiolabeled DOTA-rituximab were separately applied to the column for retention volume determination [15,16].

Radiolabeling efficiency of the lyophilized (Kit) DOTA-rituximab conjugates

The radiolabeling efficiency of the lyophilized DOTA-rituximab immunoconjugate (kit) was investigated by monthly radiolabeling with ^{111}In and ^{90}Y and ITLC analysis [15].

Determination of the stability of the lyophilized (kit) radioimmunoconjugates

For evaluation of the stability of radiolabeled DOTA-rituximab, the radiochemical purities of samples of the final solution after storage at 4°C for 4 days and at 25°C for 24 h were determined by radio-TLC analysis [15]. Integrity of radiolabeled DOTA-rituximab was checked by reducing SDS-polyacrylamide gel electrophoresis [26].

Determination of biodistribution of ^{111}In-DOTA-rituximab and ^{90}Y-DOTA-rituximab in rats

Male rates weighing 250-300 g were randomly divided into four groups. The first and second groups were administrated intravenously 0.3 mCi/kg aliquots of ^{111}In-Rituximab and ^{90}Y-rituximab solutions, respectively. The third and fourth groups were administered intravenously 250 mg/m^2 of unlabeled rituximab, 2 hours before injection 0.3 mci/kg aliquots of ^{111}In-Rituximab and ^{90}Y-rituximab, to block CD-20 positive binding sites on the B-cells in the circulation and spleen [9]. The animals were sacrificed by ether asphyxiation at the exact time intervals, and the distribution of radioactivity, represented as percent of injected dose per gram (%ID/g), was determined by measurement of radioactivity of samples from different organs using a beta-scintillator detector for ^{90}Y samples and an HPGe detector for counting the area under the curve of the 171 keV peak for ^{111}In [15,16].

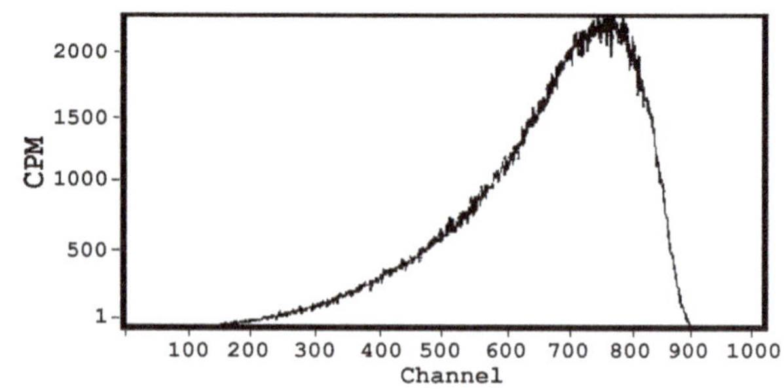

Figure 1 Beta spectrum for ^{90}Y eluted from the ^{90}Sr/^{90}Y generator sample.

Results

Preparation and quality control of radionuclides

^{111}In as $^{111}InCl_3$ solution with a specific activity of higher than1.55 GBq/μg indium at time of calibration was obtained by a non-carrier-added method. Quality control of the radionuclidic [15] showed the presence of 171 and 245 keV gamma energies, originating from ^{111}In

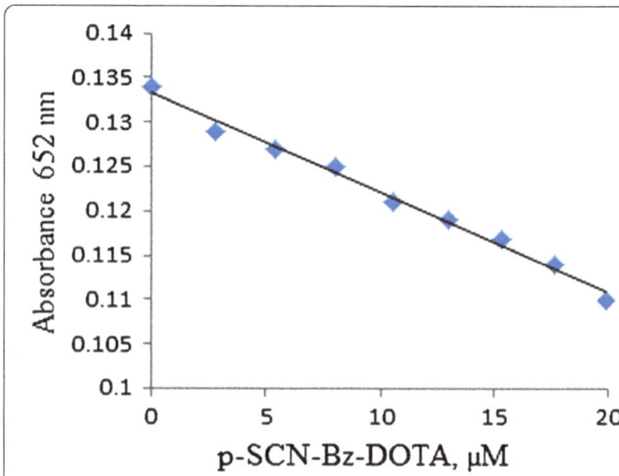

Figure 2 The relationship between the absorbance of the complex and the molarities of p-SCN-Bz-DOTA at 652 nm.

Table 1 The approximate number of DOTA molecules per rituximab molecule, radiolabeling yields, specific activity and radioimmunoreactivity of the prepared immunoconjugates and radioimmunoconjugates

Rituximab: DOTA molar ratio	Approximate number of DOTA per rituximab	Radiolabeling yield for ^{111}In (%)[a]	Radiolabeling yield for ^{90}Y (%)[a]	Specific activity (MBq/mg)[b]	
				^{111}In	^{90}Y
1:5	4	55.3	49.5	358	312
1:15	7	84	78	463	431
1:25	9	92	84	514	455

[a]Labeling conditions; 0.3 mg of immunoconjugate, 170 MBq of radioisotope, ammonium acetate buffer pH = 5.5, 37°C.
[b]Specific activity is calculated based on measured antibody concentration (UV) and radioactivity (dose calibrator).

and a purity of higher than %99. The concentrations of cadmium (from target material) and copper (from target support) were 0.1 ppm which was below the internationally accepted levels and the radiochemical purity of ^{111}In-InCl$_3$ was higher than %98.

^{90}Y was obtained from the natural decay of its parent, ^{90}Sr ($t_{1/2}$, 29 y) by an in house designed ^{90}Sr/^{90}Y generator which was developed for the research purpose. ^{90}Sr was the only radionuclide impurity resulting from the production process and in all the yttrium (^{90}Y) chloride solutions eluted from the generator the ^{90}Sr/^{90}Y ratio was $\leq 10^{-5}$. Figure 1 shows beta spectrum for Y-90 eluted from the ^{90}Sr/^{90}Y generator [24].

Determination of the number of DOTA molecules per one rituximab molecule in DOTA-rituximab conjugates

Figure 2 shows dependency of absorbance of arsenaso yttrium (III) complex at 652 nm on molarities of p-SCN-Bz-DOTA which was determined by arsenazo spectrophotometric method [25]. The solid line represents linear relationship between the absorbance, A_{652nm} and the concentration of 0–20 μM of p-SCN-Bz-DOTA. The approximate numbers of chelating group per rituximab molecule for immunoconjugates which were obtained by using different molar ratios of reactants are presented in Table 1.

Radiolabeling and quality control of the immunoconjugates

The yields for radiolabeling of immunoconjugates are presented in Table 1. In radio-TLC experiments, the best eluent system for free ^{90}Y and ^{111}In detection was 10 mM DTPA aqueous solution (R_f of 0.8). Due to the size and charge of the protein (≈150,000 D), radiolabeled DOTA-rituximab remained at the sample origin but radiolabeled DOTA showed high R_f values. Figure 3 shows the radiochromatograms of free ^{90}Y and ^{90}Y-rituximab. Free ^{111}In and ^{111}In-rituximab pair showed similar radiochromatograms.

Figure 4 shows HPLC chromatograms of free ^{111}In, ^{111}In-*P*-SCN-Bz-DOTA and ^{111}In-rituximab. Both free indium and radiolabeled DOTA eluted rapidly but ^{111}In-DOTA-rituximab was eluted at 14.8 min. ^{90}Y, ^{90}Y-*P*-SCN-Bz-DOTA and ^{90}Y-DOTA-rituximab showed similar radiochromatograms.

Results for the immunoreactivity of radioimmunoconjugates

The average immunoreactivity for radioimmunoconjugates with approximate DOTA/rituximab ratios of 4, 7 and 9 were %91.4, %72.8 and %47.3, respectively.

Results for the stability of radioimmunoconjugate against EDTA and human serum

Table 2 represents radiochemical stability of radioimmunoconjugates which were checked by radio-TLC analysis at 4°C after 4 days and at 25°C after 24 h. There was a decrease of about 1-2% in radiochemical purity of radioimmunoconjugates in the presence of EDTA, indicating of their stabilities [15].

^{111}In- and ^{90}Y-DOTA-rituximab were also stable in the presence of the fresh human serum. Analysis of

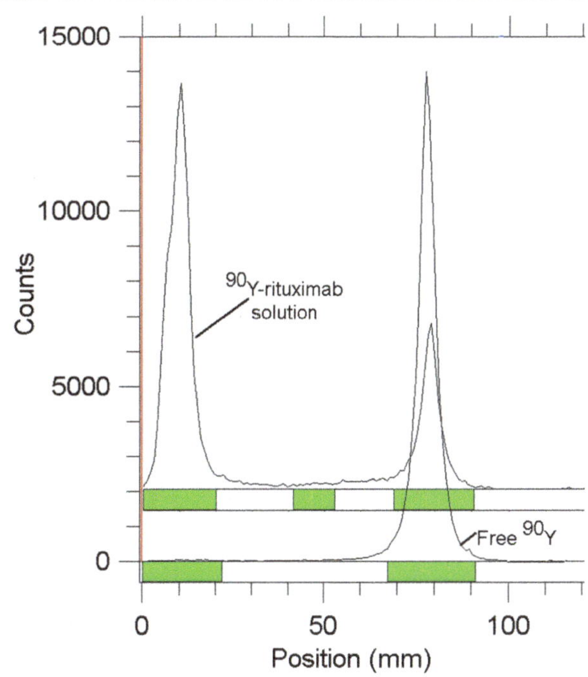

Figure 3 Radio-TLC chromatograms of ^{90}YCl$_3$ solution and ^{90}Y-DOTA-rituximab solution.

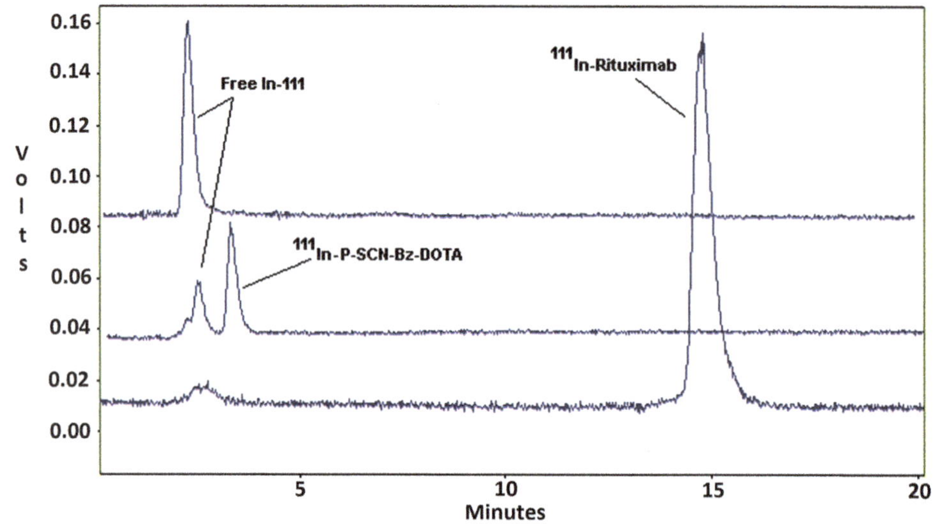

Figure 4 HPLC chromatograms of free ^{111}In, ^{111}In-DOTA and ^{111}In-rituximab.

aliquots of the samples after 24 h incubation by size exclusion chromatography showed that %96-98 of the radioactivity was associated with the radiolabeled DOTA-rituximab [13,14].

As it is shown in Figure 5, the reducing SDS-PAGE patterns for rituximab, DOTA-rituximab and ^{90}Y-DOTA-rituximab immunoconjugates were similar. Interestingly, the reducing SDS-PAGE results compared with a result for a commercially available rituximab sample showed no clear indication for antibody degradation. Similar results were obtained for monthly integrity tests on stored DOTA-rituximab immunoconjugate kits. The efficiencies of indium-111 radiolabeling of DOTA-rituximab kit (DOTA/antibody ratio = 7), measured monthly for six months, were 85.2 ± 3.1, 84.3 ± 1.7, 86.4 ± 2.8, 83.7 ± 3.4, 85.8 ± 1.9 and 84.8 ± 3.3, respectively. Reliable efficiencies also were observed for radioimmunoconjugate obtained by radiolabeling of DOTA-rituximab kit (DOTA/antibody ratio = 7) with ^{90}yttrium.

Table 2 In vitro stability of ^{111}In-DOTA-rituximab

Incubation time (h)	Radiochemical purity (%)[a]	
	25°C	4°C
0	96.4 ± 1.7	96.4 ± 1.7
6	96.1 ± 2.1	96.3 ± 1.4
12	95.7 ± 2.3	94.5 ± 2.7
24	96.6 ± 1.2	95.9 ± 1.4
48	ND[b]	94.8 ± 2.6
72	ND	95.7 ± 1.5
96	ND	96.3 ± 1.3

[a]For each time point, n = 3.
[b]Not Determined.

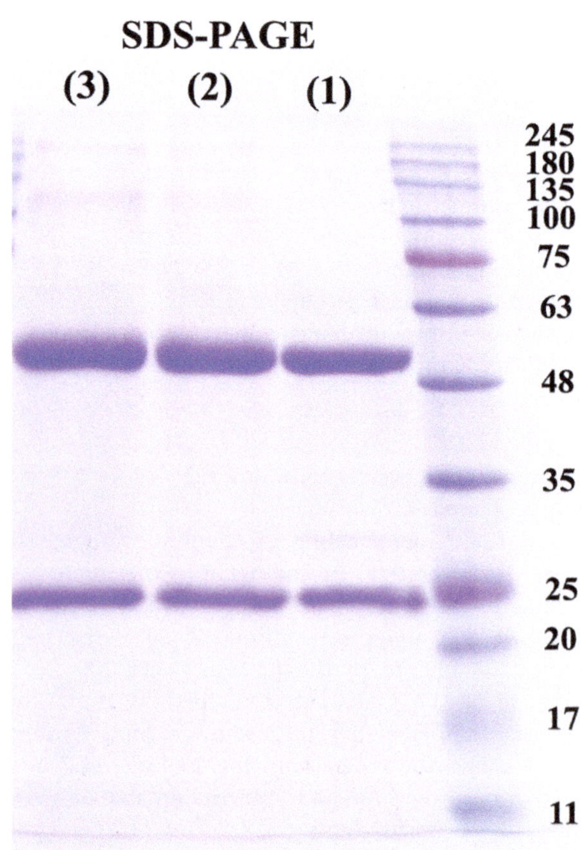

Figure 5 Reducing SDS-PAGE lane patterns for rituximab (1), DOTA-rituximab conjugate (2) and ^{90}Y-DOTA-rituximab conjugate (3).

Results for the biodistribution study

Figure 6 shows the biodistribution profiles of ^{111}In-DOTA-rituximab and ^{90}Y-DOTA-rituximab in male rats (first and second groups) which were determined by measurement of the radioactivities of the weighted samples of rat organs. Both groups showed similar biodistribution profiles. Over time, the liver and spleen uptakes were increased by reduction in the radioactivity of blood circulation. In the case of pre-injection of 250 mg/m^2 of unlabeled rituximab (third and fourth groups), a faster clearance of radioactivity from blood circulation in comparison with first and second groups was observed. Figure 7 shows the biodistribution of ^{111}In-DOTA-rituximab and ^{90}Y-DOTA-rituximab after pre-injection of unlabeled rituximab. In these two groups, also biodistribution profiles were approximately similar. Lungs uptakes in groups 3 and 4 were lower compared to groups 1 and 2. Brain and bone showed very low uptake in all groups.

Discussion

In this study preparation of a lyophilized (kit) formulation for radiolabeling of DOTA-rituximab with ^{90}Y for radioimmunotherapy of B cells lymphoma and with ^{111}In for radioimmunoscintigraphy as well as estimation of administered dose of ^{90}Y-DOTA-rituximab was investigated. ^{111} In was prepared by ^{112}Cd (p,2n)^{111}In nuclear reaction and ^{90}Y was prepared by^{90}Sr/^{90}Y generator which was developed locally for research purpose.

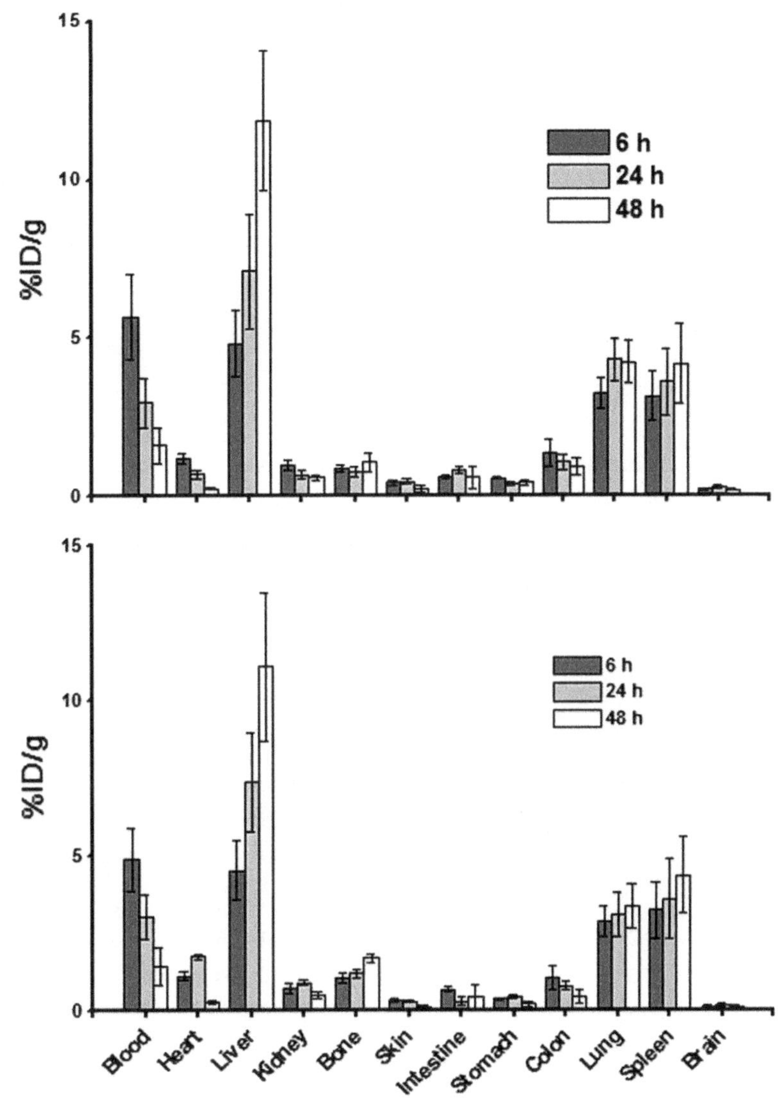

Figure 6 Percentage of injected dose per gram (%ID/g) of ^{111}In-DOTA-Rituximab (up) and ^{90}Y-DOTA-rituximab (down) with approximate DOTA/rituximab molar ratio of 7 in rat organs.

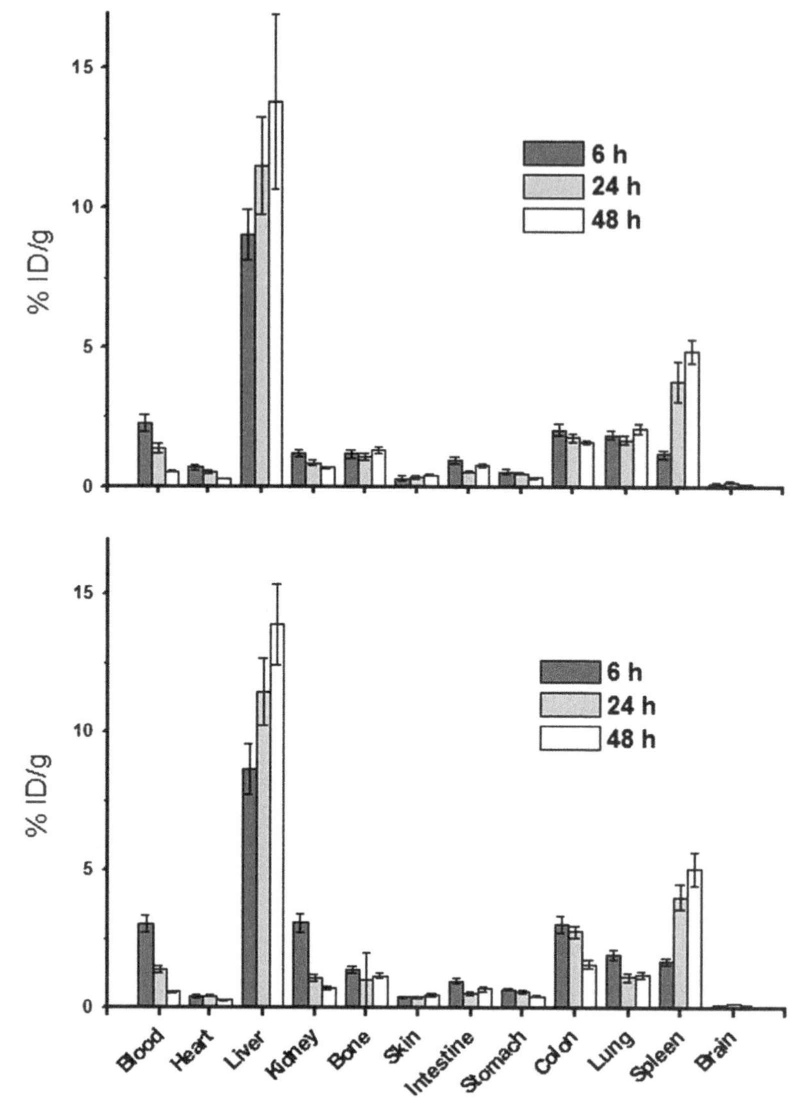

Figure 7 Percentage of injected dose per gram (ID/g%) of ^{90}Y-DOTA-rituximab (up) and ^{111}In-DOTA-rituximab (down) with approximate DOTA/rituximab molar ratio of 7 in rat organs in rat organs, 250 mg/m^2 of unlabeled rituximab was injected 2 h before injection of radioimmunoconjugates.

DOTA-rituximab immunoconjugates with approximate number of 4, 7 and 9 molecules of DOTA per one rituximab molecule were obtained by incubation of excess 5, 15 and 25 folds of p-SCN-benzyl-DOTA with rituximab using 0.2 M sodium carbonate buffer of pH = 9.5. DOTA-rituximab conjugates were successfully radiolabeled with ^{111}In and ^{90}Y, and the radiolabeling yields and efficiencies of radioimmunoconjugates which increased by increase in of DOTA/antibody molar ratios are reported in Table 1.

The immunoreactivity of radioimmunoconjugates compared to commercially available rituximab determined by Lindmo method [28] on Raji cells decreased by increase in DOTA/rituximab molar ratios and the average immunoreactivity for approximate molar ratios of 4, 7 and 9 were %91.4, %72.8 and %47.3, respectively. These findings suggest that increase in molar ratio of DOTA/antibody results to nonspecific conjugation of DOTA to antibody from antigen binding sites [29].

Due to the importance of both immunoreactivity and specific activity of radioimmunoconjugate and their oppositional behavior toward increasing the number of DOTA molecules per one antibody molecule, the immunoconjugate with approximate DOTA/antibody ratio of 7, with moderate immunoreactivity and specific activity, was selected for stability and bio-distribution studies. The selected radioimmunoconjugate showed stability when it was determined after 24 h at room temperature, after 96 h at 4°C, and after six months as lyophilized formulation. The selected radioimmunoconjugate was also stable to either EDTA or serum challenge for the duration of either experiment.

In agreement with results of studies on biodistribution of other labeled antibodies such as ^{90}Y- ibritumomab, ^{131}I-tositumomab and ^{177}Lu-Anti CD-20 [9,11,17,30], in this study after administration of ^{111}In-DOTA-rituximab and ^{90}Y-DOTA-rituximab with approximate DOTA/rituximab molar ratio of 7 in male rats the activity of blood circulation declined slowly and the activity of liver, spleen and other reticulloendothelial organs increased gradually. In the cases that rats were pre-treated with unlabeled rituximab the clearance of the radioactivity from the blood circulation was faster and the initial uptake of the activity in spleen was lower which could be attributed to blockade of CD-20 positive binding sites on B-cells in blood circulation and spleen [9]. The selected radioimmunoconjugate of this study also similar to ^{90}Y-ibritumomab did not have any significant brain uptake and compared to ^{90}Y-DTPA-rituximab of our previous investigation [14] showed significantly lower lung accumulation and ^{90}Y deposition in the bone which may be explained by possible cross-linking or cyclization of antibody with cyclic DTPA dianhydride [31] and lower stability of DTPA conjugates compared with DOTA conjugates.

Conclusion

Results of this study showed that radiolabeling of the lyophilized formulation (kit) of DOTA-rituximab having approximate DOTA/rituximab molar ratio of 7 with ^{90}Y and ^{90}In results in radioimmunoconjugates with moderate radioimmunoreactivity, and good stability and biodistribution profile. These findings suggest that further investigations may result in a kit formulation which could be easily radiolabeled with ^{111}In and ^{90}Y and to be used for radioimmunotherapy and radioscintigraphy of B cells lymphoma in Iran.

Abbreviations

DOTA: 1,4,7,10-tetraazacyclododecane-1,4,7,10-tetraacetic acid; p-SCN-Bz-DOTA: p-benzyl isothiocyanate-1,4,7,10-tetraazacyclododecane-1,4,7,10-tetraacetic acid; NHL: Non-Hodgkin's lymphoma; TLC: Thin layer chromatography; HPLC: High pressure liquid chromatography; SDS-PAGE: Sodium dodecyl sulfate-polyacrylamide gel electrophoresis.

Competing interests

The authors declare that they have no competing interests.

Authors' contributions

NG: Study design, preparing and radiolabeling of immunoconjugate, biodistribution studies and preparing of the manuscript. ARJ: Collaboration in study design, preparing of ^{111}In and the manuscript. AK: Collaboration in study design and preparing of the manuscript. FJD: Participation in radiolabeling of immunoconjugates. KY: Participation in the immunoreactivity studies. OS: Participation in the immunoreactivity studies. ARK: Participation in the preparation of yttrium-90. MA: Collaboration in study design, Participation in the preparation of the manuscript. All authors read and approved the final manuscript.

Acknowledgements

The authors wish to thank Dr. Mirzai for participating in the ^{111}In preparation and Mr. Mojarrabie Tabrizi and Mr. Salimi for participating in the ^{90}Y preparation and measurements and Mr. S. Daneshvari for participatation in the conducting animal studies and finally Mr. Naserian for participating in the integrity tests.

Author details

[1]Department of Radiopharmacy, Faculty of Pharmacy, Tehran University of Medical Sciences, P.O. Box: 14155-6451, Tehran, Iran. [2]Radiation Application Research School, Nuclear Science and Technology Research Institute, P.O. Box: 14395-836, Tehran, Iran. [3]Department of Medicinal Chemistry, Faculty of Pharmacy, Tehran University of Medical Sciences, P.O. Box: 14155-6451, Tehran, Iran. [4]Depatment of Toxicology and Pharmacology, School of Pharmacy, Tehran University of Medical Sciences, P.O. Box: 14176-14411, Tehran, Iran. [5]Research Center for Nuclear Medicine, Tehran University of Medical Sciences, P.O. Box: 14117-13137, Tehran, Iran.

References

1. Dillman RO: **Radioimmunotherapy of B-cell lymphoma with radiolabeled anti-CD20 monoclonal antibodies.** *Clin Exp Med* 2006, **6:**1–12.
2. McLaughlin P, Grillo-López AJ, Link BK, Levy R, Czuczman MS, Williams ME, Heyman MR, Bence-Bruckler I, White CA, Cabanillas F, Jain V, Ho AD, Lister J, Wey K, Shen D, Dallaire BK: **Rituximab chimeric anti-CD20 monoclonal antibody therapy for relapsed indolent lymphoma: half of patients respond to a four-dose treatment program.** *J Clin Oncol* 1998, **16:**2825–2833.
3. Hainsworth JD, Burris HA, Morrissey LH, Litchy S, Scullin DC Jr, Bearden JD 3rd, Richards P, Greco FA: **Rituximab monoclonal antibody as initial systemic therapy for patients with low-grade non-Hodgkin lymphoma.** *Blood* 2000, **95:**3052–3056.
4. Macklis RM, Pohlman B: **Radioimmunotherapy for non-Hodgkin's lymphoma: a review for radiation oncologists.** *Int J Radiat Oncol Biol Phys* 2006, **66:**833–841.
5. Leahy MF, Seymour JF, Hicks RJ, Turner JH: **Multicenter phase II clinical study of iodine-131-rituximab radioimmunotherapy in relapsed or refractory indolent non-Hodgkin's lymphoma.** *J Clin Oncol* 2006, **24:**4418–4425.
6. Skvortsova I, Popper BA, Skvortsov S, Saurer M, Auer T, Moser R, Kamleitner H, Zwierzina H, Lukas P: **Pretreatment with rituximab enhances radiosensitivity of non-Hodgkin's lymphoma cells.** *J Radiat Res* 2005, **46:**241–248.
7. Jacobs SA: **Yttrium ibritumomab tiuxetan in the treatment of non-Hodgkin's lymphoma: current status and future prospects.** *Biologics* 2007, **1:**215–227.
8. Tennvall J, Fischer M, Bischof Delaloye A, Bombardieri E, Bodei L, Giammarile F, Lassmann M, Oyen W, Brans B, Therapy Committee, EANM; Oncology Committee, EANM; Dosimetry Committee, EANM: **EANM procedure guideline for radio-immunotherapy for B-cell lymphoma with ^{90}Y-radiolabeled ibritumomab tiuxetan (Zevalin).** *Eur J Nucl Med Mol Imaging* 2007, **34:**616–622.
9. Chamarthy MR, Williams SC, Moadel RM: **Radioimmunotherapy of non-Hodgkin's lymphoma: from the 'magic bullets' to 'radioactive magic bullets'.** *Yale J Biol Med* 2011, **84:**391–407.
10. DeNardo GL: **Treatment of Non-Hodgkin's Lymphoma (NHL) with radiolabeled antibodies (mAbs).** *Semin Nucl Med* 2005, **35:**202–211.
11. Antonescu C, Bischof Delaloye A, Kosinski M, Monnin P, Schaffland AO, Ketterer N, Grannavel C, Kovacsovics T, Verdun FR, Buchegger F: **Repeated injections of 131I-rituximab show patient-specific stable biodistribution and tissue kinetics.** *Eur J Nucl Med Mol Imaging* 2005, **32:**943–951.
12. Kaminski MS, Radford JA, Gregory SA, Leonard JP, Knox SJ, Kroll S, Wahl RL: **Re-treatment with I-131 tositumomab in patients with non-Hodgkin's lymphoma who had previously responded to I-131 tositumomab.** *J Clin Oncol* 2005, **23:**7985–7993.
13. Vaes M, Bron D, Vugts DJ, Paesmans M, Meuleman N, Ghanem GE, Guiot T, Vanderlinden B, Thielemans K, Van Dongen G, Flamen P, Muylle K: **Safety and efficacy of radioimmunotherapy with ^{90}Yttrium-rituximab in patients with relapsed CD20+ B cell lymphoma: a feasibility study.** *J Cancer Sci Ther* 2012, **4:**394–400.

14. Gholipour N, Vakili A, Radfar E, Jalilian AR, Bahrami-Samani A, Shirvani-Arani S, Ghannadi-Maragheh M: **Optimization of 90 Y-antiCD20 preparation for radioimmunotherapy.** *J Can Res Ther* 2013, **9:**199–204.
15. Jalilian AR, Sardari D, Kia L, Rowshanfarzad P, Garousi J, Akhlaghi M, Shanehsazzadeh S, Mirzaii M: **Preparation, quality control and biodistribution studies of two [^{111}In]-Rituximab immunoconjugates.** *Sci Pharm* 2008, **76:**151–170.
16. Bahrami-Samani A, Ghannadi-Maragheh M, Jalilian AR, Yousefnia H, Garousi J, Moradkhani S: **Development of ^{153}Sm-DTPA-rituximab for radioimmunotherapy.** *Nukleonika* 2009, **54:**271–277.
17. Audicio PF, Castellano G, Tassano MR, Rezzano ME, Fernandez M, Riva E, Robles A, Cabral P, Balter H, Oliver P: **[^{177}Lu]DOTA-anti-CD20: labeling and pre-clinical studies.** *Appl Radiat Isot* 2011, **69:**924–928.
18. Forrer F, Chen J, Fani M, Powell P, Lohri A, Müller-Brand J, Moldenhauer G, Maecke HR: **In vitro characterization of (177)Lu-radiolabeled chimeric anti-CD20 monoclonal antibody and a preliminary dosimetry study.** *Eur J Nucl Med Mol Imaging* 2009, **36:**1443–1452.
19. Yousefnia H, Radfar E, Jalilian AR, Bahrami-Samani A, Shirvani-Arani S, Arbabi A, Ghannadi-Maragheh M: **Development of ^{177}Lu-DOTA-anti-CD20 for radioimmunotherapy.** *J Radioanal Nucl Chem* 2011, **287:**199–209.
20. Jalilian AR, Mirsadeghi L, Yari-kamrani Y, Rowshanfarzad P, Kamali-dehghan M, Sabet M: **Development of [^{64}Cu]-DOTA-anti-CD20 for targeted therapy.** *J Radioanal Nucl Chem* 2007, **274:**563–568.
21. De León-Rodríguez LM, Kovacs Z: **The synthesis and chelation chemistry of DOTA-peptide conjugates.** *Bioconjug Chem* 2008, **19:**391–402.
22. Chappell LL, Ma D, Milenic DE, Garmestani K, Venditto V, Beitzel MP: **Synthesis and evaluation of novel bifunctional chelating agents based on 1,4,7,10-tetraazacyclododecane-N, N′, N″, N‴-tetraacetic acid for radiolabeling proteins.** *Nucl Med Biol* 2003, **30:**581–595.
23. Sadeghpour H, Jalilian AR, Akhlaghi M, Kamali-dehghan M, Mirzaii M: **Preparation and biodistribution of [^{111}In]- rHu Epo for erythropoietin receptor imaging.** *J Radioanal Nucl Chem* 2008, **278:**117–122.
24. Vakili A, Jalilian AR, Yavari K, Shirvani-Arani S, Khanchi AR, Bahrami-Samani A, Salimi B, Khorrami-Moghadam AR: **Preparation and quality control and biodistribution studies of [^{90}Y]-DOTA-cetuximab for radioimmunotherapy.** *J Radioanal Nucl Chem* 2013, **296:**1287–1294.
25. Dadachova E, Chappell LL, Brechbiel MW: **Spectrophotometric method for determination of bifunctional macrocyclic ligands in macrocyclic ligand-protein conjugates.** *Nucl Med Biol* 1999, **26:**977–982.
26. Laemmli UK: **Cleavage of structural proteins during the assembly of the head of bacteriophage T4.** *Nature* 1970, **227:**680–685.
27. Jalilian AR, Akhlaghi M: **HPLC analysis of radiogallium labeled proteins using a two solvent system.** *J Liq Chromatogr Related Technol* 2013, **36:**731–739.
28. Lindmo T, Boven E, Cuttitta F, Fedorko J, Bunn PA Jr: **Determination of the immunoreactive fraction of radiolabeled monoclonal antibodies by linear extrapolation to binding at infinite antigen excess.** *J Immunol Methods* 1984, **72:**77–89.
29. Flieger D, Renoth S, Beier I, Sauerbruch T, Schmidt-Wolf I: **Mechanism of cytotoxicity induced by chimeric mouse human monoclonal antibody IDEC-C2B8 in CD20-expressing lymphoma cell lines.** *Cell Immunol* 2000, **204:**55–63.
30. Perk LR, Visser OJ, Stigter-van Walsum M, Vosjan MJ, Visser GW, Zijlstra JM, Huijgens PC, van Dongen GA: **Preparation and evaluation of (89)Zr-Zevalin for monitoring of (90)Y-Zevalin biodistribution with positron emission tomography.** *Eur J Nucl Med Mol Imaging* 2006, **33:**1337–1345.
31. Liu S: **Bifunctional coupling agents for radiolabeling of biomolecules and target-specific delivery of metallic radionuclides.** *Adv Drug Delivery Rev* 2008, **60:**1347–1370.

The effect of adipose derived stromal cells on oxidative stress level, lung emphysema and white blood cells of guinea pigs model of chronic obstructive pulmonary disease

Ahmad Ghorbani[2], Azadeh Feizpour[1], Milad Hashemzahi[1], Lila Gholami[1], Mahmoud Hosseini[3], Mohammad Soukhtanloo[4], Farzaneh Vafaee Bagheri[1], Esmaeil Khodaei[1], Nema Mohammadian Roshan[5] and Mohammad Hossein Boskabady[1*]

Abstract

Background: Chronic obstructive pulmonary disease (COPD) is a worldwide epidemic disease and a major cause of death and disability. The present study aimed to elucidate pharmacological effects of adipose derived stromal cells (ASCs) on pathological and biochemical factors in a guinea pig model of COPD. Guinea pigs were randomized into 5 groups including: Control, COPD, COPD + intratracheal delivery of PBS as a vehicle (COPD-PBS), COPD + intratracheal delivery of ASCs (COPD-ITASC) and COPD + intravenous injection of ASCs (COPD-IVASC). COPD was induced by exposing animals to cigarette smoke for 3 months. Cell therapy was performed immediately after the end of animal exposure to cigarette smoke and 14 days after that, white blood cells, oxidative stress indices and pathological changes of the lung were measured.

Results: Compared with control group, emphysema was clearly observed in the COPD and COPD-PBS groups ($p < 0.001$). Lung histopathologic changes of COPD-ITASC and COPD-IVASC groups showed non-significant improvement compared to COPD-PBS group. The COPD-ITASC group showed a significant increase in total WBC compared to COPD-PBS group but there was not a significant increase in this regard in COPD-IVASC group. The differential WBC showed no significant change in number of different types of leukocytes. The serum level of malondialdehyde (MDA) significantly decreased but thiol groups of broncho-alveolar lavage fluid (BALF) increased in both cell treated groups ($p < 0.05$ for all cases). Weight of animals decreased during smoke exposure and improved after PBS or cell therapy. However, no significant change was observed between the groups receiving PBS and the ones receiving ASCs.

Conclusion: Cell therapy with ASCs can help in reducing oxidative damage during smoking which may collectively hold promise in attenuation of the severity of COPD although the lung structural changes couldn't be ameliorated with these pharmacological therapeutic methods.

Keywords: COPD, Stromal cells, Malondialdehyde, Thiol, Emphysema, WBC, Guinea pigs

* Correspondence: boskabadymh@mums.ac.ir
[1]Neurogenic Inflammation Research Centre and Department of Physiology, School of Medicine, Mashhad University of Medical Sciences, Mashhad 9177948564, Iran
Full list of author information is available at the end of the article

Background

Chronic obstructive pulmonary disease (COPD) is a progressive lung disease. Its three most common pathological changes are chronic bronchitis, chronic obstructive bronchiolitis and emphysematous destruction of the lung parenchyma [1]. Emphysema, the main histopathologic feature of COPD, leads to a decrease in elastic recoil and therefore continuation of decrease in small airway patency during expiration causing a not fully reversible airflow limitation and increase in the lung residual volume [2]. This airway obstruction may contribute to respiratory failure and weight loss leading to cachexia [3] and eventually death. Thus, finding a fundamental and curative approach for this disease is of vital importance.

The other characteristic feature of COPD, as well as other respiratory diseases, is the oxidant-antioxidant imbalances. This imbalance is reported to be developed by the increased lipid peroxidation which is known as an index of oxidative stress and a reduction of antioxidant capacity. Decrease in plasma protein sulfhydryl concentrations in COPD patients is well documented [4]. There are also other evidences suggesting the role of reactive oxygen species in lung inflammation of COPD patients which can be a direct effect or through lipid peroxidation products [5]. Therefore, increasing the antioxidant capacity is one of the main concerns in the pharmacological treatment of COPD.

For treatment of such respiratory diseases as asthma, bronchodilating agents are helpful but the airflow limitation and accelerated loss of lung function caused by COPD cannot be reversed by this type of treatments [4,6]. The existing treatments for COPD only change the symptoms, quality of life and exacerbation frequency, while a fundamental or effective therapy is yet to be achieved. Recent advances in regenerative medicine and cell therapy have led to successful attempts to restore damaged tissues. Therefore, cell-based therapy might be a more promising therapeutic option for COPD.

Adipose tissue derived stromal cells (ASCs) and mesenchymal stem cells (MSCs), derived from ASCs or bone marrow, are readily available sources of stromal/stem cells required for cell therapy [5-10]. Many researchers such as Schweitzer et al. [5], Ahmed et al. [6], Gupta et al. [7], Baber et al. [8], Shigemura et al. [9] and Ishiazwa et al. [10] have contributed to cell therapy of lung diseases by local or systemic administration of ASCs/MSCs to the animal model of different lung injuries induced by elastase, monocrotaline or endotoxin and have observed promising pharmacological effects.

The MSCs are reported to interfere with oxidative stress and induce lung parenchymal regeneration [5,11]. Mesenchymal stem cells can ameliorate the pulmonary damages by two mechanisms. One is protecting the vascular bed endothelial cells from apoptosis by paracrine effects of several growth factors such as Hepatocyte growth factor (HGF) and Vascular endothelial growth factor (VEGF). The other mechanism is acquiring the phenotype or markers of airway or alveolar epithelial cells and vascular endothelial cells. In addition, it has been shown that transplantation of ASCs into elastase-treated emphysema models augments alveolar and vascular regeneration by enhancement of epithelial cell proliferation, inhibition of alveolar cell apoptosis and promotion of angiogenesis in lung vasculature [9,12]. Lung emphysematous destruction induced by COPD is well studied by different studies. However, MSCs ameliorative effect on COPD in guinea pigs, the main model of respiratory diseases, induced by cigarette smoking, the main cause of COPD in human was not investigated. On the other hand, some researches documented a pharmacological protective effect on the epithelial cells during oxidative damage by involvement of such cytokines as insulin-like growth factor (IGF) [7,8], HGF [9], and IL-6 [13] which raise the question if the MSCs may exert their therapeutic effect by an antioxidant function through secreting cytokines. There are few studies on the topic of antioxidant function of stem cells such as the one documenting that MSC protection of the kidneys against ischemia/reperfusion injury may be at least in part due to their antioxidant effects [14]. Another study also confirms an antioxidant along with a neuroprotective function for MSCs which have been previously approved in an *in vitro* study on neuroblastoma cells exposed to an oxidative stress [15]. However, such studies aren't formerly performed on the oxidative damage induced in the lungs of COPD model guinea pigs.

Considering the pathological changes occurring during COPD, at least three targets exist for intervention including inflammation, emphysematous destruction, and oxidative stress [5,14,15] among which the two latter ones are the focus of this study.

As far as we know, there is no study to investigate the ameliorative effect of ASCs on cigarette smoking-induced lung injury in guinea pigs, the main animal model of COPD. Therefore, the present study aimed to elucidate the pharmacological effects of local and systemic injection of ASCs on oxidative factors, lung pathology and white blood cells in cigarette smoke induced COPD in guinea pigs.

Methods

Animals and groups

Thirty one guinea pigs (600–800 g) were kept in a temperature controlled room while a 12-h on/12-h off light cycle was maintained. All animal experiments were carried out according to the ethical guidelines of the animal care of the Mashhad University of Medical Sciences. They were categorized to 5 groups as follows:

a) Control group, the animals were exposed to ambient air rather than smoke (n = 6).
b) COPD group, the animals were exposed to cigarette smoke for 3 consecutive months (n = 9).
c) COPD + PBS, the animals were exposed to cigarette smoke and then received PBS as vehicle via intratracheal injection (n = 5).
d) COPD + intratracheal delivery of ASCs (COPD-ITASC), the animals were exposed to cigarette smoke and then received 10^6 ASCs via intratracheal injection (n = 6).
e) COPD + intravenous injection of ASCs (COPD-IVASC): the animals were exposed to cigarette smoke and then received 10^6 ASCs via intravenous injection (n = 5).

Biochemical assays and lung pathological examination were done 14 days after treatment with cell or vehicle.

Exposure of animals to cigarette smoke

Exposure of guinea pigs to cigarette smoke was performed according to the method designed by Boskabady and Kiani with some modifications [16]. Briefly, the animals were placed in a special box which was divided into two parts: one held the body of the animal and the other one held its head (dimensions: 15×12×7 cm). Twenty millilitre puffs of cigarette smoke were drawn out of the cigarettes using a syringe and then exhausted at a rate of two puffs per minute into the animals' head chamber (every 30 seconds, one puff of cigarette smoke was dragged into the head chamber). Exposure of animals to each cigarette lasted for 8–9 minutes, with a 10 minutes resting period between two cigarettes. The animals were exposed initially to one cigarette per day and gradually increasing to a maximum of 5 cigarettes per day over a period of 20 days. In short, the animals were exposed to cigarette smoke (Magna: Nicotine = 5, tar = 6) for totally 3 consecutive months, 5 days per week, and 5 cigarettes per day (the cigarettes' filters weren't removed).

Preparation of stromal cells

Adipose tissues were obtained from healthy guinea pigs weighing 600–800 g. They were anesthetized by intra peritoneal injection of ketamine (150 mg/kg) and xylazine (6 mg/kg). Subcutaneous inguinal fat deposits were resected and under laminar hood, the fat tissue was minced into 1–2 mm pieces by means of a sterile scalpel [17]. The tissue pieces were incubated at 37°C for 60 minutes in PBS containing 2 mg/ml collagenase meanwhile being shaken (60 cycles/min) [18,19]. After centrifugation (300 g for 8 minutes), the floated lipid layer was discarded and the stroma-vascular fraction was collected, washed and re-suspended in DMEM medium supplemented with 10% FBS, 100 units/ml penicillin and 100 μg/ml streptomycin [19,20]. The cells were seeded into tissue culture flask and passaged when 60–80% confluent and used at passages three to six.

Differentiation of stromal cell

For differentiation to adipocyte, the stromal cells were seeded in 12-well culture plate and then incubated in DMEM supplemented with 3% FBS, 66 μM biotin, 250 μM IBMX, 1 μM dexamethasone, 34 μM d-panthothenate, 5 μM indomethacin and 0.2 μM insulin. The cells were maintained in differentiation medium for 3 days and then exposed to the adipocyte maintenance medium consisting of DMEM, supplemented with 3% FBS, 66 μM biotin, 1 μM dexamethasone, 34 μM d-panthothenate and 0.2 μM insulin. After additional 9 days of incubation, adipogenesis was confirmed by Oil Red O which stains intracellular triglyceride droplets. For staining, the cells were fixed with 10% formalin and then incubated with Oil Red O solution. Thereafter, the cells were washed three times with distilled water and photographed using inverted microscope [19].

For osteocyte differentiation, the stromal cells were incubated in DMEM supplemented with 10% FBS, 10 μg/ml ascorbic acid, 5 mM β-glycerol phosphate and 0.1 μM dexamethasone. The cells were maintained in the differentiation medium for two weeks and the culture medium was replaced every 3 days [21]. For Alizarin red staining, the cells were fixed with 10% formalin and then incubated with 2% Alizarin red solution. Thereafter, the cells were washed three times with distilled water and photographed using inverted microscope [22].

Stromal cell labeling and tracing

The cells were harvested, suspended in PBS and incubated with 2 μM cell tracker CM DiI (Invitrogen) for 5 min in 37°C and 15 min in 4°C in the absence of light. After 20 min of staining, it was centrifuged at 1500 for 5 min, washed with PBS, centrifuged again and suspended in 0.3 ml PBS. It was finally dragged to a 27 gauge insulin syringe and was prepared for injection to the animals' jugular vein or trachea. After 2 weeks of ASCs administration (either intratracheal or intravenous), the animals were euthanized and 4 μm sections were provided from different regions of their lung. Existence of the CM-DiI labeled stromal cells was detected under fluorescent microscope.

Intratracheal and systemic delivery of stromal cells

The guinea pigs of COPD-ITASC group were anesthetized and after exposing the trachea, 0.3 ml PBS containing 10^6 cells was injected under direct vision to the trachea using a 27 gauge insulin syringe. Viability of injected cells was found to be more than 90% as assessed with trypan blue staining.

In COPD-IVASC group, the animals were anesthetized and the jugular vein was exposed. Then, a volume of 0.3 ml PBS containing 10^6 cells was injected into the vein using a 27 gauge insulin syringe.

Total WBC and differential WBC measurement

Total WBC was counted in duplicate in a hemocytometer (in a Burker chamber) in blood stained with Turk solution (1:10 dilution, consisted of 1 ml of glacial acetic acid, 1 ml of gentiac vialet solution 1% and 100 ml distilled). Differential WBC was determined in blood samples stained with Turk solution and Wright-Giemsa, respectively. Briefly, differential cell counts were done on thin slide, prepared with smearing blood sample, using Wright-Giemsa stain. According to staining and morphological criteria, differential cell analysis was carried out under a light microscope by counting 100 cells, and the percentage of each cell type was calculated.

Biochemical assays

After sacrificing the guinea pigs, broncho-alveolar lavage fluid (BALF) was prepared from the lung by locating a cannula into trachea and lavage of the lungs with 2 mL of saline for 5 times (total: 10 mL). BALF was then centrifuged at 2500 × *g* for 10 min and the supernatant was collected for measurement of thiol groups' concentration.

Total thiol groups were measured using 2,2′-dinitro-5,5′-dithiodibenzoic acid (DTNB) which reacts with the SH groups to produce a yellow colored complex with peak absorbance at 412 nm [23,24]. In summary, 1 mL Tris-EDTA buffer was added to 50 μL of BALF and sample absorbance was read at 412 nm against Tris-EDTA buffer alone (A1). Then, 20 μL of DTNB reagent (10 mM in methanol) was added to the mixture and after 15 min, the sample absorbance was again read (A2). Total thiol concentration was calculated using this equation: Total thiol (mM) = (A2-A1-blank) × 1.07/0.05 × 13.6.

Five ml blood sample was collected gently from the left ventricle and placed in a citrate containing blood collection tube not to be coagulated. The blood was centrifuged and the serum was separated and kept in −70°C for further measurement of MDA concentrations. MDA level, as an index of lipid peroxidation, was measured. MDA reacts with thiobarbituric acid (TBA) as a thiobarbituric acid reactive substance (TBARS) to produce a red colored complex which has peak absorbance at 535 nm. Two mL from reagent of TBA/trichloroacetic acid (TCA)/hydrochloric acid (HCL) was added to 1 mL of serum, and the solution was heated in a water bath for 40 minutes. After cooling, the whole solutions were centrifuged at 1000 g for 10 minutes. The absorbance was measured at 535 nm [25]. The MDA concentration was calculated as follows: C (m) = Absorbance/(1.56 × 10^5).

Lung pathology

After fixation of the lung specimen in formalin and staining with H&E, the tissue sections were evaluated under a light microscope by a pathologist. The pathologic changes in the lung of COPD, COPD-PBS, COPD-ITASC and COPD-IVASC groups were evaluated according to the intensity of emphysema. Three intensities of parenchymal destruction were considered for scoring the emphysema observed in the lungs. Scoring of pathological changes was performed as previously described [16]. For this purpose, the percent of the area containing mild, moderate or severe emphysema was multiplied by the number 1, 2 or 3, respectively and the total score for each section was calculated.

Animals weight measurement

The weight of the animals of all groups was measured at the beginning of the study (week 0) and after 3 months (at the end of exposure period); but in COPD-PBS, COPD-ITASC and COPD-IVASC groups, the weight of animals was also measured after a further 2 weeks (at the end of treatment with PBS or ASC cells).

Statistical analysis

All the data were quoted as mean ± SEM and compared by means of Instat software. The data of COPD animals were compared to the control ones using unpaired "t" test. The same test was used for the comparison between PBS and either COPD + ITASC or COPD + IVASC as well as between COPD + PBS and COPD. In addition, the comparison between the weights of animals at three time points during the procedure was performed using ANOVA. Significance was accepted at $p < 0.05$.

Results

Stromal cell characterization

Figure 1A and C shows the morphology of stromal cells isolated from adipose tissue of guinea pig. The cells were adherent and showed significant expansion in the cultures (Figure 1A). After passage 3, they had a spindled, fibroblast appearance in culture that is consistent with MSCs morphology.

To determine whether the cells have pluripotent capacity, before intratracheal or intravenous injection, a number of them were cultured in differentiating media specific for adipocyte and osteocyte. Oil Red O staining showed the accumulated triglyceride droplets in the cells cytoplasm which confirms adipogenic differentiation capacity of the isolated stromal cells (Figure 1B). In addition, Alizarin Red staining revealed extracellular matrix mineralization which confirms osteogenic differentiation capacity of the stromal cells (Figure 1D).

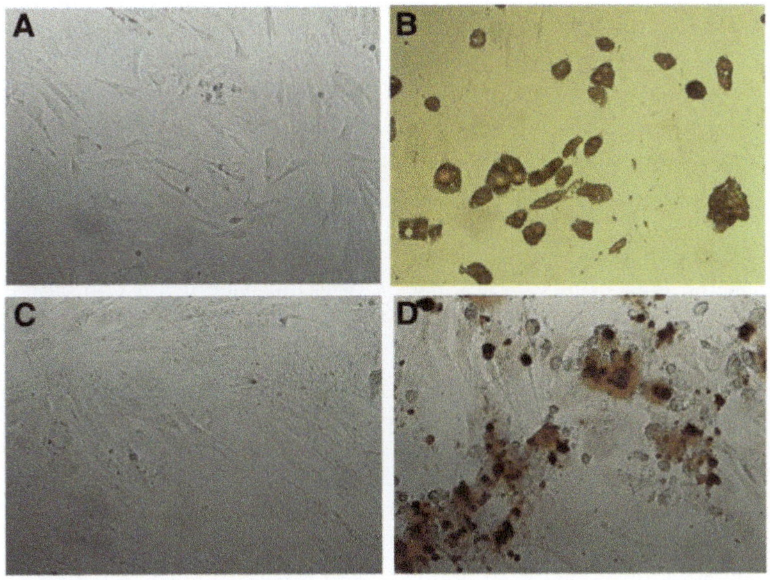

Figure 1 Differentiation of adipose derived stromal cells to adipocyte and osteocyte lineages. The stromal cells were cultured in adipogenic or osteogenic differentiating media for 12 and 14 days, respectively. **A**: Oil Red O staining of cells cultured in control media; **B**: Oil Red O staining of cultured cells in adipogenic differentiating media; **C**: Alizarin Red staining of cells cultured in control media; **D**: Alizarin Red staining of cells cultured in osteogenic differentiating media. Magnification × 100.

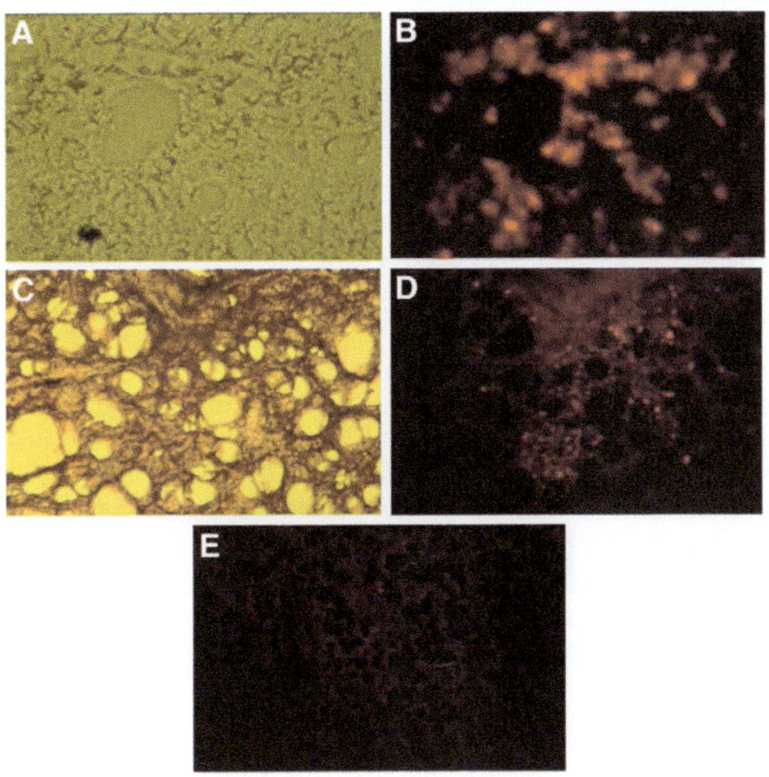

Figure 2 Fluorescence microscopic photographs of lungs after intratracheal delivery of CMDil-labeled stromal cells. **A**: Phase-contrast microscopic image of lung from normal animal harvested 2 days after injection of labeled stromal cells into trachea (Magnification × 200); **B**: The same field under fluorescent microscope. **C**: Phase-contrast microscopic image of formalin fixed lung from COPD animal harvested 14 days after injection of labeled stromal cells into trachea (Magnification × 100); **D**: The same field under fluorescent microscope; **E**: Fluorescence microscopic image of lung from COPD animal harvested 14 days after injection of PBS as vehicle (Magnification × 100).

Stromal cell detection in the lung

To detect stromal cells in airway structures, the CM-DiI labeled cells were injected to trachea. Figure 2 shows fluorescence microscopy of stromal cells after 2 or 14 days of intratracheal delivery. Two days after intratracheal injection, microscopic image of lung from normal guinea pig (guinea pig experiencing no treatment) confirmed the delivery of stromal cells into both large and small airway structures (Figure 2A and B). The CM-DiI-labeled stromal cells were also detected in the lung from COPD guinea pig 14 days after intratracheal administration (Figure 2C and D). There was no fluorescence signal in the lung harvested from COPD animal 14 days after injection of PBS as vehicle (Figure 2E).

To ensure pulmonary delivery of stromal cells after intravenous injection, fluorescence microscopy was also done on lung sections two days after cell injection. The labeled cells were detected in the lung alongside resident cells in airways and alveolar structures (Figure 3A and B). In separate homing experiments, the labeled cells were administered systemically via intravenous injection to a COPD guinea pig. Fourteen days after administration of the cells, fluorescence signals of labeled cells were still detected in the lung (Figure 3C, D and E).

Lung histopathological results

Three consecutive months of exposing animals to the cigarette smoke caused a considerable destruction of alveolar walls and consequently widespread emphysema as H&E stained sections show. The same changes were observed in the COPD-PBS group and there was no significant difference between the emphysema score in COPD-PBS and COPD groups. The change in emphysema score of COPD-ITASC and COPD-IVASC animals was non-significant compared to the COPD-PBS group (Figure 4).

Biochemical results

BALF thiol concentration had a significant decrease in COPD compared with control group ($P < 0.001$). There was also a significant reduction in this factor in COPD-PBS group compared to the COPD animals ($P < 0.05$). The thiol concentration increased in both treated groups with stromal cells, but it was only significant in COPD-IVASC compared to COPD-PBS group ($P < 0.05$), (Figure 5).

Concentration of MDA had a significant increase in the COPD group compared with the control animals ($P < 0.01$) which was not significantly different with COPD-PBS groups (Figure 6). The concentration of MDA

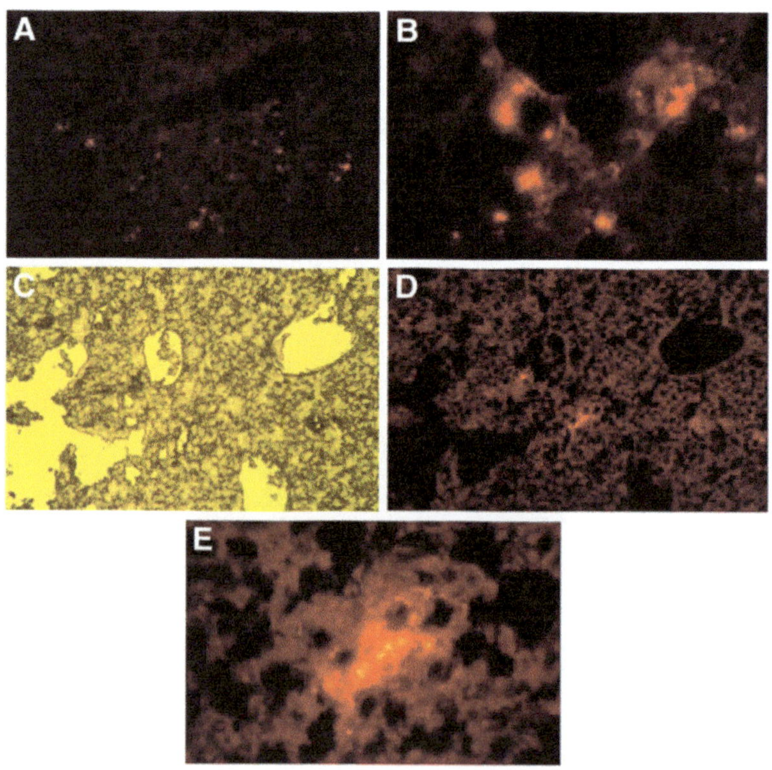

Figure 3 Fluorescence microscopic photographs of lungs after systemic delivery of CMDil-labeled stromal cells. A and **B**: Lung homing of labeled stromal cells two days after injection of cells into jugular vein of normal guinea pig (Magnification: A = ×100, B = ×400); **C**: Phase-contrast microscopic image of formalin fixed lung from COPD animal harvested 14 days after injection of labeled stromal cells into jugular vein (Magnification × 100); **D**: The same field under fluorescent microscope (Magnification × 100); **E**: The same field under fluorescent microscope with magnification of × 400.

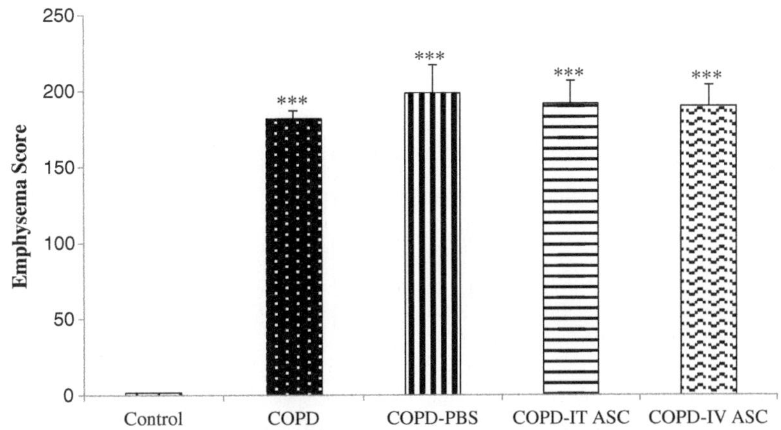

Figure 4 Effect of adipose derived stromal cells (ASCs) therapy on pathological changes of the lung according to the scoring method mentioned in the text. Data are shown as mean ± SEM. ***$P < 0.001$ as compared with control group. The animals in COPD-PBS, COPD-ITASC and COPD-IVASC groups were exposed to cigarette smoke for 3 months and then received PBS, intratracheal injection of ASCs and intravenous injection of ASCs, respectively. For scoring, the percent of the area containing mild, moderate or severe emphysema was multiplied by the number 1, 2 or 3, respectively.

in both treated groups with the stromal cells showed a significant reduction compared to the COPD-PBS animals ($P < 0.05$).

Total and differential WBC counts

There was a significant increase in total WBC in the COPD compared to the control group ($P < 0.01$). No significant difference was observed between the total WBC counts in COPD-PBS and COPD group (Figure 7A). There was a significant increase in this parameter in the COPD-ITASC group compared to COPD-PBS animals but no significant difference was observed between COPD-IVASC and COPD-PBS groups. There was no significant difference in the number of eosinophil, neutrophils, lymphocytes and monocytes between various groups (Figure 7B).

Animals weight changes

There was an increase in the weight of the animals of control group after 3 months of ambient air exposure but all the other groups showed a significant reduction in this parameter after 3 months of cigarette smoking except for COPD-IVASC group in which this increase wasn't significant (Figure 8). After the surgery and injection of stromal cells or PBS, all the three groups showed a significant increase in animals' weight during the two weeks before being euthanized.

Discussion

In many studies pertaining to asthma and COPD, the most widespread small animal species used are the mice or rats while guinea pigs are the most susceptible species and a significant airspace enlargement happens in their

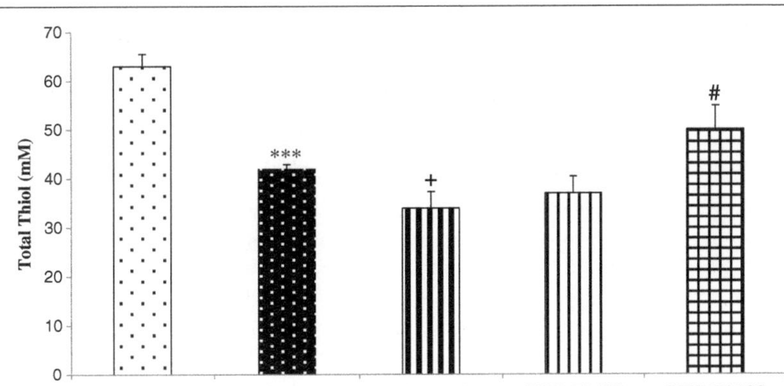

Figure 5 Thiol total concentration in broncho-alveolar lavage fluid in different groups. Data are shown as mean ± SEM. ***$P < 0.001$ as compared with control group. $^{\#}P < 0.05$ as compared with COPD-PBS group. $^{+}P < 0.05$ as compared with COPD group. The animals in COPD-PBS, COPD-ITASC and COPD-IVASC groups were exposed to cigarette smoke for 3 months and then received PBS, intratracheal injection of ASCs and intravenous injection of ASCs, respectively.

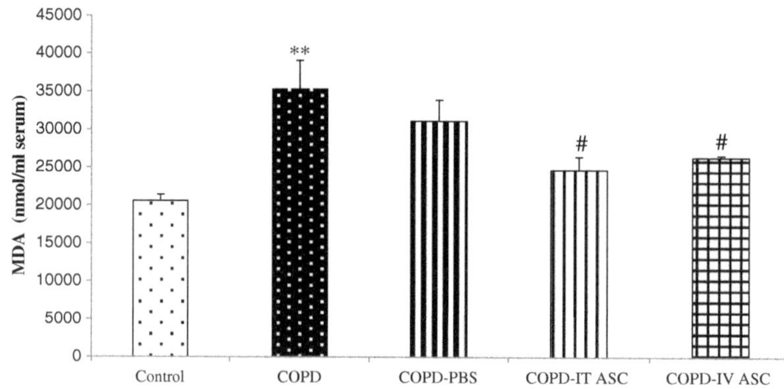

Figure 6 Serum concentration of malondialdehyde (MDA) in different groups. Data are shown as mean ± SEM. $^{**}P < 0.01$ as compared with control; $^{\#}P < 0.05$ as compared with COPD-PBS. The animals in COPD-PBS, COPD-ITASC and COPD-IVASC groups were exposed to cigarette smoke for 3 months and then received PBS, intratracheal injection of ASCs and intravenous injection of ASCs, respectively.

lungs after a few months of cigarette smoke exposure [26]. Besides, the most considerable advantage of guinea pigs, as a respiratory disease model, its airway pharmacology and physiological processes of these animals are similar to human such as the airway autonomic system, allergic reaction and responses to agonists and antagonists. The other side of the coin is that using guinea pigs in animal studies has some disadvantages too, including absence of transgenic animals, a lack of variety in guinea pig strains, and a noticeable axon reflex that is questionable whether it is present in human airways or not [27]. Therefore, despite the easier procedures and lower expenses in working with rats or mice, guinea pig was chosen as an animal model of COPD in the present study.

It is documented that the structural changes considered important in COPD are as follows: destruction of alveolar wall and existence of emphysema, alveolar space enlargement due to emphysema, increase in alveolar septum due to infiltration of leukocytes and penetration of smoke particles, elastolysis and collagen fiber deposition in alveolar septa and pulmonary vessel wall [16]. The major reasons for these changes caused by cigarette smoking are inflammatory responses, oxidative damage and changes in protease-anti protease balance. According to the results of the present study, emphysema was observed in the lungs of the smoke-exposed group of animals, so that the adjacent alveolar spaces were joined to each other due to the parenchymal destructions and air space enlargements were clearly observed. This is consistent with other studies demonstrating physiological and morphological changes induced by cigarette smoke in lung of guinea pigs [16,27,28]. In the present study, treatment of smoke exposed animals by stromal cells showed no significant improvement in the intensity of the smoke-induced emphysema. As all the procedure of familiarizing animals to the new habitat, smoke exposure and cell administrations took several months, it was assumed that higher age of the animals at the end of the study might be interfering with cell therapy. Therefore, the inconvenient histopathology result might be due to the lack of regenerative mechanisms or decreased numbers of progenitor cells in the lung parenchyma or a stromal vascular fraction of the older subjects [10]. Kasper et al. also worked on MSC properties in bone marrow; they documented that not only these cells' potential regeneration decreases with age but also their migration capability and number in bone marrow decreases as an individual grows older [29]. Furthermore, the number of systemically or locally injected cells varies from 1×10^6 to 5×10^7 in different studies on the effect of MSCs on lung injuries [9,10,30]. Accordingly, another reason of the observed result in this part of our study might be due to the inevitable low number of injected cells. The number of stromal cells was intentionally chosen to be low in this experiment because in a study, carried out by Lee et al., it was demonstrated that intravenous injection of high number of MSC into mice contributed in embolism in the lung which may be fatal [31]. Consistently, Furlani et al. documented that some of their animals died of pulmonary embolism after abdominal aorta injection of high and low doses of MSCs (1×10^6 MSCs or 0.2×10^6), while no death was observed in the present study [32]. In addition, one of the most probable reasons for the absence of improving pharmacological effects of cell therapy on structural changes of the lung is that these changes take place during a long period of development of COPD which is well known to be rarely reversible. For this reason, in further studies, the effect of cell therapy is recommended to be examined during different stages of development of COPD not at the end of the disease development.

The results of this study also showed increased total WBC in the blood of smoke exposed animal and COPD-PBS group. However, cell therapy did not affect changes in blood total WBC. The probable reasons for the absence of improving effects of cell therapy on this parameter

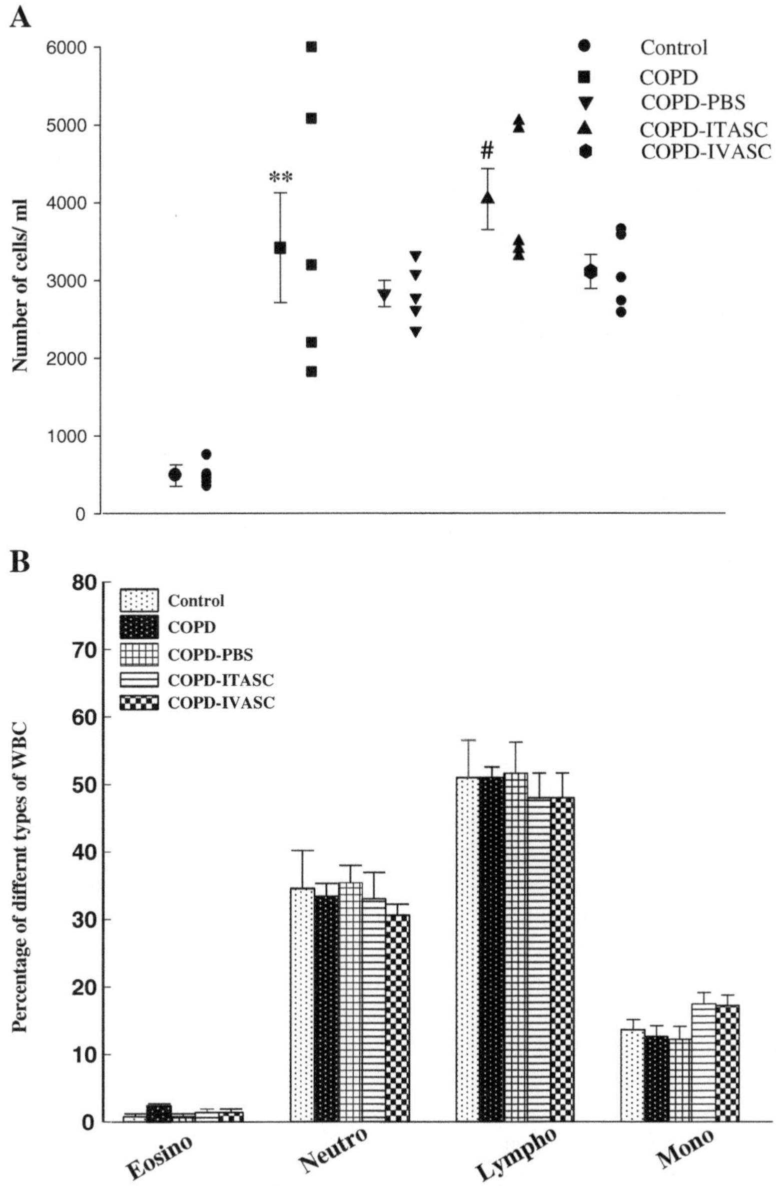

Figure 7 Effects of adipose derived stromal cells therapy on white blood cell counts in blood of different groups. Effects of adipose derived stromal cells (ASCs) on total white blood cell (WBC), **(A)** and its effect on differential WBC **(B)** counts. Data are shown as mean ± SEM. The animals in COPD-PBS, COPD-ITASC and COPD-IVASC groups were exposed to cigarette smoke for 3 months and then received PBS, intratracheal injection of ASCs and intravenous injection of ASCs, respectively.

could also be due to taking place of this change during a long period of development of COPD which is difficult to be affected by this method of therapy. However, further studies regarding the effect of cell therapy during different stages of development of COPD could be of great value. The ranges of differential WBC counts reported in this study may seem inconsistent with normal values. However, the ranges for lymphocyte, neutrophil and eosinophil number are 30-80%, 20-60% and 0-7% respectively in guinea pig which is different from human [33]. Our previous studies also showed similar range of differential WBC counts in guinea pigs [34,35].

In the present study, the cells injected into the trachea or the jugular vein of the animals were traced to confirm that they have reached the injured lung. As described before, the labeled stromal cells were detectable in the tissue even 2 weeks after cell therapy. It is consistent with another study reporting the persistence of MSCs 21 days following their injection into the trachea [8]. Schweitzer et al. also documented that systemically delivered adipose

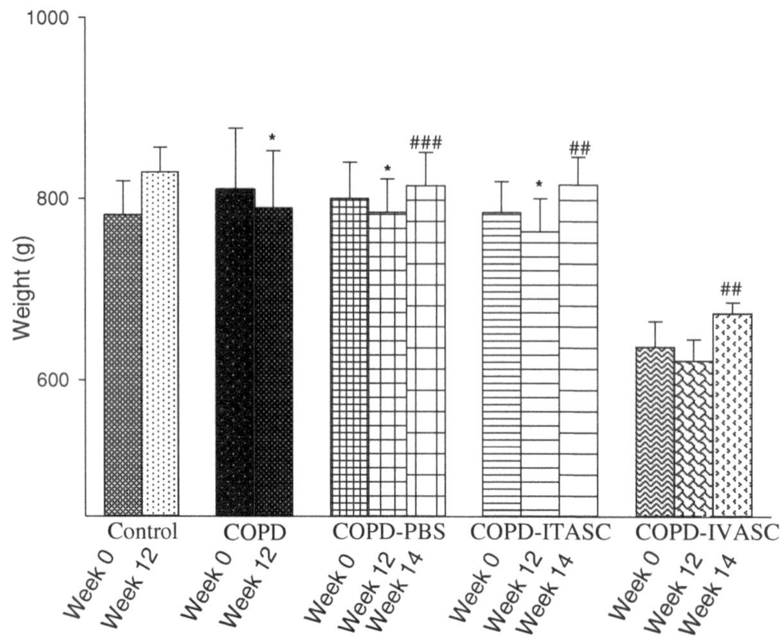

Figure 8 Body weight in guinea pigs of different groups. Data are shown as mean ± SEM values of body weight at three time points: at the first of the 3 months of inhalation (Week 0), on the last day of the 3 months of inhalation (Week 12) and 2 weeks after surgery (Week 14). $^{*}P < 0.01$ as compared with week 0; $^{\#\#}P < 0.01$ and $^{\#\#\#}P < 0.001$ as compared with week 12. The animals in COPD-PBS, COPD-ITASC and COPD-IVASC groups were exposed to cigarette smoke for 3 months and then received PBS, intratracheal injection of ASCs and intravenous injection of ASCs, respectively.

stem cells were detectable in the parenchyma and large airways of the lungs up to 21 days after injection [5]. It seems that two weeks recovery, given to the animals after administration of the cells, is a proper time for the stromal cells to exert their impact either by regeneration in the damaged tissue or by paracrine effects.

The results of the present study showed that the oxidative stress was increased in the smoke exposed group both in their BALF and serum measured by an increase in the concentration of MDA in serum and a decrease in the thiol groups in BALF. It is well documented that cigarette smoke contains stable compounds that undergo redox-cycle to form reactive oxygen species such as superoxide radicals, hydrogen peroxide, hydroxyl radicals etc. [36]. Our results are in accordance with the study carried out by Qamar et al., who reported the debility in antioxidant defenses after intratracheal instillation of cigarette smoke extract in rats [36]. Since there was no significant difference in the MDA and thiol concentration between COPD and COPD-PBS groups, it can be concluded that the PBS injection had no pharmacological effect on the parameter under investigation. BALF thiol concentration of the treated groups with intratracheal and intravenous administration of stromal cells increased significantly in COPD-IVASC group. However, both treated groups showed significant decrease in serum MDA concentration. These findings confirmed the ameliorative effect of stromal cells on the oxidative damage caused by cigarette smoke. Consistently, the antioxidant effect of mesenchymal stem cells within the stromal-vascular fraction of subcutaneous adipose tissue has been previously shown by Kim et al. documenting that these cells have potent antioxidant activity and protect HDFs from oxidative injury by decreasing apoptotic cells [11].

Considering the results, although the animals were kept in boxes with low possibility of movement and high probability of gaining weight during three months, being exposed to cigarette smoke during these months caused a considerable decrease in body weight of almost all the animals. Complied with these results, Schweitzer et al. documented that patients affected by emphysema often exhibit progressive respiratory symptoms and loss of lung function culminating in respiratory failure and systemic weight loss [5]. There are plenty of other studies demonstrating the effect of cigarette smoking on body weight loss [37,38]. In the present study, after finishing the three months of smoke exposure, the surgery and administration of the cells or PBS to the animals led to a significant increase in body weight. As Schweitzer et al. documented, therapeutic effects of adipose stem cells aren't restricted to the lung but also contains restoring the weight loss sustained by guinea pigs during cigarette smoke exposure [5]. However, the weight gain after the surgery, in the present study, can't be associated with the treatment with stromal cells because this improvement was observed in the PBS receiving groups too. Therefore, it can be concluded that smoke cessation and lower mobility of the animals due to the surgery might be the initial source of gaining weight.

In the present study, the applied method of exposing the animals to cigarette smoke resulted in exposure of all the animals to the same concentration of cigarette smoke as follows; every 30 second a twenty ml puff of smoke was dragged into the head chamber using a 20 ml syringes and duration of exposure of the animals to each cigarette was about 8 minutes with the same duration of rest between each two successive cigarettes. This protocol was maintained during the whole procedure and the smoke concentration in the head chamber was maintained the same for all the groups. This obviously leads to the similar levels of plasma nicotine and its metabolite as well as similar levels of plasma carboxyhemoglobin. Therefore, the variations observed in the results of different groups are just due to the variations in treatment protocol between them.

Conclusions

In conclusion, both intratracheal and intravenous cell therapy lead to pharmacological effect on reduction of oxidative damage and restoring the weight loss during smoking which may collectively hold promise in attenuation of the severity of the disease in the patients experiencing COPD although the lung structural changes couldn't be ameliorated with these therapeutic methods. However, more investigations are needed to further assess the pharmacological effects of adipose derived stromal cells on the microscopic structure of the damaged lung induced by cigarette smoke.

Competing interest

The authors declare that they have no competing interest.

Authors' contributions

AG: help in study design, supervision of experiments, statistical analysis and preparation of manuscript, AF: performance of experiment, help in statistical analysis and manuscript preparation, MH: help in performance of experiment, LG: help in performance of experiment, MH: help in study design and supervision of experiments, MS: Bichemichal analysis, FVB: help in performance of experiment, EK: help in performance of experiment, NMR: Patholofical evaluations, MHB: study design, supervision of experiments, help in statistical analysis and preparation of manuscript. All authors read and approved the final manuscript.

Acknowledgments

This study was financially supported by the Research Council of Mashhad University of Medical Sciences. This paper is a part of M.Sc. thesis.

Author details

[1]Neurogenic Inflammation Research Centre and Department of Physiology, School of Medicine, Mashhad University of Medical Sciences, Mashhad 9177948564, Iran. [2]Pharmacological Research Center of Medicinal Plants, School of Medicine, Mashhad University of Medical Sciences, Mashhad, Iran. [3]Neurocognitive Research Center and Department of Physiology, School of Medicine, Mashhad University of Medical Sciences, Mashhad, Iran. [4]Department of Clinical Biochemistry, School of Medicine, Mashhad University of Medical Sciences, Mashhad, Iran. [5]Department of Pathology, School of Medicine, Mashhad University of Medical Sciences, Mashhad, Iran.

References

1. Pauwels RA, Buist AS, Ma P, Jenkins CR, Hurd SS: **Global strategy for the diagnosis, management, and prevention of chronic obstructive pulmonary disease: National Heart, Lung, and Blood Institute and World Health Organization Global Initiative for Chronic Obstructive Lung Disease (GOLD): executive summary.** *Resp Care* 2001, **46**:798–825.
2. Saetta M, Ghezzo H, Kim W, King M, Angus G, Wang N, *et al*: **Loss of alveolar attachments in smokers. A morphometric correlate of lung function impairment.** *Am Rev Respir Dis* 1985, **132**:894–900.
3. Jeffery PK: **Structural and inflammatory changes in COPD: a comparison with asthma.** *Thorax* 1998, **53**:129–136.
4. Celli B, MacNee W, Agusti A, Anzueto A, Berg B, Buist A, *et al*: **Standards for the diagnosis and treatment of patients with COPD: a summary of the ATS/ERS position paper.** *Eur Respir J* 2004, **23**:932–946.
5. Schweitzer KS, Johnstone BH, Garrison J, Rush NI, Cooper S, Traktuev DO, *et al*: **Adipose stem cell treatment in mice attenuates lung and systemic injury induced by cigarette smoking.** *Am J Respir Crit Care Med* 2011, **183**:215–225.
6. Gladysheva ES, Malhotra A, Owens RL: **Influencing the decline of lung function in COPD: use of pharmacotherapy.** *Int J COPD* 2010, **5**:153–164.
7. Gupta N, Su X, Popov B, Lee JW, Serikov V, Matthay MA: **Intrapulmonary delivery of bone marrow-derived mesenchymal stem cells improves survival and attenuates endotoxin-induced acute lung injury in mice.** *J Immunol* 2007, **179**:1855–1863.
8. Baber SR, Deng W, Master RG, Bunnell BA, Taylor BK, Murthy SN, *et al*: **Intratracheal mesenchymal stem cell administration attenuates monocrotaline-induced pulmonary hypertension and endothelial dysfunction.** *Am J Physiol-Heart C* 2007, **292**:1120.
9. Shigemura N, Okumura M, Mizuno S, Imanishi Y, Nakamura T, Sawa Y: **Autologous transplantation of adipose tissue-derived stromal cells ameliorates pulmonary emphysema.** *Am J Transplant* 2006, **6**:2592–2600.
10. Ishizawa K, Kubo H, Yamada M, Kobayashi S, Numasaki M, Ueda S, *et al*: **Bone marrow-derived cells contribute to lung regeneration after elastase-induced pulmonary emphysema.** *FEBS Lett* 2004, **556**:249–252.
11. Kim W-S, Park B-S, Kim H-K, Park J-S, Kim K-J, Choi J-S, *et al*: **Evidence supporting antioxidant action of adipose-derived stem cells: protection of human dermal fibroblasts from oxidative stress.** *J Dermatol Sci* 2008, **49**:133–142.
12. Ahmed M, Katsha SO, Xin H, Kanehira M, Sun R, TNaY S: **Paracrine factors of multipotent stromal cells ameliorate lung injury in an elastase-induced emphysema model.** *ASGCT* 2010, **19**:196–203.
13. Yamamoto C, Yoneda T, Yoshikawa M, Fu A, Tokuyama T, Tsukaguchi K, *et al*: **Airway inflammation in COPD assessed by sputum levels of interleukin-8.** *CHEST J* 1997, **112**:505–510.
14. Drost E, Skwarski K, Sauleda J, Soler N, Roca J, Agusti A, *et al*: **Oxidative stress and airway inflammation in severe exacerbations of COPD.** *Thorax* 2005, **60**:293–300.
15. MacNee W: **Oxidative stress and lung inflammation in airways disease.** *Eur J Pharmacol* 2001, **429**:195–207.
16. Boskabady MH, Kiani S: **The effect of exposure of guinea pig to cigarette smoke and their sensitization in tracheal responsiveness to histamine and histamine receptor (h1) blockade by chlorpheniramine.** *Pathophysiol* 2007, **14**:97–104.
17. Ghorbani A, Varedi M, Hadjzadeh MR, Omrani GH: **Type-1 diabetes induces depot-specific alterations in adipocyte diameter and mass of adipose tissues in the rat.** *Exp Clin Endocrinol Diabetes* 2010, **118**:442–448.
18. Ghorbani A, Hadjzadeh MR, Rajaei Z, Zendehbad SB: **Effects of fenugreek seeds on adipogenesis and lipolysis in normal and diabetic rat.** *Pak J Biol Sci* 2014, **17**:523–528.
19. Ghorbani A, Jalali SA, Varedi M: **Isolation of adipose tissue mesenchymal stem cells without tissue destruction: a non-enzymatic method.** *Tissue Cell* 2014, **46**:54–58.
20. Ghorbani A, Abedinzade M: **Comparison of *in vitro* and *in situ* methods for studying lipolysis.** *ISRN Endocrinol* 2013, **2013**:205385.

21. Hsu LW, Goto S, Nakano T, Chen KD, Wang CC, Lai CY, *et al*: **The effect of exogenous histone H1 on rat adipose-derived stem cell proliferation, migration, and osteogenic differentiation *in vitro*.** *J Cell Physiol* 2012, **227**:3417–3425.
22. Raynaud C, Maleki M, Lis R, Ahmed B, Al-Azwani I, Malek J, *et al*: **Comprehensive characterization of mesenchymal stem cells from human placenta and fetal membrane and their response to osteoactivin stimulation.** *Stem Cells Int* 2012, **2012**:658356.
23. Sadeghnia HR, Yousefsani BS, Rashidfar M, Boroushaki MT, Assadpour E, Ghorbani A: **Protective effect of rutin on hexachlorobutadiene-induced nephrotoxicity.** *Ren Fail* 2013, **35**:1151–1155.
24. Sadeghnia HR, Kamkar M, Assadpour E, Boroushaki MT, Ghorbani A: **Protective effect of safranal, a constituent of Crocus sativus, on quinolinic acid-induced oxidative damage in rat hippocampus.** *Iran J Basic MedSci* 2013, **16**:73–82.
25. Khodabandehloo F, Hosseini M, Rajaei Z, Soukhtanloo M, Farrokhi E, Rezaeipour M: **Brain tissue oxidative damage as a possible mechanism for the deleterious effect of a chronic high dose of estradiol on learning and memory in ovariectomized rats.** *Arq Neuro-Psiquiat* 2013, **71**:313–319.
26. Wright JL, Churg A: **Cigarette smoke causes physiologic and morphologic changes of emphysema in the guinea pig.** *Am J Res Crit Care Med* 1990, **142**:1422–1428.
27. Boskabady MH, Kiani S, Aslani MR: **Tracheal responsiveness to both isoprenaline and beta-adrenoreceptor blockade by propranolol in cigarette smoke exposed and sensitized guinea pigs.** *Respirol* 2006, **11**:572–578.
28. Canning BJ, Chou Y: **Using guinea pigs in studies relevant to asthma and COPD.** *Pulm Pharmacol Ther* 2008, **21**:702–720.
29. Kasper G, Mao L, Geissler S, Draycheva A, Trippens J, Kühnisch J, *et al*: **Insights into mesenchymal stem cell aging: Involvement of antioxidant defense and actin cytoskeleton.** *Stem cells* 2009, **27**:1288–1297.
30. Yun Luan XZ, Kong F, Cheng G-H, Qi T-G, Zhang Z-H: **Mesenchymal stem cell prevention of vascular remodeling in high flow-induced pulmonary hypertension through a paracrine mechanism.** *Int Immunopharmacol* 2012, **14**:432–437.
31. Lee RH, Pulin AA, Seo MJ, Kota DJ, Ylostalo J, Larson BL, *et al*: **Intravenous hMSCs improve myocardial infarction in mice because cells embolized in lung are activated to secrete the anti-inflammatory protein TSG-6.** *Cell Stem Cell* 2009, **5**:54–63.
32. Furlani D, Ugurlucan M, Ong L, Bieback K, Pittermann E, Westien I, *et al*: **Is the intravascular administration of mesenchymal stem cells safe?: Mesenchymal stem cells and intravital microscopy.** *Microvas Res* 2009, **77**:370–376.
33. Suckow MA, Stevens KA, Wilson RP: *The laboratory rabbit, guinea pig, hamster, and other rodents.* San Diego: Access Online via Elsevier; 2012.
34. Boskabady MH, Keyhanmanesh R, Khamneh S, Ebrahimi MA: **The effect of *Nigella sativa* extract on tracheal responsiveness and lung inflammation in ovalbuminsensitizedguinea pigs.** *Clinics* 2011, **66**:879–887.
35. Boskabady MH, Bayrami G, Tabatabaee A: **The effect of the extract of Crocus sativus and its constituent safranal, on lung pathology and lung inflammation of ovalbumin sensitized guinea-pigs.** *Phyto Med* 2012, **19**:904–911.
36. Qamar W, Sultana S: **Farnesol ameliorates massive inflammation, oxidative stress and lung injury induced by intratracheal instillation of cigarette smoke extract in rats: an initial step in lung chemoprevention.** *Chem-BiolInteract* 2008, **176**:79–87.
37. Chen H, Hansen MJ, Jones JE, Vlahos R, Bozinovski S, Anderson GP, *et al*: **Cigarette smoke exposure reprograms the hypothalamic neuropeptide Y axis to promote weight loss.** *Am J Resp Critic Care Med* 2006, **173**:1248–1254.
38. Kubo S, Kobayashi M, Masunaga Y, Ishii H, Hirano Y, Takahashi K, *et al*: **Cytokine and chemokine expression in cigarette smoke-induced lung injury in guinea pigs.** *Eur Resp J* 2005, **26**:993–1001.

Development of a validated HPLC method for the simultaneous determination of flavonoids in *Cuscuta chinensis* Lam. by ultra-violet detection

Homa Hajimehdipoor[1], Babak Mokhtari kondori[2], Gholam Reza Amin[2], Noushin Adib[3], Hossein Rastegar[3] and Maryam Shekarchi[3*]

Abstract

Background: *Cuscuta* species known as dodder, have been used in traditional medicine of eastern and southern Asian countries as liver and kidney tonic. Flavonoids are considered as the main biologically active constituents in *Cuscuta* plants especially in *C. chinensis* Lam.

Objective: In the present study, a fast, simple and reliable method for the simultaneous determination and quantization of *C. chinensis* flavonols including hyperoside, rutin, isorhamnetin and kaempferol has been developed.

Materials and methods: The chromatographic separation was carried out on a reversed phase ACE 5 C_{18} with eluting at a flow rate of 1 ml/min using a gradient with *O*-phosphoric acid 0.25% : acetonitrile for 42 min. UV spectra were collected across the range of 200–900 nm, extracting 360 nm for the chromatograms. The method was validated according to linearity, selectivity, precision, recovery, LOD and LOQ.

Results: The method was selective for determination of rutin, hyperoside, isorhamnetin and kampferol. The calibration graphs of flavonols were linear with $r^2 > 0.999$. RSDs% of intra- and inter-day precisions were found 1.3&3.4 for rutin, 1.5&2.8 for hyperoside, 1.3&3.3 for isorhamnetin and 1.7 & 2.9 for kaempferol which were satisfactory. LODs and LOQs were calculated as 1.73 & 8.19 for rutin, 0.09 & 4.19 for hyperoside, 2.09 & 6.3 for isorhamnetin and 0.18 & 0.56 for kaempferol. The recovery averages of above-mentioned flavonols were 90.3%, 97.4%, 98.7% and 90.0%, respectively.

Conclusion: The simplicity of the method makes it highly valuable for quality control of *C. chinensis* according to quantization of flavonols.

Keywords: *Cuscuta chinensis* Lam., Hyperoside, Rutin, Isorhamnetin, Kaempferol

Introduction

Cuscuta is a genus consisted of about 100–170 species of yellow, orange, red and rarely green parasitic plants which is the only genus in the family of Cuscutaceae. *Cuscuta* Semen, a crude drug prepared from the seeds of *Cuscuta chinensis* Lam., is commonly used in traditional medicine as a liver and kidney tonic [1]. Many investigations have been established different biological activity of this plant such as improving sexual function [2], anti-cancer [3], immunostimulatory [4-7] and anti-oxidant activities [7]. The active constituents of the *C. chinensis* are including flavonoids, lignans, quinic acid derivatives and polysaccharides [1,8-10]. These compounds have been suggested to be responsible for the pharmacological activities of the plant [11,12]. Flavonoids, especially rutin, quercetin, isorhamnetin and kampferol are the main biologically active constituents in *C. chinensis* Lam. In addition, these flavonoids have exhibited various pharmacological activities, which to some extent might elucidate the mechanism of clinical

* Correspondence: shekarchim@yahoo.com
[3]Food and Drug Control Laboratories and Food and Drug Laboratory Research Center, MOH & ME, Tehran, Iran
Full list of author information is available at the end of the article

effects of this commonly used Chinese medicine. Therefore, their contents can be an important index in quality evaluation of this crude drug. Many fakes were found in the crude drug samples, which seriously influenced the drug's quality. According to FDA guide line [13], before a plant drug can be legally marketed, its spectroscopic or chromatographic finger prints and chemically assay of characteristic markers are required. Because of the complex nature of a typical botanical drug and the lack of knowledge about its active constituents, the FDA may rely on combination of tests and controls to ensure the identity, purity, quality strength, potency and consistency of these drugs. Hence, quality control of natural drugs is in great demand. Unfortunately, few studies on the quantitative determination of chemical constituents in *C. chinensis* Lam. have been reported so far. In previous papers, total flavonoids and total polysaccharides were determined by colorimetric method, but the results could not reflect the drug's quality exactly and rapidly [14,15]. In addition, these methods suffered from low resolution and sensitivity. It is known that interaction of multiple chemical compounds contributes to the therapeutics effects of herbal medicines [16]. Therefore, the analysis of multiple components is necessary and helpful to control the quality of herbal medicines. According to our knowledge, there was no report on determination of flavonols and their glycosides in *C. chinensis* Lam. by High Performance Liquid Chromatography (HPLC). So In this paper, the four major flavonols including hyperoside (1), rutin (2), isorhamnetin (3) and kaempferol (4) (Figure 1) in *C. chinensis* Lam. samples were determined simultaneously with a simple, rapid and accurate analysis by reversed phase liquid chromatography.

Materials and methods

Plant material

C.chinensis was collected from Qazvin-karaj superhighway and identified by Dr. Gh.R. Amin, Herbarium of faculty of Pharmacy, Tehran university of medicinal Sciences, Tehran, Iran, Voucher No.6737 TEH.

Instrumentation

The HPLC experiment was performed using a Waters Alliance system equipped with a vacuum degasser, quaternary detector. The UV spectra were collected across the range of 200–900 nm, extracting 360 nm for chromatograms. Empower software was utilized for instrument control, data collection and data processing. The column was an ACE C_{18} (4.6 × 250 mm, 5 μm). The mobile phase was a linear gradient with *O*-phosphoric acid 0.25% (A)- acetonitrile (B) for 42 min starting with A:B (95:5) for 2 min, changing to A:B (90:10) for 5 min, A:B (85:15) for 3 min, A:B (80:20) for 13 min, A:B (70:30) for 5 min, A:B (50:50) for 4 min with equilibrating for 10 min. The flow rate was 1 ml/min. The injection volume for all samples and standard solutions was 10 μL.

Chemicals

Hyperoside, rutin, isorhamnetin and kaempferol standard materials were purchased from ROTH (Karlsruhe, Germany). All solvents were obtained from Merck Co. (Darmstadt, Germany). Water used in all the experiments was deionized by Purelab UHQ Elga.

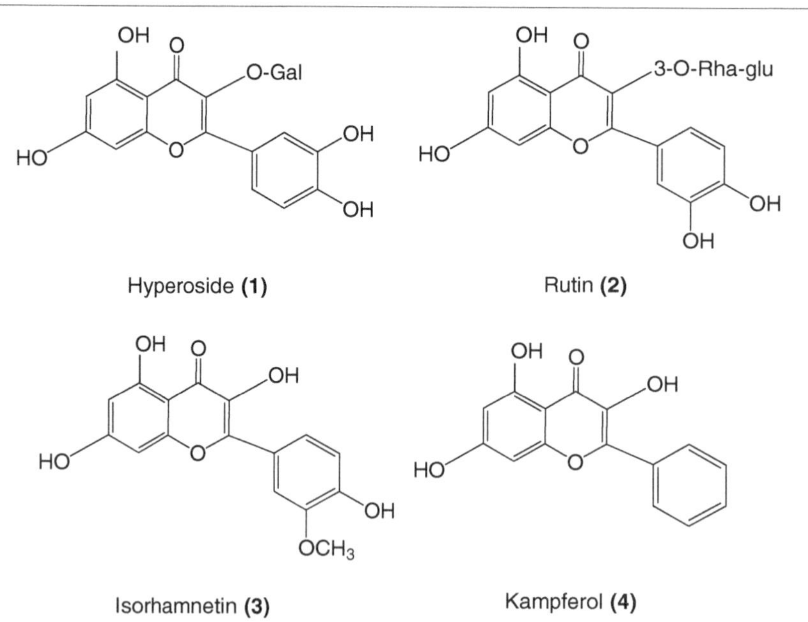

Figure 1 Chemical structure of flavonols of *C. chinensis*.

Determination of flavonols

Solvent effect

The samples were extracted with methanol, acetone and methanol–water 80:20 to determine the effect of the solvent on the extraction efficiency.

Optimization of the sample size

To evaluate the effect of the sample size on the accuracy of the flavonoids content estimation, the samples were prepared in triplicate in two sets. In the first set, 0.5 g and in the second set 1 g of powder were weighted and used for extraction.

Effect of the extraction method

To determine the effect of the procedure on the extraction, hot solvent extraction (decoction for 30 min), maceration (24 h), and ultrasonic radiation (30 min, three times) methods were compared.

Sample preparation

Powdered samples (300 μm, 0.5 g) were suspended in 80% methanol (25 ml) and extracted in an ultrasonic bath for 30 min. The suspension was filtered and the remaining powder was extracted two more times using 25 mL 80% methanol. After filtration, the filtrate was transferred to a 100 ml volumetric flask and diluted with the solvent to volume. The obtained solution was filtered through a membrane filter (0.45 μm pore size) prior to injection.

Preparation of standard solutions

Stock solutions of hyperoside, rutin, isorhamnetin and kaempferol (0.05, 0.2, 0.2 and 0.01 mg/ml) were prepared separately in methanol 80%. Standard multi flavonol solutions were made by using different amount of stock solutions (1–10, 10–60, 10–70 and 0.3-1.6 μg/ml for hyperoside, rutin, isorhamnetin and kaempferol, respectively). Stock and working standard solutions were prepared daily.

Validation

The reliability of the HPLC-method for analysis of hyperoside, rutin, isorhamnetin and kaempferol was validated through its selectivity, linearity, precision, recovery, limit of detection and limit of quantization [17].

Selectivity

For the chromatographic method, developing a separation involves demonstrating specificity, which is the ability of the method to accurately measure the analyte response in the presence of all interferences. Therefore, the extraction mixtures obtained from the sample preparation were analyzed and the analyte peaks (flavonols1-4) were evaluated for peak purity and resolution from the nearest eluting peaks.

Linearity

Due to the verification of the normal distribution of results, linearity was evaluated through the relationship between the concentration of flavonols 1–4 and the absorbances obtained from the UV-HPLC detector. The determination coefficient (r^2) was calculated by means of the least-square analysis [18,19]. The calibration lines were achieved through two replicates of each concentration of hyperoside, rutin, isorhamnetin and kaempferol (1–10, 10–60, 10–70 and 0.3-1.6 μg/mL), to identify the extent of the total variability of the response that could be explained by the linear regression model.

Precision

The precision of each method indicates the degree of dispersion within a series on the determination of the same sample. Six real samples were analyzed on the same day (intra-day) and three on consecutive days (inter-day), and then the relative standard deviations (RSDs%) were calculated. Each sample was injected to HPLC thrice.

Recovery

This parameter shows the proximity between the experimental values and the real ones. It ensures that no loss or uptake occurred during the process [18,19]. The determination of this parameter was performed during the method by studying the recovery after a standard addition procedure, with two additional levels. Three replicate amounts of plant (3 × 1.5 g) were weighted and each of them was divided into three equal portions

Table 1 The effect of different extraction procedures on recovery of *C. chinensis* flavonols

Compound	Extraction method			Solvent			Sample size	
	Decoction	*Maceration*	*Ultrasonication*	*Acetone*	*Methanol*	*Methanol 80%*	*0.5 g*	*1.0 g*
Rutin	30.11 ± 1.22*	35.23 ± 2.23	42.55 ± 0.54	21.02 ± 1.5	31.31 ± 0.41	42.55 ± 0.54	42.55 ± 0.54	35.3 ± 5.2
Hyperoside	3.12 ± 0.21	4.02 ± 0.12	6.01 ± 0.09	4.15 ± 0.22	5.23 ± 0.04	6.01 ± 0.09	6.01 ± 0.09	5.21 ± 1.2
Isorhamnetin	23.21 ± 0.18	25.30 ± 0.17	33.49 ± 0.45	34.1 ± 2.3	35.2 ± 0.25	33.49 ± 0.45	33.49 ± 0.45	34.16 ± 6.2
Kaempferol	0.26 ± 0.01	0.22 ± 0.02	0.46 ± 0.01	0.49 ± 0.02	0.45 ± 0.03	0.46 ± 0.01	0.46 ± 0.01	0.45 ± 0.03

*: Represents as μg/mL.

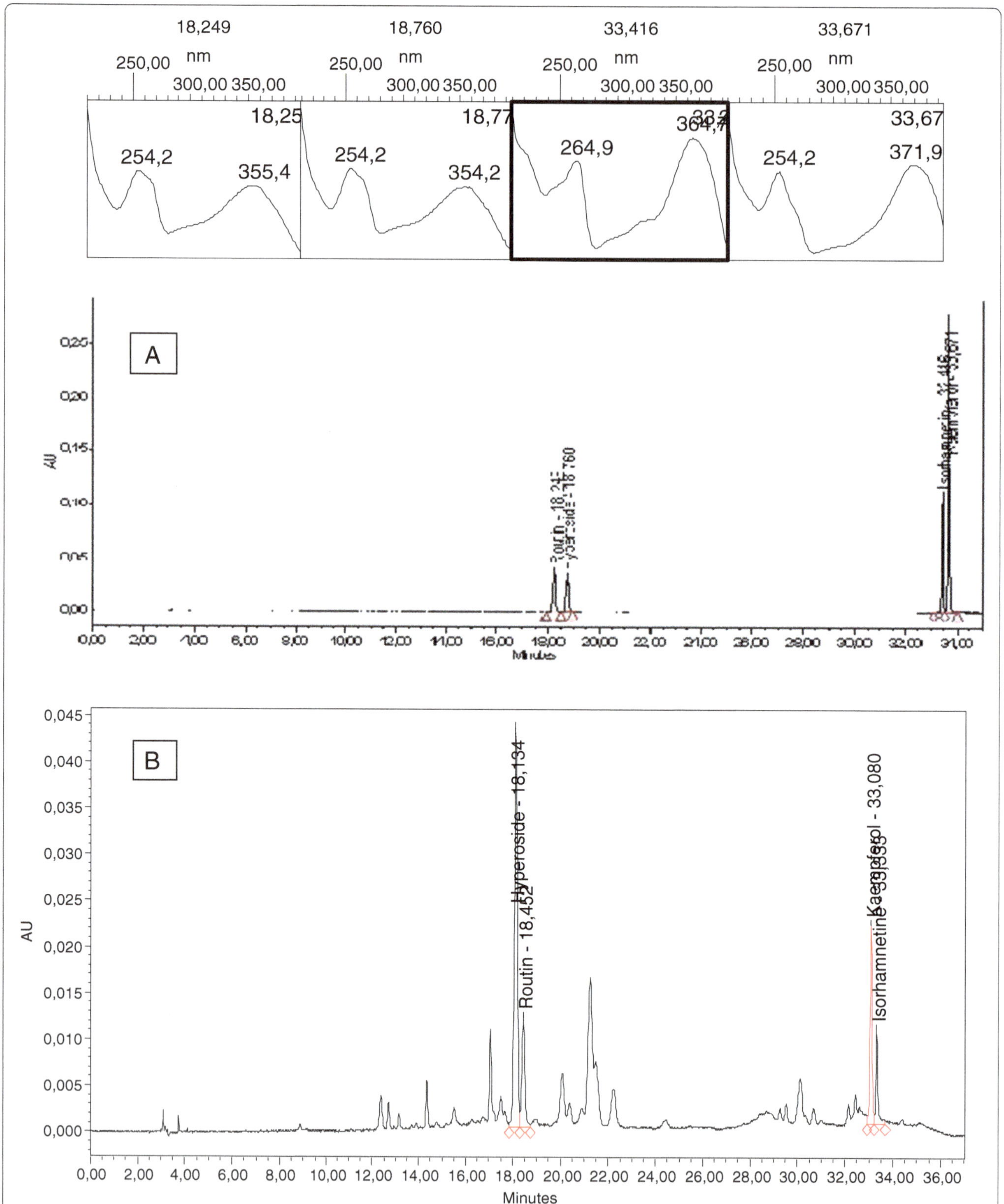

Figure 2 HPLC chromatogram of A: rutin, hyperoside, kampferol and isorhamnetin standard solution and B: *C. chinensis* sample with chromatographic UV spectra at 200–400 nm.

(0.5 g). One part was used as the real sample and others had been spiked with multi-flavonol standard solution containing hyperoside (1&3 μg/mL), rutin (5&10 μg/mL), isorhamnetin (5&10 μg/mL) and kaempferol (0.2&0.4 μg/mL) in two levels. In each additional level, three determinations were carried out and the recovery percentage was calculated in every case. Each sample was injected into HPLC three times.

Results and discussions

One of the challenging aspects of method development in quantitative analysis is the complexity of the analysis methods. The best method is the simplest one which could be conducted by different operators and in different labs. However other parameters of a quantitative method such as accuracy and precision demand more complex processes.

Extraction procedures

Extraction is the main step for the recovery and isolation of bioactive compounds from plant materials, before analysis. It is influenced by chemical nature of compounds, the extraction method employed, sample particle size, as well as the presence of interfering substances. Commonly used extraction solvents for flavonoids are alcohols (methanol, ethanol), acetone, diethyl ether, and ethyl acetate. In our experiment, very polar flavonol glycosides could not be extracted completely with pure organic solvents so 80:20 methanol–water mixture was an excellent choice. Besides the high recovery, less interfering in comparison with other solvents made it a suitable solvent for extraction of all flavonoids and preparation of standard materials. Among different methods of extraction, the ultrasonic radiation was selected in comparison with maceration and hot solvent extraction. Comparison between two experiments showed that the smaller sample size appeared to have a significant effect on the accuracy of flavonols analysis. In general, using ultrasonic radiation of the plant (0.5 g, 30 min, three times) with methanol 80% was selected as the best method for hyperoside, rutin, isorhamnetin and kaempferol analysis (Table 1).

Method development and validation

As it is shown in Figure 1, all compounds1-4 were tri- or tetra-hydroxylated flavonols, with similar structures, especially in the case of hyperoside and rutin; therefore, it was difficult to separate all components simultaneously. After comparison between the different columns such as C_8, C_{18}, CN and phenyl, the best separation efficiency was obtained by using the C_{18} column. The mobile phase investigations showed that the ratio of organic modifiers, such as the acetonitrile or methanol in the mobile phase, was the key to a good separation. The pH value played an important role in the solute ionization. In order to minimize flavonols ionization, using an acidic mobile phase was obligated. According to this, the best separation was achieved by using 0.25% *O*-phosphoric acid solution. The gradient mode of the instrument was changed to obtain the best resolution and the shortest run time. Each flavonol peak was resolved from the neighboring peaks and displayed excellent peak symmetry and separation efficiency as seen in Figure 2. These groups of compounds had a special chromophoric nature, which made them easy to identify from their UV diode-array absorption spectra. The results obtained from the method validation according to linearity, selectivity, accuracy and precision showed that the proposed method was suitable for the analysis of all four flavonols 1–4. Comparison between the purity threshold and purity angle reported in the empower software showed that the method was specific for hyperoside, rutin, isorhamnetin and kaempferol and the reported peaks were completely separated from the other interfering compounds. The linear relationship between the detector response and different concentrations of flavonols were confirmed as it was shown in Table 2. The relative standard deviations (RSDs%) of the intra-day and inter-day have been shown in Table 3. The results of intermediate precision using different analysts, different instruments, and on different days, showed that these parameters did not have any significant effect on the variation of results (data did not show). After these validation studies, the method's ability to provide good quantization in our laboratory was confirmed. The last step in the measurement of precision (reproducibility), which focused more on the bias in results, rather than

Table 2 Linearity, LOD and LOQ parameters of flavonols analysis in *C. chinensis*

Flavonols	LOD*	LOQ*	r square	Equation	Linear range*
Rutin	1.73	8.19	0.9990	Y = 8752x + 8764	10-60
Hyperoside	0.09	4.19	0.9997	Y = 17073x + 2748.7	1-10
Isorhamnetin	2.90	6.33	0.9994	Y = 3553.8x + 1305	10-70
Kaempferol	0.18	0.56	0.9990	Y = 26807x + 67263	0.3-1.6

*represents as μg/mL.

Table 3 Repeatability of flavonols analysis in *C. chinensis*

Flavonols	Mean ± SD* (Intra-day n = 6)	RSD% (Intra-day)	RSD% (Inter-day n = 3)
Rutin	42.55 ± 0.54	1.3	3.4
Hyperoside	6.01 ± 0.09	1.5	2.8
Isorhamnetin	33.49 ± 0.45	1.3	3.3
Kaempferol	0.46 ± 0.01	1.7	2.9

*: Represents as μg/mL.

Table 4 Recovery of flavonols analysis in *C. chinensis*

Flavonols	*Spiked	Found*	% Mean recovery**	Total recovery ± SD
Rutin	0.0	42.11 ± 0.71	-	90.3 ± 6.0
	5.0	46.73 ± 0.36	92.4 ± 7.2	
	10.0	50.91 ± 0.60	88.7 ± 5.1	
Hyperoside	0.0	5.80 ± 0.12	-	97.4 ± 9.1
	1.0	6.84 ± 0.10	103.0 ± 9.8	
	3.0	8.67 ± 0.20	91.7 ± 6.6	
Isorhamnetin	0.0	32.51 ± 0.68	-	98.7 ± 7.9
	5.0	37.62 ± 0.56	100.4 ± 10.9	
	10.0	42.35 ± 0.56	97.0 ± 5.5	
Kaempferol	0.0	0.45 ± 0.01	-	90.0 ± 4.1
	0.2	0.63 ± 0.01	90.0 ± 5.1	
	0.4	0.82 ± 0.02	92.5 ± 4.0	

*Represents as μg/mL, ** n = 3.

on determining the differences in precision alone, as inter-laboratory crossover studies, would be our next target. Accuracy, which was evaluated as recovery, after spiking the plant samples with standards at two concentration levels have been shown in Table 4.

As it was reported in Table 4, the careful optimization of extraction conditions caused the good recovery for each flavonols 1–4. So this method because of reaching suitable recovery and good precision can be recommended for the quantification of hyperoside, rutin, isorhamnetin and kaempferol in *C. chinensis.*

Conclusions

This work proposes a new method for simultaneous separating and determining of four flavonols of hyperoside, rutin, isorhamnetin and kaempferol. The most relevant advantage of the proposed method is the simultaneous determination of the four major flavonols in *C. chinensis* Lam. in order to reduce time required for quantitative extraction and analysis. It is a simple, fast, accurate and reliable technique in both chromatographic condition and sample preparation with minimum use of solvents. This method is suitable for quality control of *C. chinensis* Lam. and could be candidate as a routine method in quality control laboratories.

Competing interests

The authors declare that they have no competing interests.

Authors' contributions

HH carried out identification and separation of flavonols from plant. BMK prepared sample and standard solutions. GRA participated in collection and identification of the plant. NA collaborated in validation of the method. HR collaborated in validation of the method. MSh carried out method development and designing of validation protocol. All authors read and approved the final manuscript.

Author details

[1]Department of Traditional Pharmacy, School of Traditional Medicine and Traditional Medicine and Materia Medica Research Center, Shahid Beheshti University of Medical Sciences, Tehran, Iran. [2]Department of Pharmacognosy, Faculty of Pharmacy, Tehran University of Medical Sciences, Tehran, Iran. [3]Food and Drug Control Laboratories and Food and Drug Laboratory Research Center, MOH & ME, Tehran, Iran.

References

1. Du XM, Kohinata TK, Guo YT: **Components of the ether-insoluble resin glycoside-like fraction from *Cuscuta chinensis*.** *Phytochemistry* 1998, **48**:843–850.
2. Xiong YB, Zhou CH: **The effect of extracts from Herba Epimedi and Semen Cuscutae on the function of male reproduction.** *Chin Pharm J* 1994, **29**:89–90.
3. Nisa M, Akbar S, Tariq M, Hussain Z: **Effect of *Cuscuta chinensis* water extract on 7, 12-dimethylbenz [a] anthracene-induced skin papillomas and carcinomas in mice.** *J Ethnopharmacol* 1986, **18**:21–31.
4. Li GS, Chen YY, Li SC: **Immunological activity of watery extract from *Cuscuta australis*.** *China J Trad Chinese med Pharm.* 1997, **4**:256–258.
5. Xiao JS, Cui FJ, Ning TX: **Effects of the ethanol extract of *Polygonaum odoratum* and *Cuscuta australis* on immunological function of burn mice.** *China J Chin Mater Med.* 1990, **1**:557–559.
6. Pan HJ, Sun HX, Pan YJ: **Adjuvant effect of ethanol extract of *Semen Cuscutae* on the immune responses to ovalbumin in mice.** *J Ethnopharmacol* 2005, **99**:99–103.
7. Bao X, Wang Z, Fang J, Li X: **Structural features of an immunostimulating and antioxidant acidic polysaccharide from the seeds of *Cuscuta chinensis*.** *Planta Med* 2002, **68**:237–243.
8. Wang Z, Fang JN, Ge DL, Li XY: **Chemical characterization and immunological activities of an acidic polysaccharide isolated from the seeds of *Cuscuta chinensis* Lam.** *Acta Pharm Sinic.* 2000, **21**:1136–1140.
9. Ye M, Li Y, Yan Y, Liu H, Ji X: **Determination of flavonoids in *Semen Cuscutae* by RP-HPLC.** *J Pharm Biomed Anal* 2002, **28**:621–628.
10. Ye M, Yan Y, Guo DA: **Characterization of phenolic compounds in the Chinese herbal drug Tu-Si-Zi by liquid chromatography coupled to electrospray ionization mass spectrometry.** *Rapid Commun Mass Spectrom* 2005, **19**:1469–1484.
11. Williamson G, Barron D, Shimoi K, Terao J: **In vitro biological properties of flavonoids conjugates found in vivo.** *Free Radical Res.* 2005, **39**:457–469.
12. Cornwell T, Cohick W, Raskin I: **Dietary phytoestrogens and health.** *Phytochemistry* 2004, **65**:995–1016.
13. FDA Guidance for Industry: *Botanical Drug Products.* Rochville: US Food and Drug Administration; 2000.
14. Rumley AG, Paterson JR: **Analytical aspect of antioxidant and free radical activity.** *Biochem.* 1998, **35**:181–200.
15. Singleton VL, Rossi JA: **Colorimetry of total phenolics with phosphomolybdic-phosphotungstic acid reagents.** *J Enol Vitic.* 1965, **16**:144–153.
16. Shekarchi M, Hajimehdipoor H, Saeidnia S, Gohari AR: **Pirali Hamedani M: Comparative study of rosmarinic acid content in some plants of Labiatae family.** *Phcog Mag* 2012, **8**:37–41.
17. ICH Q2B: *Validation of analytical procedures.* London: methodology (CPMP/ICH/281/ 95); 1996.
18. Shekarchi M, Hajimehdipoor H, Khanavi M, Adib N, Bozorgi M, Akbari-adergani B: **A validated method for analysis of Swerchirin in *Swertia longifolia* by high performance liquid chromatography.** *Phcog Mag.* 2010, **6**:13–18.
19. Hajimehdipoor H, Shekarchi M, Khanavi M, Adib N, Amri M: **A validated high performance liquid chromatography method for the analysis of thymol and carvacrol in *Thymus vulgaris* L. volatile oil.** *Phcog Mag* 2010, **6**:154–158.

Pleurodesis by erythromycin, tetracycline, Aerosil™ 200, and erythromycin plus Aerosil™ 200 in a rat model: a preliminary study

Shahryar Hashemzadeh[1], Khosrow Hashemzadeh[2], Kamran Mamaghani[3], Elnaz Ansari[3], Raheleh Aligholipour[1], Samad EJ Golzari[4] and Kamyar Ghabili[5*]

Abstract

Background: None of the current pleurodesing agents fulfil all the criteria for best pleural sclerosant. Therefore, the search for the ideal agent for chemical pleurodesis still continues. The aim of the present study was to compare the effectiveness of erythromycin, tetracycline, Aerosil™ 200 (hydrophilic fumed amorphous silica), and erythromycin plus Aerosil™ 200 in producing pleurodesis in rats. In the present study, talc was not used as a pleurodesing agent due to an unavailability of its sterile and pure form in Iran.

Methods: Overall, 75 adult male Spraque-Dawley rats were randomized to 5 treatment groups. Each group received an intrapleural injection via 5 Fr Silastic tubes of one of the following sterile agents: 35mg/kg erythromycin in 2 ml of saline, 35mg/kg tetracycline in 2 ml of saline, 35mg/kg Aerosil™ 200 in 2ml of saline, erythromycin (35mg/kg in 2 ml of saline) plus Aerosil™ 200 (35mg/kg in 2 ml of saline), or 2 ml of saline as a control. The animals were euthanized and necropsied 30 days after injection. The pleurae were assessed for macroscopic and microscopic evidence of surrounding inflammation and fibrosis.

Results: The median macroscopic score in the Aerosil™ 200 group was significantly higher than that in the erythromycin group ($P < 0.005$). The median microscopic score in the erythromycin group was significantly lower than that in the Aerosil™ 200 and erythromycin plus Aerosil™ 200 groups ($P < 0.005$). Furthermore, maximum and minimum pleural fibrosis was observed in the erythromycin plus Aerosil™ 200 and erythromycin groups, respectively ($P < 0.05$).

Conclusion: This study suggests that Aerosil™ 200 with or without erythromycin may be more potent pleurodesis agent than erythromycin and tetracycline.

Keywords: Aerosil™ 200, Erythromycin, Pleurodesis, Silicon dioxide, Tetracycline

Background

Obliteration of the pleural space (pleurodesis) to prevent recurrent pleural effusion (mostly malignant) or pneumothorax is chiefly achieved through the use of chemical pleural sclerosants [1]. The best pleural sclerosant should be safe, inexpensive, widely available, and easily administered. However, none of the pleurodesing agents including talc, the sclerosant of choice in clinical practice, fulfil all these criteria [1-3]. Intrapleural administration of the most preferred pleurodesing agent, the talc, is believed to accompany with severe complications such as adult respiratory distress syndrome. On the other hand, parenteral tetracycline which was once the sclerosant agent of choice in clinical practice is no longer commercially available [4]. In addition, intrapleural application of some antineoplastic agents such as bleomycin is costly [5]. Therefore, the search for the ideal agent for chemical pleurodesis still continues.

Silica is the common name for silicon dioxide (SiO_2). Silica may have a crystalline or a non-crystalline (amorphous) structure. Among synthetic amorphous silicas, pyrogenic (fumed) silica is widely used as

* Correspondence: kghabili@gmail.com
[5]Physical Medicine and Rehabilitation Research Center, Tabriz University of Medical Sciences, Tabriz, Iran
Full list of author information is available at the end of the article

reinforcing filler for silicon rubber, thickening and anti-settling agents in liquid systems of coating, adhesives, printing inks and cosmetics [6]. Aerosil™ 200, a hydrophilic fumed silica, is the most widely used form of the amorphous silica. Silica-based materials have been of great interest in chemical pleurodesis. Bioglass, a silica-based biomaterial similar to the Aerosil™ 200, has been found as a pleurodesing agent as effective as talc [7,8]. The pleurodesing effect of bioglass, talc and Aerosil™ 200 may be attributed to their major content, the silicon dioxide. Interestingly, pulmonary changes following inhalation of Aerosil™ 200 have been reported in the literature [9,10]. However, pleurodesing effect of Aerosil™ 200 has not been hitherto investigated. Therefore, the aim of the present study was to compare the effectiveness of erythromycin, tetracycline, Aerosil™ 200, and erythromycin plus Aerosil™ 200 in producing pleurodesis in rats compared with saline control. We did not investigate talc as a sclerosing agent in the present study due to an unavailability of its sterile and pure form.

Methods

Adult male Spraque-Dawley rats were used in this study in accordance with the NIH Guide for the Care and Use of Laboratory Animals and local institutional guidelines for humane use of animals in research. The animals were housed three to five per cage and were provided with free access to compact food and water. Their food consisted of all essential ingredients including vitamins and minerals. The animals were kept under constant laboratory conditions with respect to humidity, illumination and temperature before and after surgery [11,12].

Overall, 75 adult male Spraque-Dawley rats, weighing 220–250 g, were anesthetized with an intramuscular injection of xylazine hydrochloride (5mg/kg) and ketamine hydrochloride (35mg/kg). Under the sterile conditions, a 1-cm incision was made over the seventh rib in the posterior axillary line on the rat's right side, and a subcutaneous tunnel was extended to the fifth intercostal space. A 5 Fr Silastic tube was inserted through the incision and placed in the right pleural cavity. The rats were randomly assigned to one of five intrapleural treatment groups as follows: fifteen rats received erythromycin ethylsuccinate (35mg/kg) in 2 ml of saline (0.9% NaCl); fifteen animals were given tetracycline (35mg/kg) in 2 ml of saline; fifteen rats were given sterile Aerosil™ 200 (35mg/kg) in 2 ml of saline; fifteen animals received erythromycin ethylsuccinate (35mg/kg in 2 ml of saline) plus sterile Aerosil™ 200 (35mg/kg in 2 ml of saline); and fifteen control animals received 2 ml of normal saline. All the sclerosing agents were given sterile. These agents were instilled into the tube and flushed with air, and the animals were rotated to assure dispersion to the entire pleural surface. The control group received normal saline in a similar approach. All residual air was aspirated from the pleural space. After a perioperative chest radiograph demonstrated a fully expanded lung, the tube was removed, and the incision was closed. All animals were left to heal with both lungs expanded.

All animals in the experimental and control groups were euthanized on 30th postoperative day by intravenous Beuthanasia-D, a pentobarbital/phenytoin commercial euthanasia solution. The thorax was removed en bloc. Lungs were fully expanded by instilling 10% formalin into trachea. After tracheal injection, the entire thorax was submerged in 10% neutral buffered formalin for 48 hours. Thereafter, a veterinary pathologist, blinded to the treatment group, performed thoracic necropsy. On macroscopic and gross observations, pleurodesis was graded as: 0 = normal pleura, 1 = multifocal fibrosis, 2 = diffuse adhesions and 3 = complete obliteration [2,13]. For microscopic evaluation, tissue sections from the lung and pleura were prepared and stained with hematoxylin and eosin (HE) and Masson's trichrome. Light microscopic assessment of the sections was performed by a pathologist blinded to the study protocol. The slides were graded for inflammation/cellularity and scored using the following system: 0 (absence of cellularity and neovascularisation), 1 (mild cellularity and neovascularisation), 2 (moderate cellularity and neovascularisation), and 3 (severe cellularity and neovascularisation) [14]. Moreover, microscopic fibrosis was defined based on the similar grading system as absent (0), mild (1), moderate (2), and severe (3).

Data were presented as mean = standard deviation (SD), median or percentage. Statistical analysis was performed with SPSS for windows version 13.0. The chi-square test ($P < 0.05$) was used to compare the incidence of pleural fibrosis, pleural cellularity and neovascularization, and pleural adhesions among the groups. The Kruskal-Wallis test ($P < 0.05$) was used to compare the median macroscopic, microscopic, cellularity, neovascularization and fibrosis scores among the groups. Thereafter, comparisons between two groups were conducted with the Mann–Whitney ranking test. In order to avoid accumulation of errors due to multiple comparisons, the significance level was modified dividing it ($P < 0.05$) by the number of comparisons made (Bonferroni correction) with $P < 0.005$ considered as significant.

Results

Gross necropsy

No deaths occurred in any of the studied groups. At 30 days, the normal saline (control) group produced no considerable adhesions or pleurodesis on gross observation. In the erythromycin group, adhesions were grossly visible between the parietal and the visceral pleurae in 66.6% (10/15) of the rats. Although Aerosil™ 200 group had the greatest number of rats with pleural adhesions (93.3%), there was no significant difference between the studied groups in this regard ($P > 0.05$, Table 1). Furthermore, Aerosil™ 200 and erythromycin plus Aerosil™ 200 groups showed higher numbers of diffuse adhesion (score 2) and complete obliteration (score 3) on gross observation ($P > 0.05$, Figure 1). The median macroscopic score in the Aerosil™ 200 group was significantly higher than that in the erythromycin group ($P < 0.005$, Bonferroni-corrected Mann–Whitney *U* test, Table 2).

Histopathology

The normal saline (control) group produced no considerable cellularity, neovascularisation, or fibrosis on microscopic observation at 30 days. Microscopically, all the erythromycin-treated rats exhibited inflammation, while only 40% (6/15) had pleural fibrosis. Pleural fibrosis was significantly lower in the erythromycin group compared with other treatment groups ($P = 0.007$, Table 1). Moreover, all rats in the treatment groups showed pleural inflammation (Table 1). In addition, pleural fibrosis was significantly higher in the erythromycin plus Aerosil™ 200 group compared with other treatment groups ($P = 0.02$, Table 1).

Figure 2 illustrates the number of each microscopic (inflammation/cellularity) score in the studied treatment groups. Accordingly, none of the treatment groups had absence of cellularity and neovascularisation in the microscopic assessment (score 0). Furthermore, Aerosil™ 200 and erythromycin plus Aerosil™ 200 groups showed higher numbers of severe cellularity and neovascularisation (score 3) on microscopic observation ($P > 0.05$, Figure 2). Overall, the median microscopic score in the erythromycin group was significantly lower than that in the Aerosil™ 200 and erythromycin plus Aerosil™ 200 groups ($P < 0.005$, Bonferroni-corrected Mann–Whitney *U* test, Table 2). On the other hand, the Aerosil™ 200 group showed higher cellularity score than erythromycin and tetracycline groups ($P < 0.005$, Bonferroni-corrected Mann–Whitney *U* test, Table 2). In addition, neovascularization and fibrosis scores in erythromycin plus Aerosil™ 200 group were significantly higher than those in the erythromycin group ($P < 0.005$, Bonferroni-corrected Mann–Whitney *U* test, Table 2).

Discussion

This rat model evaluated the effectiveness of erythromycin, tetracycline, Aerosil™ 200 and erythromycin plus Aerosil™ 200 as pleural sclerosing agents. This study demonstrated that Aerosil™ 200 with or without erythromycin was more potent pleurodesis agent both grossly and microscopically. To the best of our knowledge, the present study is the first investigation to study the pleurodesing effect of intrapleural Aerosil™ 200. However, there are a few studies on the health effects of Aerosil™ 200. In an animal investigation by Reuzel and colleagues, subchronic inhalation of Aerosil™ 200 induced the most severe changes in the lungs among other examined amorphous silicas [9]. In another study, Johnston et al. observed reversible inflammatory responses in bronchoalveolar lavage after inhalation of amorphous silica (Aerosil™ 200), while no mutagenic events were noted [10]. Likewise, recent experimental studies confirmed the pulmonary fibrogenetic effects of amorphous silica such as Aerosil™ 200 [15-17].

Chemical pleurodesis with silica-containing materials has been of utmost interest. Yeginsu and colleagues found that bioglass was as effective as talc in terms of pleurodesis [7,8]. It is believed that silicon dioxide or silica contributes to the pleurodesing effect of bioglass, talc and Aerosil™ 200. Silicon dioxide or silica exposure has been found to cause lung damage through direct cytotoxicity, generation of reactive oxygen species from alveolar macrophages, and stimulation of secretion of inflammatory cytokines, chemokines, and fibrogenic factors from alveolar macrophages and/or epithelial cells [7,18]. Although similar mechanism might be deemed for the Aerosil™ 200 particles, further investigations orchestrated on the mechanisms of Aerosil™ 200-induced pleurodesis are recommended.

Both in gross and microscopic assessments, erythromycin was less potent pleurodesis agent than the Aerosil™ 200. This finding is in contrast to that of the previous experimental study indicating that erythromycin was an ideal pleural sclerosing agent, compared with talc, doxycycline and diazepam [2]. Moreover, in a recent clinical study by Balassoulis et al., erythromycin was found as an effective and safe pleurodesing agent in patients with recurrent malignant pleural effusions [19]. However, we do not have an explanation for such a difference in the pleurodesing effect of erythromycin.

Table 1 Treatment-related microscopic and macroscopic findings, n (%)

	Saline (n = 15)	*Erythromycin (n = 15)*	*Tetracycline (n = 15)*	*Aerosil™ 200 (n = 15)*	*Erythromycin + Aerosil™ 200 (n = 15)*
Pleural fibrosis	0 (0)	6 (40%)*	11 (73.3%)	11 (73.3%)	14 (93.3%)**
Pleural inflammation	0 (0)	15 (100%)	15 (100%)	15 (100%)	15 (100%)
Pleural adhesions	0 (0)	10 (66.6%)	11 (73.3%)	14 (93.3%)	13 (86.6%)

Erythromycin treatment and erythromycin plus Aerosil™ 200 treatment significantly resulted in the minimum and maximum number of the pleural fibrosis, respectively (*$P = 0.007$; **$P = 0.02$, Chi-square test).

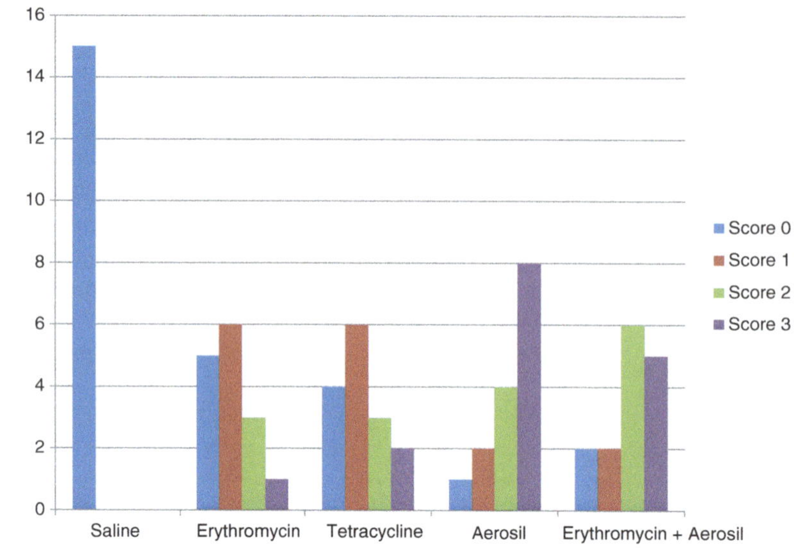

Figure 1 Frequency of macroscopic scores in the treatment groups. Microscopic scores were 0 = normal pleura, 1 = multifocal fibrosis, 2 = diffuse adhesions and 3 = complete obliteration.

Furthermore, tetracycline was not superior to the other pleurodesing agents in the present study. This finding is compatible with that of the previous reports; fibrin tissue adhesive [20], talc [21], and mitoxantrone were found as more effective sclerosing agents than tetracycline for pleurodesis [22]. In contrast, Vargas and colleagues found that tetracycline, rather than bleomycin and *Corynebacterium parvum*, was more potent pleurodesing agent in a rabbit model [23,24]. In a systematic review, tetracycline was reported to be associated with more recurrences when compared to talc [3]. The available clinical evidence supports the use of talc as the sclerosant of choice rather than other sclerosants (tetracycline, bleomycin, or mustine) [1].

This study has certain limitations. We did not investigate talc as a sclerosing agent in the present study. The rationale behind this exclusion was the lack of sterile and pure talc in Iran. Moreover, other routinely used pleurodesing agents such as bleomycin and parenteral doxycycline were not available due to their high costs. Therefore, further studies are recommended to be orchestrated in order to investigate the probable advantage of the Aerosil™ 200 over the most commonly used pleurodesis agents such as sterile and pure talc in terms of efficacy, safety, rapidity of action, mechanism of action or cost. In addition, one may consider the rabbit model as generally more established method for experimental pleurodesis. However, there are a number of experimental studies of pleurodesis on the rats [20,25-27]. Only single dose of 35 mg/kg was studied for each sclerosant, and different doses might have resulted in more favorable responses. However, the applied treatment dosages were based on those of the previous studies. Future studies with larger doses of erythromycin and tetracycline may achieve higher response rates. Furthermore, distant sequelae of the studied pleurodesing agents in

Table 2 Treatment-related macroscopic, microscopic, cellularity, neovascularization and fibrosis scores, mean ± standard deviation (median)

	Saline [a] *(n = 15)*	*Erythromycin* [b] *(n = 15)*	*Tetracycline* [c] *(n = 15)*	*Aerosil™ 200 (n = 15)*	*Erythromycin + Aerosil™ 200* [d] *(n = 15)*	*P value*
Macroscopic score	0 ± 0 (0)	1 ± 0.9 (1)	1.2 ± 1 (1)	2.3 ± 1 (3)	1.9 ± 1 (1)	<0.001
Microscopic score	0 ± 0 (0)	1.2 ± 0.4 (1)	1.5 ± 0.5 (1)	2.1 ± 0.7 (2)	2.1 ± 0.7 (2)	<0.001
Cellularity score	0 ± 0 (0)	1.2 ± 0.4 (1)	1.1 ± 0.4 (1)	2 ± 0.7 (2)	1.7 ± 0.9 (1)	<0.001
Neovascularization score	0 ± 0 (0)	0.8 ± 0.4 (1)	1.4 ± 0.5 (1)	1.1 ± 1.1 (1)	2.1 ± 0.8 (2)	<0.001
Fibrosis score	0 ± 0 (0)	0.4 ± 0.5 (0)	1.3 ± 0.9 (1)	1.5 ± 1.2 (1)	1.1 ± 0.5 (1)	<0.001

[a] All other treatment groups significantly differed from the normal saline group ($P < 0.001$, Kruskal-Wallis test).
[b] Macroscopic, microscopic and cellularity scores in erythromycin group were significantly different from Aerosil™ 200 group ($P < 0.005$, Bonferroni-corrected Mann–Whitney *U* test).
[c] Cellularity score in tetracycline group was significantly different from Aerosil™ 200 group ($P < 0.005$, test as above).
[d] Microscopic, neovascularization and fibrosis scores in erythromycin plus Aerosil™ 200 group were significantly different from the erythromycin group ($P < 0.005$, test as above).

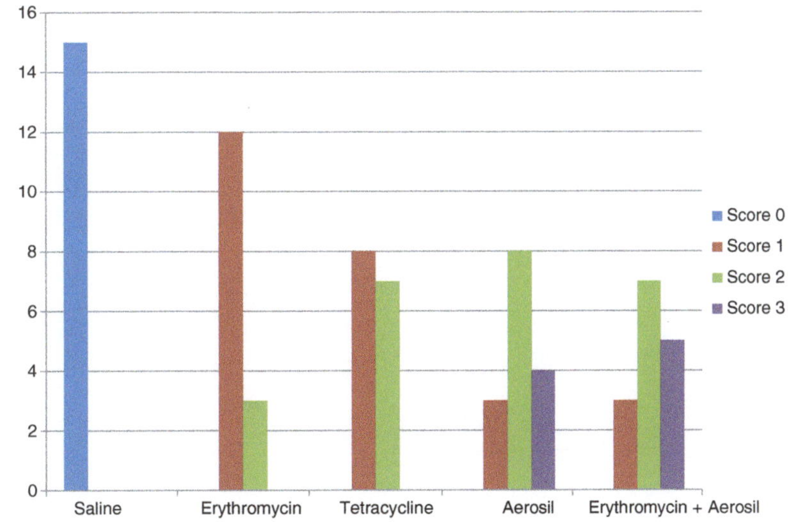

Figure 2 Frequency of microscopic (inflammation/cellularity) scores in the treatment groups. Microscopic (inflammation/cellularity) scores were 0 = absence of cellularity and neovascularisation, 1 = mild cellularity and neovascularisation, 2 = moderate cellularity and neovascularisation, and 3 = severe cellularity and neovascularisation.

the contralateral lung as well as the liver along with their systemic effects were not evaluated. Liver enzyme tests, histopathological assessment of the contralateral lung and the liver, and serum and tissue angiotensin-converting enzyme could have provided precious information regarding the toxicity of the studied pleurodesing agents, in particular the Aerosil™ 200. In addition, grading of the pleurodesis immediately after sacrificing the animals while the tissues were fresh and soft might have yielded to different results. The formalin exposure makes the tissues firm and shrunk, resulting in difficult evaluation of the pleural adhesions [8].

Conclusion

In conclusion, this preliminary study suggests that Aerosil™ 200 with or without erythromycin may be more potent pleurodesis agent than erythromycin and tetracycline. As superiority between Aerosil™ 200 alone and Aerosil™ 200 plus erythromycin could not be determined with the results of the present study, further cost-effective investigations targeting at the distant sequelae of these treatments are required.

Abbreviations

SiO_2: Silicon dioxide; HE: Hematoxylin and eosin..

Competing interests

The authors declare that they have no competing interests.

Authors' contributions

S.H., K.H., K.M., and R.A. participated in the design of study and performed the experimental parts of the research. E.A., S.G. and K.G. participated in acquisition of data, analysis and interpretation of data, drafting the article, and final approval of this version. All authors read and approved the final manuscript.

Acknowledgments

This study was financially supported by a grant from the Tuberculosis and Lung Disease Research Center, Tabriz University of Medical Sciences, Tabriz, Iran.

Author details

[1]Tuberculosis and Lung Disease Research Center, Tabriz University of Medical Sciences, Tabriz, Iran. [2]Department of Cardiovascular Surgery, Shahid Madani Hospital, Tabriz University of Medical Sciences, Tabriz, Iran. [3]Department of General and Thoracic Surgery, Tabriz Branch, Islamic Azad University, Tabriz, Iran. [4]Cardiovascular Research Center, Tabriz University of Medical Sciences, Tabriz, Iran. [5]Physical Medicine and Rehabilitation Research Center, Tabriz University of Medical Sciences, Tabriz, Iran.

References

1. Shaw P, Agarwal R: **Pleurodesis for malignant pleural effusions.** *Cochrane Database Syst Rev* 2004, **1**:CD002916.
2. Miller Q, Meschter C, Neumaster T, Pratt J, Moulton M, Downey D, Harre J: **Comparison of pleurodesis by erythromycin, talc, doxycycline, and diazepam in a rabbit model.** *J Surg Educ* 2007, **64**:41–45.
3. Tan C, Sedrakyan A, Browne J, Swift S, Treasure T: **The evidence on the effectiveness of management for malignant pleural effusion: a systematic review.** *Eur J Cardiothorac Surg* 2006, **29**:829–838.
4. Marchi E, Teixeira LR, Vargas FS: **Management of malignancy-associated pleural effusion: current and future treatment strategies.** *Am J Respir Med* 2003, **2**:261–273.
5. Dikensoy O, Light RW: **Alternative widely available, inexpensive agents for pleurodesis.** *Curr Opin Pulm Med* 2005, **11**:340–344.
6. Merget R, Bauer T, Küpper HU, Philippou S, Bauer HD, Breitstadt R, Bruening T: **Health hazards due to the inhalation of amorphous silica.** *Arch Toxicol* 2002, **75**:625–634.
7. Yeginsu A, Filiz NO, Köseoğlu D, Etikan I: **Bioglass as a pleurodesing agent as effective as talc in rabbits.** *Turkish J Thorac Cardiovasc Surg* 2005, **13**:386–391.
8. Yeginsu A, Ergin M, Ozyurt H, Bassorgun CI: **Pleurodesic effect of bioglass in experimental rabbits.** *Iran Red Crescent Med J* 2009, **11**:254–258.
9. Reuzel PG, Bruijntjes JP, Feron VJ, Woutersen RA: **Subchronic inhalation toxicity of amorphous silicas and quartz dust in rats.** *Food Chem Toxicol* 1991, **29**:341–354.

10. Johnston CJ, Driscoll KE, Finkelstein JN, Baggs R, O'Reilly MA, Carter J, Gelein R, Oberdörster G: **Pulmonary chemokine and mutagenic responses in rats after subchronic inhalation of amorphous and crystalline silica.** *Toxicol Sci* 2000, **56**:405–413.
11. Jouyban A, Shoja MM, Ardalan MR, Khoubnasabjafari M, Sadighi A, Tubbs RS, Agutter PS, Ghabili K: **The effect of quince leaf decoction on renal injury induced by hypercholesterolemia in rabbits: a pilot study.** *J Med Plants Res* 2011, **5**:5291–5295.
12. Ashrafi H, Ghabili K, Alihemmati A, Jouyban A, Shoja MM, Aslanabadi S, Adl FH, Ghavimi H, Hajhosseini L: **The effect of quince leaf (Cydonia oblonga Miller) decoction on testes in hypercholesterolemic rabbits: a pilot study.** *Afr J Tradit Complement Altern Med* 2013, **10**:277–282.
13. Mitchem RE, Herndon BL, Fiorella RM, Molteni A, Battie CN, Reisz GR: **Pleurodesis by autologous blood, doxycycline, and talc in a rabbit model.** *Ann Thorac Surg* 1999, **67**:917–921.
14. Hurewitz AN, Lidonicci K, Wu CL, Reim D, Zucker S: **Histologic changes of doxycycline pleurodesis in rabbits. Effect of concentration and pH.** *Chest* 1994, **106**:1241–1245.
15. Chen Y, Chen J, Dong J, Jin Y: **Comparing study of the effect of nanosized silicon dioxide and microsized silicon dioxide on fibrogenesis in rats.** *Toxicol Ind Health* 2004, **20**:21–27.
16. Choi M, Cho WS, Han BS, Cho M, Kim SY, Yi JY, Ahn B, Kim SH, Jeong J: **Transient pulmonary fibrogenic effect induced by intratracheal instillation of ultrafine amorphous silica in A/J mice.** *Toxicol Lett* 2008, **182**:97–101.
17. Costantini LM, Gilberti RM, Knecht DA: **The phagocytosis and toxicity of amorphous silica.** *PLoS One* 2011, **6**:e14647.
18. Castranova V, Vallyathan V: **Silicosis and coal workers' pneumoconiosis.** *Environ Health Perspect* 2000, **108**:675–684.
19. Balassoulis G, Sichletidis L, Spyratos D, Chloros D, Zarogoulidis K, Kontakiotis T, Bagalas V, Porpodis K, Manika K, Patakas D: **Efficacy and safety of erythromycin as sclerosing agent in patients with recurrent malignant pleural effusion.** *Am J Clin Oncol* 2008, **31**:384–389.
20. Cetin B, Atalay C, Arzu Koçkaya E, Turan Akay M: **The efficacy of fibrin tissue adhesives in pleurodesis in rats.** *Exp Lung Res* 2005, **31**:713–718.
21. Mourad IA, Abdel Rahman AR, Aziz SA, Saber NM, Fouad FA: **Pleurodesis as a palliative treatment of advanced lung cancer with malignant pleural effusion.** *J Egypt Natl Canc Inst* 2004, **16**:188–194.
22. Light RW, Wang NS, Despars JA, Gruer SE, Sassoon C, Vargas FS: **Comparison of mitoxantrone and tetracycline as pleural sclerosing agents in rabbits.** *Lung* 1996, **174**:373–381.
23. Vargas FS, Wang NS, Lee HM, Gruer SE, Sassoon CS, Light RW: **Effectiveness of bleomycin in comparison to tetracycline as pleural sclerosing agent in rabbits.** *Chest* 1993, **104**:1582–1584.
24. Vargas FS, Wang NS, Teixeira LR, Carmo AO, Silva LM, Light RW: **Corynebacterium parvum versus tetracycline as pleural sclerosing agents in rabbits.** *Eur Respir J* 1995, **8**:2174–2177.
25. Gözübüyük A, Ozpolat B, Ciçek AF, Caylak H, Yücel O, Kavaklı K, Gürkök S, Genç O: **Comparison of side effects of oxytetracycline and talc pleurodesis: an experimental study.** *J Cardiothorac Surg* 2010, **5**:128.
26. Ozpolat B, Gazyagci S, Gözübüyük A, Ayva S, Atinkaya C: **Autologous blood pleurodesis in rats to elucidate the amounts of blood required for reliable and reproducible results.** *J Surg Res* 2010, **161**:228–232.
27. Fraticelli A, Robaglia-Schlupp A, Riera H, Monjanel-Mouterde S, Cau P, Astoul P: **Distribution of calibrated talc after intrapleural administration: an experimental study in rats.** *Chest* 2002, **122**:1737–1741.

Fungal transformation of androsta-1,4-diene-3, 17-dione by *Aspergillus brasiliensis*

Tahereh Hosseinabadi[1], Hossein Vahidi[1], Bahman Nickavar[1] and Farzad Kobarfard[2*]

Abstract

Background: The biotransformation of steroids by fungal biocatalysts has been recognized for many years. There are numerous fungi of the genus *Aspergillus* which have been shown to transform different steroid substances. The possibility of using filamentous fungi *Aspergillus brasiliensis* cells in the biotransformation of androsta-1,4-diene-3,17-dione, was evaluated.

Methods: The fungal strain was inoculated into the transformation medium which supplemented with androstadienedione as a substrate and fermentation continued for 5 days. The metabolites were extracted and isolated by thin layer chromatography. The structures of these metabolites were elucidated using ^{1}H-NMR, broadband decoupled ^{13}C-NMR, EI Mass and IR spectroscopies.

Results: The fermentation yielded one reduced product: 17β-hydroxyandrost-1,4-dien-3-one and two hydroxylated metabolites: 11α-hydroxyandrost-1,4-diene-3,17-dione and 12β-hydroxyandrost-1,4-diene-3,17-dione.

Conclusions: The results obtained in this study show that *A. brasiliendsis* could be considered as a biocatalyst for producing important derivatives from androstadienedione.

Keywords: *Aspergillus brasiliensis*, Fungi, Androsta-1, 4-diene-3, 17-dione, Steroid, Biotransformation

Background

Microbial biotransformation by the whole cell microorganisms is economically and ecologically a competitive tool for the biotechnological professionals in search of new techniques to manufacture valuable chemicals, pharmaceutical and agrochemical compounds [1,2]. The production of steroid drugs and hormones is one of the best examples of the successful application of microbial technology in large scale industrial processes [3]. A large number of bacterial and fungal species are able to biotransform steroid compounds [4]. Among them, there are numerous fungi of the genus *Aspergillus* including *A. wentti, A. niger, A. nidulans, A. ochraceus, A. parasiticus, A. oryzae, A. flavus, A. tamari, A. parasiticus* and *A. fumigatus* which have been used for the biotransformation of many steroids and shown to mediate hydroxylation, oxidation, reduction, double bond formation and epoxidation of various steroid substances [5-7]. Insertion of a hydroxyl group to a steroid molecule is one of the most important steps in the production of steroidal derivatives which is carried out by many of filamentous fungi. Several positions in the steroid molecules can be hydroxylated by various microbial strains via their hydroxylase enzyme [8].

The filamentous fungi, *Aspergillus brasiliensis* is a biseriate black species, described and named within *Aspergillus* section *Nigri*, by Varga et al. in 2007. It is differentiable from the other black aspergilla because of its unique morphology, extrolite profiles and genotypic features [9]. Literature review shows that there is no report indicating the ability of this filamentous fungus to modify the structure of steroids. In the present work, the capability of *A. brasiliensis* was evaluated for the biotransformation of androsta-1,4-diene-3,17-dione (ADD) as an exogenous substrate. ADD is one of the most important steroids, which is used as a precursor for preparing some pharmaceutically-interesting steroids. It is commercially produced by the microbiological transformation of β-sitosterol and cholesterol [8]. It is presently used in the industrial synthesis of estradiol or estrone [4,10].

* Correspondence: farzadkf@yahoo.com
[2]Department of Medicinal Chemistry, School of Pharmacy, Shahid Beheshti University of Medical Sciences, Vali-e Asr Ave., Niayesh Junction, Tehran 1996835113, Iran
Full list of author information is available at the end of the article

Biotransformation of this substrate, has already been reported by some other fungi, such as *Mucor racemosus, Acremonium strictum, Cephalosporium aphidicola* and *Neurospora crassa* leading to the production of different compounds [11-14].

Experimental

Materials

ADD was purchased from Sigma- Aldrich. All other chemicals and reagents used, were of analytical grade and commercially available.

Microorganism

The fungal strain *A. brasilliensis* PTCC 5298 was purchased From Iranian Research Organization for Science and Technology (IROST).

Cultures of fungi were grown at 26°C for 5 days until good sporulation was obtained on Czapec medium, consisting of 30 g sucrose, 2.0 g $NaNO_3$, 1.0 g K_2HPO_4, 0.50 g $MgSO_4$, 0.50 g KCl, 0.01 g $FeSO_4$, 15 g Agar and 1000 ml DW, based on IROST catalogue for this fungus [15]. Stock cultures were maintained at 4°C on Czapec medium slopes and freshly subcultured before use in transformation experiments. The organism was transferred to fresh medium and refreshed every two weeks.

Inoculum preparation and biotransformation process

Spores freshly obtained from Czapec slopes were washed with distilled water (DW) containing Tween-80 and transferred aseptically into 500 ml flasks containing 100 ml sterile medium, in a biological safety cabinet (pH of the medium was adjusted to 7.4 before sterilization).

Volume of inoculums, containing 1×10^6 spores, was used in all experiments unless otherwise stated. After cultivation at 26°C for 2 days on a rotary shaker (125 rpm) and pellet formation, ADD (100 mg) was dissolved in 1 ml acetone and aseptically added to each flask. A parallel control without substrate and also a culture medium, containing substrate but no microorganism were run concurrently (as control cultures). Biotransformation was carried out under above condition for further 5 days.

Sampling was carried out every 24 h. The samples were extracted with three volumes of chloroform and the transformation was then checked using thin layer chromatography (TLC).

After detecting the transformation on TLC plate, the fermentation was conducted on the larger scale.

Ten 1000 ml-Erlenmeyer flasks were filled with 200 ml cultivation medium. The culture media were incubated under the same conditions and then 1000 mg of substrate, (dissolved in 10 ml acetone) was distributed evenly among the flasks and process continued for 5 days.

All the experiments were performed in duplicate.

Product isolation and analyses

At the end of incubation, the fungus mycelium was separated from the broth by filtration and the mycelium was rinsed with DW. Mycelia and the filtrate were separately extracted with chloroform (3 volumes), dried over anhydrous sodium sulfate and concentrated under vacuum. The residue was analyzed by TLC, then loaded on chromatography plates and fractionated with chloroform/acetone (6.5:3.5 v/v) as the eluent solvent. The metabolites were then separated from silica gel using a mixture of methanol/chloroform/acetone (three times). The transformation products were analyzed and identified using different spectroscopic data (^{13}C NMR, ^{1}H NMR, FTIR and MS).

Instruments

Melting points (mp) were determined on thermoscientific 9200 apparatus and were uncorrected.

^{1}H and ^{13}C nuclear magnetic resonances (NMR) spectra were recorded using a Bruker DRX (Avance 500) spectrometer (Rheinstetten, Germany) at 500 and 125 MHz, respectively, in $CDCl_3$ with tetramethylsilane (TMS) as the internal standard. Chemical shifts (δ) are given in parts per million (ppm) relative to TMS. The coupling constants (J) are given in hertz (Hz). Infrared (IR) spectra were recorded on a Perkin-Elmer 843 spectrometer with KBr as a diluent. Mass spectra (MS) were obtained using Agilent 6410 Triple Quadrupole mass spectrometer. TLC was conducted on 0.25 mm thick layers of silica gel G (Kieselgel 60 $HF_{254+366}$, Merck). Chromatography plates were developed with chloroform/acetone (3.5:6.5, v/v) and visualized by spraying the plates with a mixture of methanol/ sulfuric acid (6:1, v/v) and heating them in an oven at 100°C for 3 min until the colors developed. The compounds were also visualized under a UV lamp (Strstedt– Gruppe HP-UVIS) at 254 nm.

Results

Microbial transformation of ADD by *A. brasiliensis* in 5 days resulted in the formation of three hydroxysteroid-1,4-dien-3-one derivatives (II to IV), presented in Figure 1. No transformation occurred in the control media. Steroid products were characterized using different spectroscopic data (^{13}C NMR, ^{1}H NMR, FTIR and MS) and melting points.

The analytical data for compounds II–IV are mentioned in a respective order. ^{13}C NMR assignments for the substrates and metabolites are listed in Table 1.

17β-hydroxyandrost-1, 4-diene-3-one (Boldenone) (II)

Colorless crystalline compound; yield 24.5%; mp 169–172°C; R_f (acetone/chloroform 3.5:6.5, v/v): 0.71; IR ν_{max} 3489, 1666, 1619 cm^{-1}; MS (EI) m/z: 286 (M^+, $C_{19}H_{26}O_2$), 227, 159, 147, 121, 91, 77; ^{1}H NMR ($CDCl_3$, 500 MHz) δ 7.07 (1H, d, J = 10 Hz, H-1), 6.22 (1H, d, J = 10 Hz, H-2), 6.07

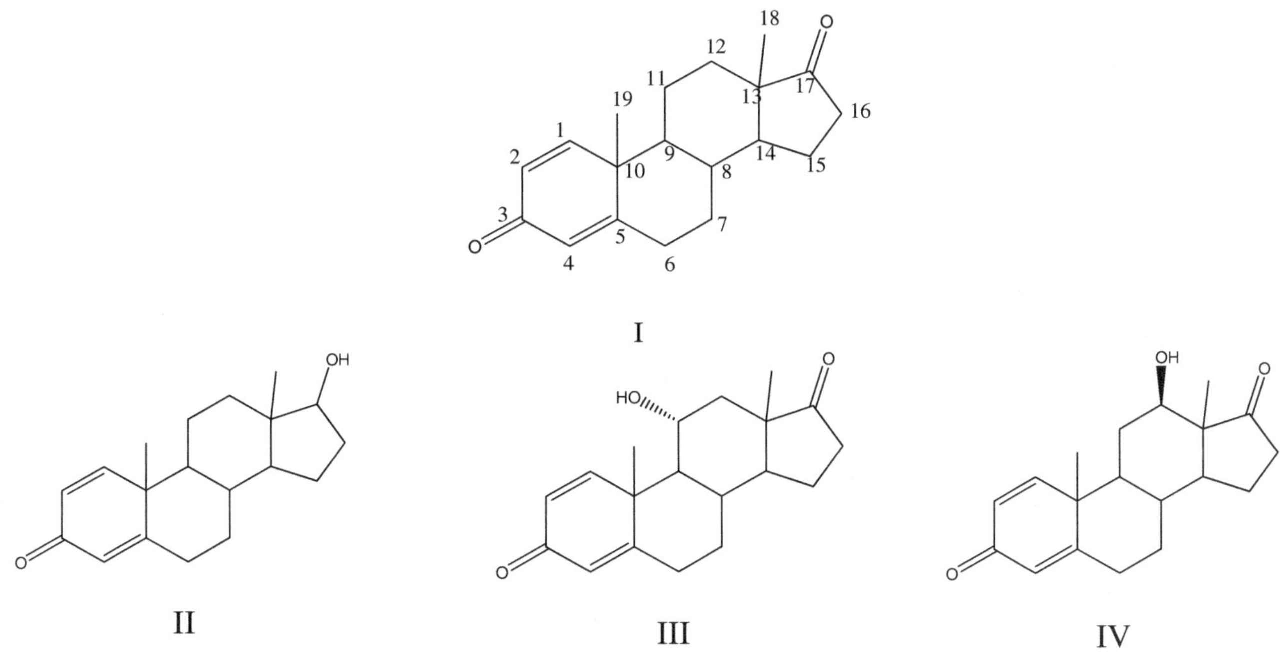

Figure 1 The structure of androstadienedione (I) and its metabolites; 17β-Hydroxyandrost-1,4-diene-3-one (II), 11α-Hydroxyandrost-1, 4-diene-3,17-dione (III) and 12β-Hydroxyandrost-1,4-diene -3,17-dione (IV).

Table 1 ^{13}C NMR data determined in $CDCl_3$ at 500 MHz for compounds I-IV

Carbon atom	I	II	III	IV
1	155.20	156.00	158.81	155.35
2	127.60	127.46	128.80	127.66
3	186.00	186.45	186.77	186.28
4	124.08	123.83	124.71	124.10
5	168.19	169.30	167.66	168.33
6	32.29	32.78	32.85	32.48
7	31.21	33.14	29.70	33.32
8	35.08	35.56	33.96	34.35
9	52.31	52.44	60.48	52.13
10	43.39	43.6	43.0	43.48
11	22.07	22.50	67.69	36.03
12	32.51	36.30	42.29	85.97
13	47.62	43.1	47.85	42.64
14	50.41	50.09	49.59	44.13
15	21.88	23.53	21.85	22.16
16	35.58	30.32	35.79	35.53
17	219.66	81.41	218.25	216.31
18	13.80	11.17	14.59	11.50
19	18.70	18.72	18.65	18.72

(1H, s, H-4), 3.64 (1H, t, $J_{17\alpha,16\alpha\beta}$ = 8.5 Hz, H-17α), 2.06 (1H, m, H-16α), 1.55 (1H, m, H-16β), 1.24 (3H, s, H-19), 0.82 (3H, s, H-18); ^{13}C NMR ($CDCl_3$) δ 186.4 (C-3), 169.3 (C-5), 156.0 (C-1), 127.5 (C-2), 123.8 (C-4), 81.4 (C-17), 18.7 (C-19), 11.1(C-18).

11α-hydroxyandrost-1,4-diene-3,17-dione (III)

Colorless crystalline compound; yield 9.6%; mp 210–214°C; R_f (acetone/chloroform 3.5:6.5, v/v): 0.29; IR ν_{max} 3456, 1737, 1663, 1622 cm^{-1}; MS (EI) m/z: 300 (M^+, $C_{19}H_{24}O_3$), 282 , 231, 161, 124, 109, 84, 55; ^{1}HNMR ($CDCl_3$, 500 MHz): δ 7.27 (1H, d, J = 10 Hz, H-1), 6.15 (1H, d, J = 10 Hz, H-2), 6.08 (1H, s, H-4), 4.12 (1H, m, H-11$_\beta$), 2.31(1H, m, H-12$_\beta$), 1.54 (1H, m, H-12$_\alpha$), 1.24 (3H, s, H-19), 0.96 (3H, s, H-18); ^{13}CNMR ($CDCl_3$) δ 218.2 (C-17), 186.7 (C-3), 167.6 (C-5), 158.8 (C-1), 128.8 (C-2), 124.7 (C-4), 67.69 (C-11), 18.6 (C-19), 14.5 (C-18).

12β-hydroxyandrost-1,4-dien-3,17-dione (IV)

Colorless crystalline compound; yield 10.3%; mp 164–167°C; R_f (acetone/chloroform, 3.5:6.5 v/v): 0.60; IR ν_{max} 3408, 1741, 1661, 1618 cm^{-1}; MS (EI) m/z 300 (M^+, $C_{19}H_{24}O_3$), 161, 147, 134, 122, 91, 55; ^{1}H NMR ($CDCl_3$, 500 MHz) δ 7.06 (1H, d, J = 10 Hz, H-1), 6.24 (1H, d, J = 10 Hz, H-2), 6.07 (1H, s, H-4), 3.74 (1H, s, H-12), 2.03, 1.45 (1H, m, H-11), 1.25 (3H, s, H-19), 0.79 (3H, s, H-18); ^{13}C NMR ($CDCl_3$) δ 216.3 (C-17), 186.3 (C-3), 168.3 (C-5), 155.3 (C-1), 127.6 (C-2), 124.1 (C-4), 85.97 (C-12), 18.7 (C-19), 11.50 (C-18).

Spectra interpretation

The EI-MS spectrum of compound II showed the M^+ at m/z 286 which corresponds to the molecular formula $C_{19}H_{26}O_2$, 2 a.m.u. higher than the molecular weight of parent compound and thus indicated a possible hydrogenation of compound I. The IR spectrum showed an absorbance at 3489 cm^{-1}, characteristic of a hydroxyl group. The lack of absorption band at 1736 cm^{-1} (17-ketone) and the existence of a peak at 3489 cm^{-1}, verify the reduction of the carbonyl group to a hydroxyl group at C-17 position. The ^{1}H-NMR spectrum of II showed an additional methine proton signal at δ 3.64 that is assigned to 17-H. This modification is confirmed by the appearance of a new methine carbon signal at δ 81.41 in ^{13}C-NMR spectra. The stereochemistry of the newly formed hydroxyl group was deduced to be β, based on the chemical shift of 17-H (δ 3.64), its coupling constant (J = 8.5 Hz) and splitting pattern (triplet) which is in agreement with the published data for a C-17α proton in 17β-hydroxysteroids [13,16]. This pattern is often seen when the 17β position is substituted with a hydroxyl group (e.g. pregnan-20-ones7 or androstan-17β-ols) [17]. In the case of 17α-hydroxy steroids, the splitting of H-17 β is generally a doublet [18].

The EI-MS spectrum of the transformed product III, showed the M^+ at m/z 300 (calcd for $C_{19}H_{24}O_3$ 300.1749), which was 16 a.m.u. higher than the molecular weight of compound I, thus suggesting the possible hydroxylation of it. The IR spectrum displayed hydroxyl signal at 3456 cm^{-1}. ^{1}H- and ^{13}C-NMR spectra were very similar to those of the substrate, except for a new downfield methine proton signal at δ 4.12 (ddd, $J_{11\beta,12\beta}$ = 12.2 Hz, $J_{11\beta,9\alpha}$ = 10.3 Hz, $J_{11\beta,12\alpha}$ = 5.4 Hz) which was assigned to the methine H-11 geminal to OH and with a downfield methine carbon signal at δ 67.69. This finding is also confirmed by the data reported in literature for this compound [13].

The mass spectrum for compound IV, showed the molecular ion peak at *m/z* 300 ($C_{19}H_{24}O_3$), which suggested the possible insertion of one oxygen atom in the structure of the substrate (I). The IR spectrum, showed two carbonyl absorption bands at 1741 and 1661 cm^{-1} for C-17 and C-3 respectively. The absorbance at 3408 cm^{-1}, confirmed the existance of a hydroxyl group. Melting point, ^{13}C-NMR and ^{1}H-NMR spectral data, assignments and chemical shifts for this compound were in agreement with those which have been reported by Zafar et al. in 2013 for 12β-hydroxyandrost-1,4-dien-3,17-dione [19].

Discussion

In light of the results obtained in this study, it appears that the *A. brasiliensis* transformation of ADD led to the formation of three major bioproducts. The bioconversion characteristics observed were 17-ketone reduction, 11α and 12β-hydroxylation.

ADD is one of the important intermediates for producing some valuable pharmaceutical steroid compounds and has been used in many studies as a substrate of the biotransformation experiments [20]. Compound II, Boldenone, also called 1-dehydrotestosterone or androsta-1, 4-dien-17β-ol-3-one, is a steroid which only differs from testosterone by one double bond at position 1. Reduction of 17-keto group of ADD results in formation of boldenone. Boldenone with its low androgenic characteristics but strong anabolic characteristics allows improving anabolic processes like growth and development of muscle mass without any undesired side-effects [21].

Reduction of 17-carbonyl group of ADD has been reported previously by *Mucor racemosus* and *Acremonium strictum* and *Cephalosporium aphidicola* fermention [11,12]. 11α-hydroxyandrost-1,4-diene-3,17-dione (III) which is used in the preparation of anti-osteoporosis active compounds, has been previously obtained by ADD biotransformation in *Cephalosporium aphidicola, Rhizopus arrhizus* and *Aspergillus ochraceus* culture media [13,20,22]. It has also been reported by fermentation of dihydrotestosterone (DHT) with *Gibberella fujikuroi.* This compound which is significant and specific inhibitor of butyrylcholinesterase (BChE), in comparison to standard drug, galanthamine. 12β-hydroxyandrost-1,4-diene-3,17-dione (IV) was also another hydroxylated steroid which has been obtained from DHT biotransformation by *G. fujikuroi* [19]. Although hydroxylation of steroidal substrates is common by filamentous fungi, hydroxylation at C-12 position is relatively rare [6]. The 12β-hydroxylation is proprietary reaction for filamentous fungi and is unknown in humans [23]. Introduction of a C-12 substituent and especially a β C-12 substituent into glucocorticoids improves their usefulness as topical anti-inflammatories by increasing their topical activity relative to their systemic activity [24]. Therefore from an industrial viewpoint, the ability of *A. brasiliensis* to carry out 12β-hydroxylation on ADD substrate may be interesting as a process for production of glucocorticoids.

Conclusion

The present research shows that the transformation of androstendienedione using *A. brasiliensis* whole cells yielded interesting transformation products. The observed modifications included hydroxylation at C-11α, C-12β and 17-carbonyl reduction into the related C-17β hydroxyl forms. These products were separated and characterized on the basis of their spectral data. To the best of our knowledge, there are only few reports for ADD biotransformation by microorganisms and also no report for *A. brasiliensis.* Therefore *A. brasiliensis* could be considered as efficient biocatalyst for preparation of new steroids with commercial significance.

Abbreviations

ADD: Androsta-1,4-diene-3,17-dione; DHT: Dihydrotestosterone; TLC: Thin layer chromatography; NMR: Nuclear magnetic resonances.

Competing interests

The authors declare that they have no competing interests.

Authors' contributions

All authors contributed to developing the study protocol. In addition, TH participated in project proposal and design, literature search, carried out whole analytic experiments, involved in analysis some part of data and interpretation of spectral data and drafted the manuscript. HV contributed to fermentation technique and supported the culture of microorganism. FK contributed to interpretation of the spectral data, structure elucidation and revising the manuscript. BN participated in project proposal and design, separation techniques and analysis of some part of data. All authors approved the final manuscript.

Acknowledgements

The authors would like to thank Research Deputy of Shahid Beheshti University of Medical Sciences in Iran for the financial support for this research. This study was a part of PhD thesis of Tahereh Hosseinabadi, proposed and approved in Faculty of Pharmacy, Shahid Beheshti University of Medical Sciences, Tehran, Iran.

Author details

[1]Department of Pharmacognosy and Biotechnology, School of Pharmacy, Shahid Beheshti University of Medical Sciences, Vali-e Asr Ave., Niayesh Junction, Tehran 1996835113, Iran. [2]Department of Medicinal Chemistry, School of Pharmacy, Shahid Beheshti University of Medical Sciences, Vali-e Asr Ave., Niayesh Junction, Tehran 1996835113, Iran.

References

1. Carballeira J, Quezada M, Hoyos P, Simeó Y, Hernaiz M, Alcantara A, Sinisterra J: **Microbial cells as catalysts for stereoselective red–ox reactions.** *Biotechnol Adv* 2009, **27**:686–714.
2. Luo J, Liang Q, Shen Y, Chen X, Yin Z, Wang M: **Biotransformation of bavachinin by three fungal cell cultures.** *J Biosci Bioeng* 2014, **117**:191–196.
3. Mohamed SS, El-Refai AMH, El-Raoof Sallam LA, Abo-Zied KM, Hashem AGM, Ali HA: **Biotransformation of progesterone to hydroxysteroid derivatives by whole cells of *Mucor racemosus*.** *Malay J Microbiol* 2013, **9**:237–244.
4. Bhatti HN, Khera RA: **Biological transformations of steroidal compounds: a review.** *Steroids* 2012, **77**:1267–1290.
5. Fernandes P, Cruz A, Angelova B, Pinheiro HM, Cabral JMS: **Microbial conversion of steroid compounds: recent developments.** *Enzyme Microb Tech* 2003, **32**:688–705.
6. Mahato SB, Garai S: **Advances in microbial steroid biotransformation.** *Steroids* 1997, **62**:332–345.
7. Hunter AC, Coyle E, Morse F, Dedi C, Dodd HT, Koussoroplis SJ: **Transformation of 5-ene steroids by the fungus *Aspergillus tamarii* KITA: mixed molecular fate in lactonization and hydroxylation pathways with identification of a putative 3β-hydroxy-steroid dehydrogenase/Δ5-Δ4 isomerase pathway.** *BBA - Mol Cell Biol L* 2009, **1791**:110–117.
8. Donova MV, Egorova OV: **Microbial steroid transformations: current state and prospects.** *Appl Microbiol Biot* 2012, **94**:1423–1447.
9. Varga J, Kocsubé S, Tóth B, Frisvad JC, Perrone G, Susca A, Meijer M, Samson RA: ***Aspergillus brasiliensis* sp. nov., a biseriate black *Aspergillus* species with world-wide distribution.** *Int J Syst Evol Micr* 2007, **57**:1925–1932.
10. Sripalakit P, Wichai U, Saraphanchotiwitthaya A: **Biotransformation of various natural sterols to androstenones by *Mycobacterium* sp. and some steroid-converting microbial strains.** *J Mol Catal B Enzym* 2006, **41**:49–54.
11. Faramarzi MA, Zolfaghary N, Yazdi MT, Adrangi S, Rastegar H, Amini M, Badiee M: **Microbial conversion of androst-1,4-dien-3,17-dione by *Mucor racemosus* to hydroxysteroid-1,4-dien-3-one derivatives.** *J Chem Technol Biot* 2009, **84**:1021–1025.
12. Faramarzi MA, Yazdi MT, Jahandar H, Amini M, Monsef-Esfahani HR: **Studies on the microbial transformation of androst-1,4-dien-3,17-dione with *Acremonium strictum*.** *J Ind Microbiol Biot* 2006, **33**:725–733.
13. ChoudHary MI, Musharraf SG, Shaheen F, Atta-Ur-Rahman: **Microbial transformation of (+)-androsta-1, 4-diene-3, 17-dione by *Cephalosporium aphidicola*.** *Nat Prod Lett* 2002, **16**:377–382.
14. Faramarzi MA, Hajarolasvadi N, Yazdi MT, Amini M, Aghelnejad M: **Microbiological hydroxylation of androst-1,4-dien-3,17-dione by *Neurospora crassa*.** *Biocatal Biotransform* 2007, **25**:72–78.
15. Atlas RM: *Handbook of Microbiological Media.* 3rd edition. Florida: CRC press; 2004.
16. Bridgeman J, Cherry P, Clegg A, Evans J, Jones ER, Kasal A, Kumar V, Meakins G, Morisawa Y, Richards E: **Microbiological hydroxylation of steroids. Part I. Proton magnetic resonance spectra of ketones, alcohols, and acetates in the androstane, pregnane, and oestrane series.** *J Chem Soc C: Organic* 1970, **2**:250–257.
17. Kirk DN, Harold C, Robert W: **A survey of the high-field 1H NMR spectra of the steroid hormones, their hydroxylated derivatives, and related compounds.** *J Chem Soc, Perkin Transactions* 1990, **2**:1567–1594.
18. Choudhary MI, Sultan S, Hassan Khan MT, Yasin A, Shaheen F, Atta-Ur-Rahman: **Biotransformation of (+)-androst-4-ene-3, 17-dione.** *Nat Prod Res* 2004, **18**:529–535.
19. Zafar S, Choudhary MI, Dalvandi K, Mahmood U, Ul-Haq Z: **Molecular docking simulation studies on potent butyrylcholinesterase inhibitors obtained from microbial transformation of dihydrotestosterone.** *Chem Cent J* 2013, **7**:164.
20. Holland HL, Chenchaiah PC: **Microbial hydroxylation of steroids. 11. Hydroxylation of A-nor-, B-homo-Δ1-, and Δ1-testosterone acetates by *Rhizopus arrhizus*.** *Can J Chem* 1985, **63**:1127–1131.
21. Verheyden K, Noppe H, Zorn H, Van Immerseel F, Bussche JV, Wille K, Bekaert K, Janssen C, De Brabander H, Vanhaecke L: **Endogenous boldenone-formation in cattle: alternative invertebrate organisms to elucidate the enzymatic pathway and the potential role of edible fungi on cattle's feed.** *J Steroid Biochem Mol Biol* 2010, **119**:161–170.
22. Bird TGC, Fredericks PM, Jones ER, Meakins GD: **Microbiological hydroxylation. Part 23. Hydroxylations of fluoro-5α-androstanones by the fungi *Calonectria decora*, *Rhizopus nigricans*, and *Aspergillus ochraceus*.** *J Chem Soc, Perkin Transactions* 1980, **1**:750–755.
23. Ye M, Qu G, Guo H, Guo D: **Specific 12β-hydroxylation of cinobufagin by filamentous fungi.** *Appl Environ Microbiol* 2004, **70**:3521–3527.
24. Avery MA, Detre G, Tanabe M, Yasuda D: **Topically active steroidal anti-inflammatory agents.** U.S. Patent 4,910,192, issued March 20, 1990.

Silymarin effect on amyloid-β plaque accumulation and gene expression of APP in an Alzheimer's disease rat model

Parichehreh Yaghmaei[1*], Katia Azarfar[1], Mehrooz Dezfulian[2] and Azadeh Ebrahim-Habibi[3,4*]

Abstract

Background: The deposition of amyloid peptides is associated with Alzheimer's disease (AD). These amyloid peptides are derived from the amyloid protein precursor (APP). Silymarin, a standardized extract of milk thistle, which is currently used in liver diseases, may be effective in the inhibition of amyloid formation. However, its effect has not been assessed on APP expression.

Results: In this study, first, the effect of silymarin was examined on the passive avoidance learning in a rat model of AD. This model was induced by the intracerebroventricular injection of Aβ peptide ($A\beta_{1-42}$) in Wistar rats. Rats were treated with 70 and 140 mg/kgof the extract, once a day, for 4 weeks. Memory function that was evaluated in a shuttle-cage test, showed improvement upon administration of this extract. Brain amyloid plaques had also decreased upon administration of the extract. Furthermore, APP gene expression was compared in treated and untreated groups. The result showed that silymarin was able to suppress APP expression.

Conclusion: Our results are in accordance with the *in vitro* tests concerning the positive antiamyloidogenic property of the main component of silymarin, namely silibinin. We suggest that the beneficial effect of sylimarin in the AD model is related to its capacity to disaggregate amyloid plaques and to suppress APP expression. Considering the limited side effects of silymarin, this compound could be of use in AD therapy.

Keywords: Silymarin, RT-PCR, Passive avoidance learning, Alzheimer's disease, Beta amyloid

Background

Alzheimer's disease (AD) is a progressive neurodegenerative disorder which has been characterized by the existence of extraneuronal aggregates of amyloid β (Aβ) peptide as well as intraneuronal deposits of hyperphosphorylated tau [1]. It is usually assumed that Aβ (abeta) aggregation in the brain is the starting trigger of a pathological cascade which ultimately leads to synaptic dysfunction and loss, neuronal death, and eventually cognitive dysfunction [2]; the process includes also oxidative stress and inflammatory response, which play their roles in neuronal dysfunction [3,4]. It is suggested that the reactive microglia and astrocytes that surround the Aβ plaques in the AD brain may release reactive oxygen species and proinflammatory molecules [5].

Various isoforms of Aβ peptide with lengths varying from 14 to 42 aminoacids have been characterized which are derivated from "APP", the amyloid precursor protein (APP) [6,7]. However, it is generally accepted that the main dominant forms of Aβ (40 and 42 aminoacids) are the toxic species involved in AD pathophysiology, as for example, it has been shown that the presence of Aβ 42 in cerebrospinal fluid could be a reliable predictor of AD progression [8].

The intracerebroventricular administration of Aβ peptide into rodent brain has been used as a mean to simulate AD disease, since this injection could induce histological and biochemical changes as well as oxidative damage and inflammatory responses which result into memory deficits [9,10]. With this animal model, *in vivo* studies could be performed to test potential new candidates for AD therapy.

* Correspondence: yaghmaei_p@srbiau.ac.ir; aehabibi@sina.tums.ac.ir
[1]Department of Biology, Science and Research Branch, Islamic Azad University, Tehran, Iran
[3]Biosensor Research Center, Endocrinology and Metabolism Molecular-Cellular Sciences Institute, Tehran University of Medical Sciences, Tehran, Iran
Full list of author information is available at the end of the article

The flavonoid silibinin (or sylibin) [(2*R*,3*R*)-3,5,7-trihydroxy-2-[(2*R*,3*R*)-3-(4-hydroxy-3-methoxyphenyl)-2-(hydroxy-methyl)-2,3-dihydrobenzo[*b*][1,4]doxin-6-yl] chroman-4-one] is the main compound of the herb milk thistle (*Silybum marianum*) extract (silymarin) [11]. This compound possess anti-inflammatory and antioxidative effects [12]. It has also been reported that silymarin has protective effects against ethanol-induced brain injury [13], and neurotoxicity induced by lipopolysaccharide (LPS) [14]. In this study, we investigated the effect of silymarin on the memory impairment induced by Aβ1-42 injection in rats. We also examined its effect on changes in APP gene expression in the rats' brain.

Materials and methods

Animals

Male Wistar rats weighing 250 ±300 g were housed at six per cage (42 × 26 cm), 23 ± 0.5°C, under a 12/12-h light/dark cycle (lights on from 8:00 AM to 8:00 PM). Animals had free access to standard pellet food and water. Behavioral experiments were carried out in a sound-attenuated room, to which the rats were habituated for at least 1 hour. All experiments were performed in accordance with to the international guidelines set out in the *Guide for the Care and Use of Laboratory Animals* (Institute of Laboratory Animal Resources, 1996) and approved by the Research and Ethics Committee of Science and Research Branch, Azad University.

Inducing Alzheimer's disease in animals and used compound

Aβ1-42 (Sigma, St Louis, MO, USA), was dissolved in PBS and incubated at 37°C for 7 days, after which bilateral surgery and injection of Aβ1-42 peptide was done in rats hippocampus with the help of a stereotaxic apparatus (SR-6 N Narishig, Japan) [15]. Ketamine and xylazin (Alfasan,Woerden-Holland) were used to anesthetize the rats. Injection was performed slowly into the CA1 region of the hippocampus at both sides of the brain as mentioned in the Paxinos atlas [16].

Silymarin tablets, containing ethyl acetate extracted Silymarin, were purchased from Goldaru Pharmaceutical Laboratory, (Isfahan, Iran) and suspended in a distilled water solution. Treatment group was administered two different dosages of the compound (70 and 140 mg/kg/day P.O.) for 4 weeks after the injection with Aβ*1–42*. A volume of 0.1 ml/10 g body weight was used.

Animals were divided into four groups with n = 6: the control group did not undergo surgery, the sham group underwent surgery (AD inducing) and ws given distilled water 7 days after surgery, the experimental groups Exp1 and Exp2 received 70 and 140 mg/kg/day of the compound respectively (7 days after surgery).

Testing the treatment efficacy

a. Passive avoidance test
A shuttle-cage consisting of two compartments of equal size (26 × 26 cm) separated by a sliding door (8 × 8 cm) was used. The shock compartment was dark in contrast to the starting compartment. Each experiment started with a pre-training trial, where the rat was placed in the starting compartment for 5 seconds, after which the sliding door was raised, and the rat was allowed to stay in the dark compartment for 10 seconds. The rat was then put back in its cage and stayed there for 30 minutes after which it was again put into the shuttle box, and this time, after entering the dark compartment, a footshock (50 Hz, 1 mA, and 5 s) was delivered. The rat was then put back into cage and stayed there for 120 seconds. When put back in the shuttle box, if a latency (in the order of 120 seconds) is observed before entering the dark compartment, successful acquisition of passive avoidance is recorded. A similar procedure was used 24 hours after training sessions to make a retention test for evaluating long-term memory. Higher or lower latencies are taken as indicative of increase or decrease in memory retention [17].
b. Histological studies of brain tissue
At the end of experiment animals were decapitated under anesthesia and their brain removed for histological assessments. First, the brains were fixed in 10% formalin and later processed for embedding with paraffin, after which serial sections in 6 mm of thickness were prepared. For staining of hippocampus cells, Thioflavin-S method which is detected by fluorescent microscopy was used [18].
c. Assessing amyloid precursor protein (APP) expression
Semi-quantitative RT-PCR was performed to assess APP expression. RNA was extracted from the homogenized brain tissue of the rats by use of RNX plus kit (CinnaGen, Iran). Isolated RNA was reverse-transcribed using the following gene-specific primers: 5′-GGA TGC GGA GTT CGG ACA TG −3′ (forward) and 5′-GTT CTG CAT CTG CTC AAA G −3′(reverse). GAPDH was used as housekeeping gene as a control [5′- GACATGCCGCCTGGAGAAAC −3 ' (forward) and 5′- AGCCCAGGATGCCCTTTAGT −3′ (reverse)]. The difference in threshold cycles between APP gene and GAPDH gives the standardized expression level. PCR were performed using the One-Step SYBR PrimeScript RT-PCR kit (Cinagen,Tehran-Iran). The reaction profile consisted of a first round at 95°C for 3 min and then 40 cycles of denaturation at 95°C for 30 s, annealing at 57°C for 30 s, and extension at 72°C for30 s, with a final extension reaction carried out at

72°C for 10 min. The RT-PCR products were loaded onto agarose gels and the resulting bands from electrophoresis were photographed with a UV transillumnator.

Statistical analyses

The results are expressed as the mean ± S.E.M. Statistical significance was determined with the one-way ANOVA followed by Tukey's multiple comparisons test. A Pearson correlation analysis was performed to elucidate the relationships. $p < 0.05$ was taken as a significant level of difference.

Results

Passive avoidance test

Both experimental groups showed significantly longer step-through latency compared to control group ($p < 0.05$) both in the training (Figure 1A) and test (Figure 1B) days.

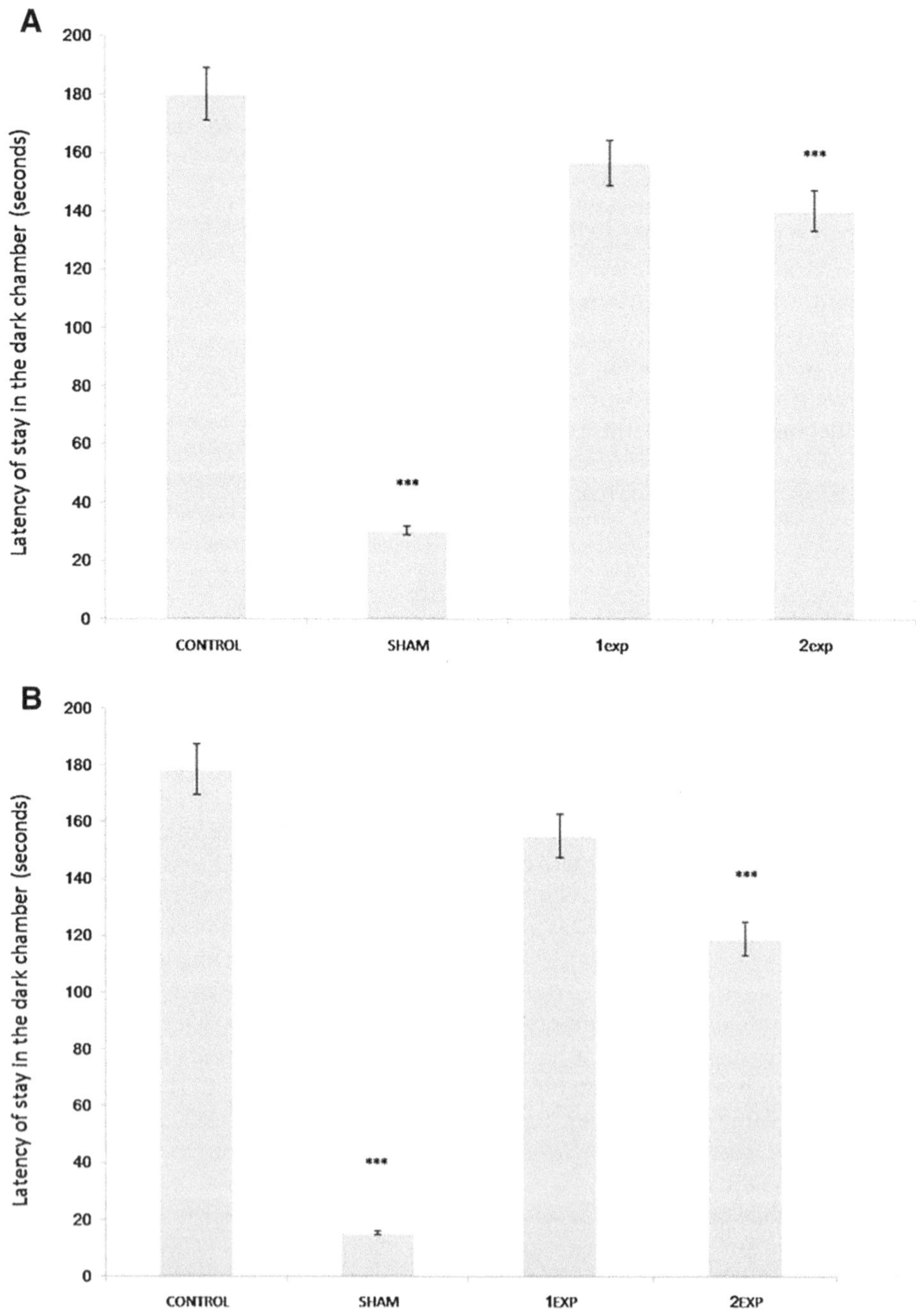

Figure 1 The mean latency to enter the dark chamber on the training (A) and test day (B). *** is indicative of ($P < 0.001$). 1Exp group was treated with 70 mg/kg Silymarinan and 2Exp group had received 140mg/kg Silymarin.

However, it is interesting to note that the 2Exp group, which had received a higher dose of silymarin showed slightly lower results in comparison with the 1Exp group. The 1Exp group has no significant difference in the step-through latency compared with the control group.

Histological studies of brain tissue

ThT staining was used to show the formation of plaques in the abeta-treated brain tissues. Usually, amyloid plaques could be detected in different areas of the brain, including the hippocampus and cortex (for an example of whole brain sections showing plaques distribution see Figure three A,B in reference # [19]). In the present study, both these areas were observed separately with regard to plaques concentration. The normal hippocampus and cortex tissues are showed in Figure 2A. Upon injection of abeta, plaques are formed in both tissues and observed as lighter areas (Figure 2B and C showing the cortex and hippocampus respectively). Treatment with silymarin is effective in diminishing the plaques amount, but here too, administration of 70 mg/Kg of the compound (Figure 2D and E) has a better effect than the higher used dose of 140 mg/Kg (Figure 2F and G).

Amyloid precursor protein (APP) expression

Results of electrophoresis are shown in Figure 3. When the housekeeping gene GAPDH is seen in all samples, APP expression is detected in the sham group, which had only received the compound solvent, and is absent in both experimental groups.

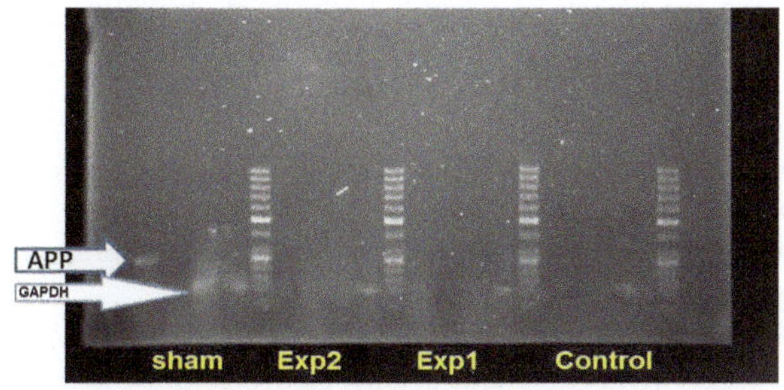

Figure 3 RT-PCR results comparing gene expression of control, sham and experimental groups. The locations of the housekeeping gene and APP are indicated by arrows.

Discussion

From the different theories that try to explain AD pathology, two have been more focused on: the cholinergic theory, which points to the decrease of acetyl choline as the main cause of the disease [20,21] and the amyloid hypothesis, which considers the aggregation of different derivatives of APP as having an important role in the pathophysiology of AD [22]. Therapeutic approaches may

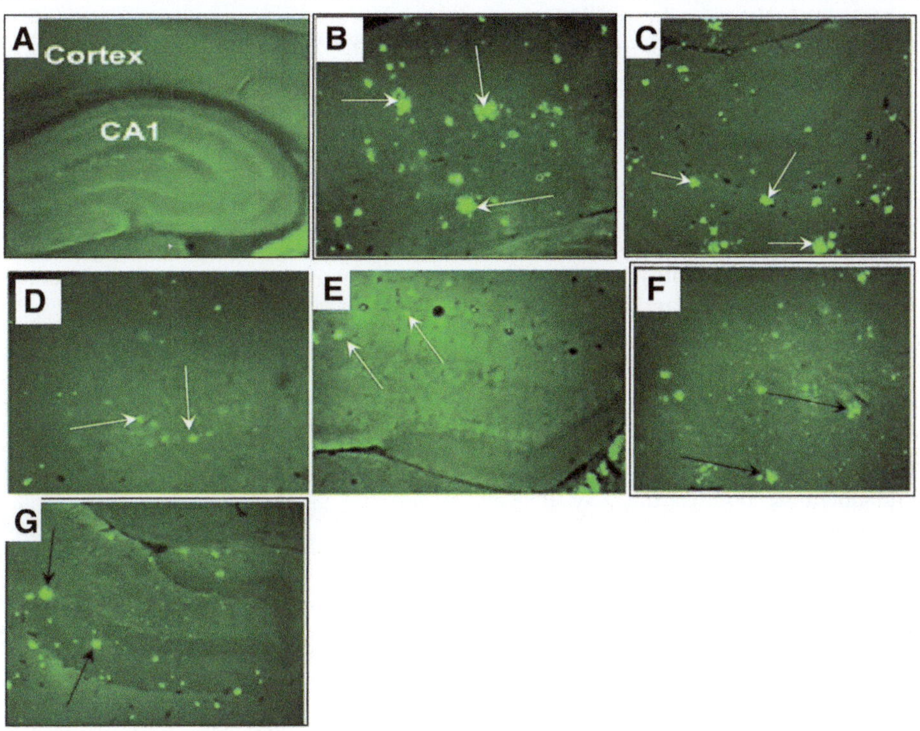

Figure 2 Brain slices from the frontal cortex &hippocampus with a magnification of 40. (A), control group, **(B,C)**, sham group: arrows indicate positions where abeta plaques accumulation has occured, **(D,E)** 1Ex group which was treated with 70 mg/kg silymarin and **(F,G)** 2Ex group which was treated with 140mg/kg silymarin. **B,D,** and **E** correspond to the cortex whereas **C,E,** and **G** correspond to the hippocampus.

include the design of acetyl cholinesterase inhibitors [23] as well as efforts toward finding Aβ aggregation blockers [24], or compounds that would inhibit secretases, i.e. enzymes which cleave APP to Aβ peptides of various length [25]. Some researchers have also tried to employ two or more therapeutic approaches simultaneously, or to find molecules that could affect more than one therapeutic target [26].

Abeta deposits are directly associated with AD. Various isoforms of abeta are derived from the precursor APP, including Aβ25–35 which is one of the most toxic species detected in the brain of AD patients [27,28]. At any rate, administration of abeta variants has led to cognitive impairement [9,29,30] which has also been observed in the present study. The hippocampus is known to be the part of the brain which is first affected by AD [31] and the result of this damage shows itself by cognitive impairement [32] that has been assessed here by the shuttle-box test.

Silymarin, the extract of *Silybum marianum* that contains flavonolignans, has been shown to possess multiple therapeutic properties, including protective effect against nerve damage and brain aging [33,34]. This extract may act via its antioxidant which could protect cells from oxidative stress damage [33], as it has been shown that silymarin effect against oxidative stress may be the result of an increase in reduced glutathione, ascorbic acid and superoxide dismutase levels [35]. Silymarin had also a neuroprotective effect in diabetic mice brains [36], and in mice treated with the brain damaging drug metamphetamine [37]. Previous studies have also reported the beneficial effect of silymarin on Aβ plaques formation, and the effect was suggested to be related to microglial inflammation reduction and direct effect on Aβ accumulation by blocking its aggregation in an Alzheimer's disease model of transgenic mice [19].

As a matter of fact, silibinin has the ability to inhibit the amyloid structure formation of various model or pathogenic proteins *in vitro*, including $A\beta_{1-42}$ [38] human islet amyloid polypeptide [39], and human insulin and albumin [40]. This may be suggestive of a generic anti-amyloidogenic effect for this compound, as it has been suggested/observed for various other aromatic/polyphenolic molecules [41,42]. It should be pointed out that in the present study, what has been observed is a disaggregative effect of silymarin on Aβ plaques, since the decrease of plaques was observed *after* they had been formed. This is an important fact, which is directly suggestive of a potential therapeutic effect for the compounds that are able to act on existing fibrils. The current view in the search for AD therapeutic compounds is preferably directed toward compounds that could preserve the native conformation of peptides that may form amyloid structure [43] or to focus on compounds that inhibit the formation of intermediate structures in the course of amyloid formation [44,45]. However, it could make sense to include the compounds that have destabilizing effect on pre-formed fibrils into the spectra of potential AD therapies.

Flavonoids are able to cross the blood brain barrier [46], a fact that should also be true about silymarin, given its established neuroprotective effect [47]. Furthermore, this extract presents few side effects and drug interactions [48] which makes it a quite interesting potential drug for AD. Silymarin is already used as adjuvant therapy in liver insufficiency [49], which is another positive point for a potential drug candidate.

The beneficial effect of silymarin on the short term memory of rats is thus related with less abeta plaques, but also, as demonstrated in the present study, with a negative regulatory effect on the APP gene expression. Increased expression of APP has been detected in the ageing brain [50], and specifically related to AD pathophysiology [51]. Furthermore, the overexpression of APP that is present in the established transgenic mouse model of AD is definitely linked to the pathological characteristics of the model [52].

As far as we know, this should be a first report about the extract effect on APP, which is expanding our knowledge about the mechanism of action of silibinin in attenuating AD symptoms.

Competing interests
The authors declare that they have no competing interest.

Authors' contributions
PY has designed and supervised the project, analyzed the data and advised on writing the paper. This report is part of the results of KA MSc thesis project who performed experiments and wrote the first draft of the manuscript. MD has been an advisor to the thesis, supervised studies and analyzed data. A.E-H. advised on the project, analyzed data, and finalized the manuscript. All authors read and approved the final manuscript.

Author details
[1]Department of Biology, Science and Research Branch, Islamic Azad University, Tehran, Iran. [2]Department of Microbiology, College of Science, Islamic Azad University, Karaj Branch, Karaj, Iran. [3]Biosensor Research Center, Endocrinology and Metabolism Molecular-Cellular Sciences Institute, Tehran University of Medical Sciences, Tehran, Iran. [4]Endocrinology and Metabolism Research Center, Endocrinology and Metabolism Clinical Sciences Institute, Tehran University of Medical Sciences, North Kargar Avenue, 1411413137 Tehran, Iran.

References
1. Blennow K, de Leon MJ, Zetterberg H: **Alzheimer's disease.** *Lancet* 2006, **368**(9533):387–403.
2. Walsh DM, Selkoe DJ: **Deciphering the molecular basis of memory failure in Alzheimer's disease.** *Neuron* 2004, **44**(1):181–193.
3. Butterfield DA, Reed T, Newman SF, Sultana R: **Roles of amyloid beta-peptide-associated oxidative stress and brain protein modifications in the pathogenesis of Alzheimer's disease and mild cognitive impairment.** *Free Radic Biol Med* 2007, **43**(5):658–677.
4. Farfara D, Lifshitz V, Frenkel D: **Neuroprotective and neurotoxic properties of glial cells in the pathogenesis of Alzheimer's disease.** *J Cell Mol Med* 2008, **12**(3):762–780.

5. Combs CK, Karlo JC, Kao S-C, Landreth GE: **Beta-amyloid stimulation of microglia and monocytes results in TNF alpha dependent expression of inducible nitric oxide synthase and neuronal apoptosis.** *J Neurosci* 2001, **21**(4):1179–1188.
6. Portelius E, Brinkmalm G, Tran AJ, Zetterberg H, Westman-Brinkmalm A, Blennow K: **Identification of novel APP/Abeta isoforms in human cerebrospinal fluid.** *Neurodegener Dis* 2009, **6**(3):87–94.
7. Portelius E, Mattsson N, Andreasson U, Blennow K, Zetterberg H: **Novel a isoforms in Alzheimers disease-their role in diagnosis and treatment.** *Curr Pharm Des* 2011, **17**(25):2594–2602.
8. van Harten AC, Visser PJ, Pijnenburg YA, Teunissen CE, Blankenstein MA, Scheltens P, van der Flier WM: **Cerebrospinal fluid Abeta42 is the best predictor of clinical progression in patients with subjective complaints.** *Alzheimers Dement* 2013, **9**(5):481–487.
9. Frautschy SA, Baird A, Cole GM: **Effects of injected Alzheimer beta-amyloid cores in rat brain.** *Proc Natl Acad Sci U S A* 1991, **88**(19):8362–8366.
10. Maurice T, Lockhart BP, Privat A: **Amnesia induced in mice by centrally administered beta-amyloid peptides involves cholinergic dysfunction.** *Brain Res* 1996, **706**(2):181–193.
11. Kvasnicka F, Biba B, Sevcik R, Voldrich M, Kratka J: **Analysis of the active components of silymarin.** *J Chromatogr A* 2003, **990**(1–2):239–245.
12. Kren V, Walterova D: **Silybin and silymarin–new effects and applications.** *Biomed Pap Med Fac Univ Palacky Olomouc Czech Repub* 2005, **149**(1):29–41.
13. la Grange L, Wang M, Watkins R, Ortiz D, Sanchez ME, Konst J, Lee C, Reyes E: **Protective effects of the flavonoid mixture, silymarin, on fetal rat brain and liver.** *J Ethnopharmacol* 1999, **65**(1):53–61.
14. Lu P, Mamiya T, Lu LL, Mouri A, Zou LB, Nagai T, Hiramatsu M, Ikejima T, Nabeshima T: **Silibinin prevents amyloid β peptide-induced memory impairment and oxidative stress in mice.** *Br J Pharmacol* 2009, **157**(7):1270–1277.
15. Cetin F, Dincer S: **The effect of intrahippocampal beta amyloid (1–42) peptide injection on oxidant and antioxidant status in rat brain.** *Ann N Y Acad Sci* 2007, **1100**:510–517.
16. Paxinos G, Watson C: *The rat brain in stereotaxic coordinates: hard cover edition.* The Netherlands: Academic Press, Elsevier; 2006.
17. Guaza C, Borrell J: **Prolonged ethanol consumption influences shuttle box and passive avoidance performance in rats.** *Physiol Behav* 1985, **34**(2):163–165.
18. Gandy S: **The role of cerebral amyloid beta accumulation in common forms of Alzheimer disease.** *J Clin Invest* 2005, **115**(5):1121–1129.
19. Murata N, Murakami K, Ozawa Y, Kinoshita N, Irie K, Shirasawa T, Shimizu T: **Silymarin attenuated the amyloid beta plaque burden and improved behavioral abnormalities in an Alzheimer's disease mouse model.** *Biosci Biotechnol Biochem* 2010, **74**(11):2299–2306.
20. Boller F, Forette F: **Alzheimer's disease and THA: a review of the cholinergic theory and of preliminary results.** *Biomed Pharmacother* 1989, **43**(7):487–491.
21. Robbins T, McAlonan G, Muir J, Everitt B: **Cognitive enhancers in theory and practice: studies of the cholinergic hypothesis of cognitive deficits in Alzheimer's disease.** *Behav Brain Res* 1997, **83**(1):15–23.
22. Selkoe DJ: **Toward a comprehensive theory for Alzheimer's disease. Hypothesis: Alzheimer's disease is caused by the cerebral accumulation and cytotoxicity of amyloid beta protein.** *Ann N Y Acad Sci* 2000, **924**(1):17–25.
23. Wilkinson DG, Francis PT, Schwam E, Payne-Parrish J: **Cholinesterase inhibitors used in the treatment of Alzheimer's disease.** *Drugs Aging* 2004, **21**(7):453–478.
24. Cheng B, Gong H, Xiao H, Petersen RB, Zheng L, Huang K: **Inhibiting toxic aggregation of amyloidogenic proteins: a therapeutic strategy for protein misfolding diseases.** *Biochimica et Biophysica Acta (BBA)-General Subjects* 2013, **1830**(10):4860–4871.
25. Citron M: **Beta-Secretase inhibition for the treatment of Alzheimer's disease-promise and challenge.** *Trends Pharmacol Sci* 2004, **25**(2):92–97.
26. Bajda M, Guzior N, Ignasik M, Malawska B: **Multi-Target-Directed ligands in Alzheimer's disease treatment.** *Curr Med Chem* 2011, **18**(32):4949–4975.
27. Pike CJ, Walencewicz-Wasserman AJ, Kosmoski J, Cribbs DH, Glabe CG, Cotman CW: **Structure-activity analyses of beta-amyloid peptides: contributions of the beta 25–35 region to aggregation and neurotoxicity.** *J Neurochem* 1995, **64**(1):253–265.
28. Kubo T, Nishimura S, Kumagae Y, Kaneko I: **In vivo conversion of racemized beta-amyloid ([D-Ser 26]A beta 1–40) to truncated and toxic fragments ([D-Ser 26]A beta 25-35/40) and fragment presence in the brains of Alzheimer's patients.** *J Neurosci Res* 2002, **70**(3):474–483.
29. Alkam T, Nitta A, Mizoguchi H, Itoh A, Nabeshima T: **A natural scavenger of peroxynitrites, rosmarinic acid, protects against impairment of memory induced by Abeta(25–35).** *Behav Brain Res* 2007, **180**(2):139–145.
30. Tsunekawa H, Noda Y, Mouri A, Yoneda F, Nabeshima T: **Synergistic effects of selegiline and donepezil on cognitive impairment induced by amyloid beta (25–35).** *Behav Brain Res* 2008, **190**(2):224–232.
31. Busche MA, Chen X, Henning HA, Reichwald J, Staufenbiel M, Sakmann B, Konnerth A: **Critical role of soluble amyloid beta for early hippocampal hyperactivity in a mouse model of Alzheimer's disease.** *Proc Natl Acad Sci* 2012, **109**(22):8740–8745.
32. Sabuncu MR, Desikan RS, Sepulcre J, Yeo BTT, Liu H, Schmansky NJ, Reuter M, Weiner MW, Buckner RL, Sperling RA: **The dynamics of cortical and hippocampal atrophy in Alzheimer disease.** *Arch Neurol* 2011, **68**(8):1040.
33. Raza SS, Khan MM, Ashafaq M, Ahmad A, Khuwaja G, Khan A, Siddiqui MS, Safhi MM, Islam F: **Silymarin protects neurons from oxidative stress associated damages in focal cerebral ischemia: a behavioral, biochemical and immunohistological study in Wistar rats.** *J Neurol Sci* 2011, **309**(1):45–54.
34. Galhardi F, Mesquita K, Monserrat JM, Barros DM: **Effect of silymarin on biochemical parameters of oxidative stress in aged and young rat brain.** *Food Chem Toxicol* 2009, **47**(10):2655–2660.
35. Nencini C, Giorgi G, Micheli L: **Protective effect of silymarin on oxidative stress in rat brain.** *Phytomedicine* 2007, **14**(2):129–135.
36. Marrazzo G, Bosco P, la Delia F, Scapagnini G, di Giacomo C, Malaguarnera M, Galvano F, Nicolosi A, Li Volti G: **Neuroprotective effect of silibinin in diabetic mice.** *Neurosci Lett* 2011, **504**(3):252–256.
37. Lu P, Mamiya T, Lu L, Mouri A, Niwa M, Kim HC, Zou LB, Nagai T, Yamada K, Ikejima T, *et al*: **Silibinin attenuates cognitive deficits and decreases of dopamine and serotonin induced by repeated methamphetamine treatment.** *Behav Brain Res* 2010, **207**(2):387–393.
38. Yin F, Liu J, Ji X, Wang Y, Zidichouski J, Zhang J: **Silibinin: a novel inhibitor of Abeta aggregation.** *Neurochem Int* 2011, **58**(3):399–403.
39. Cheng B, Gong H, Li X, Sun Y, Zhang X, Chen H, Liu X, Zheng L, Huang K: **Silibinin inhibits the toxic aggregation of human islet amyloid polypeptide.** *Biochem Biophys Res Commun* 2012, **419**(3):495–499.
40. Chinisaz M, Ghasemi A, Larijani B, Ebrahim-Habibi A: **Amyloid formation and inhibition of an all-beta protein: a study on fungal polygalacturonase.** *J Mol Struct* 2014, **1059**:94–100.
41. Ono K, Yoshiike Y, Takashima A, Hasegawa K, Naiki H, Yamada M: **Potent anti-amyloidogenic and fibril-destabilizing effects of polyphenols in vitro: implications for the prevention and therapeutics of Alzheimer's disease.** *J Neurochem* 2003, **87**(1):172–181.
42. Choi Y-T, Jung C-H, Lee S-R, Bae J-H, Baek W-K, Suh M-H, Park J, Park C-W, Suh S-I: **The green tea polyphenol (−)-epigallocatechin gallate attenuates β-amyloid-induced neurotoxicity in cultured hippocampal neurons.** *Life Sci* 2001, **70**(5):603–614.
43. Johnson SM, Petrassi HM, Palaninathan SK, Mohamedmohaideen NN, Purkey HE, Nichols C, Chiang KP, Walkup T, Sacchettini JC, Sharpless KB: **Bisaryloxime ethers as potent inhibitors of transthyretin amyloid fibril formation.** *J Med Chem* 2005, **48**(5):1576–1587.
44. Hafner-Bratkovič I, Gašperšič J, Šmid LM, Bresjanac M, Jerala R: **Curcumin binds to the α-helical intermediate and to the amyloid form of prion protein–a new mechanism for the inhibition of PrPSc accumulation.** *J Neurochem* 2008, **104**(6):1553–1564.
45. Liu D, Xu Y, Feng Y, Liu H, Shen X, Chen K, Ma J, Jiang H: **Inhibitor discovery targeting the intermediate structure of β-amyloid peptide on the conformational transition pathway: implications in the aggregation mechanism of β-amyloid peptide.** *Biochemistry* 2006, **45**(36):10963–10972.
46. Youdim KA, Shukitt-Hale B, Joseph JA: **Flavonoids and the brain: interactions at the blood–brain barrier and their physiological effects on the central nervous system.** *Free Radic Biol Med* 2004, **37**(11):1683–1693.
47. Baluchnejadmojarada T, Roghanib M, Mafakheria M: **Neuroprotective effect of silymarin in 6-hydroxydopamine hemi-parkinsonian rat: involvement of estrogen receptors and oxidative stress.** *Neurosci Lett* 2010, **480**(3):206–210.
48. Jacobs BP, Dennehy C, Ramirez G, Sapp J, Lawrence VA: **Milk thistle for the treatment of liver disease: a systematic review and meta-analysis.** *Am J Med* 2002, **113**(6):506–515.
49. Feher J, Lengyel G: **Silymarin in the prevention and treatment of liver diseases and primary liver cancer.** *Curr Pharm Biotechnol* 2012, **13**(1):210–217.
50. Lukiw WJ: **Gene expression profiling in fetal, aged, and alzheimer hippocampus: a continuum of stress-related signaling.** *Neurochem Res* 2004, **29**(6):1287–1297.

51. Theuns J, Brouwers N, Engelborghs S, Sleegers K, Bogaerts V, Corsmit E, de Pooter T, van Duijn CM, de Deyn PP, van Broeckhoven C: **Promoter mutations that increase amyloid precursor-protein expression are associated with Alzheimer disease.** *Am J Hum Genet* 2006, **78**(6):936–946.
52. Howlett DR, Richardson JC: **The pathology of APP transgenic mice: a model of Alzheimer's disease or simply overexpression of APP?** *Histol Histopathol* 2009, **24**(1):83–100.

Permissions

All chapters in this book were first published in DARU-JPS, by BioMed Central; hereby published with permission under the Creative Commons Attribution License or equivalent. Every chapter published in this book has been scrutinized by our experts. Their significance has been extensively debated. The topics covered herein carry significant findings which will fuel the growth of the discipline. They may even be implemented as practical applications or may be referred to as a beginning point for another development.

The contributors of this book come from diverse backgrounds, making this book a truly international effort. This book will bring forth new frontiers with its revolutionizing research information and detailed analysis of the nascent developments around the world.

We would like to thank all the contributing authors for lending their expertise to make the book truly unique. They have played a crucial role in the development of this book. Without their invaluable contributions this book wouldn't have been possible. They have made vital efforts to compile up to date information on the varied aspects of this subject to make this book a valuable addition to the collection of many professionals and students.

This book was conceptualized with the vision of imparting up-to-date information and advanced data in this field. To ensure the same, a matchless editorial board was set up. Every individual on the board went through rigorous rounds of assessment to prove their worth. After which they invested a large part of their time researching and compiling the most relevant data for our readers.

The editorial board has been involved in producing this book since its inception. They have spent rigorous hours researching and exploring the diverse topics which have resulted in the successful publishing of this book. They have passed on their knowledge of decades through this book. To expedite this challenging task, the publisher supported the team at every step. A small team of assistant editors was also appointed to further simplify the editing procedure and attain best results for the readers.

Apart from the editorial board, the designing team has also invested a significant amount of their time in understanding the subject and creating the most relevant covers. They scrutinized every image to scout for the most suitable representation of the subject and create an appropriate cover for the book.

The publishing team has been an ardent support to the editorial, designing and production team. Their endless efforts to recruit the best for this project, has resulted in the accomplishment of this book. They are a veteran in the field of academics and their pool of knowledge is as vast as their experience in printing. Their expertise and guidance has proved useful at every step. Their uncompromising quality standards have made this book an exceptional effort. Their encouragement from time to time has been an inspiration for everyone.

The publisher and the editorial board hope that this book will prove to be a valuable piece of knowledge for researchers, students, practitioners and scholars across the globe.

List of Contributors

Majid Eshghpour
Dental Research Center, Department of Oral and Maxillofacial, Mashhad University of Medical Sciences, Mashhad, Iran

Hamed Mortazavi
Department of Oral Medicine, Dental School, Shahid Beheshti University of Medical Sciences, Tehran, Iran

Naser Mohammadzadeh Rezaei
Mashhad University of Medical Sciences, Mashhad, Iran

AmirHossein Nejat
Member of Student Research Committee, School of Dentistry, Mashhad University of Medical Sciences, Mashhad, Iran

Niayesh Mohebbi
Department of Clinical Pharmacy, Faculty of Pharmacy, Tehran University of Medical Sciences, Tehran, Iran

Alireza Khoshnevisan
Department of Neurosurgery, Tehran University of Medical Sciences, Tehran, Iran

Soheil Naderi
Department of Neurosurgery, Tehran University of Medical Sciences, Tehran, Iran

Sina Abdollahzade
Department of Neurosurgery, Tehran University of Medical Sciences, Tehran, Iran

Jamshid Salamzadeh
Department of Clinical Pharmacy, Shahid Beheshti University of Medical Sciences, Tehran, Iran

Mohammadreza Javadi
Department of Clinical Pharmacy, Faculty of Pharmacy, Tehran University of Medical Sciences, Tehran, Iran

Mojtaba Mojtahedzadeh
Department of Clinical Pharmacy, Faculty of Pharmacy, Tehran University of Medical Sciences, Tehran, Iran

Kheirollah Gholami
Department of Clinical Pharmacy, Faculty of Pharmacy, Tehran University of Medical Sciences, Tehran, Iran

Mohammad Hashem Hashempur
Research Center for Traditional Medicine and History of Medicine, Shiraz University of Medical Sciences, Shiraz, Iran
Essence of Parsiyan Wisdom Institute, Traditional Medicine and Medicinal Plant Incubator, Shiraz University of Medical Sciences, Shiraz, Iran

Kaynoosh Homayouni
Department of Physical Medicine and Rehabilitation, Shiraz University of Medical Sciences, Shiraz, Iran
Shiraz Geriatric Research Center, Shiraz University of Medical Sciences, Shiraz, Iran

Alireza Ashraf
Department of Physical Medicine and Rehabilitation, Shiraz University of Medical Sciences, Shiraz, Iran
Shiraz Burn Research Center, Shiraz University of Medical Sciences, Shiraz, Iran

Alireza Salehi
Research Center for Traditional Medicine and History of Medicine, Shiraz University of Medical Sciences, Shiraz, Iran

Mohsen Taghizadeh
Research Center for Biochemistry and Nutrition in Metabolic Disease, Kashan University of Medical Sciences, Kashan, Iran

Mojtaba Heydari
Essence of Parsiyan Wisdom Institute, Traditional Medicine and Medicinal Plant Incubator, Shiraz University of Medical Sciences, Shiraz, Iran

Mohammad Mahdi Rezaee
Department of Pharmacology, Babol University of Medical Sciences, Babol, Iran

Sohrab Kazemi
Department of Pharmacology, Babol University of Medical Sciences, Babol, Iran
Cellular and Molecular Biology Research Centre, Babol University of Medical Sciences, Babol, Iran

Mohammad Taghi Kazemi
Department of Pharmacology, Babol University of Medical Sciences, Babol, Iran

Saeed Gharooee
Department of Pharmacology, Babol University of Medical Sciences, Babol, Iran

Elham Yazdani
Department of Pharmacology, Babol University of Medical Sciences, Babol, Iran

Hoda Gharooee
Department of Pharmacology, Babol University of Medical Sciences, Babol, Iran

Mohammad Reza Shiran
Department of Pharmacology, Mazandaran University of Medical Sciences, Sari, Iran

Ali Akbar Moghadamnia
Department of Pharmacology, Babol University of Medical Sciences, Babol, Iran
Cellular and Molecular Biology Research Centre, Babol University of Medical Sciences, Babol, Iran

Anahita Johari
Department of Medicinal Chemistry, Faculty of Pharmacy and Pharmaceutical Sciences Research Center, Tehran University of Medical Sciences, Tehran, Iran
Institute of Biochemistry and Biophysics, University of Tehran, Tehran, Iran

Ali Akbar Moosavi-Movahedi
Institute of Biochemistry and Biophysics, University of Tehran, Tehran, Iran

Massoud Amanlou
Department of Medicinal Chemistry, Faculty of Pharmacy and Pharmaceutical Sciences Research Center, Tehran University of Medical Sciences, Tehran, Iran

Sahabjada Siddiqui
Molecular Endocrinology Laboratory, Department of Zoology, University of Lucknow, Lucknow 226007, India

Mohammad Arshad
Molecular Endocrinology Laboratory, Department of Zoology, University of Lucknow, Lucknow 226007, India

Gilda Kianimehr
Psychiatric Research Center, Roozbeh Hospital, Tehran University of Medical Sciences, Tehran 13337, Iran

Farzad Fatehi
Shariati Hospital, Neurology Department, Tehran University of medical Sciences, Tehran, Iran

Sara Hashempoor
Razi Psychiatric Hospital, University of Social Welfare and Rehabilitation, Tehran, Iran

Mohammad-Reza Khodaei-Ardakani
Razi Psychiatric Hospital, University of Social Welfare and Rehabilitation, Tehran, Iran

Farzin Rezaei
Qods Hospital, Kurdistan University of Medical Sciences, Sanandaj, Iran

Ali Nazari
Qods Hospital, Kurdistan University of Medical Sciences, Sanandaj, Iran

Ladan Kashani
Infertility Ward, Arash Hospital, Tehran University of Medical Sciences, Tehran, Iran

Shahin Akhondzadeh
Psychiatric Research Center, Roozbeh Psychiatric Hospital, Tehran University of Medical Sciences, South Kargar Street 13337, Tehran, Iran

Abolfazl Akbari
Department of Molecular Medicine, School of Advanced Medical Technologies, Tehran University of Medical Sciences, Tehran, Iran

Saeid Amanpour
Cancer Research Center, Cancer Institute of Iran, Tehran University of Medical Sciences, Tehran, Iran

Samad Muhammadnejad
Cancer Research Center, Cancer Institute of Iran, Tehran University of Medical Sciences, Tehran, Iran

Mohammad Hossein Ghahremani
Department of Molecular Medicine, School of Advanced Medical Technologies, Tehran University of Medical Sciences, Tehran, Iran
Department of Pharmacology and Toxicology, Faculty of Pharmacy, Tehran University of Medical Sciences, Tehran, Iran

Seyed Hamidollah Ghaffari
Hematology, Oncology and Stem Cell Transplantation Research Center, Shariati Hospital, Tehran University of Medical Sciences, Tehran, Iran

Ahmad Reza Dehpour
Department of Pharmacology, School of Medicine, Tehran University of Medical Sciences, Tehran, Iran

Gholam Reza Mobini
Department of Molecular Medicine, School of Advanced Medical Technologies, Tehran University of Medical Sciences, Tehran, Iran

Fatemeh Shidfar
Department of Molecular Medicine, School of Advanced Medical Technologies, Tehran University of Medical Sciences, Tehran, Iran

Mahdi Abastabar
Invasive Fungi Research Center, Department of Medical Mycology and Parasitology, School of Medicine, Mazandaran University of Medical Sciences, Sari, Iran

Ahad Khoshzaban
Stem Cells Preparation Uinte, Farabi Eye Hospital, Tehran University of Medical Sciences, Tehran, Iran

Ebrahim Faghihloo
Department of Virology, School of Public Health, Tehran University of Medical Sciences, Tehran, Iran

Abbas Karimi
Department of Molecular Medicine, Faculty of Advanced Technologies in Medicine (FATiM), Iran University of Medical Sciences, Tehran, Iran

Mansour Heidari
Stem Cells Preparation Uinte, Farabi Eye Hospital, Tehran University of Medical Sciences, Tehran, Iran
Department of Medical Genetics, School of Medicine, Tehran University of Medical Sciences, Tehran, Iran

Monireh Afzali
Department Toxicology & Pharmacology, Faculty of Pharmacy, Toxicology & Poisoning Research Center, Tehran University of Medical Sciences, 14155/ 6451 Tehran, Iran

Padideh Ghaeli
Department Clinical Pharmacy, Faculty of Pharmacy & Rational Drug Use Research Center, Tehran University of Medical Sciences, 14155/6451 Tehran, Iran

Mahnaz Khanavi
Department Pharmacognosy, Faculty of Pharmacy, Tehran University of Medical Sciences, 14155/6451 Tehran, Iran

Maliheh Parsa
Department Toxicology & Pharmacology, Faculty of Pharmacy, Toxicology & Poisoning Research Center, Tehran University of Medical Sciences, 14155/ 6451 Tehran, Iran

Hamed Montazeri
Department Toxicology & Pharmacology, Faculty of Pharmacy, Toxicology & Poisoning Research Center, Tehran University of Medical Sciences, 14155/ 6451 Tehran, Iran

Mohammad Hossein Ghahremani
Department Toxicology & Pharmacology, Faculty of Pharmacy, Toxicology & Poisoning Research Center, Tehran University of Medical Sciences, 14155/ 6451 Tehran, Iran

Seyed Nasser Ostad
Department Toxicology & Pharmacology, Faculty of Pharmacy, Toxicology & Poisoning Research Center, Tehran University of Medical Sciences, 14155/ 6451 Tehran, Iran

Songhee Jeon
Dongguk University Research Institute of Biotechnology, Seoul 100-715, Republic of Korea

Chia-Hung Lee
Department of Neuropsychiatry, Graduate School of Oriental Medicine, Dongguk University, Gyeongju, Republic of Korea

Quan Feng Liu
Department of Neuropsychiatry, Graduate School of Oriental Medicine, Dongguk University, Gyeongju, Republic of Korea

Geun Woo Kim
Department of Korean Neuropsychiatry, Dongguk University Bundang Oriental Hospital, Sungnam, Republic of Korea

Byung-Soo Koo
Department of Korean Neuropsychiatry, Dongguk University Ilsan Oriental Hospital, Goyang, Republic of Korea

Sok Cheon Pak
School of Biomedical Sciences, Charles Sturt University, Bathurst, NSW 2795, Australia

Massoud Amanlou
Department of Medicinal Chemistry, Faculty of Pharmacy, Pharmaceutical Sciences Research Center, Tehran University of Medical Sciences, Tehran, Iran

Ali-akbar Saboury
Institute of Biochemistry and Biophysics, University of Tehran, Tehran, Iran

Roya Bazl
Institute of Biochemistry and Biophysics, University of Tehran, Tehran, Iran

Mohammad Reza Ganjali
Institute of Biochemistry and Biophysics, University of Tehran, Tehran, Iran

Shokoofeh Sheibani
Center of Excellence in Electrochemistry, Faculty of Chemistry, University of Tehran, Tehran, Iran

Clarence S. Yah
Department of Biochemistry and Microbiology, Nelson Mandela Metropolitan University, Port Elizabeth, South Africa Department of Epidemiology, Johns Hopkins Bloomberg School of Public Health, E7146, 615 N. Wolfe Street, Baltimore 21205, MD, USA

Geoffrey S. Simate
School of Chemical and Metallurgical Engineering, University of the Witwatersrand, P/Bag 3, Wits 2050, Johannesburg, South Africa

Amir Ghaderi
Department of Addiction studies, School of Medical Kashan University of Medical Sciences, Kashan, Iran

Naser Vahdati-Mashhadian
Departments of Pharmacodynamics and Toxicology, School of Pharmacy, Mashhad University of Medical Sciences, Mashhad, Iran

Zohreh Oghabian
Department of Clinical Toxicology, Kerman University of Medical Sciences, Kerman, Iran

Valiallah Moradi
Departments of Pharmacodynamics and Toxicology, School of Pharmacy, Mashhad University of Medical Sciences, Mashhad, Iran

Reza Afshari
Addiction Research Centre, Mashhad University of Medical Sciences, Imam Reza Hospital, Ibn-e-Sina Street, Mashhad 91735-348, Iran
British Columbia Center for Disease Control, Vancouver, Canada

Omid Mehrpour
Atherosclerosis and Coronary Artery Research Center, Birjand University of Medical Science, Birjand, Iran

Fatemeh Attari
Department of Neuroscience, School of Advanced Technologies in medicine, Tehran University of Medical Sciences, Tehran, Iran
Shefa Neuroscience Research Center, Khatamolanbia Hospital, Tehran, Iran

Maryam Zahmatkesh
Department of Neuroscience, School of Advanced Technologies in medicine, Tehran University of Medical Sciences, Tehran, Iran

Hadi Aligholi
Department of Neuroscience, School of Advanced Technologies in medicine, Tehran University of Medical Sciences, Tehran, Iran
Shefa Neuroscience Research Center, Khatamolanbia Hospital, Tehran, Iran

Shahram Ejtemaei Mehr
Department of Pharmacology, School of Medicine, Tehran University of Medical Sciences, Tehran, Iran

Mohammad Sharifzadeh
Faculty of Pharmacy, and Pharmaceutical Sciences Research Center, Tehran University of Medical Sciences, Tehran, Iran

Ali Gorji
Shefa Neuroscience Research Center, Khatamolanbia Hospital, Tehran, Iran
Epilepsy Research Center, WestfälischeWilhelms-UniversitätMünster, Münster, Germany

Tahmineh Mokhtari
Department of Anatomy, School of Medicine, Tehran University of Medical Sciences, Tehran, Iran

Mojtaba Khaksarian
Department of Physiology, Medical College, Lorestan University of Medical Sciences, Khorramabad, Iran

Gholamreza Hassanzadeh
Department of Neuroscience, School of Advanced Technologies in medicine, Tehran University of Medical Sciences, Tehran, Iran
Department of Anatomy, School of Medicine, Tehran University of Medical Sciences, Tehran, Iran

Mohsen Zeeb
Department of Applied Chemistry, Faculty of science, Islamic Azad University, South Tehran Branch, Tehran, Iran

Behrooz Mirza
Department of Applied Chemistry, Faculty of science, Islamic Azad University, South Tehran Branch, Tehran, Iran

Arezou Lari
Students Research Committee, Faculty of Pharmacy, Kermanshah University of Medical Sciences, Kermanshah, Iran

Isaac Karimi
Laboratory of Molecular and Cellular Biology, School of Veterinary Medicine, Razi University, Kermanshah, Iran

Hadi Adibi
Novel Drug Delivery Research Center, Faculty of Pharmacy, Kermanshah University of Medical Sciences, Kermanshah, Iran

Alireza Aliabadi
Novel Drug Delivery Research Center, Faculty of Pharmacy, Kermanshah University of Medical Sciences, Kermanshah, Iran

Loghman Firoozpour
Drug Design and Development Research Center, Tehran University of Medical Sciences, Tehran, Iran

Alireza Foroumadi
Drug Design and Development Research Center, Tehran University of Medical Sciences, Tehran, Iran
Neuroscience Research Center, Institute of Neuropharmacology, Kerman University of Medical Sciences, Kerman, Iran

Darshana S Jain
Department of Pharmaceutics, C.U. Shah College of Pharmacy, SNDT Women's University, Juhu Tara Road, Santacruz (West), Mumbai 400 049, India

Rajani B Athawale
Department of Pharmaceutics, C.U. Shah College of Pharmacy, SNDT Women's University, Juhu Tara Road, Santacruz (West), Mumbai 400 049, India

Amrita N Bajaj
SVKM's Dr. Bhanuben Nanavati College of Pharmacy, Vileparle, Mumbai 400 056, India

Shruti S Shrikhande
Department of Pharmaceutics, C.U. Shah College of Pharmacy, SNDT Women's University, Juhu Tara Road, Santacruz (West), Mumbai 400 049, India

Peeyush N Goel
Gude Lab, Advanced Centre for Treatment, Research & Education in Cancer (ACTREC), Tata Memorial Centre, Kharghar, Navi Mumbai 410 210, India

Yuvraj Nikam
Gude Lab, Advanced Centre for Treatment, Research & Education in Cancer (ACTREC), Tata Memorial Centre, Kharghar, Navi Mumbai 410 210, India

Rajiv P Gude
Gude Lab, Advanced Centre for Treatment, Research & Education in Cancer (ACTREC), Tata Memorial Centre, Kharghar, Navi Mumbai 410 210, India

Rasool Haddadi
Student Research Committee, Tabriz University of Medical Sciences, Tabriz, Iran
Department of Pharmacology and Toxicology, Faculty of Pharmacy, Tabriz University of Medical Sciences, Tabriz, Iran

Alireza Mohajjel Nayebi
Drug Applied Research Center, Tabriz University of Medical Sciences, Tabriz, Iran
Department of Pharmacology and Toxicology, Faculty of Pharmacy, Tabriz University of Medical Sciences, Tabriz, Iran

Safar Farajniya
Drug Applied Research Center, Tabriz University of Medical Sciences, Tabriz, Iran

Shahla Eyvari Brooshghalan
Drug Applied Research Center, Tabriz University of Medical Sciences, Tabriz, Iran

Hamdolah Sharifi
Urmia University of Medical Science, Urmia, Iran

Monia Deghrigue
Laboratoire de développement chimique, galénique et pharmacologique des médicaments (LR12ES09). Equipe de Pharmacologie marine, Faculté de pharmacie de Monastir, Université de Monastir, Monastir, Tunisie

Carmen Festa
Department of Pharmacy, University of Naples "Federico II", via D. Montesano 49, I- 80131 Napoli, Italy

Lotfi Ghribi
Laboratoire de chimie hétérocyclique, produits naturels et réactivité. Equipe de chimie médicinale et produits naturels (LR11ES39), Faculté des sciences de Monastir, Université de Monastir, Monastir, Tunisie

Maria Valeria D'auria
Department of Pharmacy, University of Naples "Federico II", via D. Montesano 49, I- 80131 Napoli, Italy

Simona de Marino
Department of Pharmacy, University of Naples "Federico II", via D. Montesano 49, I- 80131 Napoli, Italy

Hichem Ben Jannet
Laboratoire de chimie hétérocyclique, produits naturels et réactivité. Equipe de chimie médicinale et produits naturels (LR11ES39), Faculté des sciences de Monastir, Université de Monastir, Monastir, Tunisie

Rafik Ben Said
Institut National des Sciences et Technologie de la Mer (INSTM), Salambo, Tunis, Tunisie

Abderrahman Bouraoui
Laboratoire de développement chimique, galénique et pharmacologique des médicaments (LR12ES09). Equipe de Pharmacologie marine, Faculté de pharmacie de Monastir, Université de Monastir, Monastir, Tunisie

Vahid Ramezani
Department of Pharmaceutics, Faculty of Pharmacy, Tehran University of Medical Sciences, Tehran, Iran
Department of Pharmaceutics, Faculty of Pharmacy, Shahid Sadoughi University of Medical Sciences, Yazd, Iran

Alireza Vatanara
Department of Pharmaceutics, Faculty of Pharmacy, Tehran University of Medical Sciences, Tehran, Iran

Abdolhossein Rouholamini Najafabadi
Department of Pharmaceutics, Faculty of Pharmacy, Tehran University of Medical Sciences, Tehran, Iran

Mohammad Ali Shokrgozar
National Cell Bank of Iran, Pasteur Institute of Iran, Tehran, Iran

Alireza Khabiri
Department of Mycology, Pasteur Institute of Iran, Tehran, Iran

Mohammad Seyedabadi
Department of Molecular Imaging, The Persian Gulf Biomedical Sciences Research Institute, Bushehr University of Medical Sciences, Bushehr, Iran

Mehdi Esfandyari-Manesh
Nanotechnology Research Centre, Faculty of Pharmacy, Tehran University of Medical Sciences, Tehran, Iran
Novel Drug Delivery Lab, Department of Pharmaceutics, Faculty of Pharmacy, Tehran University of Medical Sciences, Tehran, Iran

Seyed Hossein Mostafavi
Novel Drug Delivery Lab, Department of Pharmaceutics, Faculty of Pharmacy, Tehran University of Medical Sciences, Tehran, Iran
Department of Bioengineering, University of California, Riverside, CA, USA
Medical Nanotechnology Department, School of Advanced Technologies in Medicine, Tehran University of Medical Sciences, Tehran, Iran

Reza Faridi Majidi
Medical Nanotechnology Department, School of Advanced Technologies in Medicine, Tehran University of Medical Sciences, Tehran, Iran

Mona Noori Koopaei
Novel Drug Delivery Lab, Department of Pharmaceutics, Faculty of Pharmacy, Tehran University of Medical Sciences, Tehran, Iran

Nazanin Shabani Ravari
Nanotechnology Research Centre, Faculty of Pharmacy, Tehran University of Medical Sciences, Tehran, Iran
Novel Drug Delivery Lab, Department of Pharmaceutics, Faculty of Pharmacy, Tehran University of Medical Sciences, Tehran, Iran

Mohsen Amini
Department of Medicinal Chemistry, Faculty of Pharmacy, Tehran University of Medical Sciences, Tehran, Iran

Behrad Darvishi
Nanotechnology Research Centre, Faculty of Pharmacy, Tehran University of Medical Sciences, Tehran, Iran
Medical Nanotechnology Department, School of Advanced Technologies in Medicine, Tehran University of Medical Sciences, Tehran, Iran

Seyed Nasser Ostad
Department of Toxicology and Pharmacology, Faculty of Pharmacy, Tehran University of Medical Science, Tehran, Iran

Fatemeh Atyabi
Nanotechnology Research Centre, Faculty of Pharmacy, Tehran University of Medical Sciences, Tehran, Iran
Novel Drug Delivery Lab, Department of Pharmaceutics, Faculty of Pharmacy, Tehran University of Medical Sciences, Tehran, Iran

Rassoul Dinarvand
Nanotechnology Research Centre, Faculty of Pharmacy, Tehran University of Medical Sciences, Tehran, Iran
Novel Drug Delivery Lab, Department of Pharmaceutics, Faculty of Pharmacy, Tehran University of Medical Sciences, Tehran, Iran

Somayeh Rajabi
Cell and Molecular Biology Departments, Pharmaceutical Sciences Branch, Islamic Azad University, Tehran, Iran

Ali Ramazani
Cell and Molecular Biology Departments, Pharmaceutical Sciences Branch, Islamic Azad University, Tehran, Iran
Biotechnology Departments, School of Pharmacy, Zanjan University of Medical Sciences, Zanjan, Iran

Mehrdad Hamidi
Zanjan Pharmaceutical Nanotechnology Research Center, Zanjan University of Medical Sciences, Zanjan, Iran

Tahereh Naji
Cell and Molecular Biology Departments, Pharmaceutical Sciences Branch, Islamic Azad University, Tehran, Iran

Fatemeh Sadat Hoseini
Department of Anatomy and Reproductive Biology, School of Medicine, Tehran University of Medical Sciences, Tehran, Iran

Seyed Mohammad Hossein Noori Mugahi
Departments of Histology, School of Medicine, Tehran University of Medical Sciences, Tehran, Iran

Firoozeh Akbari-Asbagh
Department of Obstetrics and Gynecology, Tehran Women General Hospital, School of Medicine, Tehran University of Medical Sciences, Tehran, Iran

Poopak Eftekhari-Yazdi
Department of Embryology at Reproductive Biomedicine Research Center, Royan Institute for Reproductive Biomedicine, ACECR, Tehran, Iran

Behrouz Aflatoonian
Lab director Assisted Conception Units, Laleh Hospital, Tehran, Iran and Madar Hospital, Yazd, Iran

Seyed Hamid Aghaee-Bakhtiari
Department of Molecular Biology and Genetic Engineering, Stem Cell Technology Research Center, Tehran, Iran and Molecular Medicine Department, Biotechnology Research Center, Pasteur Institute of Iran, Tehran, Iran

Reza Aflatoonian
Department of Endocrinology and Female Infertility at Reproductive Biomedicine Research Center, Royan Institute for Reproductive Biomedicine, ACECR, Tehran, Iran

Nasser Salsabili
Department of Physiotherapy, School of Rehabilitation of Tehran University of Medical Sciences, Tehran, Iran; Lab director Assisted Conception Unit, Tehran Women General Hospital, Tehran University of Medical Sciences, Tehran, Iran

Seyedeh Sara Mirfazli
Department of Medicinal Chemistry, Faculty of Pharmacy and Pharmaceutical Sciences Research Center, Tehran University of Medical Sciences, Tehran, Iran

Farzad Kobarfard
Department of Medicinal Chemistry, School of Pharmacy, Shahid Beheshti University of Medical Sciences, Tehran, Iran
Phytochemistry Research Center, Shahid Beheshti University of Medical Sciences, Tehran, Iran

Loghman Firoozpour
Drug Design and Development Research Center, Tehran University of Medical Sciences, Tehran, Iran

Ali Asadipour
Neuroscience Research Center, Institute of Neuropharmacology, Kerman University of Medical Sciences, Kerman, Iran

Marjan Esfahanizadeh
Department of Medicinal Chemistry, School of Pharmacy, Shahid Beheshti University of Medical Sciences, Tehran, Iran

Kimia Tabib
Department of Medicinal Chemistry, School of Pharmacy, Shahid Beheshti University of Medical Sciences, Tehran, Iran

Abbas Shafiee
Department of Medicinal Chemistry, Faculty of Pharmacy and Pharmaceutical Sciences Research Center, Tehran University of Medical Sciences, Tehran, Iran

Alireza Foroumadi
Department of Medicinal Chemistry, Faculty of Pharmacy and Pharmaceutical Sciences Research Center, Tehran University of Medical Sciences, Tehran, Iran
Neuroscience Research Center, Institute of Neuropharmacology, Kerman University of Medical Sciences, Kerman, Iran

Nazila Gholipour
Department of Radiopharmacy, Faculty of Pharmacy, Tehran University of Medical Sciences, P.O. Box: 14155-6451, Tehran, Iran

Amir Reza Jalilian
Radiation Application Research School, Nuclear Science and Technology Research Institute, P.O. Box: 14395-836, Tehran, Iran

Ali Khalaj
Department of Medicinal Chemistry, Faculty of Pharmacy, Tehran University of Medical Sciences, P.O. Box: 14155-6451, Tehran, Iran

Fariba Johari-Daha
Radiation Application Research School, Nuclear Science and Technology Research Institute, P.O. Box: 14395-836, Tehran, Iran

Kamal Yavari
Radiation Application Research School, Nuclear Science and Technology Research Institute, P.O. Box: 14395-836, Tehran, Iran

Omid Sabzevari
Depatment of Toxicology and Pharmacology, School of Pharmacy, Tehran University of Medical Sciences, P.O. Box: 14176-14411, Tehran, Iran

Ali Reza Khanchi
Radiation Application Research School, Nuclear Science and Technology Research Institute, P.O. Box: 14395-836, Tehran, Iran

Mehdi Akhlaghi
Research Center for Nuclear Medicine, Tehran University of Medical Sciences, P.O. Box: 14117-13137, Tehran, Iran

Ahmad Ghorbani
Pharmacological Research Center of Medicinal Plants, School of Medicine, Mashhad University of Medical Sciences, Mashhad, Iran

Azadeh Feizpour
Neurogenic Inflammation Research Centre and Department of Physiology, School of Medicine, Mashhad University of Medical Sciences, Mashhad 9177948564, Iran

Milad Hashemzahi
Neurogenic Inflammation Research Centre and Department of Physiology, School of Medicine, Mashhad University of Medical Sciences, Mashhad 9177948564, Iran

Lila Gholami
Neurogenic Inflammation Research Centre and Department of Physiology, School of Medicine, Mashhad University of Medical Sciences, Mashhad 9177948564, Iran

Mahmoud Hosseini
Neurocognitive Research Center and Department of Physiology, School of Medicine, Mashhad University of Medical Sciences, Mashhad, Iran

Mohammad Soukhtanloo
Department of Clinical Biochemistry, School of Medicine, Mashhad University of Medical Sciences, Mashhad, Iran

Farzaneh Vafaee Bagheri
Neurogenic Inflammation Research Centre and Department of Physiology, School of Medicine, Mashhad University of Medical Sciences, Mashhad 9177948564, Iran

Esmaeil Khodaei
Neurogenic Inflammation Research Centre and Department of Physiology, School of Medicine, Mashhad University of Medical Sciences, Mashhad 9177948564, Iran

Nema Mohammadian Roshan
Department of Pathology, School of Medicine, Mashhad University of Medical Sciences, Mashhad, Iran

Mohammad Hossein Boskabady
Neurogenic Inflammation Research Centre and Department of Physiology, School of Medicine, Mashhad University of Medical Sciences, Mashhad 9177948564, Iran